Modern Trends in Human Leukemia II
Biological, Immunological, Therapeutical and Virological Aspects

Hämatologie und Bluttransfusion

Herausgegeben von W. Stich, G. Ruhenstroth-Bauer und H. Heimpel

Sonderbände zu Blut · Zeitschrift für die gesamte Blutforschung
Organ der Deutschen Gesellschaft für Hämatologie
Organ der Deutschen Gesellschaft für Bluttransfusion

Band 19

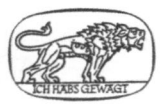

J. F. Lehmanns Verlag München

Modern Trends in Human Leukemia II

Biological, Immunological, Therapeutical and Virological Aspects

Edited by

Rolf Neth
Molekularbiologisch-hämatologische Arbeitsgruppe
Universitäts-Kinderklinik
Hamburg-Eppendorf, W. Germany

Robert C. Gallo
Laboratory of Tumor Cell Biology
Division of Cancer Treatment
National Cancer Institute
National Institutes of Health
Bethesda, Maryland, USA

Klaus Mannweiler
Heinrich-Pette-Institut für experimentelle Virologie
und Immunologie an der Universität Hamburg
Hamburg-Eppendorf, W. Germany

William C. Moloney
Harvard Medical School
Department of Medicine
Hematology Division
Boston, Massachusetts, USA

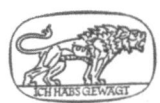

J. F. Lehmanns Verlag München

We should like to thank all those in Germany and the USA who made this work-shop possible:

Stiftung Volkswagenwerk, Hannover

National Cancer Institute, National Institutes of Health, Bethesda, Maryland, USA

Deutsche Gesellschaft für Hämatologie

Hamburgische Wissenschaftliche Stiftung, Hamburg

Hertha-Grober-Stiftung, Hamburg

Paul-Martini-Stiftung, Frankfurt

Universitäts-Gesellschaft Hamburg

We thank the Behörde für Wissenschaft und Kunst der Freien und Hansestadt Ham-burg, the lord mayor of Lüneburg, the Stiftung F. V. S. zu Hamburg and the Amerikahaus in Hamburg for their generous hospitality.

We thank Miss D. Dirks for proof-reading of the manuscripts and translational help.

We thank the publisher J. F. Lehmanns Verlag and the Druckerei Poeschel & Schulz-Schomburgk for prompt and conscious collaboration.

Gesamtherstellung: Druckerei Poeschel & Schulz-Schomburgk, 344 Eschwege/Werra

ISBN 978-3-540-79785-2   ISBN 978-3-642-87524-3 (eBook)
DOI 10.1007/978-3-642-87524-3

Frederick Stohlmann Workshop: Modern Trends in Human Leukemia II
"De Emhoff" in Wilsede, Naturschutzpark Lüneburger Heide
June 23rd to 27th, 1975

On behalf of the Deutsche Gesellschaft für Hämatologie
and the National Cancer Institute
the workshop was organized by

Rolf Neth
Molekularbiologisch-hämatologische Arbeitsgruppe
Universitäts-Kinderklinik
Hamburg-Eppendorf, W. Germany

Robert C. Gallo
Laboratory of Tumor Cell Biology
Division of Cancer Treatment
National Cancer Institute
National Institutes of Health
Bethesda, Maryland, USA

Klaus Mannweiler
Heinrich-Pette-Institut für experimentelle Virologie und Immunologie an der
Universität Hamburg
Hamburg-Eppendorf, W. Germany

Frederick Stohlmann, Jr. †
St. Elizabeth's Hospital of Boston
Tufts University Medical School
Boston, Massachusetts, USA

Contents

Cell Biology of Leukemia

Immunology of Leukemia

Therapy of Leukemia

Oncogenic Viruses in Leukemia

RNA Synthesis and Translation in Leukemic Cells

Preface

We are glad that you have all come to this small village and I hope that you will feel at home here for the next few days. The special atmosphere of the surroundings will probably have a good influence on our discussions, and you will perhaps remember this when you are back home again. It takes hard work to save this little piece of nature for man in our highly industrialized world, and we should all be grateful to the Verein Naturschutzpark e. V. (founded in 1909), Alfred Toepfer and his associates for their efforts.

We intend to discuss modern trends in human leukemia in this workshop, but we should also take the opportunity to reflect on the trends of the past, which might still be modern.

Rudolf VIRCHOW was the first using the name "leukemia" to express that this was a disease sui generis. About 125 years ago VIRCHOW wrote the following words:

"This is what we know about leukemia: During normal blood cell production the cells differentiate into specific types. In a pathologic situation the differentiation into specific cells is blocked. This disturbance of normal differentiation – so called leukemia – is a disease sui generis. We know the sequels of this disease, but we don't know its origin. As yet there has been no successful case of complete cure."

It is perhaps depressing and certainly a challenge that these words are today as true as they were in 1849, when they were written. In fact, the origins of human organic sickness are now as unknown as before. We can, however, help the patient better than we could a few years ago. Besides cytostatic therapy and supportive care, the personal efforts of the doctors themselves are the most important factor of therapy.

As long as there is no leukemia-specific therapy as well as a specific therapy of other cancers, early diagnosis of the disease appears to be very important. Despite of the progress in morphologic techniques, the sensitivity of leukemia diagnosis is not much better than 80 years ago, when Paul EHRLICH developed his staining technique.

Leukemia is usually diagnosed when it can be recognized in the bone marrow, i. e. when there are more than 10^{12} leukemic cells in the patient. But this is already too late. The reason for this late diagnosis is that leukemic cells cannot be distinguished morphologically from normal stem cells.

Two years ago, when we had our first workshop on modern trends in human leukemia, we could give no answer how to find a more sensitive leukemia specific signal, and we learnt that molecular biologic techniques failed and could not offer a successful way to help the patient directly.

In the meantime various groups have tried to find leukemic cell membrane specific antibodies and to use them as a diagnostic signal. The molecular biologists have critically revised their results. And we hope for a successful virologic research. Apart from this the clinicians developed during the last years more effective and promising therapeutic methods – without having a leukemia specific cell marker and without any knowledge about the origin of the disease.

Our workshop's aim is to think about the practical application of our research and about its use for the patient. It was one of Frederick Stohlman's persuasions to ask for this practical approach, and he also did when we started together planning this workshop. I think we should all together try to realize this plan, and to remind us of this aim the second Wilsede meeting will be named "Frederick Stohlman Workshop". Moreover, all further Wilsede meetings will comprise a "Frederick Stohlman lecture".

Rolf Neth

Frederick Stohlman, Jr. in the garden of "De Emhoff" during a personal discussion (first workshop, June 1973). Foto: Moldvay (STERN-Magazin) ▶

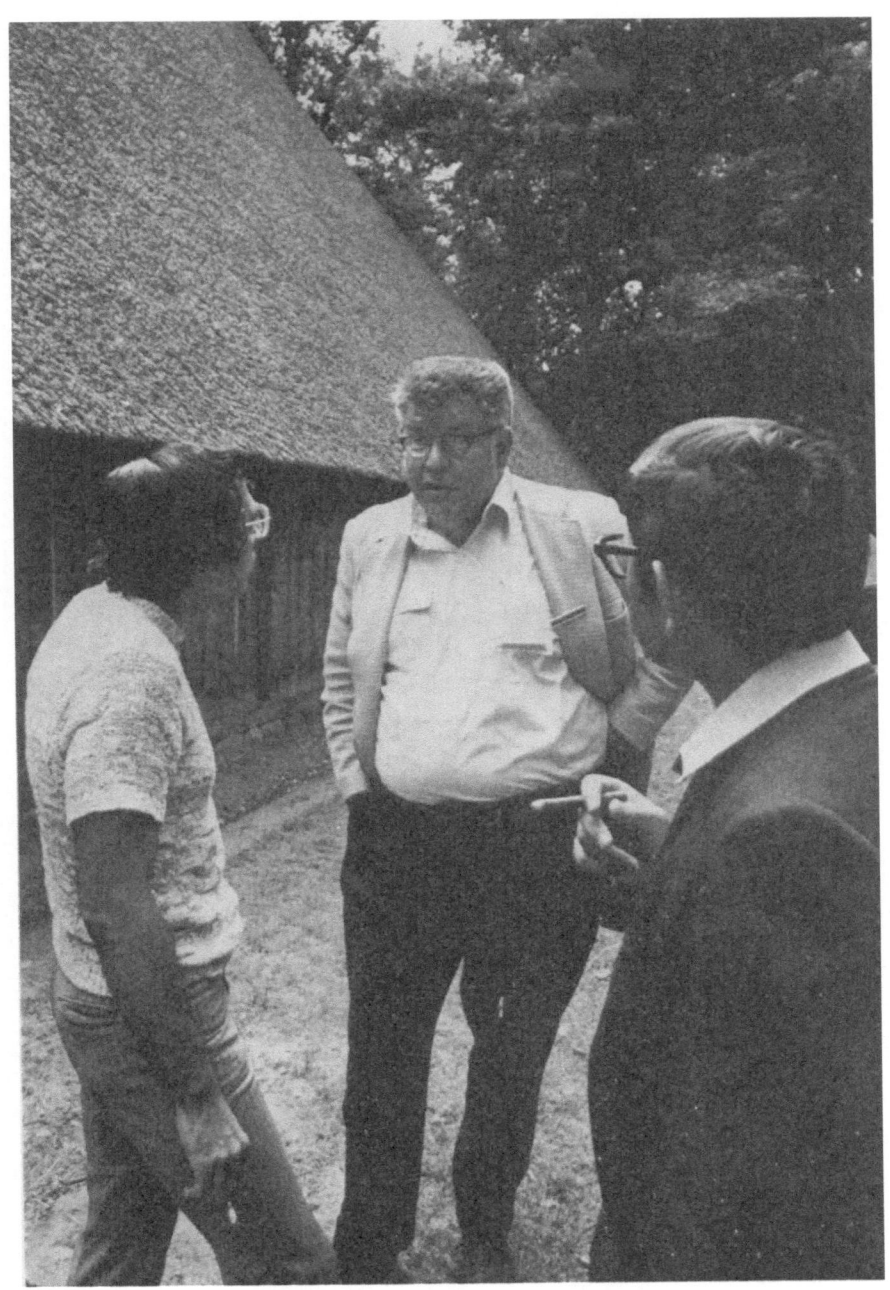

Notions About the Hemopoietic Stem Cell*

Eugene P. Cronkite, M. D.

Medical Department
Brookhaven National Laboratory
Upton, New York 11973

The intent of this presentation is to present a notion that the *in vitro* bone marrow and blood culture system does not truly measure the dimensions of the committed stem cell pool.

The measure of stem cell reserve – preferably the pluripotent and the committed stem cell pools is not a trivial, clinical problem. In the course of disease, chemotherapy, radiotherapy, one could much better guide management if there were a reliable reproducible method to assay for the stem cell reserve. In addition, a stem cell assay for man is critical to an understanding of normal hematopoiesis and its full characterization. At first look, the *in vitro* bone marrow culture combined with tritiated thymidine suicide appeared to be an answer to the problem. This can now be questioned. The diffusion chamber culture technique measures both pluripotent and committed stem cells but it also is capricious and poorly reproducible although some technical progress is being made (1, 2).

The concept of stem cells in hemopoiesis is several decades old. Maximow and Bloom (3) have expressed their thoughts clearly. They divided hemopoiesis into homoplastic and heteroplastic hemopoiesis. Homoplastic hemopoiesis is defined as the production of mature cells by young elements of the same type. They believe that under physiological conditions the needs of the adult organism are supplied generally by homoplastic hemopoiesis. When requirements for blood cells were increased, as after hemorrhage, during infection, during regeneration from injury, homoplastic hemopoiesis was insufficient and new erythroblasts and myelocytes then developed from a pluripotent stem cell and this they called heteroplastic hemopoiesis. Modern parlance divides the stem cells into the pluripotent and the committed stem cells (4, 5).

Pluripotent hemopoietic stem cell can only be studied directly in the mouse. It is measured by the capability of hemopoietic cell suspensions to produce splenic colonies. The cell that produces the colony is called the CFU-S. The CFU-S derived from the bone marrow and spleen of the mouse has a capability of producing erythrocytic, granulocytic, and megakaryocytic lines, respectively (6). Becker et al. (7) have clearly shown that colonies are formed from a single CFU-S, demonstrating the clonal nature of the spleen colonies. Till et al. (8) in studying the growth rates of splenic colonies developed a stochastic model for stem cell proliferation, in

* Research supported by the U. S. Energy Research and Development Administration.

which they feel that the birth process or replication of the stem cell and the death process (differentiation into a cell no longer able to replicate the CFU-S) appear at random in the population of the colony forming cells proliferating in the splenic colony. Becker et al. (9) have determined the fraction of the CFU-S that are in DNA synthesis by treating suspensions of stem cells with high concentrations of ^{3}HTdR to kill the cells in DNA synthesis. When the hemopoietic system is expanding a large fraction of the CFU-S (as much as 60–70 %) may be in DNA synthesis. In the steady state proliferation of the adult marrow and spleen the fraction of CFU-S in DNA synthesis is barely perceptible. Vassort et al. (10) have shown that the CFU-S has a ^{3}HTdR suicide varying from 9–20 % depending upon the strain of the adult mouse.

Only a fraction of the CFU-S produce splenic colonies upon transplantation. The fraction of these that produce splenic colonies is called the f-factor (11); this is roughly 0.17. There is considerable variation in the f-factor depending upon the period of time that the cell will circulate in the blood and many other factors of biological and statistical nature that may operate at any given time.

As of the moment there is no way of detecting the pluripotent stem cell in man or mammals other than the mouse, and to a lesser extent, the rat.

Pluripotent stem cells migrate through the blood. Two clear-cut experiments showed this years ago. Brecher and Cronkite (12) showed that when one member of a parabiotic pair is shielded while the other is receiving fatal irradiation, the irradiated one is protected from radiation lethality, thus showing the migration of the pluripotent hemopoietic stem cell from the nonirradiated into the irradiated twin. Swift et al. (13) showed the protection against radiation is conferred if one half the body only is exposed, followed in a matter of minutes by exposure of the remaining half and shielding of the previously exposed portion, thus showing migration of the pluripotent hemopoietic stem cell during this interval. Goodman and Hodgson (14) and Trobaugh and Lewis (15) showed that the PHSC circulate in the peripheral blood under normal steady state conditions. In mice the concentration of the CFU-S is 10–30 cells/ml (16). Their half-time in the blood, however, is reported to be only about 6 minutes (17). Accordingly, one can estimate in the 30 g mouse that the PHSC daily turnover rate is equal to:

$$\text{PHSCTR} = \frac{\text{PHSC}_T \times 0.693}{\text{T } 1/2} = \frac{20 \times 0.693 \times 60 \times 24}{6} \sim 3.3 \times 10^3/\text{day}$$

Where:

PHSC_T = total number of PHSC in blood
= blood volume (ml) x concentration PHSC (ml)
T 1/2 = half time of PHSC in blood = 6 min.
PHSCTR = daily PHSC turnover rate in mouse

If the human being has the same concentration in the blood as the mouse and similar rate of clearance (T 1/2, 6 minutes) the turnover rate in the standard man will be 1.7×10^7/day or 2×10^5/kg/day. Thus, this line of logic leads one to believe that a number of stem cells pass through the blood per day equivalent to about 1/10 the number of PHSC estimated in the bone marrow. It is presumed that a dynamic equilibrium between blood and marrow exists.

Of considerable interest is the flow of pluripotent stem cells through the alveolar capillaries. The number passing through the capillaries is equal to the concentration in the blood times the cardiac output. In man this amounts to $\sim 10^5$/min. Thus, pluripotent hemopoietic stem cells are brought to within one to a very few micrometers of the gaseous external environment. This is of potential importance in pulmonary toxicology in considering the hazards of inhaled toxic gases such as ozone, the nitrogen oxides, etc. thus submitting pluripotent hemopoietic to potential inhaled leukemogenic agents.

Committed stem cell pool

In man the abundance of the committed stem cells is generally considered to be measured by the *in vitro* bone marrow culture of colony forming units-culture (CFU-C). In man their abundance is about 0.1 to $1/10^4$ blood cells and 0.1 to $1/10^3$ bone marrow cells (18). Their thymidine suicide is of the order of 0.35, representing the fraction in DNA synthesis (19).

A study of the human stem cell is very difficult. Human cells do not produce spleen colonies in mice. It has been suggested by several investigators that the colonies formed in culture of human peripheral blood or bone marrow by CFU-C are the committed stem cells since they produce differentiated cells (erythrocytic, granulocytic, and macrophagic colonies).

Since one cannot measure human stem cells satisfactorily, an approach to the study of the human stem cell pool is to start from the peripheral blood, where the turnover rates of erythrocytes and granulocytes are well known. From the sum of these turnover rates, the structure of human bone marrow (amplification from stem cell to nondividing stem cell), absolute cellularity, DNA synthesis time, and the fraction of cells in DNA synthesis, the minimum flux of committed stem cells into the erythrocytic and granulocytic differentiated pools of the marrow can be estimated. The data from which the calculations are made have been reviewed (20) and are summarized as follows:

1. Erythrocyte average life span = 120 days
2. Erythrocyte turnover rate (RTR) = 12×10^7/kg/hr (288×10^7/day)
3. Granulocyte life span (random loss) half time of 6.8 hrs. (21)
4. Granulocyte turnover rate (GTR) = 6.8×10^7/kg/hr
5. RTR + GTR = 18.8×10^7/kg/hr
6. Erythroid marrow cellularity (N^E) = 536×10^7/kg (22, 23)
7. Granulocytis marrow (N^G) = 1140×10^7/kg (22, 23)
8. $N^E + N^G = 1,676 \times 10^7$/kg
9. DNA synthesis time in human bone marrow is about 12 hours for erythrocytic and granulocytic proliferating pool. (24)
10. Amplification from the committed stem cell to the nondividing erythrocytic and granulocytic cell averages 16.

This is shown schematically in Figure 1.

$$(N^{PHSC} + N^{CSC} + N^E + N^G + ALL\ OTHER\ CELLS = 1800 \times 10^7/kg)$$

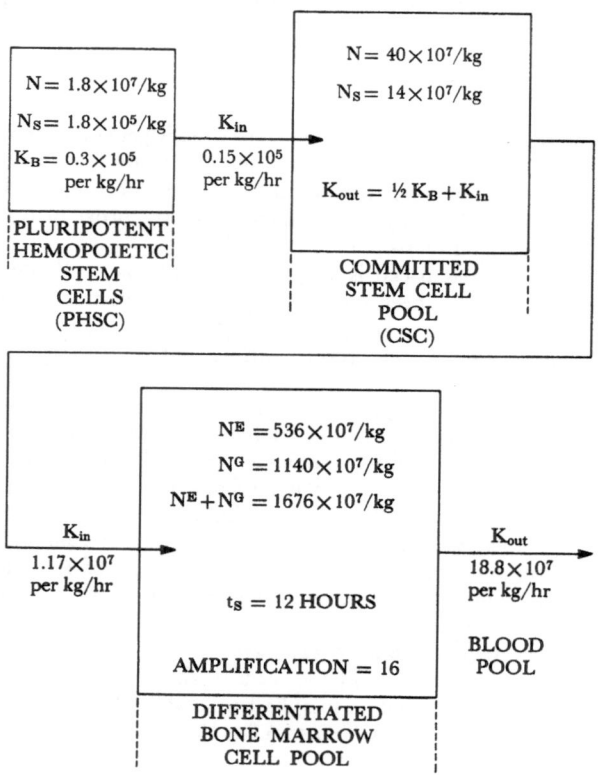

Fig. 1*: Schematic presentation of human bone marrow structure, proliferation and possible quantitation of the stem cell compartments.
Marrow cellularity from Donohue et al (23)
Amplification from Cronkite and Vincent (20)
DNA synthesis time from Stryckmans et al (24)
It is assumed that 1 per 1000 bone marrow cells are pluripotent and that 1 % are in DNA synthesis.

If it is assumed that detection of the most immature erythrocytic and granulocytic precursor establishes the cytologic boundary between the committed stem cell pool, an estimate can then be made of flux of committed stem cells into the differentiated pool (red and white) by dividing the sum of the red cell turnover rate and granulocyte turnover rate in the blood by the average amplification of 16. The

* This figure published by courtesy of Appleton-Century-Crofts.

total turnover rate in the blood is 18.8 x 10⁷/kg/hr. Thus with an amplification of 16 in the bone marrow the input of committed stem cells into the cytologically differentiated bone marrow pool is 1.17 x 10⁷/kg/hr.

In a stem cell pool the birth rate (K_B) must be twice the exit from the stem cell pool in order to maintain its steady state size. Thus birth rate is 2.35 x 10⁷/kg/hr. By assuming that the DNA synthesis time of committed stem cells is the same as that which has been measured in the differentiated pool of 12 hours, one can then simply calculate the number of cells that must be in DNA synthesis from the product of the DNA synthesis time and the birth rate. Thus, there are 28 x 10⁷/kg in DNA synthesis. If one uses the ³HTdR suicide of 0.35 as an estimate of the fraction of the committed stem cells that are in DNA synthesis, then the quotient of the number of cells in DNA synthesis by the fraction in DNA synthesis gives the absolute number or 80 x 10⁷/kg. Referring to Figure 1 one sees that the total number of differentiated erythrocytic and granulocytic cells is 1676 x 10⁷/kg. The ratio of the committed stem cells to the differentiated stem cells is therefore 1:21. Thus 4.8 % of the total marrow is committed stem cells and one can on a priori grounds say that the *in vitro* marrow culture system does not measure the committed stem cell pool.

One can ask whether this approach is valid. Does the thymidine suicide for the colony forming unit in culture apply to all the committed stem cell pool? If the fraction in DNA synthesis is smaller, the fraction of the total marrow occupied by committed stem cells becomes larger. If the time for DNA synthesis is overestimated, the number is overestimated. If the DNA synthesis time is really less than the measured time for differentiated marrow cells, the estimate of the number in DNA synthesis is too high. Even reducing time for DNA synthesis to a probably unrealistic low value of 1 hour for man reduces the number of committed stem cells to 6.6 x 10⁷/kg or still 1 in 300 marrow cells are committed stem cells. The above line of logic and assumption leads to a ratio of committed stem cells to total marrow cells that is completely incompatible with the *in vitro* bone marrow culture of 5/10⁴ colony forming cells in human bone marrow. It can be argued that the culture technique does not have sufficient stimulatory power to switch all the colony stimulating cells into proliferation. This is an attractive thought since the ratio has tended to increase as more potent sources of colony stimulating factor are developed and culture techniques are thus "souped up."

Let us take another line of argument and accept that the *in vitro* colony forming techniques do, in fact, accurately measure the number of committed stem cells in the bone marrow. If one then goes through the arithmetic as before and calculate on the basis of the DNA synthesis time of 12 hours, thymidine suicide of 0.35 and an absolute marrow cellularity of 1800 x 10⁷/kg, it is simple to show that the flux of the committed stem cells into the differentiated pool is such that an amplification of 520 would be required. Such an amplification would require about 9 serial mitoses in the proliferating granulocytic pool alone. In the granulocytic series it is reasonably well established that the time from the myeloblast to the myelocyte is 130 hours (20). If there is equal time for each successive multiplicative cell cycle there would be a generation time of 14 hours. The mitotic time is 0.75 hours (25). The mitotic index would be about 5 % or 5 times that observed by Killmann et al. (26). With a DNA synthesis time of 12 hours (24) the fraction of granulocytic proliferating cells in DNA synthesis would be 0.85 compared to the observations in man of

5

0.15–0.30 (26) and become incompatible with the number of myelocytes known to have a diploid DNA content. From these lines of reasoning and calculations based on experimentally determined data the notion of 9 serial mitoses in the granulocytic proliferating pool must be rejected along with the notion that the present *in vitro* methods of culturing bone marrow determines the fraction of committed stem cells in human bone marrow.

In addition, one can argue that knowledge on the cell turnover rate in the peripheral blood is incorrect. However, this is unlikely. Other arguments are that calculations based on average values are misleading and that there is a small fraction of stem cells that are dividing very rapidly or that the proliferation rate in the differentiated pool is grossly underestimated by averages and a small fraction of rapidly dividing cells will enable on one to "balance the books". The answer is not evident and for the moment this autohor feels compelled to question whether the *in vitro* culture bone marrow methods really estimate the fraction of the bone marrow that consists of committed stem cells.

References

1. Boyum, A., Carsten, A. L., Laerum, O. D. and Cronkite, E. P. Kinetics of cell proliferation of murine bone marrow cells cultured in diffusion chambers: effect of hypoxia, bleeding, erythropoietin injections, polycythemia, and irradiation of the host. Blood *40*:174, 1972.
2. Cronkite, E. P., Boecker, W., Carsten, A. L., Chikkappa, G., Joel, D., Laissue, J. and Ohl, S. The use of diffusion chamber cultures in the study of normal and leukemic cell proliferation in man. *In* Robinson, W. A. (ed.) Hemopoiesis in Culture, DHEW Publ. No. (NIH) 74–205, Bethesda, 1973, P. 185.
3. Maximow, A. A. and Bloom, W. (eds) Text Book of Histology, Philadelphia, W. B. Saunders, 1935.
4. Stohlman, F., Jr. The Kinetics of Cellular Proliferation, Grune and Stratton, New York, 1959.
5. Stohlman, F., Jr. (ed) Symposium on Hemopoietic Cellular Proliferation. St Elizabeth's Hospital Centennial 1869–1969, Boston, Massachusetts, Nov. 5–6 1969, Grune and Stratton, New York, 1970.
6. Till, J. E. and McCulloch, E. A. A direct measurement of the radiation sensitivity of normal mouse bone marrow cells. Radiat. Res. *14*:213, 1961.
7. Becker, A. J., McCulloch, E. A. and Till, J. E. Cystological demonstration of the clonal nature of spleen colonies derived from transplanted mouse marrow cells. Nature *197*:452, 1963.
8. Till, J. E., McCulloch, E. A. and Siminovitch, L. A. stochastic model of stem cell proliferation, based on the growth of spleen colony-forming cells. Proc. Nat. Acad. Sci. *51*:29, 1964.
9. Becker, A. J., McCulloch, E. A., Siminovitch, L. and Till, J. E. The effect of differing demands for blood cell production on DNA synthesis by hemopoietic colony-forming cells of mice. Blood *26*:296, 1965.
10. Vassort, F., Winterholer, M., Frindel, E. and Tubiana, M. Kinetic parameters of bone marrow stem cells using *in vivo* suicide by tritiated thymidine or by hydroxyurea. Blood *41*:789, 1973.

11. Till, J. E. and McCulloch, E. A. The "f-factor" of the spleen colony assay for hemopoietic stem cells. Series Hematology 5:15–21, 1972.
12. Brecher, G. and Cronkite, E. P. Postradiation parabiosis in survival in rats. Proc. Soc. Exper. Biol. Med. 77:292, 1951.
13. Swift, M. N., Taketa, F. T. and Bond, V. P. Regionally fractionated x-irradiation equivalent in dose to total body exposure. Rad. Res. 1:241, 1954.
14. Goodman, J. E., Hodgson, G. S. Evidence for stem cells in the peripheral blood of mice. Blood 19:702, 1962.
15. Trobaugh, F. E., Lewis, J. P., Jr. Repopulating potential of blood and marrow. J. Clin. Invest. 43:1306, 1964.
16. Hellman, S. and Grate, H. E. Kinetics of circulating haemopoietic colony-forming units in the mouse. In Doyle, E. (ed.) Effects of Radiation on Cellular Proliferation and Differentiation. Vienna, International Atomic Energy Agency, 1968(a), p. 187.
17. Hodgson, G., Guzman, E. and Herrera, C. Characterization of the stem cell population of phenylhydrazine-treated rodents In: Doyle, E. (ed.) Effects of Radiation on Cellular Proliferation and Differentiation. Vienna, International Atomic Energy Agency, 1968, p. 163.
18. Senn, J. S. and McCulloch, E. A. Radiation sensitivity of human bone marrow cells measured by a cell culture method. Blood 35:56, 1970.
19. Moore, M. A. S. and Williams, N. Functional, morphologic, and kinetic analysis of the granulocyte-macrophage progenitor cell. In Robinson, W. A. (ed) Hemopoiesis in Culture, DHEW Publication No. (NIH) 740205, Bethesda, 1973, p 17.
20. Cronkite, E. P. and Vincent, P. C. Granulocytopoiesis. Ser. Haemat. Vol. II, 4, 1969, 3–43.
21. Cartwright, G. E., Athens, J. W. and Wintrobe, M. M. The kinetics of granulopoiesis in normal man. Blood 24:780, 1964.
22. Donohue, D. M., Reiff, R. H., Hanson, M. L., Betson, Y and Finch, C. A. Quantitative measurements of the erythrocytic and granulocytic cells of the marrow and blood. J. Clin. Invest. 37:1571, 1958.
23. Donuhue, D. M., Gabrio, B. W. and Finch, C. A. Quantitative measurement of hematopoietic cells of the marrow. J. Clin. Invest. 37:1564, 1958.
24. Stryckmans, P., Cronkite, E. P., Fliedner, T. M. and Tamos, J. DNA synthesis time of erythropoietic and granulopoietic cells in human beings. Nature 211:717, 1966.
25. Odartchenko, N., Cottier, H., Feinendegen, L. E. and Bond, V. P. Evaluation of mitotic time in vivo using tritiated thymidine as a cell marker: Successive labeling with time of separate mitotic phases. Exp. Cell. Res. 35:402, 1964.
26. Killmann, S. A., Cronkite, E P., Fliedner, T. M. and Bond, V. P. Mitotic index of human bone marrow cells I. Number and cytologic distribution of mitoses. Blood 19:743, 1962.

Productivity in Normal and Leukemic Granulocytopoiesis*

T. M. Fliedner, D. Hoelzer and K. H. Steinbach

Department of Clinical Physiology
University of Ulm
D 79 Ulm (Donau)
Germany

1. Introduction

At the request of the organizers of this workshop on "Modern Trends in Human Leukemia II" we have been asked to review briefly some aspects of the physiology and pathophysiology of myelopoiesis, focusing mainly on the problems of the obvious deficiency of this system in case of acute myelocytic leukemia to provide an adequate number of granulocytes. A vast amount of information has been collected during the last 1 or 2 decades on the possibilities and limitations of cell production and differentiation in normal and leukemic myelopoieses. In spite of this, we have to confess today that there are many more open questions than solved problems. It probably is correct to state that "we are still quite ignorant about normal and leukemic cell production and differentiation but at a higher level" than 17 years ago, when the first cell kinetic study utilizing tritiated thymidine as a specific DNA label was performed in Dr. Cronkite's laboratory (1, 2, 3).

It is therefore the purpose of this presentation to outline the present concept of normal and leukemic cell proliferation and differentiation using granulocyte kinetics as a model. This will lead to the conclusion that the obvious deficiency of granulocyte production in acute leukemia is a consequence of a highly ineffective cell proliferation and differentiation in the appropriate precursor compartments and points to the stem-cell pool as the major site of leukemic cell transformation.

2. Efficient granulocyte production: a property of the normal granulocytic cell renewal system

The normal granulocytic cell renewal system (Fig. 1) maintains in the peripheral blood of man a granulocyte concentration that appears to be constant from day to day, although detailed studies may indicate a cyclic pattern with a phase length of some twenty days, the amplitude of which may increase in certain diseases such as cyclic neutropenia (4, 5). The extravascular portion, the function of which guarantees a sufficient blood granulocyte concentration, is normally located ecxlusively in the bone marrow, distributed in many bones throughout the body, but nevertheless acting as one organ. The regulatory mechanisms responsible for this unity

* Research work supported by the Deutsche Forschungsgemeinschaft through the Sonderforschungsbereich 112 (Zellsystemphysiologie).

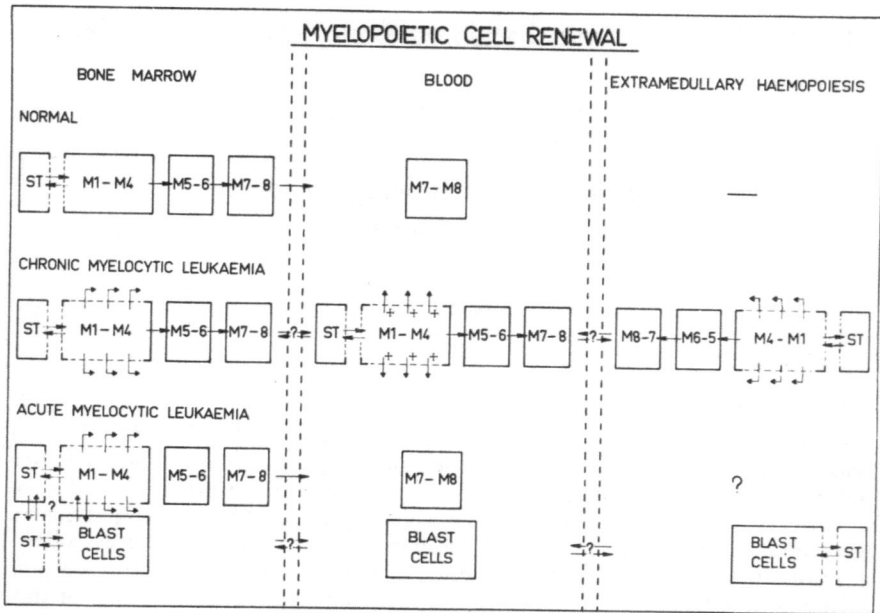

Fig. 1: Schematic representation of the functional structure of the myelopoietic cell renewal system in normal conditions, in chronic myelocytic leukemia and in acute myelocytic leukemia.

of function, in spite of topographic diversity, are far from being understood in detail but should include humoral as well as neural factors and may well be associated with stem-cell migration via the blood stream. The functional structure of the granulocytic cell renewal system can be described as a number of catenated cell compartments. The granulocytes of the blood – segmented forms and band forms, M 8 and M 7 respectively, – represent the *functional pool* of cells. It is known since the work of the Salt Lake City Group (6) that the half-life of the mature cells is in the order of 7 hours. The mature granulocytes leave the blood either by emigration or after death due to senescence (7, 8). This pool is fed continuously by the M 7/M 8 *storage pool* in the marrow. This is considered to be a part of the *maturation-only pool* in the marrow, but with a variable "time delay": it is known through the work of the Brookhaven Group that the time of granulocytes between the last division of myelocytes and their release into the blood as mature granulocytes may vary and can be as short as 2 days (instead of 4 days) in cases of infection (7, 8). It is this pool that contains a large amount of reserve cells that can be released into the blood after appropriate stimulation and may increase the blood granulocyte concentration several times within a few hours (9). This pool in turn is fed by the *maturing-only pool* of metamyelocytes and juvenile cells – M 5 and M 6. Furthermore, there is a *dividing-maturing pool* of granulocyte precursors, the myeloblasts, promyelocytes and myelocytes (M 1 – M 4). These cells are considered

10

to be capable of division but not of self-replication. On the basis of morphological, cell-kinetic and cinematographic studies, the number of cell divisions in this pool has been estimated to be 2–4 in normal marrow (10–13). The maintenance of a homeostatic equilibrium between production and utilization in this system is maintained by a *stem-cell pool* which has the dual function of maintaining its own size and at the same time responding to specific stimuli, such as erythropoetin or a still hypothetical granulopoietin (14) (which may or may not be identical to CSF (15), with differentiation into the well-known hematopoietic cell lineages. Dr. Cronkite, in this conference, has indicated the present state of knowledge about this cell pool and its conceptual difficulties (16). Nevertheless, it appears justified to assume that this pool contains at least 2 sub-populations of cells which may be denoted as "committed and uncommitted", or "determined and undetermined" (14, 17, 18), depending on the author. These expressions are meant to indicate that this pool contains cells that have to undergo a certain process of physiological "development" or "maturation" in order to proceed from a pluripotent stage – in which most cells appear to be in a cytokinetically resting phase called G_0 (19) – to a stage of being "committed" to respond to specific stimuli with irreversible differentiation, resulting in a catenated process of cell multiplication and/or maturation. In the human, various methods have been developed in recent years to elucidate one or the other aspect of this pool. In diffusion chambers implanted into irradiated recipients (goats (20), rats and mice (21, 22)), human bone marrow cells and blood mononuclear cells have been shown to be able to form granulocytes, erythroblasts and megakaryocytes and, hence, to be indicative of the presence of a population of pluripotent cells. In cell cultures with appropriate media and stimulation factors, one has been able to trigger stem-cells into granulocytic, erythropoietic and megakaryocytic differentiation, thus looking – presumably – at the "committed" cell population of the stem-cell pool (23, 24). In spite of such efforts, it appears that it is not yet possible to characterize the stem-cell pool completely in terms of quantitative and qualitative properties, but one is "recognizing" only certain aspects and is limited by the inherent constraints of the methods used to approach the problem. It may be of interest at this point to say a few words about the regulatory mechanisms of the granulocytic cell-renewal system. Its particular structure led several investigators to the hypothesis that it can be considered as a cell system, regulated by a negative feed-back mechanism and that it must have oscillatory properties (25, 26). It is assumed that there are factors that are capable of inducing a release of granulocytes into the blood stream in case of need and that there are other factors, both inhibiting as well as stimulating factors, that trigger cells into differentiation at the stem-cell level or prevent them from differentiating (27, 28, 29).

In *conclusion*, the characteristic blood granulocyte concentration appears to be the result of a feed-back controlled cell-renewal system. This is capable of lifelong granulocyte production without exhaustion and can adapt itself to increased demands by an appropriate increase in production. Further research has to explore the degree of efficiency under the conditions of the normal steady state. A maximum degree of efficiency would be reached when all cells triggered into the granulopoietic pathway undergo an equal number of cell divisions and all reach the blood as mature cells without cell death along the dividing-maturing pathway by intrinsic deficiencies. It may well be, however, that there is normally a "death function" at all levels of granulopoietic proliferation and maturation, the extent of which would be highest in the functional cell pool (30).

3. Inefficient granulocyte production: a consequence of leukemic transformation of the granulopoietic cell system

In leukemia, both in the chronic myelocytic and in the acute myelocytic forms, the granulocyte production is drastically altered (Fig. 1). In *chronic myelocytic leukemia* (CML), one observes in the blood and in extramedullary sites the presence of granulocyte precursors. In a recent article, Drs. Vincent and Cronkite and associates presented a wealth of information on the cell kinetics of this disease and came to the conclusion "that increased myelocyte proliferation as well as an increased stem-cell input must contribute to the expansion in granulocytopoiesis seen in chronic myelocytic leukemia. Myelocytes in CML divide 3–4 times, compared with twice in normal marrow, thus increasing the amplification of the stem-cell input. The size of the total myelocyte mass in the patients studied was estimated to be 3 and 25 times normal (12)". Further studies have to explore the extent of cell death of the myelocytes so produced and hence the degree of efficiency or inefficiency of cell production in the system.

In *acute myelocytic leukemia,* the blood picture is characterized by the presence of some mature granulocytes and of "blast-cells" (Fig. 1). There is evidence in the bone marrow of some proliferation and maturation of myelocytes and promyelocytes, resulting in the appearance of some normal-looking and functioning granulocytes in the blood. However, the bulk of cells usually is comprised of "blast-cells" showing a spectrum of morphological appearance. There is also today a fair amount of information on the kinetics of such blast-cells in bone marrow and blood and, more recently, some evidence about the developmental potential of the leukemic blast-cells. Usually, the blast-cells in the bone marrow show a low tritiated thymidine (^{3}H-TdR) labeling index as compared to normal myeloblasts or promyelocytes, when exposed to ^{3}H-TdR in vitro or in vivo. The labeling index of blood blast-cells is still lower (31). If leukemic blast-cells are labeled in vitro with tritiated cytidine (^{3}H-Cyt) and autotransfused, the calculated blood transit times are between *3.7 and 8.5 days,* much longer than those of granulocytes (32). Hoelzer and Kurrle in our group (33) have studied the fate of leukemic blast-cells in diffusion chambers implanted intraperitoneally into irradiated mice. They came to the conclucion that some leukemic blast-cells appear to have the potential to differentiate into granulocytic precursors and to mature into granulocytes. Thus, it may well be that the accumulation of blast-cells in human acute myelocytic leukemia can be taken to indicate the extreme of inefficiency: the bulk of cells accumulates in the form of "blast-cells" that, in principle, may have the potential for differentiation and production of granulocytes, but rarely do so in the phase of full-blown acute leukemia. It is, therefore, of interest to ask whether there is any normal rest function of granulocytopoiesis and, if so, with what characteristics, or whether granulocyte production arises from leukemic precursor cells, some of which exercise their potential to differentiate, proliferate and mature.

In many patients, both in Brookhaven and in Ulm, the kinetics of granulocyte production was studied by means of tritiated thymidine labeling (7, 8). The typical,

LABELING INDEX OF GRANULOCYTES

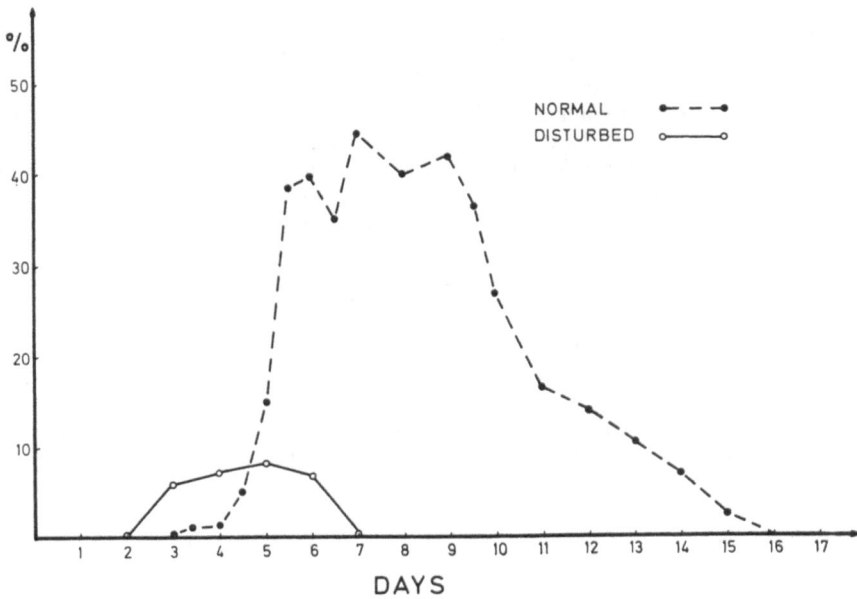

Fig. 2: Labeling index of blood granulocytes as a function of time after administration of 3H-TdR.
○ person with undisturbed hemopoiesis.
● patient with acute myelocytic leukemia.

normal labeling pattern of blood granulocytes after thymidine labeling shows the appearance of the first labeled, segmented forms in the blood after a lag-phase of about 4 days (maturation time from the last division to release) followed by a rise of the labeling index to about 60 % and a subsequent decline (Fig. 2). The same labeling pattern is seen for granulocytes removed from the mucous membranes, indicating that they had migrated onto these surfaces, and for the pycnotic granulocytes, the latter delayed, however, by some 24–30 hours, indicating the upper limit of life in the blood stream. In various forms of acute leukemia, the labeling pattern of blood granulocytes in acute leukemia is markedly different. Although the first appearance of labeled granulocytes may be normal or somewhat shortened – as seen also in cases of infection – there is a labeling pattern with several abnormal features. The labeling indices never reach the normal values but are below 30 %, in many cases not exceeding 10–20 percent. The labeled cells disappear again quite rapidly, so that, after 6 days, many or all may have disappeared. In other cases, a few may be seen until 12 days after 3H-TdR injection (7, 8).

The attempt to answer the question as to the reasons for the low labeling indices combined, usually, with a granulocytopenia in spite of a normal blood emergence time for labeled granulocytes, leads one to the problem of the efficiency or

13

inefficiency of cell production and/or maturation in the various precursor pools of blood granulocytes.

In Fig. 2, the labeling pattern of blood granulocytes is shown for a patient with undisturbed hemopoiesis (34) and for a patient with acute myelocytic leukemia. It is clear that the labeling pattern of the leukemic patient is markedly different with respect to the maximum labeling index achieved and to the duration of the presence of labeled cells. In order to try to formulate questions for further studies on the efficiency of cell production in leukemic patients, we approached the problem by trying to simulate the labeling curve on a computer using the GPSS (general purpose simulation system) language (35). In order to simulate the labeling curve, the following experimental data had to be recognized (one patient):

1. The labeling index of the bone marrow cells (M 2–M 4) 1 hour after ^{3}H-Tdr was found to be 14 %.
2. The relationship of the relative proportion of the dividing-maturing (M 2–M 4) cells to the maturing-only cells (M 5–M 7) and hence, the absolute numbers of these cells, was 18:1.
3. The DNA-synthesis time of the dividing cells was estimated to be 24 hours.
4. In the circulating pool of granulocytes, there were 123 cells per μl.

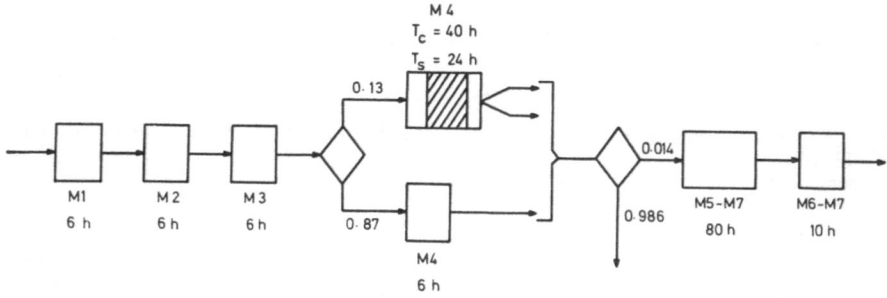

DISTURBED GRANULOPOIESIS

Fig. 3: The model of the granulocytic cell renewal system in a patient with AML.

A model that allows the approximate reconstruction of the labeling pattern of blood granulocytes in this patient with acute leukemia and still recognizes all the conditions specified in points 1–4 is given in Fig 3. In this model, one has to assume that cells entering the M 1, M 2 and M 3 compartments do so without synthesizing DNA and dividing. The compartment transit time must be taken to be 6 hours for each. After leaving the M 3 compartment, a divergence of the cell "stream" occurs. About 87 % of the cells enter an "ineffective" M 4 compartment which they leave after 6 hours of further maturation. The remaining 13 % of cells coming from M 3 synthesize (in M 4) DNA and divide. The DNA synthesis time was determined to be 24 hours, the cell cycle time 40 hours. In such a system, a labeling

14

index of 14 % is found. In order to find now a relationship of 18:1 between M 2–M 4 cells and M5–M 7 cells and in order to fill the circulating compartment with 123 granulocytes per µl, 98.6 % of the cells coming from the two M 4 compartments must leave the system (by cell death) and only 1.4 % of the cells enter the maturation-only compartment to stay in it for an average of 80 hours. The functional pool, with a transit time of 10 hours, and a marginal and circulating pool of equal size is the last compartment of such a simulated system. To maintain a concentration of 246 granulocytes per µl in the last compartment an efflux-rate of 1580 cells/h from the stem-cell pool must be provided.

As already stated, the computer language used was the GPSS. The particular advantage of this language is seen in the fact that the inevitable variabilities of experimental data can be fully recognized.

LABELING INDEX OF GRANULOCYTES

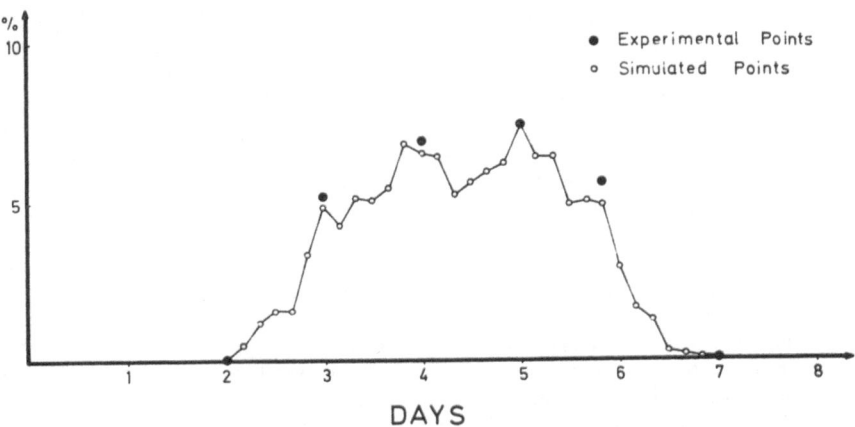

Fig. 4: The computer simulated labeling index in the functional pool in comparison to the experimental points.

Fig. 4 shows the labeling index pattern in the functional pool as it was simulated by the computer system in comparison to the experimental points. There is evidence that there is reasonable agreement between the experimental points and the simulated curve. In the simulation system, the time parameters of the system were assumed to follow a normal distribution with a standard error of 50 % of the mean. It was assumed that there is a steady state for the duration of the experimental study.

In order to obtain the labeling indices as shown in Figure 4 and with recognition of conditions 1–4 (see above), several mean values for the different system-parameters were obtained and are given in Table 1.

Of course, the information obtained from computer system simulation on one patient is far from being sufficient to draw general conclusions. Furthermore, results of system simulation models cannot be taken as evidence that they reflect

Table I: Computer derived cell kinetic parameters in the patient with acute myelocytic leukemia

Time of cell cycle	40 h
Compartment transit time (M 1 – M 4)	6 h
Fraction of maturing cells	1.4 %
Kinetic (Stem-Cell pool)	1580 h^{-1}
Multiplication factor M 1 – M 4	1.13

4. Leukemic granulocytopoiesis: a consequence of inefficient productivity

Of course, the information obtaine from computer system simulation on one patient is far from being sufficient to draw general conclusions. Furthermore, results of system simulation models cannot be taken as evidence that they reflect biological facts, processes or dynamic events. They can help, however, to pose questions and to focus on experimental approaches for obtaining information on the biological mechanisms underlying the observed sequence of events.

In the present system-simulation of one patient with acute leukemia, it appears of interest to note that the labeling pattern observed points to several possible deviations from normal in the dividing-maturing pool of granulocyte precursors. First of all, there appears to be decreased degree of proliferation; the cells, originating in an undefined stem-cell pool, cannot undergo the normal sequence of doubling divisions. The presence of leukemic blast-cells in marrow and blood may thus be regarded as an accumulation of cells that cannot make full use of their potential to divide and mature. The facts that some of them can be labeled by means of tritiated thymidine and that they show a turnover – when studied after retransfusion, labeled with ^{3}H-cytidine – are indications of some renewal which, however, remains totally inept with respect to granulocyte formation. The information obtained from leukemic patients with respect to granulocyte turnover, on the other hand, shows that some granulocyte formation is possible. It is to be asked whether this granulocyte formation is a reflection of a resting of normal hemopoiesis or whether it is the inefficient responce of a leukemic blast population for differentiation and maturation (as may be observable in diffusion chambers) or both. The results of the simulation model could be interpreted to mean an overwhelming disturbance of the normal process of proliferation and maturation and would be more compatible with the notion of a leukemic cell population with a resting or maturing-only capacity. In other leukemic patients, the granulocyte labeling pattern resembles more that of a normal hemopoiesis. Thus, it may well be that the clinical diversity of hematological findings is due to the wide spectrum of differentiation potentialities that may be presented in leukemia: at the one end of the spectrum may be seen a complete block of differentiation for granulocyte formation and an accumulation of "blast-cells" unresponsive to differentiation signals; at the other end (in remission) may be a "leukemic" population that is practically normal in its capability to differentiate, to proliferate and to mature. Between these two extremes may be all degrees of lack of differentiation, proliferation and maturation; certainly, in the overt cases of leukemia, there is a high degree of inefficiency of granulocyte production and, at best, an abortive attempt to respond to the demands of the periphery in terms of increased granulocyte production. The data obtained from the granulocyte kinetic study of leukemic patients also indicate a lack of responsiveness for differentiation at the level of the stem-cell pool. Normally, granulocyte removal from the blood results in a feed-back mechanism resulting in an increase in cell production. In leukemia, the demand is clearly there, but the appropriate proliferative pool is not able to respond with normal production and maturation.

From all these considerations, it may be concluded that the basic defect in leukemia must be sought in the stem-cell pool. It is here that one must locate a defect in the normal response to differentiate into a granulocyte lineage with subsequent proliferation and maturation. One must ask whether there is a complete transformation of all normal cells into leukemic cells without a residual normal population (even though suppressed) or whether there is a normal population remaining in conjunction with the leukemic population with a certain "growth advantage" which is, however, insufficient to produce normal cells.

References

1. Cronkite, E. P., T. M. Fliedner, J. R. Rubini, V. P. Bond and W. L. Hughes: Dynamics of proliferating cell systems of man studied with tritiated thymidine. J. Clin. Investigation 37, 887, 1958.
2. Cronkite, E. P., V. P. Bond, T. M. Fliedner and J. R. Rubini: The use of tritiated thymidine in the study of DNA synthesis and cell turnover in hemopoietic tissues. Laboratory Investigation 8, 263–275, 1959.
3. Cronkite, E. P., T. M. Fliedner, V. P. Bond and J. R. Rubini: Dynamics of hemopoietic proliferation in man and mice studied by ^{3}H-thymidine incorporation into DNA. Ann. N.Y. Acad. Sci. 77, 803–830, 1959.
4. King-Smith, E. A. and Morley, A.: Computer simulation of granulopoiesis: normal and impaired granulopoiesis. Blood 36, 254–262, 1970.
5. Meuret, G. und Fliedner, T. M.: Zellkinetik der Granulozytopoese und des Neutrophilensystems bei einem Fall von zyklischer Neutropenie. Acta Haemat. (Basel) 43, 48–63, 1970.
6. Athens, J. W., Haab, O. P., Raab, S. O., Maurer, A. M., Ashenbrucker, H., Cartwright, G. E. und Wintrobe, M. M.: Leukokinetic studies: IV. The total blood, circulating and marginal granulocyte pools and the granulocyte turnover rate in normal subjects. J. Clin. Invest. 40, 989–995, 1961.
7. Fliedner, T. M., E. P. Cronkite, and Robertson, J. S.: Granulocytopoiesis. I. Senescence and random loss of neutrophilic granulocytes. Blood 24, 402–414, 1964.
8. Fliedner, T. M., E. P. Cronkite, S. A. Killmann and V. P. Bond: Granulocytopoiesis. II. Emergence and pattern of labelling of neutrophilic granulocytes in humans. Blood 24, 683–699, 1964.
9. Stodtmeister, R. und T. M. Fliedner: Die akute Streß-Situation des Knochenmarkes. Med. Klinik 52, 2225–2227, 1967.
10. Boll, I. and A. Kühn: Granulocytopoiesis in bone marrow cultures, studied by means of kinematography. Blood 26, 449, 1965.

11. Cronkite, E. P. and T. M. Fliedner: Granulocytopoiesis. New England Journal of Medicine, 270, 1347–1352, 1964.
12. Vincent, P. C., E. P. Cronkite, T. M. Fliedner, M. L. Greenberg, C. Hunter, W. Kirsten, J. S. Robertson, L. M. Schiffer and P. A. Stryckmans: Leukocyte kinetics and chronic myeloid leukemia: II. Size distribution of myelocytes and initial labelling pattern of cells in blood and marrow. To be published 1975.
13. Killmann, S. A., E. P. Cronkite, T. M. Fliedner, V. P. Bond and G. Brecher: Mitotic indices of human bone marrow cells. II. The use of mitotic indices for estimation of time parameters of proliferation in serially connected multiplicative cellular compartments. Blood 21, 141–163, 1963.
14. McCulloch, E. A. and J. E. Till: Cellular interactions in the control of hemopoiesis. In: F. Stohlman jr. (Edit.): Hemopoietic cellular proliferation. Grune and Stratton, New York/London, 1970.
15. Metcalf, D. and Moore, M. A. S.: Haemopoietic cells. North-Holland Publishing Company, Amsterdam/London, 1971.
16. Cronkite, E. P.: Hemopoietic stem cells: An analytical review of hemopoiesis. To be published in the Year Book of Pathology, edited by Joachim.
17. Stohlman, F. jr.: Regulation of red cell production. In: Greenwalt, T. J. and Jamieson, G. A. (Editors): Formation and destruction of blood cells. Philadelphia, J. B. Lippincott, 1970.
18. Lajtha, L. G.: Stem cell kinetics. In: A. S. Gordon (Edit.): Regulation of hemopoiesis. Appleton-Century-Crofts. Educational Division/Meredith Corporation, New York, 1970.
19. Lajtha, L. G., Oliver, R. and Gurney, C. W.: Kinetic model for a bone marrow stem cell population. Brit. J. Haemat. 8, 442, 1962.
20. Cronkite, E. P., A. L. Carsten, G. Chikkappa, J. A. Laissue and S. Öhl: Culture of normal and leukemic cells in diffusion chambers. In: Prognostic Factors in Human Acute Leukemia. Advances in the Biosciences 14, Pergamon Press, Oxford, New York, Toronto, Sydney, 1975.
21. Benestad, H. B.: Formation of granulocytes and macrophages in diffusion chamber cultures of mouse blood leukocytes. Scand. J. Haematology 7, 279–288, 1970.
22. Bøyum, A., Boecker, W., Carsten, A. L. and Cronkite, E. P.: Proliferation of human bone marrow cells in diffusion chambers implanted into normal or irradiated mice. Blood 40, 163–173, 1972.
23. Bradley, T. R. and Metcalf, D.: The growth of mouse bone marrow cells invitro. Austral. J. exp. Biol. med. Sci. 44, 287–300, 1966.
24. Robinson, W. A. (Edit.): Haemopoiesis in culture. DHEW publication number (NIH 74–205), 1974.
25. Morley, A., King-Smith, E. A. and Stohlman, F. jr.: The oscillatory nature of hemopoiesis. In: F. Stohlman jr. (Edit.): Hemopoietic cellular proliferation. Grune and Stratton, New York, 1970.
26. Morley, A., Baikie, A. G. and Galton, D. A. G.: Cyclical leukocytosis as evidence for retention of normal homeostatic control in chronic granulocytic leukemia. Lancet II, 1320, 1970.
27. Gordon, A. S., Handler, E. S., Siegel, Ch. D., Dornfest, B. S. and Lo Bue, J.:

Plasma factors influencing leukocyte release in rats. Ann. N. Y. Acad. Sci. 113, 766–789, 1964.

28. Bierman, H. R., Marshall, G. J., Maekawa, T. and Kelly, K. H.: Granulocytic activity of human plasma. Acta haemat. (Basel) 27, 217–228, 1962.

29. Rytömaa, T. and Kiviniemi, K.: Control of granulocyte production. II. Mode of action of chalone and antichalone. Cell and Tissue Kinet. 1, 341–350, 1968.

30. Patt, H. M. and M. A. Maloney: A model of granulocyte kinetics. In: H. Biermann (Edit.): Leukopoiesis in Health and Disease Ann. N.Y. Acad. Sci., 113, 515–522, 1964.

31. Killmann, S. A.: Acute leukemia. The kinetics of leukemic blast-cells in man. Ser. Haematol. 1, 38, 1968.

32. Hoelzer, D., E. B. Harriss, T. M. Fliedner and H. Heimpel: The turnover of blast cells in peripheral blood after in-vitro ³H-cytidine labelling and re-transfusion in human acute leukemia. Europ. J. Clinical Investigation 2, 259–268, 1972.

33. Hoelzer, D., E. B. Harriss and E. Kurrle: Prognostic indications of diffusion chamber and agar culture studies in human acute leukemia. In: Prognostic factors in human acute leukemia, Advances in the Biosciences 14. Pergamon Press, Oxford, New York, Toronto, Sydney, 1975.

34. Fliedner, T. M., Cronkite, E. P. and Bond, V. P.: Die Proliferationsdynamik der Blutzellbildung, autoradiographisch untersucht mit tritiummarkiertem Thymidin. Schweiz. med. Wschr. 89, 1061, 1959.

35. General Purpose Simulation System V. User's Manual, IBM, SH 20–0851–1.

Cytologie and Cytochemistry of Colony Cells in Soft Agar Gel Culture from Normal and Leukemic Bone Marrow

H. Beckmann[1], R. Neth[1], H. Soltau[1], R. Mertelsmann[2],
K. Winkler[3], K. Hausmann[4], H. Hellwege[1] and G. Skrandies[4].

[1] Molekularbiologisch-hämatologische Arbeitsgruppe
[3] Abteilung für Gerinnungsforschung und Onkologie
Universitätskinderklinik
[2] 1. Medizinische Universitätsklinik
[4] Hämatologische Abteilung, Allgemeines Krankenhaus
St. Georg,
Hamburg, West Germany

Summary

In order to judge differentiation of cells in soft agar colonies, cytological and cytochemical classification of single cells within these colonies is necessary. In this study, 1,026 colonies from 15 normal and 95 leukemic bone marrows have been evaluated using cytological, cytochemical, and immunocytochemical techniques. In 180 colonies from 15 normal controls no segmented neutrophils have been observed. The colonies mostly consisted of monocytes and macrophages, rarely pure eosinophil colonies were observed. The number of monocyte/macrophage colonies in untreated AML and the percentage of pure eosinophil colonies in AML and ALL in remission are reduced, as compared to normal controls.

In 174 colonies from a total of 926 colonies derived from bone marrows of leukemic patients, plasma cells and in 20 colonies, blast cells have been observed. In contrast to normal colonies, growth of colonies containing blast cells does not depend upon the conditioned medium of the leukocyte feederlayer.

This investigation has demonstrated the necessity of cytological and cytochemical classification in addition to quantiative evaluation of soft agar colonies when studying the effect of factors on proliferation and differentiation of normal and leukemic stem cells.

Supported by a grant from the Deutsche Forschungsgemeinschaft

Acknowledgment: The authors are indepted to Professor H. Busch, director of the blood bank of the University Hospital Hamburg-Eppendorf, who kindly supported us by research material, and to Miss B. Heinisch, B. Schaeffer and H. Stührk for their excellent technical assistance.

21

Introduction

Human bone marrow contains cells which form – dependent on specific interactions with diffusible factors – leukocyte and erythrocyte colonies in soft agar (1–6). On the base of published data, most authors assume that each colony arises from one single cell. Leukemic bone marrow cells exhibit a nearly total failure of colony formation in vitro (7–14), which is most probably due to the blocked differentiation. Recent results have shown that cells from untreated AML and from AML in relapse could be stimulated with PHA to form colonies in soft agar in the absence of diffusible factors, i. e. without feeder layer (8). GALLAGHER et al. reports proliferation and differentiation of AML cells in suspension cultures after stimulation with conditioned medium from embryonal tissues (15). These data suggest that some of the organizational and regulatory features of normal hemopoiesis persist in leukemic hemopoiesis. In order to judge differentiation of cells in soft agar colonies, a cytological and cytochemical classification of single cells within these colonies appears necessary. Simple quantitative evaluation of colony formation does not yield enough information regarding differentiation patterns. As a first step towards the evalutation of the effect of specific differentiation factors on normal and leukemic bone marrow cells in soft agar, more than 1,000 colonies from normal and leukemic bone marrows have been classified according to cytological and cytochemical criteria (16–19).

MaterialandMethods

a) Source of Material

Normal bone marrow was obtained by aspiration from the iliac crest or sternum, taken during the hematologic examination of 13 children and two adults. Six of these patients were defined as normal, and the other nine showed no evidence of hemoblastosis or granulopoietic abnormalities. For cytological and cytochemical classification of bone marrow cells the usual criteria were used.

ALL patients received the same chemotherapy described by PINKEL et al (20), including vincristine (VCR) and prednisone (PRED), followed by central nervous system (CNS) leukemia prophylaxis with CNS irradiation and intrathecal methotrexate (MTX). For maintenance a combination of cyclophosphamide, MTX, and 6-mercaptopurine (6-MP) was given. Patients with AML were treated with a combination of 6-thioguanine and cytosine arabinoside.

b) Cell Separation

For the separation of leukocytes the method of BÖYUM (21) was used. The resulting buffy coat was suspended in culture medium. The nucleated cells were counted with a hemocytometre. For the preparation of feeder layers, granulocytes and monocytes were counted. The cell layer was prepared by suspending two or three drops of aspirated bone marrow into the culture medium, followed by a hypertonic shock, repeated twice for lysis of erythrocytes, and by counting the number of mononucleated bone marrow cells, omitting non-deviding cells like metamyelocytes and polymorphs.

22

c) Culture Technique

Agar cultures were prepared using the double layer agar technique of PIKE and ROBINSON (22). McCoy's 5A medium containing 15 % fetal calf serum and supplemented with amino acids and vitamins, was mixed in a 9:1 ratio with boiled 5 % agar (Difco). After addition of the appropriate number of leukocytes (1.5 – 1.8 x 10^6), 1 ml of this agar cell medium mixture was pipetted into 35 mm plastic Petri Dishes (Falcon Plastics). These prepared feeder layers were stored at 37 °C in a humidified incubator continously flushed with 8 % CO_2. The washed bone marrow cells were mixed with culture medium and boiled 3 % agar, in a ratio of 9:1; of this, 1 ml aliquots were then pipetted onto the feeder layer. The final concentration of the cell layer was 1 x 10^5 mononucleated bone marrow cells per ml. Following this preparation, no aggregates, clumps, or tissue fragments were found in bone marrow suspensions or in agar. The dishes were incubated for three weeks. During this time, at intervals of 12 to 14 days, the number of colonies was counted with an inverted microscope (Diavert) at 40x magnification. Only those colonies containing 50 or more cells were counted. For each experiment, at least four plates with, und two plates without feeder layer were examined; the counts were expressed as the mean result of these plates. The number of colonies in two plates never varied more than 10 % for bone marrow cells, and maximally 100 % for peripheral blood leukocytes.

d) Source of Colony Stimulating Factor

A feeder layer of peripheral blood leukocytes was used as source of colony stimulating factor (CSF). Since the induction of proliferation of colonies depends on the age of the feeder layer, the feeder layer was used during the day of preparation or only few days later. After seven days of incubation, the feeder layer had lost about 50 % of its original stimulating activity (23).

Mature granulocytes inhibit the proliferation of colonies (24). Therefore the number of granulocytes in the feeder layer was not allowed to exceed 1 x 10^6 cells per ml (23). At this concentration of granulocytes the feeder layer contained nearly 1–2 x 10^5 monocytes per ml.

c) Cytologic Analysis of Colonies

For cytologic analysis, colonies were picked out of the agar under the inverted microscope with an angled (ca 110°) micro-hematocrit. They were put on slides and incubated for 10 minutes in a humidified chamber wit a 1 % solution of agarase (Calbiochem., Los Angeles). The colonies were prepared according to the method of TESTA and LORD (25). After incubation, the agarase was drawn off carefully, and the colonies were fixed according to the cytochemical reaction necessary (10 % formalin alcohol for peroxidase reaction, 60 % cold acetone for acid phosphatase reaction). Fixation solution was dropped onto the slide. Then a coverslip was placed on top of the drop. This in turn was covered with a piece of filter paper and gently pressed. The slide was frozen on dry ice for 10 minutes, the cover slip was removed quickly, and the slide immediately dried. The colony cells were stained with May-Grünwald-Giemsa, respectively for peroxidase (16), or acid phosphatase (26).

f) Demonstration of Immunoglobulins

To demonstrate immunoglobulin within plasma cells, some colonies were fixed as described above, stained for 30 minutes with FITC conjugated anti-human immunoglobulins (Table 2), and then washed three times with PBS.

The colonies were investigated with a Leitz ortholux microscope equipped with an Opak-Fluor vertical illuminator.

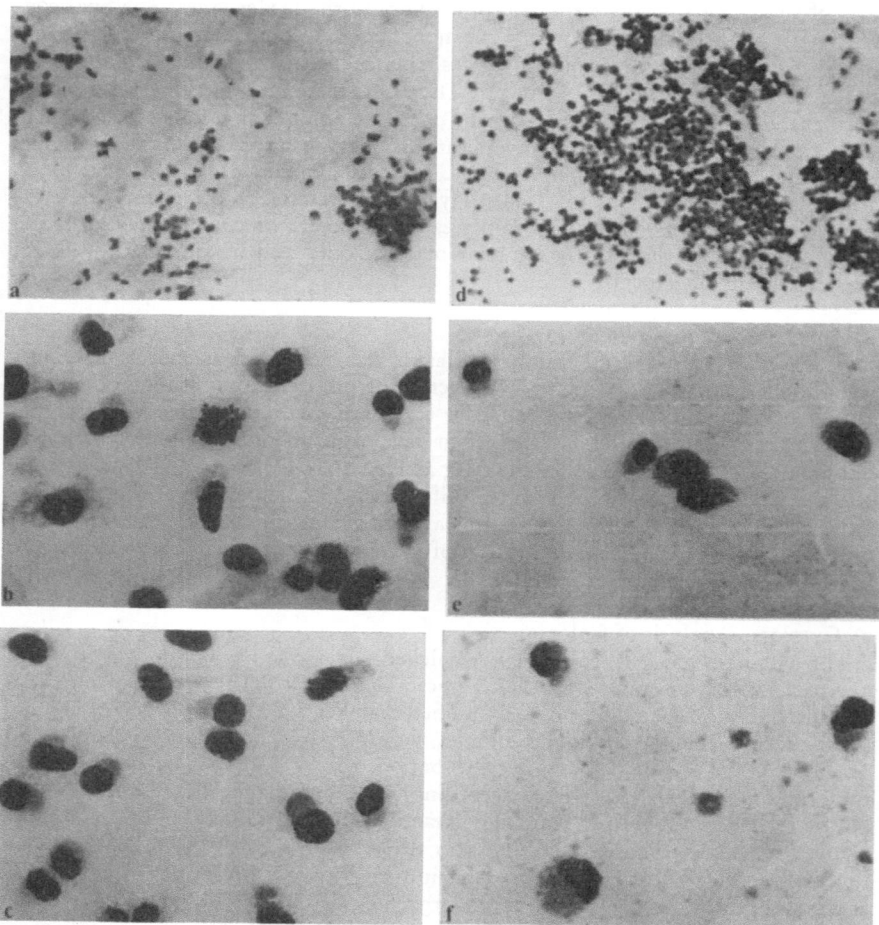

Fig. 1: Peroxidase negative monocyte colony (a) and peroxidase positive eosinophil colony (d), counterstained with Giemsa stain.
b, c: Monocytes in mitosis,
e, f: peroxidase positive eosinophils.

Results

1,026 colonies from 15 normal and 95 leukemic bone marrows have been evaluated using cytochemical and cytological techniques (Table 1). Quantitative analysis of colony formation confirmed the well-known reduction of colony formation in untreated ALL and AML and the increased colony formation in CML as compared to normal controls (4, 5, 7, 10–14). Cytological and cytochemical methods allow further differentiation of colony formation by analyzing the cellular composition of these colonies (Fig. 1–3). In untreated AML or AML in relapse there is a significant reduction of monocyte/macrophage colonies as compared to ALL and an increase of pure eosinophil colonies (Table 1). During remission, fewer pure eosinophil colonies are observed in both, ALL and AML, as compared to nor-

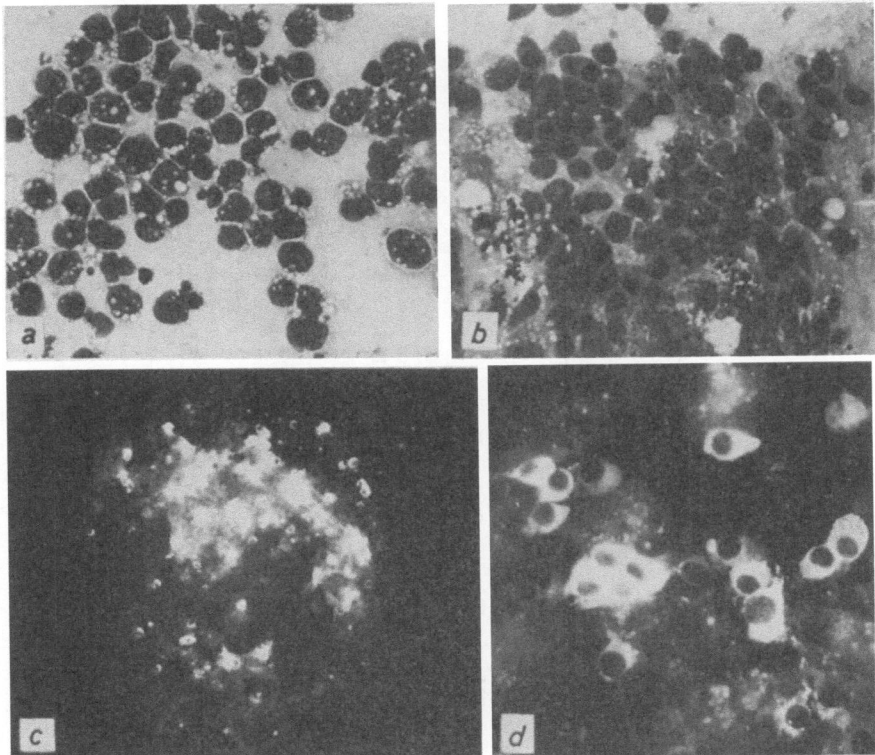

Fig. 2: Cells of isolated colonies from patients with AML.
a: blast cells of a peroxidase negative colony, counterstained with Giemsa stain,
b: a group of macrophages and plasma cells, Giemsa stain,
c: plasma cells of a colony with positive fluorescence in the cytoplsma, spread between several negative cells,
d: plasma cells with positive fluorescence, the positive background reaction is a result of immunoglobulin phagocytosed by macrophages.

Table I: Cytological Classifikation of Colonies (%)

diagnosis	number of patients	number of colonies analyzed	mon	mac	mon mac	eos	mon eos	mac eos	mon mac eos	mon mac eos neu	pc mon mac	pc mon mac eos	pc bc mon mac	bc mon mac
ALL untreated All	21	164	70,5	8.	12	2	2	–	0,5	–	4	–	0,5	0,5
CR ALL	33	331	53	9	6	2	4,5	4	5	3	7	6	0,5	–
PR AML	5	97	44	10	4	–	4	–	1	–	29	1	6	1
untreated AML	12	74	18,5	–	–	16,5	5	1	5	4	27	14	6,5	2,5
CR AML	5	76	64	5	2,5	2,5	6,5	–	–	–	–	17	2,5	–
PR CML	7	21	58	4,5	4,5	–	–	–	–	–	9	24	–	–
remission normal	2	83	59	2,5	21	1	2,5	–	–	–	5	10	–	–
bone marrow	15	180	76	2,5	6	5,5	5	1	4	–	–	–	–	–
	n = 110	n = 1,026												

CR = complet remission, PR = partial remission, mon = monocyt, mac = macrophag, eos = eosinophil, neu = neutrophil, pc = plasma cells, bc = blast cells mal controls while the sum of pure eosinophil colonies and mixed colonies with eosinophils is of the same order as in normal bone marrow (Table 1).

The most remarkable observation is the presence of plasma cells in 174 colonies and of blast cells in 20 colonies of a total of 926 colonies derived from the bone marrows of leukemic patients. Neither plasma cells nor blast cells were observed in any of 180 colonies from normal bone marrow. Using immunofluorescence techniques we were able to demonstrate that these plasma cells produce immunoglobulins in vitro (10). Plasma cells in isolated colonies exhibited positive immunofluorescence after incubation with goat FITC-anti-human-globulin (Fig. 2, Table 2). In colonies from five patients, additional labelling was carried out with specific antisera against IgG, IgA, and IgM heavy chains. Some plasma cells showed positive immunofluorescence with only one, others with all three antisera used. In addition, plasma cells from these colonies were incubated with anti-kappa and anti-lambda sera. The plasma cells of all colonies studied were labelled by both antisera (Table 2).

In order to study the effect of diffusible factors, produced by the feeder layer, on proliferation of leukemic cells, we investigated colony formation with and without feeder layer in various leukemias during remission and relapse. Bone marrows from patients in complete remission yield fewer colonies as compared to

Table II: Demonstration of Immunoglobulins in Plasma Cells from Soft Agar Colonies

patient	diagnosis	anti-Ig	anti-IgG	anti-IgM	anti-IgA	anti-kappa	anti-lambda
D.	ALL untreated	nt	+ (2)	nt	nt	+ (1)	+ (2)
B.	ALL partial remission	+ (1)	+ (1)	nt	− (2)	+ (6)	+ (6)
Z.	AML partial remission	nt	+ (3)	+ (1)	+ (3)	+ (3)	+ (3)
H.	AML partial remission	+ (5)	− (2)	− (2)	nt	nt	nt
	complete remission	nt	nt	− (1)	+ (1)	+ (1)	+ (1)
Wa.	AML complete remission	+ (4)	nt	nt	nt	+ (1)	+ (1)
We.	AMML untreated	+ (4)	+ (2)	− (1)	nt	nt	nt
O.	AMML untreated	nt	nt	nt	nt	nt	+ (1)

demonstration of immunoglobulins using FITC coupled anti-human-immunoglobulin (goat), and anti-IgG, anti-IgM, anti-IgA (H-chain specific; rabbit), anti-kappa, anti-lambda (rabbit)
+ = positive immunofluorescence / / − = negative immunofluorescence / / nt = not tested / / ( ) = number of colonies studied

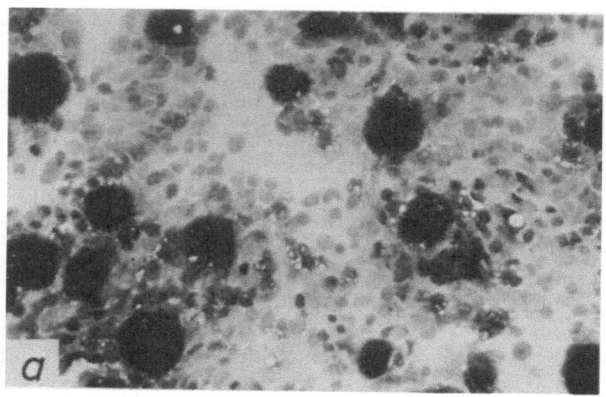

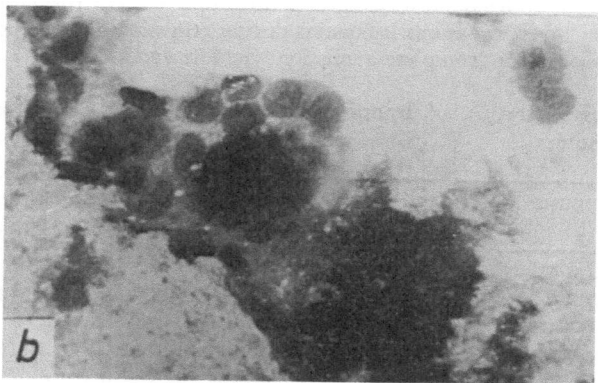

Fig. 3: Mixed colonies of macrophages, blast cells, and plasma cells (acid phosphatase reaction). Strongly positive reaction in macrophages (a, b), granular positive reaction in plasma cells (b), negative reaction in blast cells (a, b).

normal controls with and without leukocyte feeder layer (Table 3). While hardly any normal colonies have been observed without feeder layer, colonies consisting of blast cells only or of blast cells in combination with normal cells (Fig. 2, 3) have been detected in equivalent quantities with and without feeder layer.

Discussion

The results described (Table 1) demonstrate that under the culture conditions used (of Materials and Methods), normal bone marrow cells mainly produce colonies consisting of monocytes and macrophages. In addition, pure eosinophil colonies and mixed colonies of monocytes and eosinophils are observed. In all 180 colonies from 15 normal controls investigated so far, no segmented neutrophils

Table III: Dependence of Normal and Leukemic Colony Formation on CSF

patient	diagnosis	number of colonies[1] / 1 x 10^5 mononuclear bone marrow cells			
		with feeder layer		without feeder layer	
		normal	pathologic	normal	pathologic
P.	ALL	1,3	0,3	∅	∅
D.	ALL				
	untreated	0,8	9	∅	14
	untreated	0,8	0,3	∅	∅
W.	AMML				
	untreated	∅	1	∅	2
O.	AMML				
	untreated	∅	0,4	∅	1
B.	ALL				
	PR	78	0,7	∅	∅
H.	AML				
	PR	96	1,8	∅	2
	CR	95	0,5	∅	0,3
Z.	AML				
	PR	7	1,5	∅	0,3
	PR	31	1	∅	1,5
	CR	55	1,2	2	0,5
D.	AML				
	PR	224	0,2	∅	0,3
K.	AMoL				
	PR	238	1,5	∅	1,3
H.	AMoL				
	PR	1,5	1,3	∅	2,5
W.	AML				
	CR	59	1	∅	1

[1] = mean of five plates
CR = complete remission – PR = partial remission

have been observed. These data are in good agreement with the only other systematic cytologic study of colony formation in soft agar we are aware of. This study has been carried out by SHOHAM et al. (27), who used spleen cells as source of conditioned medium.

The reduced number of monocyte/macrophage colonies in untreated AML and AML in relapse is probably a result of the reduced number of normal myeloid precursor cells during the active stages of AML. The relatively high percentage of pure eosinophil colonies would then represent the differentiated stages of a residual population of normal stem cells. Cytochemical analysis using the N-ASD-chloracetate reaction, which shows a positive reaction in leukemic eosinophils only (28, 29), as well as comparative cytogenetic studies in these colonies from leukemias with chromosomal aberrations will give some important information regarding this hypothesis. Since macrophages are regarded to play an important role in the afferent limb of the immune system, the reduced number of monocyte/macrophage colonies in AML as compared to ALL and normal bone marrow might be of relevance for the clinical course of the disease. The relatively low percentage of pure eosinophil colonies from bone marrow of patients with AML and ALL in remission as compared to normal controls could be the result of a persisting differentiation defect in these cells, since eosinophils have to be regarded as the most differentiated myeloid cell in soft agar colonies. This hypothesis would also explain the increased number of mixed monocyte/macrophage/eosinophil colonies in these patients. Further studies are necessary to investigate the role of pure eosinophil colonies as a marker of marrow differentiation capacity and the possible correlation with the clinical course of the disease.

The presence of plasma cells in colonies derived from leukemic patients and their absence in normal colonies cannot be explained so far. These plasma cells could be present accidentally in a colony containing blast cells. A specific interaction between immunologically competent B cells and blast cells would then explain the persistence of plasma cells in abnormal colonies only. Due to the limited supply of plasma cells as yet no investigations have been carried out regarding the specificity of the antibodies produced, e. g. against leukemic blast cells. The alternative explanation would be that macrophages, monocytes, eosinophils and plasma cells, are derived from one pluripotent stem cell in presence of leukemic blast cells. The demonstrated presence of both, kappa- and lambdachains, in colonies containing plasma cells does not favour the hypothesis of a monoclonal origin of these plasma cells since the simultaneous presence of both, kappa- and lambda-chains, is observed in 1–2 % of all plasma cells only. The demonstration of colonies containing blast cells derived from leukemic bone marrows suggest the presence of factors inducing proliferation and in some cases even differentiation of blast cells under our cultural conditions. The experiments described by GALLAGHER (15) and DICKE (8, 30) also prove that these factors do exist. Our data, however, demonstrate that these factors do not originate from the leukocyte feeder layer, since there was the same number of pathologic colonies with and without feeder layer, while normal colonies were almost completely missing (Table 3). If it were possible to enhance growth of pathologic colonies from AML remission bone marrow with PHA, this technique allowed better evaluation of the residual leukemic stem cells during clinical remission.

Our investigation has demonstrated the necessity of cytological and cytochemical classification in addition to quantitative evaluation of soft agar colonies when studying the effect of factors on proliferation and differentiation of normal and leukemic stem cells. Differentiation patterns should only be interpreted after careful cytological and cytochemical identification of the cell.

References

1. Cronkite, E. P.: in: Modern Trends in Human Leukemia II. J. F. Lehmanns Verlag, München 1976.
2. WU, A. M., Gallo, R. C.: in: Modern Trends in Human Leukemia I. Grune & Stratton, New York and J. F. Lehmanns Verlag, München 1974, p. 148.

3. WU, A. M., Gallo, R. C.: in: Modern Trends in Human Leukemia II. J. F. Lehmanns Verlag, München 1976.
4. Stohlman, F., Jr.: in: Modern Trends in Human Leukemia I. Grune & Stratton, New York and J. F. Lehmanns Verlag, München 1974, p. 50.
5. McCulloch, E. A., Mak, T. W., Price, G. B., Till, J. E.: Biochim. biophys. Acta *355*, 260 (1974).
6. Paran., M., Sachs, L., Barak, Y., Resnitzky, R.: Proc. nat. Acad. Sci., USA *67*, 1542 (1970).
7. Moore, M. A. S.: in: Modern Trends in Human Leukemia II. J. F. Lehmanns Verlag, München 1976.
8. Dicke, K. A., Spitzer, G., Scheffers, H. M., Cork, A., Ahearn, M. J., Lowenberg, B., McCredie, K. B.: in: Modern Trends in Human Leukemia II. J. F. Lehmanns Verlag, München 1976.
9. Till, J. E., Mak, T. W., Price, G. B., Senn, J. S., McCulloch, E. A.: in: Modern Trends in Human Leukemia II. J. F. Lehmanns Verlag, München 1976.
10. Beckmann, H., Neth, R., Soltau, H., Ritter, J., Winkler, K., Garbrecht, M., Hausmann, K., Rutter, G.: in: Progress in Differentiation Research. Elsevier/North Holland Biomedical Press B. V., Amsterdam 1976, p. 383.
11. Moore, M. A. S., Metcalf, D.: in: In Vitro Culture of Hemopoietic Cells. Radiolobiological Institute TNO, Rijswijk 1972, p. 334.
12. Moore, M. A. S., Williams, N., Metcalf, D.: J. nat. Canc. Inst. *50*, 603 (1973).
13. Robinson, W. A., Kurnick, J. E., Pike, B. L.: Blood *38*, 500 (1971).
14. Duttera, M. J., Bull, J. M., Northup, J. D., Henderson, E. S., Stashick, E. D., Carbone, P. P.: Blood *42*, 687 (1973)
15. Gallagher, R. E., Salahuddin, S. Z., Hall, W. T., McCredie, K. B., Gallo, R. C.: Proc. nat. Acad. Sci. USA *72*, 4137 (1976).
16. Undritz, E.: Hämatologische Tafeln Sandoz. – II. Auflage, Sandoz 1972.
17. Hayhoe, F. G. J., Qualigno, D., Doll, R.: Her Myjesty's Stationery Office, London 1964.
18. Löffler, H.: in: Chemo- und Immunotherapie der Leukosen und malignen Lymphome. Bohmann, Wien 1969, p. 120.
19. Beckmann, H., Neth, R., Gaedicke, G., Landbeck, G., Wiegers, U., Winkler, K.: in: Modern Trends in Human Leukemia I. Grune & Stratton, New York and J. F. Lehmanns Verlag, München 1974, p. 26.
20. Aur, R. J., Husta, H. O., Verzosa, M. S., Wood, A. Simone, J. V.: Blood *42*, 349 (1973).
21. Böyum, A.: J. clin. Lab. Invest. (Suppl. 97) *21*, 1 (1968).
22. Pike, B. L., Robinson, W. A.: J. cell. Physiol. *76*, 77 (1970).
23. Beckmann, H., Soltau, H., Garbrecht, M., Winkler, K.: Klin. Wschr. *52*, 603 (1974).
24. Bruch, Ch.: personal communication.
25. Testa, N. G., Lord, B. J.: Blood *36*, 586 (1970).
26. Leder, L. D.: Der Blutmonocyt. Springer-Verlag, Berlin–Heidelberg–New York 1967.
27. Shoham, D., Ben David, E., Rozenszajn, L. A.: Blood *44*, 221 (1974).
28. Löffler, H.: in: Leukämie. Springer-Verlag, Berlin–Heidelberg–New York 1972, p. 119.

29. Wulfhekel, U., Döllmann, D., Bartels, H., Hausmann, K.: Virch. Arch. A, path. Anat. Hist. *365*, 289 (1975).
30. Dicke, K. A., Spitzer, G., Ahearn, M. J.: Nature *259*, 129 (1976).

Cellular Subclasses in Human Leukemic Hemopoiesis

J. E. Till, T. W. Mak, G. B. Price, J. S. Senn and E. A. McCulloch

Ontario Cancer Institute and Sunnybrook Medical Centre
University of Toronto
Toronto, Canada.

Abstract

Cellular organization and communication in leukemic hemopoiesis may be compared with its counterpart in normal hemopoiesis. Results obtained using cell culture methods have provided some support for the view that leukemic hemopoiesis, like normal hemopoiesis, may involve 3 levels of differentiation: leukemic stem cells, committed leukemic progenitors, and more mature cells. Evidence is also beginning to emerge that leukemic populations may be regulated by messages from the environment in a manner analogous to normal hemopoiesis. The apparent similarities between leukemic and normal hemopoiesis raise the possibility that the target cell for leukemic transformation is the normal pluripotent stem cell. The development of culture methods for the production of leukovirus-like particles from human leukemic cells provides a possible first step toward the direct identification of leukemic target cells.

Indrotuction

The purpose of this paper is to discuss leukemic hemopoiesis in relation to its normal counterpart. The approaches being used to investigate leukemic hemopoiesis are analogous to those that have, over the last decade, provided information about cellular organization and communication in the normal hemopoietic system. These approaches, principally using developmental methods based on colony formation either *in vivo* or in culture, have led to a generally accepted view of interrelationships among normal hemopoietic progenitors (1, 2). The earliest identified class is the pluripotent stem cells, whose proliferative potential includes sufficient capacity for self-renewal to maintain the system (3). The next position in hemopoietic lineage is occupied by populations of progenitor cells each committed to a specific differentiation pathway such as granulopoiesis, erythropoiesis or megakaryocytopoiesis. These committed progenitor cells, while probably lacking sufficient proliferative potential for self-maintenance, permit subpopulations of cells within the different pathways of differentiation to expand independently of each other, giving rise to a variety of functional cells in appropiate numbers.

Each stage in hemopoietic differentiation represents a potential site of regulation. It has been proposed (4) that distinct classes of "managerial" cells with specialized regulatory functions coexist with the classes of cells subject to their control. A defect in the function of one such managerial cell class has been detected in genetically anemic Sl/Sl^d mice (5). Recently developed cell culture methods have greatly extended the study of regulatory mechanisms. Extensive studies on granulopoiesis in culture have shown that diffusible substances derived from another coexistent cell class can promote the production of granulocytes (6, 7). Although extrapolation from events observed in cell culture to the corresponding events *in vivo* must be done with great caution, the analytical power of cell culture techniques provides justification for their use to study regulation.

This background of conceptual and methodological information about normal hemopoiesis makes it feasible to examine leukemic hemopoiesis. Specifically, one can ask whether or not some of the organizational and regulatory features of normal hemopoiesis persist in human leukemia. Some evidence that this is the case, based on results obtained using cell culture methods, will be summarized below.

Heterogeneity in leukemia

Leukemic cell populations might be considered to retain features of normal hemopoiesis if they were, like normal hemopoietic populations, composed of heterogeneous cell classes interrelated as cell lineages and responsive to regulatory messages. Initial evidence in favor of this view came from the application to leukemic cell populations of methods for growing granulopoietic colonies in cell culture. Reports from a number of laboratories indicated that marrow specimens from patients with apparently similar clinical forms of leukemia behaved very differently in culture. For example, in some patients with acute myelogenous leukemia (AML), colony formation was greatly diminished or absent, while in other patients it exceeded normal levels (8, 9). Thus, cell populations from different leukemic patients showed heterogeneous behaviour in cell culture. In addition, it was evident that marrow from some patients with acute leukemia contained cells capable of differentiation in culture and, like their counterparts in normal marrow, were dependent for growth in culture on the presence of appropriate stimulatory factors (see, for example, refs. 10, 11). Thus, these initial observations were compatible with the view that analogies might be found between leukemic and normal hemopoiesis.

More clear-cut evidence for heterogeneity in leukemic cell populations has emerged from studies of leukemic cells in liquid cultures (12, 13). Large quantities of morphologically identified blasts may be obtained from the peripheral blood of patients; repeated experiments can be done on cells from a single source by storage of the cell populations at -70 °C in 5 % dimethyl sulfoxide. When such cells are placed in fluid cultures in appropriate media, little change in cell number is usually observed over a period of many days. Nonetheless, active proliferation is occurring; when cultures are pulse-labelled at different times with ^{3}H-thymidine, extensive increases are observed in the incorporation of the label into acid-insoluble material (12). This incorporation is associated with increased numbers of labelled cells as detected by autoradiography. The increase in ^{3}H-thymidine incorporation is sensitive to ionizing radiation and survival curves have been obtained with parameters characteristic of mammalian cell proliferation (Fig. 1) (14). Recent studies based on the technique of limiting dilution indicate that the proliferative subpopulation detected by ^{3}H-thymidine incorporation is a minority one, con-

34

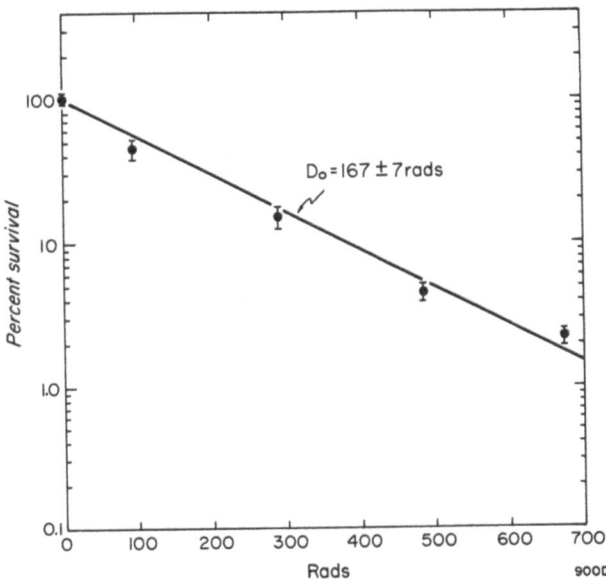

Fig. 1: Radiation survival curve for the incorporation of ^{3}H-thymidine by cells in liquid culture, derived from a patient with AML. Ordinate: percent survival of ^{3}H-thymidine incorporation over 45 min by 10^5 cells per ml in 3 ml liquid cultures, 4 cultures per point. The cells were exposed to ^{3}H-thymidine 8 days after irradiation and initiation of the cultures. Abscissa: dose of ^{137}Cs gamma radiation. The D_0 value is the dose required to reduce the percent survival to 37 ^{0}/o of the initial value. The errors indicated are standard errors.

sisting of between 1:100 and 1:1000 of the total cells (14). If it is assumed that at least a portion of the proliferating subpopulation consists of leukemic cells (15), then these results are compatible with the view that a minority population of leukemic cells is able to proliferate and contribute to the numbers of a larger leukemic population with a modified capacity for proliferation. Such a situation would be analogous to that found in normal hemopoietic differentiation where a minority population of stem cells proliferates and gives rise to a large population of progeny, most of which have lost stem cell properties.

Regulation in populations of leukemic cells

Two of the major properties of stem cells are the capacity for extensive proliferation including self-renewal, and the capacity to give rise to cells with different characteristics. Approaches to the identification of cells with these properties in a minority subpopulation in leukemia were outlined above. The third major property of stem cells is their sensitivity to control mechanisms (16). Some evidence for cellular interactions of a regulatory nature has also been obtained from studies of leukemic peripheral blood cells in fluid cultures. When the usual synthetic culture

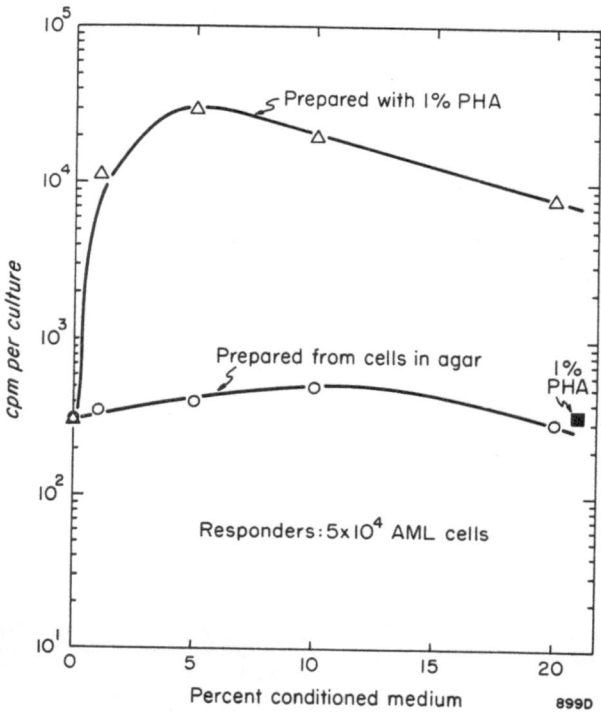

Fig. 2: Stimulation of ^{3}H-thymidine incorporation into AML cells in liquid culture by various concentrations of leukocyte-conditioned medium. Triangles: an active conditioned medium prepared in liquid culture in the presence of 1 % phytohemagglutinin (PHA) (12). Circles: a conditioned medium prepared from cells immobilized in agar, in the absence of PHA (47); this conditioned medium showed little or no activity when assayed on these particular responder cells. Closed square: the same conditioned medium as for the results shown as circles, but with 1 % PHA added to the cultures of responder cells together with the conditioned medium.

medium supplemented with fetal calf serum was supplemented further by the addition of supernatants from cultures of normal or leukemic leukocytes, incorporation of ^{3}H-thymidine into peripheral blood cells from some patients increased at a more rapid rate. Although considerable patient-to-patient variation has been observed, it is usually possible under conditions of limiting dilution to demonstrate that the leukemic populations contain cells that proliferate only in the presence of an active leukocyte-conditioned medium (Fig. 2). Using cell separation methods, preliminary evidence has been obtained that leukemic populations not only contain cells capable of responding to growth-promoting factors, but also another class of cells capable of producing these growth-promoting factors, either spontaneously or in response to phytohemagglutinin (13). Thus, evidence is available that the third major stem cell property, sensitivity to control mechanisms, may be retained by leukemic stem cells. This implies that a basic feature of normal granulopoiesis in culture, regulation by cellular interaction, is also found in leukemic populations.

Committed progenitor cells in leukemia

Progenitor cells committed to granulópoiesis can be detected readily by their capacity to form granulopoietic colonies in culture (6). The granulopoietic progenitors detected using this assay in the marrow or blood of patients with leukemia might belong either to the leukemic population or to a co-existing normal population. Convincing evidence for the existence of leukemic committed progenitors has been obtained for patients with chronic myelogenous leukemia (CML). The Philadelphia chromosome has been identified in colonies formed by cells from some but not all patients with Ph[+] CML (11, 17–20). Analogous evidence is available for acute myelogenous leukemia (AML) in that characteristic chromosomal abnormalities found in direct marrow preparations have been identified in pooled cultures (21) and in individual colonies (10, 11) derived from the marrow or peripheral blood of leukemic patients. These results indicate that at least some committed progenitors found in leukemic cell populations are of leukemic origin. In some patients, therefore, leukemic stem cells give rise to progeny as detected by the culture assay for granulopoietic progenitors. Although the differentiation processes occurring in cultures derived from leukemic granulopoietic progenitors may be abnormal (10, 22, 23), these progenitors are, like their normal counterparts, dependent for their growth in culture on diffusible factors derived from either normal or leukemic cells (8–11). We conclude that, in addition to cellular heterogeneity in leukemia of the kind to be expected if leukemic stem cells are present, evidence for parent-to-progeny lineage relationships also exists and that leukemic committed granulopoietic progenitors respond in culture to factors similar to those that regulate differentiation in culture by their normal counterparts.

Erythropoietic differentiation from pluripotent leukemic stem cells has been demonstrated in CML on the basis of chromosomal evidence (24–26). Analogous though less extensive evidence is also available for acute leukemia (27, 28). Colony techniques are now available for human erythropoietic progenitors (29, 30); as these are applied to cells from patients with leukemia it will become possible to investigate the potential for differentiation of leukemic erythropoietic progenitors in a manner similar to the studies already carried out on leukemic granulopoietic progenitors (10, 11, 21).

Diffusible regulators of cell growth in culture

Granulopoietic colony formation in culture is dependent on the presence of a suitable source of certain diffusible factors. These factors, collectively termed colony stimulating activity (CSA) have been studied extensively in the serum and urine of patients with leukemia. Studies on sera have been complicated by the presence of inhibitors (31) and even when these were removed, correlation of CSA serum levels with clinical status was not observed (32). These CSA measurements have generally been complicated by the use of mouse marrow cells rather than human marrow cells in the assay procedure. Evidence is available that CSA

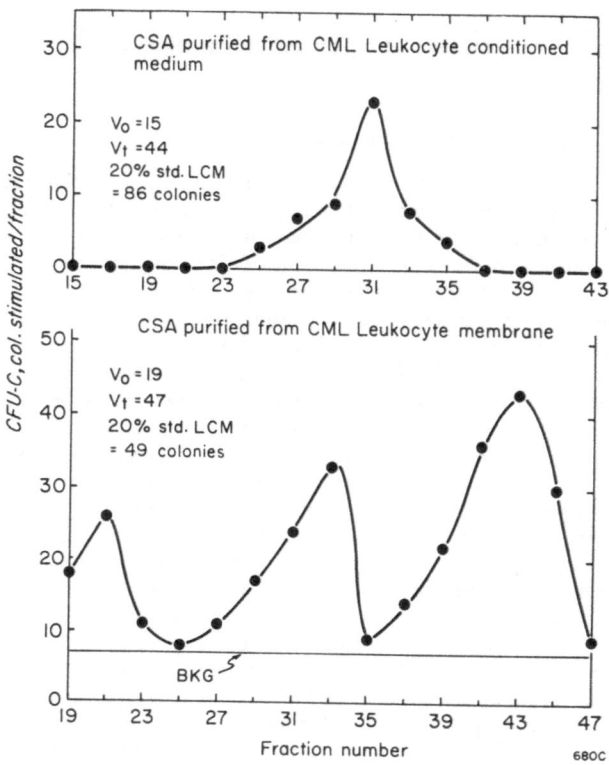

Fig. 3: Gel filtration on Sephadex G-150 of CSA assayed by stimulation of colony formation by granulopoietic progenitor cells (CFU-C). Upper panel: CSA purified from leukocyte-conditioned medium (LCM) prepared from peripheral leukocytes of a patient with chronic myelogenous leukemia (CML). Lower panel: CSA purified from surface membranes of leukocytes from the same CML patient, after solubilization of the membranes in 2 % sodium dodecyl sulfate. The methods used for isolation of membranes and purification of CSA have been described (34, 36).

detected by the mouse assay need not be the same as CSA detected using human cells (33). For this reason, much of the work on CSA in leukemia is difficult to interpret.

More recent studies using cells of human origin to assay for either CSA or CSA-producing cells have yielded a more consistent pattern. A convenient source of CSA active on human granulopoietic progenitors is medium in which normal or leukemic leukocytes have been cultured for 3–7 days. Purification of CSA from such leukocyte conditioned media has revealed four apparent molecular species; of these, three are nondialyzable and have molecular weights of approximately 93,000, 36,500 and 14,700 (34). The fourth species is dialyzable, hydrophobic and has a molecular weight of less than 1300 (35). The cellular location of the three high molecular weight species of CSA has been investigated and they have been found in assiciation with cell surface membranes (36).

Leukemic cells also add CSA to culture media. However, when peripheral leukocytes from newly-diagnosed leukemic patients are used to prepare conditioned media, and the same purification procedure as that used for media conditioned by normal leukocytes is applied, only one of the three species of high molecular weight CSA is detected in the leukocyte conditioned media (34).

The difference in number of high molecular weight species of CSA detectable in media conditioned by normal and leukemic leukocystes does not appear to be simply the result of differences in the relative numbers of various cell classes in the two populations. Evidence supporting this view is presented in Figure 3, which shows results from a direct comparison of high molecular weight CSA in media conditioned by cells from a patient with CML and high molecular weight CSA obtained from the surface membranes of cells from the same patient. The leukocyte conditioned medium yielded only a single species of high molecular weight CSA, even though the cells in the peripheral blood of this same patient contained all three species, and the cell classes present included all those found in normal blood.

This approach has also been applied to cells from patients with idiopathic sideroblastic anemia, a condition known to be associated with a high incidence of leukemic transformation. Leukocyte conditioned media were prepared from peripheral leukocytes of six patients with idiopathic sideroblastic anemia. Although the distribution of cell classes in the blood of these patients was not abnormal, in three instances only a single species of high molecular weight CSA was detected in the leukocyte conditioned media (37). Two of these three patients subsequently developed leukemia while the third died of myocardial infarction three months after his cells were assessed. None of the patients whose leukocytes released all three high molecular weight species of CSA have developed leukemia (5–12 months of follow-up to date). The controls in these studies consisted of four patients with secondary or congenital sideroblastic anemia. Leukocyte conditioned media prepared from their leukocytes contained the usual three species of high molecular weight CSA.

These data are consistent with the view that the capacity of leukocytes to release these particular bioactive molecules into culture media is an expression of their phenotype. The findings in sideroblastic anemia support the hypothesis that a reduced capacity of leukemic leukocytes to release certain species of CSA in culture may be related to the leukemic phenotype rather than a secondary manifestation of disordered cell metabolism or altered distribution of cellular populations. Since high molecular weight CSA species are located in or near cell membranes the proposal that their abnormal release in leukemia is part of the leukemic phenotype is consistent with other evidence suggesting membrane changes in this disease and reminiscent of the model proposed for regulation of normal granulopoiesis by membrane interactions (36, 38, 2). If the molecular species that are essential for proliferation and differentiation in culture are also physiologically active *in vivo*, the decreased ability of leukemic leukocytes to release such bioactive membrane components may contribute to abnormal cell regulation in leukemia. In any event, the findings provide further support for the view that leukemic populations retain some of the regulatory features of normal hemopoiesis.

Leukemic Target Cells

The cell culture data summarized above provide clues that leukemic populations may be heterogeneous, with a hierarchy of cell classes linked by lineage relationships and responsive to regulatory mechanism in a manner analogous to the relationships found in normal hemopoiesis. These results, however, do not bear directly on the relationship between leukemic stem cells and their normal counterparts. The evidence for both granulopoietic and erythropoietic differentiation in CML and AML makes it attractive to consider that the target cell for leukemic

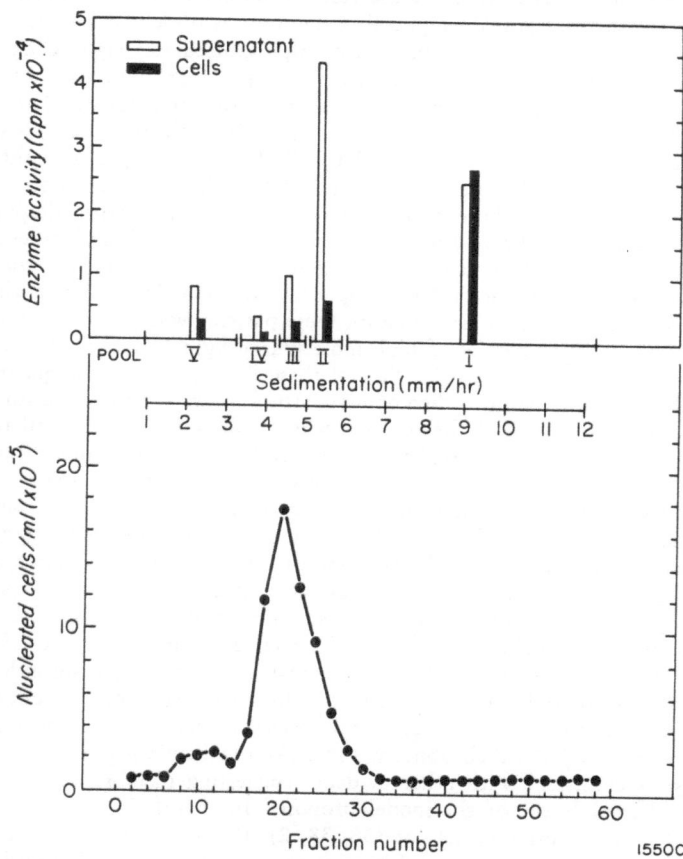

Fig. 4: Velocity sedimentation profile of marrow cells from a patient with acute lymphocytic leukemia (ALL). Lower panel: profile of nucleated cells. Upper panel: distribution of reverse transcriptase activity in pools of cells cultured for 5 days. The total enzyme activities in the supernatant medium and the cells from each pool are shown as bars. Reverse transcriptase activity as stimulated by poly rC(dG)$_{12-18}$ was assayed after the cells and supernatant medium were fractionated in sucrose gradients, as described (39, 40, 46).

transformation is the normal pluripotent stem cell. If this view is correct, then the various types of leukemia recognized morphologically must be determined by the transforming events rather than by the cell class in which they occur.

If the normal pluripotent stem cells are the target cells for leukemic transformation, then methods for studying this transformation are required in order to make a direct identification of the leukemic target cells. A start toward this goal has been taken wtih the development of culture methods which result in the production of particles with many of the physical, biochemical and morphological properties of leukoviruses (39–43). The biological significance of the production of these virus-like particles by leukemic cells is still unclear; in particular, it is not known whether or not they are able to cause a leukemic transformation of normal hemopoietic cells. However, if the cellular heterogeneity in leukemic populations is related, as in the normal, to patterns of growth, it might be anticipated that any cell properties with functional significance would be associated with specific subpopulations rather than with all cells in the leukemic populations. From this viewpoint, the capacity to produce leukovirus-like particles may be regarded simply as a functional property of cells, and one may test whether or not only a subpopulation of leukemic cells exhibit this particular function. On the basis of this reasoning, leukemic populations were separated by velocity sedimentation, and fractions were pooled to yield suspensions of approximately equal cell numbers. These were then tested for their capacity to release virus-like particles, using as the criterion of particle release the presence of RNA-dependent DNA polymerase (reverse transcriptase) whose acitivity is stimulated by poly $rC(dG)_{12-18}$ and is associated with densities from 1.17 to 1.22 gm/ml. This criterion was chosen because poly $rc(dG)_{12-18}$ is considered to be a specific template for viral-related reverse transcriptase (44, 45) and because assays for enzyme activity revealed peaks of activity in density regions characteristic of intact virus or viral cores (1.17 and 1.22 gm/ml respectively). For cells from 6 of 12 patients, including patients with AML, ALL, CML, and AMML, particle release was associated with pools containing rapidly sedimenting (large) cells. An example of data from a typical experiment is shown in Figure 4. Cell populations from 6 other patients provided no evidence of particle release in cultures from any of the cell pools (46).

As controls, marrow from 11 patients without leukemia were separated by velocity sedimentation and pools of cells of appropriate sedimentation velocities were examined for particle release using the same criterion. In 4 of these experiments small but significant amounts of enzyme activity were detected, although at lower levels than those found for the 6 cases of leukemia where particle release was detected. In contrast to the leukemic populations, however, enzyme activity was always associated with pools of slow sedimentation velocity (small cells).

As emphasized earlier, the criterion for particle release used in these experiments was limited to the detection of reverse transcriptase activity in association with appropriate densities on sucrose gradients and stimulated by the artificial template poly $rC(dG)_{12-18}$. In the absence of more detailed characterization, particularly of the material obtained from normal cells, the relationship of the enzyme-containing particles to known viruses or to preparations from different patients can be only a matter of speculation. However, the cellular specificity of particle release is consistent with the view that this property reflects functionally important aspects of the phenotypes of specific cell populations in normal and leukemic hemopoiesis. The relationship of these particle-releasing subpopulations to the other normal or leukemic cellular subpopulations remains to be determined.

Concluding Remarks

Information about leukemic populations is much too limited to permit the construction of a detailed model of cell lineage relationships. It is reasonable only to postulate the existence of leukemic stem cells capable of extensive proliferation, including self renewal, and of giving rise to other cell classes with different properties. The latter cell classes include leukemic progenitors committed to granulopoiesis and other leukemic progenitors committed to erythropoiesis. In acute leukemia, the major morphologically-recognizable population consists of blast cells, whose relationship to the leukemic stem cells is unknown. For example, the blast cells might be at an early level of differentiation analogous to that of normal committed progenitors, but prevented by the leukemic lesion from further maturation. Alternatively, they might be cells that have progressed along another pathway unique to the leukemic population. The limited amount of information that is available does, however, provide some support for the view that leukemic populations may be organized into cell lineages and regulated by messages from the environment in a manner analogous to normal hemopoiesis. If this viewpoint is correct, it should be possible to identify a class of "managerial cells" in leukemia. At present, it is not known whether messages able to modulate leukemic growth originate from cells within the leukemic population, or from normal managerial cells, or both. For leukemic leukocytes in culture, the release of a single species of high molecular weight CSA into culture medium, in contrast to the three high molecular weight species of CSA released by normal leukocytes, could be a direct manifestation in culture of the defective regulation characteristic of leukemic populations. Alternatively, the differences may arise from surface membrane changes in leukemic cells which are part of the leukemic phenotype, but not directly related to the defective regulation characteristic of leukemia. We have proposed (36, 38, 2) that these molecular species of CSA represent a novel class of surface membrane-associated bioactive macromolecules. From this viewpoint, they represent a means to detect surface membrane differences between normal and leukemic cells. To date, the only circumstances in which a reduction in numbers of high molecular weight species has been observed were for leukemic patients and for patients proven to be pre-leukemic (37). Thus, the shift from three high molecular weight species of CSA to one species may prove to be a very useful marker of leukemic or pre-leukemic cell populations.

Another very intriguing question concerns the possible significance of the capacity of a rapidly-sedimenting subpopulation of leukemic cells to release virus-like particles. Is the capacity of this particular subpopulation to produce particles a property only of leukemic stem cells? Should this be the case, it need not necessarily imply an etiologic role of such virus-like particles in human leukemia. Instead, it might be a reflection of a more extensive capacity for gene expression in the leukemic stem cells compared with other cell types present in leukemic populations. Such a marker for leukemic stem cells, whatever its functional role, would be of great value. However, the basis for the enzyme activity detected in pools of slowly sedimenting cells derived from non-leukemic marrow needs to be clarified; it remains to be demonstrated that the particles produced by the normal and leukemic subpopulations are different enough to be useful as specific markers. Also, it should be stressed that the culture conditions used to obtain release of particles are unlikely to be representative of events occurring *in vivo*.

Taken together, the areas of ignorance greatly outnumber those where firm information is available. Nevertheless, the elucidation of the organization and regulation of leukemic cell populations should lead to novel therapeutic modalities; one can visualize, in addition to the toxic agents used to inactivate leukemic stem cells, a second generation of non-toxic agents able to modify regulatory mechanisms and thus control, in a more selective way, the proliferation and differentiation of cells in leukemic populations.

References

1. Discussion Group 2, Dahlem Workshop on Myelofibrosis-Osteosclerosis Syndrome, Berlin, November 13–15, 1974. *In:* Advances in the Biosciences, Vol. 16, Burkhardt, R., Adler, S. S., Conley, C. L., Pincus, T., Lennert, K. and Till, J. E., eds. Pergamon Press, Oxford, pp. 255–271.
2. Till, J. E., Price, G. B., Mak, T. W. and McCulloch, E. A. (1975). *Federation Proc., 34:* 2279–2284.
3. Siminovitch, L., McCulloch, E. A. and Till, J. E. (1963). *J. Cell. Comp. Physiol. 62:* 327–336.
4. McCulloch, E. A., Gregory, C. J. and Till, J. E. (1973). *In:* Haemopoietic Stem Cells, Ciba Foundation Symposium, Vol. 13, ASP, Amsterdam, pp. 183–199.
5. McCulloch, E. A., Siminovitch, L., Till, J. E., Russell, E. A. and Bernstein, S. E. (1965). *Blood 26:* 399–410.
6. Metcalf, D. and Moore, M. A. S. (1971). Haemopoietic Cells. North-Holland, Amsterdam.
7. McCulloch, E. A., Mak, T. W., Price, G. B. and Till, J. E. (1974). *Biochim. Biophys. Acta 355:* 260–299.
8. Van Bekkum, D. W. and Dicke, K. A., eds. (1972). In Vitro Culture of Hemopoietic Cells. Radiobiological Institute TNO, Rijswijk, Netherlands.
9. Robinson, W. A., ed. (1974). Hemopoiesis in Culture, Second International Workshop. U.S. Government Printing Office, Washington, D.C.
10. Aye, M. T., Till, J. E. and McCulloch, E. A. (1974). *Exp. Hemat. 2:* 362–371..
11. Moore, M. A. S. and Metcalf, D. (1973). *Int. J. Cancer 11:* 143–152.
12. Aye, M. T., Niho, Y., Till, J. E. and McCulloch, E. A. (1974). *Blood 44:* 205–219.
13. Aye, M. T., Till, J. E. and McCulloch, E. A. (1975). *Blood 45:* 485–493.
14. McCulloch, E. A., unpublished.
15. Aye, M. T., Till, J. E. and McCulloch, E. A. (1972). *Blood 40:* 806–811.
16. Becker, A. J., McCulloch, E. A., Siminovitch, L. and Till, J. E. (1965). *Blood 26:* 296–308.
17. Chervenick, P. A., Ellis, L. D., Pan, S. F. and Lawson, A. L. (1971). *Science 174:* 1134–1136.

18. Shadduck, R. K. and Nankin, H. R. (1971). *Lancet 2:* 1097–1098.
19. Aye, M. T., Till, J. E. and McCulloch, E. A. (1973). *Exp. Hemat. 1:* 115–118.
20. Moore, M. A. S., Ekert, H., Fitzgerald, M. G. and Carmichael, A. (1974). *Blood 43:* 15–22.
21. Duttera, M. J., Bull, J. M. C., Whang-Peng, J. and Carbone, P. P. (1972). *Lancet 1:* 715–717.
22. Moore, M. A. S., Spitzer, G., Williams, N. and Metcalf, D. (1974). *In:* Hemopoiesis in Culture, Second International Workshop. Robinson, W. A., ed. U.S. Government Printing Office, Washington, D.C., pp. 303–311.
23. Morley, A. and Higgs, D. (1974). *Cancer 33:* 716–720.
24. Tough, I. M., Jacobs, P. A., Court Brown, W. M., Baikie, A. G. and Williamson, E. R. D. (1963). *Lancet 1:* 844–846.
25. Whang, J., Frei, E., Tjio, J. H., Carbone, P. P. and Brecher, G. (1963). *Blood 22:* 664–673.
26. Rastrick, J. M. (1969). *Brit. J. Haemat. 16:* 185–191.
27. Jensen, M. K. and Killman, S. (1967). *Acta. Med. Scand. 181:* 47–53.
28. Blackstock, A. M. and Garson, O. M. (1974). *Lancet 2:* 1178–1179.
29. Axelrad, A. A., McLeod, D. L., Shreeve, M. M. and Heath, D. S. (1974). *In:* Hempoiesis in Culture, Second International Workshop.
    Robinson, W. A., ed., U. S. Government Printing, Office Washington, D.C., pp. 226–234.
30. Iscove, N. N. and Sieber, F. (1975). *Exp. Hemat. 3:* 32–43.
31. Chan, S. H., Metcalf, D. and Stanley, E. R. (1971). *Brit. J. Hemat. 20:* 329–341.
32. Metcalf, D., Chan, S. H., Gunz, F. W., Vincent, P. and Ravich, R. B. M. (1971). *Blood 38:* 143–152.
33. Lind, D. E., Bradley, M. L., Gunz, F. W. and Vincent, P. C. (1974). *J. Cell. Physiol. 83:* 35–42.
34. Price, G. B., Senn, J. S., McCulloch, E. A. and Till, J. E. (1975). *Biochem. J. 148:* 209–217.
35. Price, G. B., McCulloch, E. A. and Till, J. E. (1973). *Blood 42:* 341–348.
36. Price, G. B., McCulloch, E. A. and Till, J. E. (1975). *Exp. Hemat. 3:* 227–233.
37. Senn, J. S., Pinkerton, P. H., Price, G. B., Mak, T. W. and McCulloch, E. A. (1976). *Brit. J. Cancer,* in press.
38. Price, G. B. (1974). *In:* The Cell Surface: Immunological and Chemical Approaches. Kahan, B. D. and Reisfeld, R. A. (eds.). Plenum Press, New York, pp. 237–239.
39. Mak, T. W., Manaster, J., Howatson, A. F., McCulloch, E. A. and Till, J. E. (1974). *Proc. Nat. Acad. Sci. U.S.A. 71:* 4336–4340.
40. Mak, T. W., Kurtz, S., Manaster, J. and Housman, D. (1975). *Proc. Nat. Acad. Sci. U.S.A. 72:* 623–627.
41. Gallagher, R. E. and Gallo, R. C. (1975). *Science 187:* 350–353.
42. Panem, S., Prochownik, E. V., Reale, F. R. and Kirsten, W. H. (1975). *Science 189:* 297–299.
43. Vosika, G. J., Krivit, W., Gerrard, J. M., Coccia, P. F., Nesbit, M. E., Coalson, J. J. and Kennedy, B. J. (1975). *Proc. Nat. Acad. Sci. U.S.A. 82:* 2804–2808.

44. Baltimore, D. and Smoler, D. (1971). *Proc. Nat. Acad. Sci. U.S.A. 68:* 1507–1511.
45. Scolnick, E. M., Parks, W. D., Todaro, G. J. and Aaronson, S. A. (1972). *Nature New Biol. 235:* 35–40.
46. Mak, T. W., Price, G. B., Niho, Y., Miller, R. G., Senn, J. S., Curtis, J., Till, J. E. and McCulloch, E. A. (1976), in preparation.
47. Iscove, N. N., Senn, J. S., Till, J. E. and McCulloch, E. A. (1971). *Blood 37:* 1–5.

Characterisation of normal and Pathological Growth of Human Bone Marrow Cells by Means of a New System Cell Assay

by

F. Walther, J. C. F. Schubert and K. Schopow[1]
Universitätskliniken Frankfurt/Main,
Abteilung für Hämatologie
6000 Frankfurt/Main
West Germany

The disturbance in growth of hemopoietic cells in human leukemia takes place at the stem cell level. In order to characterize the leukemic cell populations attention has been focused on first steps of the development of the hemopoietic system.

The stem cell level can be understood as a compartment of cell populations which are distinguished by their capacity of growth and differentation. Normally, the system is in a steady state. Little, however, is known about the precise relationship between the cells within this compartment (Lajtha 75). The variety of these cells complicates considerably a detailed study. Therefore attempts were made to cope with this problem by using isolated cell classes (Moore 72, Quesenberry 74).

Besides cell density (Leif 70) and cell volume (Miller 67) cell surface specific parameters are used for cell separation procedures since it has been shown that the cell surface is involved in various cell functions as maturation (Lichtmann 72), antigenicity (Sandford 67), malignant transformation or metastasizing (Abercombie 62). The negative electric surface charge of mammallian cells is one of the cell surface specific parameters which can be used to discriminate between functionally defined cells (Ruhenstrodt-Bauer 61). The preparative continuous free flow cell electrophoresis enables additionally the functional testing after the separation (Hannig 61). The successful application of this method on mammallian cell mixtures has been shown by several investigators (Hannig 69, Zeiller 72a, 72b, Schubert 73, v. Boehmer 74). It is the purpose of this presentation to show that preparative cell electrophoresis combined with the diffusion chamber assay contributes to further characterisation of the human stem cell compartment.

For the isolation of human bone marrow cells the electrophoretic cell separator FF5 (Bender and Hobein, München) was used. The separation conditions were described elsewhere (Schubert 73, Zeiller 75). After separation the single fractions were tested for their capacity of growth and differentiation by the conventional diffusion chamber method (Benestad 70, Boyum 72). NMRI mice were used as hosts. In order to stimulate erythropoiesis the animals were kept at 0.5 atm.

The work was supported by Deutsche Forschungsgemeinschaft grant 157/Schu.
[1] Holder of scholarship of Kind-Philipp-Stiftung.

47

immediately after chamber implantation (Schopow 75, Walther 76). Each chamber was filled with 750,000 nucleated cells. Harvesting was done on day nine.

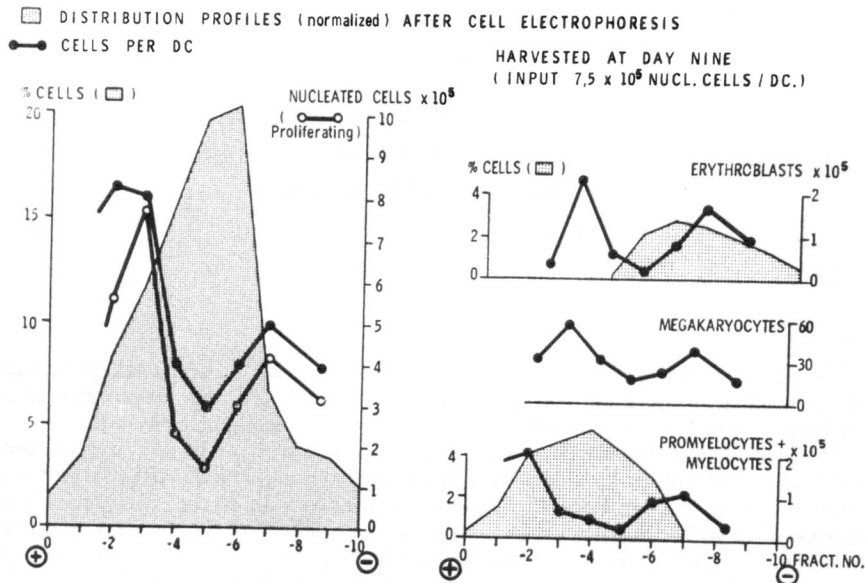

Fig. 1: For explanation see text.

The results of the analysis of normal human bone marrow are shown in Fig. 1. The number of nucleated cells grown in the diffusion chamber are plotted against electrophoretic migration. Each point represents the mean value of up to six chamber contents. It is evident that two different stem cell populations based on their electrophoretic migration are existent with comparable growth capacity. The maxima are in fraction –3 and –6 repsectively. On the right side of Fig. 1 the morphological analysis of the chamber output into erythroblasts, megacaryocytes and immature granulocytes is shown. Again a bimodal distribution is also exhibited by the subpopulations. The cellular composition in both maxima is nearly identical. Besides the cell types described mature granulocytes, unknown blasts and macrophages have also been classified. No correlation exists between the cellular composition filled originally into the chambers (shaded areas Fig. 1) and that harvested on day nine. This gives evidence that the cells grown in the diffusion chambers are newly generated from stem cells which are not accessible to a precise morphological characterisation within the bone marrow cell mixture. The application of this method to human acute leukemia shows a striking difference of the growth behaviour in comparison to normal conditions as shown in Fig. 2 (The graphic presentation is in accordance to Fig. 1). On day nine only those cells caused progeny in the chambers which originated from the region of slow electrophoretic migration (fraction –5 to –10). The lack of cell growth in the fast migrating region which contained originally the myeloblasts of the bone marrow can be due to very different growth kinetics or insufficient proliferation capacity. Both statements are not in accordance with observations made with unseparated peripheral human blood myeloblasts (Hoelzer 74).

If these results with bone marrow cells of human acute leukemia are specific must be proven in further experiments. With the presented experimental approach it might be possible to seize upon disturbances at the stem cell level and contribute to further insight into the pathogeneses of human leukemias.

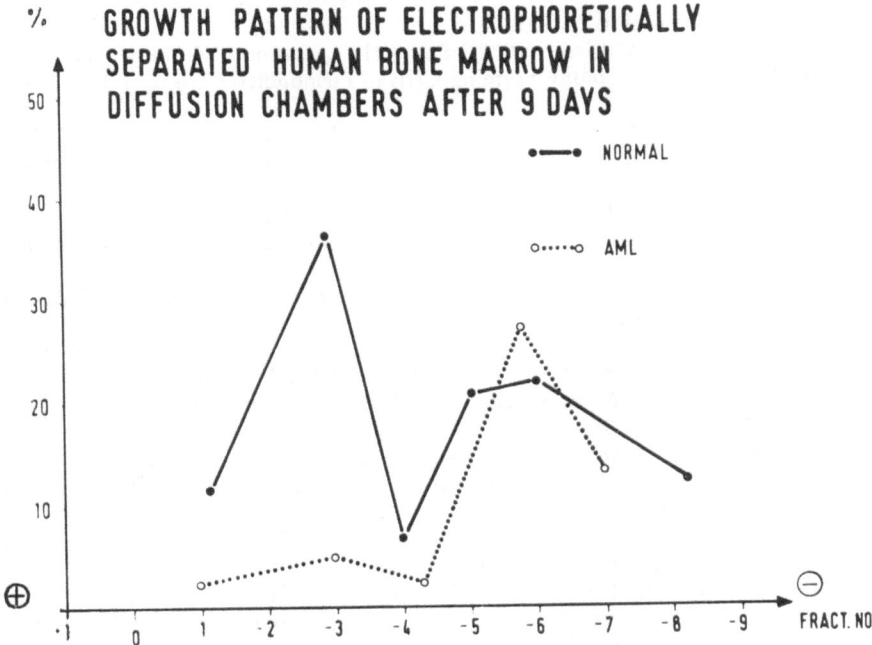

Fig. 2: Nucleated cells normalized grown in DC on day nine plotted against electrophoretic migration. (Myeloblasts subtracted).

References

Abercombie, M. and E. J. Ambrose (1962): The Surface Properties of Cancer Cells: A Review. Cancer Rex. 22, 525.

Hannig, K. (1961): Die trägerfreie kontinuierliche Elektrophorese und ihre Anwendung. Z. Anal. Chem., 181, 244.

Hannig, K., K. Zeiller (1969): Zur Auftrennung und Charakterisierung immunkompetenter Zellen mit Hilfe der trägerfreien Ablenkungselektrophorese. Hoppe-Seyler's Z.-Physiol. Chem. 350, 467.

Hoelzer, D., E. Kurrle and E. B. Harris (1974): Diffusion Chamber Technique

Applied in Human Acute Leukemia. Modern Trends in Human Leukemia, J. F. Lehmanns Verlag München p. 78 (eds. R. Neth, R. C. Gallo, S. Spiegelmann, F. Stohlman, jr.).

Lajtha, L. G. (1975): Hemopoietic Stem Cells. Brit. J. Haematol. *29*, 529.

Leif, R. C. (1970): Automated Cell Identification and Cell Sorting, Acad. Press Nr. 4 (G. L. Wied and G. F. Bahr, eds.).

Lichtmann, M. A. and J. R. Weed (1972): Alteration of the Cell Periphery during Maturation. Blood *39*, 301.

Miller, G. R. and R. A. Phillips (1969): Separation of Cells by Velocity Sedimentation. J. Cell. Physiol. *73*, 791.

Moore, M. A. S., N. Williams (1972): Physical Separation of Colony Stimulating Cells from In Vitro Colony Forming Cells in Hemopoietic Tissue. J. Cell. Phys. *80*, 195.

Quesenberry, P., E. Niskanen, M. Symann, D. Howard, M. Ryan, J. Halpern and F. Stohlman, jr. (1974): Growth of Stem Cell Concentrates in Diffusion Chambers (DC). Cell Tissue Kinet. *7*, 227.

Ruhenstroht-Bauer, G., E. Straub, P. Sachtleben, G. F. Fuhrmann (1961): Die elektrophoretische Beweglichkeit von Blutzellen beim Gesunden und beim Kranken. Münchener Med. Wschr. *103*, 794.

Sandford, B. H. (1967): An Alteration in Tumor Histocompatibility Induced by Neuramidases. Transplantation *5*, 1273.

Schopow, K., J. C. F. Schubert and F. Walther (1975): Demonstration of Human Erythropoietic Precursor Cells by a Diffusion Chamber Assay. Third Meeting of the European and African Division of the International Society of Haematology 24.–28. August 1975.

Schubert, J. C. F., F. Walther, E. Holzberg, G. Pascher and K. Zeiller (1973): Preparative Electrophoretic Separation of Normal and Neoplastic Human Bone Marrow Cells. Klin. Wschr. *51*, 327.

Walther, F., K. Schopow, J. C. F. Schubert and K. Zeiller (1976): Stimulation of Human Erythropoiesis in DC. In preparation.

Zeiller, K., R. Löser, G. Pascher and K. Hannig (1975): "Free Flow Electrophoresis" Analysis of the Method with Respect to Preparative Cell Separation. Hoppe-Seyler's Z. Phys. Chem. *353*, 95.

Zeiller, K., K. Hannig and G. Pascher (1971): Free-Flow Electrophoretic Separation of Lymphocytes. Separation of Graft Versus Host Reactive Lymphocytes of Rat Spleens. Hoppe-Seyler's Z. Phys. Chem. *352*, 1168.

The Phenotypic Abnormality in Leukemia:
A Defective Cell-Factor Interaction?

A. M. Wu[1] and R. C. Gallo[2]

[1] Department of Molecular Biology Bionetics Research
Laboratory
[2] Laboratory of Tumor Cell Biology National Cancer Institute
National Institutes of Health Bethesda, Maryland 20014 U.S.A.

Abstract

Differentiation of hemopoietic cells appears to depend upon specific interactions of certain cell-factors. The phenotypic abnormality in leukemia may involve an impairment in these interactions. In this report we present some of our views of leukemogenesis with respect to cell-factor interaction and the feasibility of experimental approaches to this problem. In culture, the interaction of myelogenous cells with factor(s) leading to differentiation can be measured either with a suspension mass culture method or by a solid (semi-soft) clonal method. The protein factors that support the growth of hemopoietic cells in suspension culture are termed growth stimulating factors (GSA) and in semi-solid culture, colony stimulating factors (CSA). Studies using conditioned medium prepared from phytohemagglutinin stimulated human lymphocytes (PHA-LyCM) and whole human embryo cells (WHE) revealed that GSA and CSA were not identical for growth of either normal human or leukemic leukocytes. In some cases maturation of leukemic leukocytes was observed. Fractionation of PHA-LyCM showed that there are three peaks for CSA. Each peak contains different fractions for supporting cellular proliferation, differentiation, and self-renewal of precursor cells in suspension culture. Apparently, each contains heterogenous species of protein factors some of which functionally overlap, while others do not.

Introduction

In order to carry out the normal function of hempoietic tissue, it is essential to have a continuous supply of mature functional cells, granulocytes, erythrocytes, megakaryocytes and plasma cells. These mature cells are derived from some progenitor cells which are committed for a particular pattern of differentiation, for example, granulocytes derived from a granulocytic cell progenitor (1, 2) and erythrocytes from an erythrocytic cell progenitor (3). The committed progenitor cells are in turn derived from some multipotent stem cells (4, 5, 6). The transition from precursor cells to differentiated cells requires some protein factors. Colony stimulating activity (CSA) and erythropoietin are examples of factors required for the transition from progenitor cells to differentiated cells (1–3). Little is known about the factors required for the transition from stem cells to progenitor cells (7). Specific interactions between factors and factor responsive cells appears to be required for normal differentiation and proliferation. Disturbances in these interactions may impair the normal differentiation process. The phenotypic change in leukemia probably involves changes in the normal interaction between factors and the factor responsive cells, leading to a block in the normal maturation process (8, 9, 10). In this paper we wish to present our concepts of leukemogenesis with respect to cell-factor interactions and, more importantly, to present some preliminary results which illustrate the feasibility of experimental approaches to this problem.

Defectiveness of cell-factor interaction:

There are at least three means by which cell-factor interactions can be blocked (see Table 1). *First,* defectiveness in differentiation could be, and most likely is, in

Table 1: Defects in Cell-Factor Interactions

Defect	Response to factors *in vitro*
Factor responsive cells	_*
Factor	+
Factor producing cells	+

* Sometimes a positive response could be obtained either because of artificial conditions *in vitro* (there is less stringent control(s) *in vitro*) or because of the presence of some other factor for the specific abnormal situation.

the factor responsive cells. For example, if the membrane or factor receptor sites of the responsive cells is altered as a result of viral infection or treatment with physical or chemical agents, these cells may no longer respond to normal concentrations of factor (11). *Secondly,* defectiveness in differentiation could be due to the production of abnormal factors or to the presence of inhibitors. This situation would result in an insufficient concentration of factors for normal differentiation. *Thirdly,* the defect could be due to alteration(s) in the factor producing cells. For example, if the factor producing cells are infected by a virus, inadequate production of the factor might result. Among the three possibilities just described, the first is intrinsic to the factor responsive cells, while the other two are extrinsic to the responsive cells. Both the intrinsic and extrinsic causes may result in either an accumulation of early immature cells (such as in polycythemia vera and leukemia) and/or in a deficiency in the mature cell population (such as in neutropenia, aplastic anemia and pancytopenia).

The response of the factor responsive cells to exogenous factors in culture is different in each of the situations described (Table 1). In the first, most of the target cells cannot respond to factors, and therefore no growth and differentiation will be observed in culture. However, sometimes these defective cells might respond to factors under artificial *in vitro* conditions or respond to some specific factors. In the second and the third situations, one would predict that the factor responsive cells will proliferate and differentiate in culture if proper exogenous factors are provided. In fact, results from many studies strongly suggest that *some* acute myelocytic leukemic cells from *some* patients grow and differentiate in culture while some apparently do not (12–16). This type of response or non-response has also been observed in some cases of neutropenia (17–19).

Measurement of factor-cell interactions:

Cell-factor interactions are expressed in three processes: proliferation, differentiation, and self-renewal. In granulocytic differentiation, these processes are conventionally measured in culture by two methods (Table 2). One is the colony

Table 2: Measurement of Cell-Factor Interaction

Methods	Factors Involved	Measurements/[1]
Semi-soft medium (agar or methylcellulose)	CSA	Colonies
Suspension culture	GSA	Cell counts and morphology [³H]dThd Number of colony-forming cells

[1] The procedures for these measurements are described in the Legend to Figure 1.

forming assay in semi-soft agar (1, 2) or methylcellulose (20, 21). The factors involved in this assay are called colony stimulating activity (CSA) or colony stimulating factor (CSF). This method provides a quantitative measurement of the number of progenitor cells and also the differentiation and proliferation capacity of the progenitor cells (21, 22, 23). The other method is by suspension culture assay. By counting the cell number or by measuring thymidine uptake, it is possible to measure the proliferative capacity of the target cells. By observing the morphology of the cells, it is possible to determine the degree of differentiation. One can also measure the process of self-renewal by measuring the growth of colony-forming cells in suspension culture using the above mentioned colony technique in culture. The protein factors that stimulate these activities in a suspension culture are called growth stimulating activity (GSA). It is worth emphasizing that both CSA and GSA are defined according to their function as they might contain a pool of many activities. Identification of the protein factors corresponding to each functional entity is obviously critical in achieving an unambiguous understanding of the nature of these factor-cell interactions.

Conditioned medium from human lymphocytes:

Conditioned medium was prepared from normal human blood lymphocytes (24, 25). We have previously demonstrated that conditioned medium from this source is specific for human and subhuman primates, and it is relatively easy to prepare

53

(24). The procedure for preparation has previously been described in detail (24) but is also summarized here. 10^7 cells per ml are incubated in serum free Dulbecco's Modified Eagle's Medium for four to six days. When conditioned medium is prepared in the presence of phytohemagglutinin (PHA), the culture contains 10^6 lymphoid cells per ml, 1 % PHA-M (Difco), and 1 % homologous plasma in RPMI-1629 medium. The cells are incubated at 37 °C with 10 % CO_2. The medium is harvested the third day after incubation. The conditioned medium obtained in the presence of PHA (PHA-LyCM) contains CSA for human and monkey target cells but not mouse cells (Table 3 and Reference 24). Another advantage of

Table 3: Species Specificity and Colony Size from LCM and LyCM in the Presence and Absence of PHA

Source of Condition Medium	PHA	Colony Formation/[1]			Colony Size (Human Cells)
		Human	Primate	Mouse	
Leukocytes (LCM)	−	++		++	Medium to cluster/[2]
	+	++++		±	Large to medium
Lymphocyte (LyCM)	−	++		±	Medium to cluster
	+	++++	+++	±	Large to medium

[1] The procedure for the agar colony assay is described in the Legend to Figure 1.
[2] Cluster: less than 50 cells; small colony: about 50 to 200 cells; and large colony: more than 200 cells.

using PHA for factor production is that the size of colonies stimulated by this factor is much larger than those stimulated by conditioned medium without PHA stimulation. Very often the colonies contain several thousand cells. Conditioned medium prepared from buffy coat leukocytes in the presence of PHA are similar to those prepared from the lymphocyte enriched fraction with respect to species specificity and colony size (Table 3). In the studies described here, the experiments were mostly done with conditioned medium prepared from lymphocyte-enriched fraction in the presence of PHA. We found that CSA is produced both from B and T lymphocyte populations. While the B lymphocyte fraction is able to produce CSA without PHA stimulation, the T cell population requires PHA stimulation. It has been reported that CSA for human cells are produced from human monocytes (26, 27) or adherent cells (28). Our findings would suggest that CSA are produced from more than one type of cell. Alternatively, the factor producing cells may be co-fractionated with both adherent and non-adherent cells.

CSA activity in PHA-LyCM:

As discussed above, PHA-LyCM contained CSA that stimulates the formation of large size colonies in semi-soft agar medium. Six types of colonies can be distinguished by morphology (Wu, Glick and Gallo, manuscript in preparation). Some have been described before (21, 23). Type-1 colonies are compact with uneven rigid edges. They contain mainly eosinophilic granulocytes which are peroxidase positive. Type-2 colonies look compact in the center with cells loosely distributed in the periphery. This type of colony consists mainly of neutrophilic granulocytes or monocytes which are peroxidase positive. Type-3 colonies are those with cells evenly and loosely distributed. These are peroxidase negative macrophage cells. Type-4 are colonies that are scattered with clumps of cells. Each clump contains less than 10 cells. Each cell in the clump is relatively large compared with other colony cells. It will be of interest to determine if these cells are megakaryocytes. Type-5 colonies are the clusters which contain less than 50 cells. They could look like type-1 or type-2 except for their smaller cell numbers. Finally, type-6 colonies are those which contain an aggregation of several clusters (less than 50 cells per cluster). This type of colony resembles the "burst" formation in erythrocytic colony formation in the plasma clot system (34). This type of colony sometimes is difficult to distinguish betwenn single-cell origin or multi-cell origin. At the conclusion of morphological identification, one should point out that the correlation between colony morphology and histochemical properties of colony cells is a relatively rough one. For precise study, the identification of the nature of colonies still requires histochemical staining.

The CSA described here are relatively heat stable. They are active after treatment at 70 °C for one hour (Table 4). After treatment at 90 °C for an

Table 4: Some Properties of LyCM

Treatment/[1]	Colonies/10^5 Cells/[2]
None (37 °C)	41
56 °C	50
70 °C	49
90 °C	0
Trypsin (100 µg/ml)	0
Neuraminidase (100 µg/ml)	0
0.5 M NaCl	0

[1] LyCM are treated at 37 °C, 56 °C, 70 °C and 90 °C respectively for one hour. Trypsin treatment was performed at 37 °C for one hour. Neuraminidase treatment was performed at 37 °C for one hour.
[2] Average of 4 plates.

hour, all type-1, 2, 3, and 5 colonies disappear, but type-4 and 6 colonies are not significantly affected. This suggests that there are different types of CSA with respect to heat sensitivity. All CSA are sensitive to trypsin and neurominidase treatment, suggesting that CSA are glycoproteins. Another feature of CSA from PHA-LyCM is that they are sensitive to high salt treatment. The activity can be completely restored after removal of the salt by a dialysis against phosphate buffered saline (PBS), but dilution of the high salt treated CSA with PBS is not sufficient to restore the activity. This observation suggests that an active form of CSA is formed during the dialysis, for example, the formation of a polymer.

GSA in PHA-LyCM

GSA in PHA-LyCM are measured by three procedures in suspension culture, namely, viable cell number, [³H] thymidine uptake and number of CFC following culture. The suspension culture technique is similar to that described by Aye *et al.* (29). Three ml of cell suspension containing 20 % fetal calf serum in medium 10⁶ nucleated cells and 20 % of PHA-LyCM is placed in a T30 plastic flask. When PHA-LyCM is omitted, an equivalent amount of PHA is included in the culture medium. The number of viable cells is estimated by the trypan blue exclusion technique. [³H] thymidine uptake is performed by labelling cells with 5 μc/

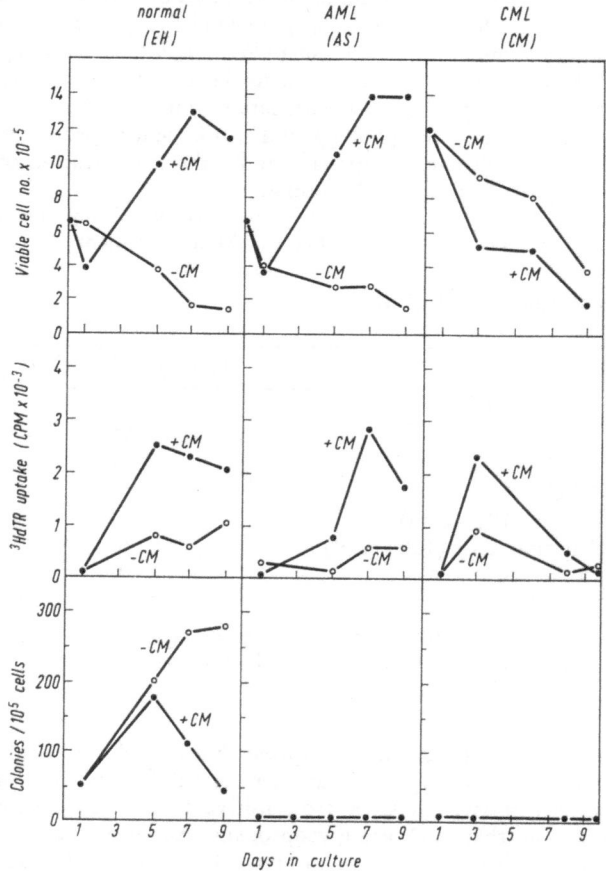

Fig. 1: *Growth of Normal and Leukemic Leukocytes in Suspension Culture.*
Non-adherent cells (NAC) are prepared according to the procedures described by Messner *et al.* (28). Bone marrow cells from a normal woman (EH), a woman with acute myelogenous leukemia (AML), patient (A. S.), and a woman with chronic myelogenous leukemia (CML), patient (OM), were separately placed on petri dishes (Falcon plastic) and incubated

at 37 °C with 10 % CO_2 for one hour. Those cells that did not adhere to the dishes were decanted onto an dish and the incubations were repeated for $2^{1/2}$ hours. These NAC were then used for all of the experiments. The suspension culture contained 1.6 x 10^6 nucleated cells/ml, 60 % α medium, 20 % fetal calf serum, and 20 % LyCM. Since LyCM contained 1 % PHA-M, the 1 % PHA-M was used for control culture without LyCM. Three ml of this culture were placed in a T60 flask and were incubated at 37 °C with 10 % CO_2. Samples were harvested at different days and viable cell number, [^3H]dThd uptake, and number of colony forming cells were measured. Viable cell count was performed with a standard trypan blue exclusion technique. For [^3H]dThd uptake, 15 μc of [^3H]dThd were added to 3 ml of suspension culture for four hours before the harvest of cells. The harvested cells were washed twice with phosphate buffered saline (PBS) and twice with high pH buffer (0.01 M Tris; pH 8.8, 0.14 M NaCl, 0.02 M $MgCl_2$) at 4 °C. The cell pellet was then lysed with 1 ml of the same buffer containing 1 % Triton X-100. Aliquots (50 and 100 μl) of lysate were precipitated with 10 % trichloroacetic acid (TCA) at 4 °C. The acid precipitable count was the determined. The number of colony forming cells was measured by an agar colony assay according to the procedures we have previously described (24). Briefly, the assay consisted of two layers of soft agar medium in a 60 mm petri dish. The upper layer contained 0.8 ml of 0.3 % agar in McCoy's 5A medium containing 20 % fetal calf serum and 10^5 nucleated NAC, and the lower layer 2.5 ml of 0.5 % agar in McCoy's 5A medium containing 20 % fetal calf serum and 25 % LyCM. Cultures were incubated at 37 °C with 10 % CO_2. Colonies were examined between 12 to 14 days after incubation. When more than 50 cells were found, they were scored as positives as a colony.

ml of [^3H] thymidine for 4 hours. The number of CFC in suspension culture is measured by plating 10^5 viable cells in an upper layer of agar medium in a 60 mm petri dish containing 20 % of PHA-LyCM in the lower layer of the petri dish. Under these conditions, colony formation is still dependent on CSA, suggesting that CSA is still required for colony formation although these cells were exposed to CSA in suspension culture.

Figure 1 shows that the growth of non-adherent cells from normal human bone marrow cells is stimulated by the PHA-LyCM measured both by viable cell count and by DNA synthesis. However, CFC from normal non-adherent cells increased even in the absence of PHA-LyCM. This GSA independent self-renewal process is inhibited by PHA-LyCM in the later period of the culture. We observed that when unfractionated or adherent marrow cells were used for this study, no stimulation of cell growth was observed. Results from assays of bone marrow cells from a patient with AML and one from CML are also shown in Figure 1. PHA-LyCM produces an exponential increase in the number of viable cells in the case of AML while there is no detectable effect on the cell number in the case of CML, although DNA synthesis is stimulated in both. Cells from both are not able to replicate CFC nor respond to stimulation with conditioned medium. These results clearly demonstrate that PHA-LyCM contains GSA and that these GSA are heterogenous with respect to the three activities measured in this study. The GSA responsible for each activity appear to be separable, although it is still questionable whether PHA-LyCM contains activity sufficient for self-renewal. However, we would like to emphasize that these results are given to stress the heterogeneity among GSA and CSA and not to be generalized as a specific pattern of response of a specific leukemia to PHA-LyCM.

CSA and GSA are not identical:

Protein species may exist which contain overlapping CSA and GSA, but the major protein sources of these activities are clearly not identical. For example, as illustrated in Table 5, factors A, B, C, D, and E are required for the formation

Table 5: Model of Relationship Between CSA and GSA

activity	protein species*
CSA	A. B. C. D. E.
GSA	C. D. E. F. G.

* The number and name of protein species are hypothetical.

of one type of colony in a semi-soft agar medium, while factors C, D, E, F, and G are required for the growth and maturation of hemopoietic cells in suspension culture. Factors C, D, and E are required for both assays but factor A, B, F, or G are required only for one particular assay. Some observations shown in Table 6 illustrate this point. Bone marrow cells from a patient with AML (AS) are grown in suspension culture containing either PHA-LyCM or WHE-1 CM (conditioned medium prepared from a particular cell line of whole human embryo),

Table 6: Some Results which Differentiate CSA and GSA

Source of Factor Responsive Cells	Contitioned Medium	Colony Formation in Semi-Soft Agar Medium/[3]	Proliferation in Suspension Culture/[4]
AML (AS)	none	–	–
	LyCM	–	+++
	WHE-1 CM/[2]	–	+++
AMML (JC)	none	–	+++
NA/[1]	LyCM	+++	±
	WHE-1 CM	+++	+
Normal (EH)	none	+	–
NA	LyCM	+++	++
	WHE-1 CM	+	–

[1] NA: non-adherent cells. These are prepared according to the procedure of Messner *et al.* (28).
[2] WHE-1 CM denotes conditioned medium prepared from whole human embryo cell strain no. 1 in our laboratory. The conditioned medium was harvested 48 hours after WHE-1 cells reached stationary phase.
[3] The procedures for the agar colony assay are described in the Legend to Figure 1. – = no colony formation; + = one colony per 10^4 nucleated cells; +++ = one colony per 10^3 nucleated cells.
[4] This is based on results obtained from viable cell count. – = no stimulation of cell proliferation; + = slight stimulation of cell growth; ++ = moderate stimulation of cell growth; +++ = exponential growth of the factor responsive cells.

but the same cells do not form any agar colonies in the presence of either factor. Conversely, marrow cells from a case of AMML (acute monomyelocyte leukemia) (JC) form agar colonies in the presence of the conditioned medium, but no growth was observed in the suspension culture, although the growth of these cells is observed in the absence of exogenous conditioned medium. It is likely that these leukemic cells produced some unique protein factors that support the growth of leukemic cells, and these factors are ineffective in the presence of protein factors isolated from normal cells. Normal marrow cells grow both in agar medium culture and suspension culture in the presence of PHA-LyCM, but WHE-1 CM supports the growth of normal cells in agar medium culture but not in suspension culture. Apparently, WHE-1 CM is able to support the growth of some leukemic cells in suspension culture in an exponential manner but not normal cells. In this aspect, this is similar to the factor(s) described by Gallagher et al. (30). These results not only show that CSA and GSA are not identical, but also that the ability of GSA in supporting the growth of normal and some leukemic leukocytes could be different.

Fractionation of PHA-LyCM:

An attempt was made to separate various activities in PHA-LyCM. Conditioned medium was fractionated by conventional biochemical procedures, including ammonium sulfate precipitation, sephadex gel filtration (G200) and DEAE cellulose chromatography. Table 7 summarizes the result of this fractionation pro-

Table 7: Summary of Purification of PHA-CSF

Purification step/[1]	Volume (ml)	Activity/[2] (units/ml)	Protein (mg/ml)	Specific Activity (units/mg)	Purification	Yield
I. Unpurified	15000	120	0.78	153	1	
II. ASP (45–65 %)/[3]	200	18000	100	280	1.8	100
III. Sephadex G 200						
Peak I	460	2000	1.53	1310	8.5	16.4
Peak II	640	6300	0.48	13120	85.8	71.4
IV. DEAE Cellulose						
Peak I	380	4900	0.76	6400	42.1	33.9
Peak II	225	10400	0.60	17600	113	41.1
Peak III	175	9600	0.36	26700	175	30.4

[1] The details of purification procedures will be described elsewhere (31).
[2] Unit is defined as colony number per 10^5 cells stimulated by 1 % increment of CSF (in a linear region).
[3] Inhibitory activity is detected in the ammonium sulfate precipitate (ASP) (45–65 %).

cedure; the details of which will be described elsewhere (31). After DEAE cellulose chromatography, three peaks of CSA are obtained with estimated molecular weights of 70,000, 40,000 and 25,000 respectively. Peak I predominantly stimulates type-3 colony growth, and Peak II and III stimulate all types of colonies. An attempt was made to distinguish their colony stimulatory ability, but clear results were not obtaned probably because Peaks II and III were not well separated. The GSA in each CSA peak were measured with normal cells and are shown in Table 8. Peak I sti-

Table 8: GSA in Purified CSA Preparation

| Factors [1] | Viable Count (x 10^{-6} cell/ml) | Suspension Culture/[2] (normal marrow cells) | | Semi-soft/[3] Agar Medium Colony Formation (units x 10^{-3}/ml) |
		[³H]dThd Uptake (cpm x 10^{-3})	CFC in Culture (colonies/10^5 cells)	
None	2.3	2.6	105	0
D I	2.1	5.0	105	4.9
D II	2.2	2.8	165	10.4
D III	2.2	4.5	125	9.6

[1] DI, DII and DIII represent Peak I, II and III CSA after DEAE cellulose chromatography shown in Table 7. For all experiments only 2 % of each fraction was used.
[2] The procedures for the suspension culture are described in the Legend to Figure 1.
[3] These results were the same as those shown in Table 7.

mulates [³H] thymidine uptake, but it does not enhance the number of viable cells nor of CFC. Peak II enhances the growth of CFC but not of viable cells nor [³H] thymidine uptake. Peak III is similar to Peak I in that only [³H] thymidine uptake is enhanced in the suspension culture. Although these results are preliminary, they suggest that it is feasible to study a specific interaction between protein factors and their specific target cells with fractionated defined factors. We are currently looking for some peak activities containing the self-renewal activity. Success in the isolation of this activity will be important for establishing measurements of multipotent stem cells in culture.

Conclusions

We believe that a generalized statement regarding leukemia as a stem cell disease is unwarranted. It is more likely that stem cells are one cell type that can be transformed. Other cell types may also be target cells, but the term leukemic transformation should not be loosely used since it is difficult and sometimes impossible to distinguish between the accumulation of normal immature cells and the accumulation of abnormal blood cells. Elucidation of cell-factor interactions should be very useful in making the distinction.

To study specific cell-factor interactions, well-defined quantitative assays are required. At present, the literature concerning CSA and GSA for myeloid cell differentiation describe many activities which are ill-defined. Even the growth of erythroid colonies in culture stimulated by erythropoietin (3, 32, 33) are not well defined. To obtain quantitative measurements of each cell-factor interaction we need: 1) fractionation and purification of protein factors that promote the growth and differentiation of hemopoietic cells; 2) determination of the interrelationship among various factors; 3) fractionation and identification of target cells for specific protein factors; and 4) identification of specific biochemical events in cells associated with a particular cell-factor interaction. The studies presented in this paper represent some of our initial attempts in pursuing these goals.

Acknowledgment

The authors wish to thank Ellen Hambleton and Dr. Frank Ruscetti for useful discussions and Ellen Hambleton and Vicky Baer for excellent technical assistance. This work was in part supported by a contract from the Virus Cancer Program, National Cancer Institute.

References

1. Bradley, J. R. and Metcalf, D. (1966). Aust. J. Expt. Biol. Med. Sci. *44:* 287.
2. Pluznik, D. H. and Sachs, L. (1965). J. Cell Comp. Physiol. *66:* 319.
3. Stephenson, J. R., Axelrad, A. A., Mclead, D. L. and Shreeve, M. M. (1971). Proc. Nat. Acad. Sci., U.S.A. *69:* 1542.
4. Till, J. E. and McCulloch, E. A. (1961). Rad. Res. *14:* 213.
5. Fowler, J. H., Wu, A. M., Till, J. E., Siminovitch, L. and McCulloch, E. A. (1967). J. Cell Physiol. *69:* 65.
6. Wu, A. M., Till, J. E., Siminovitch, L. and McCulloch, E. A. (1967). J. Cell Physiol. *69:* 177.
7. McCulloch, E. A., Gregory, C. J. and Till, J. E. (1973). *In:* Hemopoietic stem cells. Ciba Foundation Symposium 13 ASP, Amsterdam, pp. 183–199.
8. Ginsburg, H. and Sachs, L. (1965). J. Cell Comp. Physiol. *66:* 199.
9. Perry, S. and Gallo, R. C. (1970). *In:* Regulation of hemopoiesis, A. Gordon (ed.), Appleton-Century-Crofts, N.Y., p. 1221.
10. McCulloch, E. A. and Till, J. E. (1971). Amer. J. Path. *65:*737.
11. Gallo, R. C. (1973). On the Etiology of Human Acute Leukemia, Med. Clin. of North America *57:* 343.
12. Paran, M., Sachs, L., Barak, Y., Resnitzky, P. (1970). Proc. Nat. Acad. Sci., U.S.A. *67:* 1542.
13. Robinson, W. A., Kurnick, J. E., Pike, B. L. (1971). Blood *38:* 500.
14. Moore, M. A. S., Spitzer, G., Williams, N., Metcalf, D. and Buckley, J. (1973). Blood *42:* 331.
15. Greenberg, P. L., Nichols, W. C. and Schrier, S. L. (1971). New England J. Med. *184:* 1225.
16. Moore, M. A. S., Williams, N. and Metcalf, D. (1975). J. Nat. Cancer Inst. *50:* 591.
17. Mintz, U. and Sachs, L. (1973). Blood *41:* 745–751.

18. Senn, J. S., Messner, H. A. and Stanley, E. R. (1973). *In:* "Hemopoiesis in Culture", 2nd Int. Workshop, Robinson, W. A. (ed.), published NIH, p. 367.
19. Greenberg, P. L. and Schrier, S. L. (1973). Blood *41*: 753.
20. Worton, R. G., McCulloch, E. A. and Till, J. E. (1969). J. Cell Physiol. *74*: 171.
21. Iscove, N. N., Senn, J. S., Till, J. E. and McCulloch, E. A. (1971). Blood 37:1.
22. Paran, M. and Sachs, L. (1969). J. Cell Physiol. *73*: 91.
23. Shoham, D., David, E. B. and Rozenszaju, L. A. (1974). Blood *44*:221.
24. Prival, J., Paran, M., Gallo, R. C. and Wu, A. M. (1974). J. Nat. Cancer Inst. *53*: 1583.
25. Cline, M. J. and Golde, D. W. (1974). Nature *248*: 703.
26. Golde, D. W. and Cline, M. J. (1972). J. Clin. Invest. *51*: 2981.
27. Chervenick, P. A. and LoBuglio, A. F. (1972). Science *178*: 164.
28. Messner, H. A., Till, J. E. and McCulloch, E. A. (1973). Blood *42*: 701.
29. Aye, M. T., Till, J. E. and McCulloch, E. A. (1974). Blood *44*: 205.
30. Gallagher, R. E., Salahuddin, S. Z., Hall, W. T., McCredie, K. B. and Gallo, R. C. (1976). Proc. Nat. Acad. Sci., U.S.A. 72:4137
31. Wu, A. M. and Gallo, R. C. In preparation.
32. Iscove, N. N., Sieber, F. and Winterhalter, K. H. (1974). J. Cell Physiol. *83*: 309.
33. Iscove, N. N. and Sieber, F. (1975). Expt. Hemat. 3: 32.
34. Axelrad, A. A., Mcleod, D. L., Shreeve, M. M. and Heath, D. S. (1974). *In:* Hemopoiesis in Culture, W. A. Robinson (ed.), U. S. Government Printing Office, Washington, D. C , p. 226.

In Vitro Colony Growth of Acute Myelogenous Leukemia

K. A. Dicke*
G. Spitzer
P. H. M. Scheffers
A. Cork
M. J. Ahearn
B. Löwenberg
K. B. McCredie

University of Texas System Cancer Center, M. D. Anderson
Hospital and Tumor Institute
Houston, Texas 77025, USA.

Summary

Colony formation in vitro by marrow cells from patients with untreated acute myelogenous leukemia (AML) and from patients in AML relapse is infrequent using the standard Robinson assay. A newly developed culture system has been described in which marrow from AML patients in these disease stages form leukemic cell colonies. In this in vitro system, phytohaemagglutinin is the essential stimulator for colony formation. The leukemic origin of the colonies has been proven by ultrastructural morphology and cytogenetics. It appears that colony formation by leukemic cells in this system is predominantly independent from the leukocyte factor which is the main stimulator in the Robinson assay for growing colonies of marrow cells from haematologically normal individuals.

Bone marrow cells in untreated acute myelogenous leukemia (AML) demonstrate abnormal growth in vitro in the Robinson assay (Robinson et al., 1971; and Bull et al., 1973). Characteristically, there is a near total failure of colony formation; pre dominantly clusters are formed containing 20 cells or less (Bull et al., 1973; Greenberg et al., 1971; Moore et al., 1973 and 1974, and van Bekkum et al., in press). The absence of colonies has been shown to be due to a marked decrease of the normal myeloid precursor cell population in untreated AML. The small aggregate formation of AML cells has been attributed to the suboptimal response of leukemic cells to the leukocyte stimulation factor. Because this poor proliferation in vitro might not represent the maximal in vitro and in vivo proliferation potential of the leukemic cells, we studied a number of modifications of the in vitro culture system. A number of factors were studied which may have some influence on cell pro-

* Visiting Professor from the Radiobiological Institute TNO, Rijswijk, The Netherlands.
** Supported by Public Health Service Research Grant No. CA 12687, from the National Cancer Institute, Bethesda, Maryland 20014, USA.

liferation in general, notably phytohaemagglutinin (PHA), which induces lymphocyte colonies in vitro (Rozenszajn et al., 1974), and endotoxin which has been demonstrated to increase the labelling index of leukemic cells in vivo (Golde et al.).

In this paper an in vitro system is described in which marrow cells from untreated AML and AML in relapse were stimulated by phytohaemagglutinin (PHA) to form leukemic cell colonies in soft agar. These (similar) cells predominantly formed small aggregates (20 cells or less) in the presence of the normal leukocyte feeder layer alone. Moreover, in the course of the experiments, it appeared that by adding low concentrations of endotoxin to the cultures, the stimulating effect of PHA could be amplified.

Materials and Methods

Patients with acute myelogenous leukemia

The clinical diagnosis and the haematological findings of 13 patients with leukemia included in the study have been listed in Table I. Cases both untreated and

Table I: Differentials and Cytrochemistry of Marrow Cells from Untreated AML and AML in Relapse

Patient	Blast	Promye-locytes	Lympho-cytes	Mono-cytes	Auer Rods	Perox-idase	Es-terase**	P. A. S.
Ca	84	1	1	2		+	+	−
Fl	83	1	13	0.5		+		
He	84	0.8	6.5	0.2	+	+	−	−
St	75	3	5	0	+			
Tu	82	7	4	0	+			
Kr	53	6	1	0.2		+	−	−
Sal	70	0.4	5	0	+	+	−	−
San	6.1	52.4	11	0	+	+	−	−
Se	85	1	4.8	0		+	−	−
Ka	93	0.2	0.6	0.8		+	+	−
Ne	74	0.6	2.1	0	+	+	−	−
Pa	91	1	3	0.4		+	−	−
Po	72	2.8	3.2	0	+	+	−	−
Wo***	38.5	2	20	15.5		+	−	−
Be***	91	2	2	1		+	−	−
El***	55	2	15	0		+	−	−
Fr***	73	0	16	0		+	−	−

Header for table:
Bone Marrow Differential* / Wright-Giemsa Staining / Cytochemistry

* 500 cells per slide counted.
** Non-specific esterase.
*** Patients in relapse.

in relapse had greater than 50 % leukemic blast cells on bone marrow differentials (Table I). The leukemia was diagnosed morphologically and cytochemically by the same criteria as described by Hayhoe et al. (1964). Leukemic relapses as presented in Table I, all occurred after previous treatment with combination chemotherapy plus immunotherapy according to the protocol documented by McCredie et al. (1975) and Gutterman et al. (1974).

Haemopoietic cell culture in vitro using a leukocyte feeder layer as source of stimulation (Robinson assay)

The technique used in these studies only differed in minor details from that described by Pike and Robinson (1970). The basic components of the Robinson system is a feeder layer of peripheral leukocytes and an overlay of human bone marrow cells. Peripheral leukocytes were obtained from peripheral blood from healthy volunteers, collected by venipuncture into heparinized tubes. Methyl cellulose (final concentration 0.1 %) was added to the blood sample and the red cells were allowed to sediment by gravity for 20 minutes. The buffy coat was then collected, and after centrifugation, the cells were resuspended in Dulbecco's modified Eagle's medium (MEM) to which 20 % serum plus agar was added (the final agar concentration was 0.5 %). The serum was a mixture of 1 volume fetal calf serum (FCS), 1 volume horse serum, and 1 volume 3 % trypticase soy broth. From this cell suspension 1 x 10^6 cells were pipetted into a 35 mm plastic petri dish (Falcon) (final volume: 1 ml agar medium) and the medium was allowed to gel. Bone marrow cells were obtained by aspiration from the posterior iliac crest and collected into heparinized tubes. After removing the erythrocytes by the buffy coat method (Dicke et al., 1969), the cells were incorporated into the same medium used for the feeder cells with the exception of using 0.25 % agar. One hundred thousand cells in a volume of 0.2 ml agar medium were then pipetted gently over the solidified feeder layer and allowed to gel. The plates were incubated at 37 °C in a humidified atmosphere of 7.5 % CO_2 in air. At the end of seven days, a cluster estimate was performed, and after 14 days of incubation, the plates were removed and the colonies scored visually. Aggregates containing 50 cells or greater were scored as colonies. Aggregates containing less than 50 cells were scored as clusters. All cultures were scored in triplicate.

The in vitro PHA + E assay

Basically, the technique consists of two phases: an initial liquid phase of 15 hours at 37 °C, and a semi-solid phase of seven days incubation at 37 °C. In the liquid phase 2 x 10^6 cells per ml medium (Dulbecco's MEM + 20 % serum) were cultured in pyrex glass tubes to which 0.05 ml PHA (Difco, PHAM) per ml medium and endotoxin (Difco, Lipopolysaccharide W. E. coli, 0111:B4) 10^7 g/m were added. After 15 hours of incubation, the cells were washed X 2 using HBSS (305 mOsm) and resuspended in agar medium (final concentration agar 0.25 %, medium Dulbecco's MEM + 20 % serum). After resuspension in agar medium, the cells (1 x 10^5 0.2 ml per dish) were pipetted into Falcon plastic petri dishes containing 1 ml agar medium (final concentration agar 0.5 %, medium Dulbecco's MEM + 20 % serum) to which 1×10^6 peripheral blood leukocytes from normal individuals were added using the method as detailed for the Robinson assay. Simultaneously, the cells were plated in petri dishes containing agar underlayers without leukocytes. After seven days of incubation in a 7.5 % CO_2 gas controlled humidified incubator at 37 °C, colonies were visible microscopically. These colonies were counted using an inverted microscope. Aggregates containing 50 cells or more were considered colonies. Aggregates containing 50 cells or less were considered to be clusters. The number of colonies and clusters presented in this paper is the mean value of triplicate petri dish cultures.

Electronmicroscopical procedure

Soft agar colonies for morphological observation were fixed in their petri dishes for 12 hours at 37 °C with 2.5 % Sorensen's buffered glutaraldehyde, pH 7.2, for 30 minutes each and then incubated in the dark with 33' diaminobenzidine tetrahydrochloride reagent for two hours at room temperature. The staining solution for endogenous peroxidase was removed with three additional rinses of Sorensen's phosphate buffer and postfixed in 1 % osmium tetroxide, pH 7.2, for one hour at 4 °C. Following three distilled H_2O rinses the agar disks were removed to flat covered glass dishes for the acetone dehydration and Epon infiltration steps. Final embedding of the agar disks was accomplished in foil weighing cups. After Epon polymerization at 80 °C, the aluminum foil was removed from the specimen, and the colonies of interest marked under a dissecting microscope. Those colonies selected for observation were cut from the specimen disk and mounted on plastic rods for ultramicrotomy. Alternate thick and thin serial sections were cut for light and electron microscopic study of the entire colony. Epon sections for light microscopy were stained with Paragon's stain for frozen sections. For ultrastructural observation, thin sections were stained with 0.5 % uranyl acetate and Reynold's Lead Citrate prior to their examinations with a Siemens' Elmiskop IA at 80 kV.

Cytogenetic procedure

Chromosome studies were performed on cells from both the liquid phase and from the colonies which had formed after seven days in culture. The cells obtained from the liquid phase, following the 15 hours incubation with PHA + E, were placed in 10 ml Ham's F 10 tissue culture medium supplemented with 20 % fetal calf serum and incubated overnight at 37 °C. The following day the cells were arrested in metaphases with 0.01 mg/ml Colchicine, submitted to hypotonic treatment with 0.075 M KC1 and fixed in methanol : acetic acid (3:1) mixture. Air-dry slide preparations were made, stained with Giemsa and scanned for well spread metaphases using a Zeiss microscope.

To obtain dividing cells from the colonies which were formed after seven days in culture, 0.1 μg colcemid was added to the petri dishes and incubated for an additional 3 hours. The colonies were collected with a fine Pasteur pipette and pooled in 0.2 ml Hank's Balanced Salt Solution (HBSS). The harvesting and slide preparations were completed as above and the slides scanned for analyzable metaphases.

Results

Colony formation in vitro

Colony formation by marrow cells from leukemic patients was obtained by exposing the cells to PHA and endotoxin (E). As has been mentioned already in materials and methods, the culture system consisted of two stages. An initial liquid phase (15 hrs), in which the cells were cultured in the presence of the two stimuli and a semi-solid phase (7 days) in which the cells were immobilized in an agar containing medium. In the second phase, the actual colony formation occurred. In the PHA + E assay used for analyzing the marrow of the patients, listed in Table I, on colony formation, PHA and endotoxin were only added in the liquid phase and were not present in the semi-solid phase.

Figure 1 shows a logarithmic plot of the relationship between the number of colonies and the number of cells, plated in dishes which contained agar without leukocytes. The 12 data points as depicted in Figure 1 were obtained from one individual in two experiments on two successive days. The data were consistent between experiments and so the data were combined. The calculated slope of the least

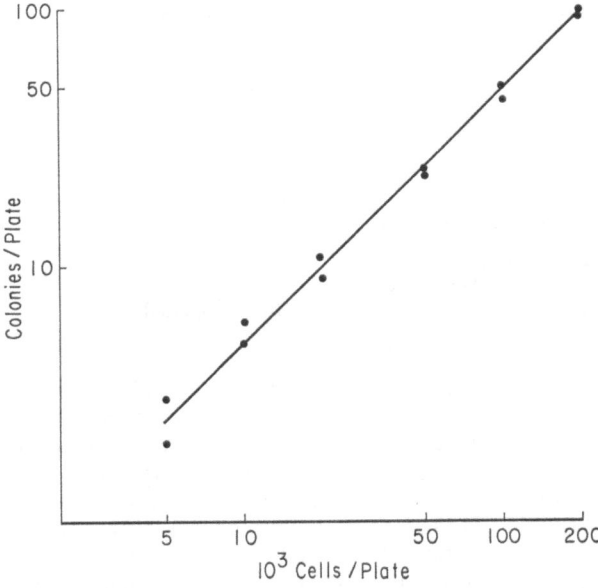

Fig. 1: Relationship between number of colonies per plate scored at seven days and number of cells cultured per plate. The data of two experiments were combined and have been depicted. Each point represents the mean value of colony number of 5–10 plates. The coefficient of variations at the different cell levels per plate ranged from 10–25 %. The stimulated slope of the least squares regression line is 0.98 ± 0.03, which is consistent with a slope of one.

squares regression line is 0.98 ± 0.03, which is consistent with a slope of one and shows that the number of colonies produced is proportional to the number of cells plated (Iscove et al., 1975). In these experiments, colony incidence was approximately 1 per 1,640 bone marrow cells.

Table II: Comparison between Number of CFU-c in the Robinson Assay and the PHA+E Assay of Marrow from Untreated Acute Myeloid Leukemics and Normals*

	Patient Name	Leukocyte Feeder	Agar**	Leukocyte Feeder	Agar**
	Knt	1***	n. d.****	75	n. d.
	San	0	n. d.	68	n. d.
	Sal	0	n. d.	290	n. d.
	Se	0	0	280	440
AML	He	0	0	29	30
	Ka	0	0	59	43
	Ne	0	0	50	54
	Pa	0	0	14	22
	Po	0	0	22	16
	1	30	n. d.	25	n. d.
	2	25	n. d.	30	n. d.
Normal	3	40	1	35	0
	4	44	2	34	0
	5	32	1	22	0

    * See materials and methods.
   ** Agar underlayer without leukocytes.
  *** Figure represents number of colonies per 10^5 cells plated.
**** n. d. = not done.

In Table II, the results of experiments have been listed in which bone marrow cells from untreated AML patients and from haematologically normal individuals were cultured in the Robinson assay, and the PHA + E assay. It can be noted that in the Robinson system, no colonies were present when marrow from untreated AML patients were cultured, which is in contrast to the presence of colonies in the PHA + E assay. Even in those cases in which no leukocytes had been added to the agar underlayer on which the bone marrow cells were plated after the liquid phase in the PHA + E assay, a distinct number of colonies could be grown from AML marrow cells. In the majority of cases, this number was equivalent to or exceeded the number of colonies present in cultures to which leukocytes were added, which clearly demonstrates that colony formation of leukemic marrow in the PHA + E system is independent of the presence of leukocyte feeder layers. This is in contrast with the results obtained with marrow cells from normal individuals which show that colony formation by normals is clearly leukocyte dependent, both in the Robinson system and the PHA + E assay. Moreover, no additional effect of the PHA + E on colony growth by normal marrow has been obtained.

Table III: Comparison between Number of CFU-c in the Robinson Assay and the PHA+E Assay of Marrow from AML in Relapse and from AML in Remission

	Patient Name	Robinson Assay Leukocyte Feeder	Agar**	PHA + E Assay* Leukocyte Feeder	Agar**
	Wo	2***	n. d.****	52	0
AML	Be	0	0	150	130
Relapse	El	0	0	160	103
	Bo	17	n. d.	8	1
	We	36	n. d.	20	0
AML	Ja	24	0	20	0
Remission	Ba	44	0	46	0
	Br	6	0	0	0
	Mo	5	0	0	0

   * See materials and methods.
  ** Agar underlayer without leukocytes.
 *** Figure represents number of colonies per 10^5 cells plated.
**** n. d. = not done.

In Table III, the results of growth of marrow cells from AML relapse and from AML remission have been listed. It can be observed that the behavior of marrow cells from AML relapse in the two in vitro systems was identical to that of marrow cells from untreated AML patients, whereas the in vitro growth characteristics of marrow cells from patients in complete remission resembled that of haematologically normal marrow.

In order to make sure that colony formation was not an artifact due to clumping of cells by phytohaemagglutinin in the liquid phase of the PHA + E assay, the total number of colonies and clusters per plate were counted. It was reasoned that colony formation is unlikely to be caused by clumping in experiments in which the total number of colonies and clusters in the PHA + E assay is equivalent to or exceeds the number of aggregates in the in vitro systems to which PHA + E was not added. In Table IV, results have been documented of cultures in which the total number of aggregates were counted. It is evident from these results that the total number of aggregates in the cultures to which PHA + E were added to the liquid phase was highly increased. Furthermore, close observation at the time of plating in the semi-solid phase, after 15 hours of PHA + E incubation, did not reveal any higher degree of clumping than that observed in the cell suspension used for plating in the Robinson system which did not involve previous PHA incubation.

A summary of the results has been listed in Table V, in which the mean values

Table IV: **Total Number of Aggregates in the Robinson Assay and the PHA+E Assay of Bone Marrow Cells from Untreated AML**

Patient	Robinson Assay Leukocyte Feeder	Agar	Without PHA+E* Leukocyte Feeder	Agar	With PHA+E** Leukocyte Feeder	Agar
Tu	0***/330****	0/0	0/45	0/0	166/590	144/530
Fl	0/827	0/1867	0/840	14/885	80/1800	300/3200
He	0/157	0/3	0/3	0/3	29/220	30/226
Ca	0/20	0/20	0/90	0/140	66/280	60/360
St	0/360	0/0	0/47	0/0	38/460	20/440

    * Incubation of cells in liquid medium without PHS and endotoxin before plating on leukocyte feeders and agar underlayers without leukocytes.
    ** See materials and methods; PHA+E assay.
    *** Figure represents number of colonies per 10^5 plated marrow cells.
    **** Figure represents number of clusters per 10^5 plated marrow cells, the size of the clusters is predominantly smaller than 20 cells.

of the number of colonies per 10^5 plated cells from marrow obtained from AML and haematologixally normal patients has been documented. As has been already mentioned, no increase in number of colonies produced by normal marrow has

Table V: **Mean Number of Marrow Colonies from AML Patients and Haematologically Normal Individuals in the Robinson Assay and the PHA+E Assay**

Bone Marrow***	Robinson Assay Leukocyte Feeder	PHA+E Assay* Leukocyte Feeder	Agar Feeder	Ratio** PHA+E Leukocyte Feeder	Robinson Assay
Haematologically Normal	34****(25-44)****	29 (22-35)	0 (0)		0.85
Remission AML	22 (5-44)	16 (8-46)	0.16 (0-1)		0.72
Untreated AML	0.0 (0-1)	99 (14-290)	113 (22-440)		1187
Relapse AML	0.5 (0-2)	125 (52-160)	95 (0-130)		250

    * See materials and methods.
    ** Ratio between number of CFU-c in the PHA+E assay with leukocyte feeders, and in the Robinson assay.
    *** Normals are listed in Table II. AML patients are listed in Tables I and II.
    **** Mean number of CFU-c per 10^5 marrow cells plated. Figures in parentheses represent the range of colonies obtained.

been observed by adding PHA + E to the system, resulting in a ratio of the number of colonies between the PHA + E assay and the Robinson assay of < 1. The same ratio holds for marrow from AML in remission. These results are in contrast with the results obtained from marrow cultured from AML in relapse and from untreated AML patients. In those cultures, the colony ratio between the two in vitro systems is markedly increased, demonstrating the need for PHA and endotoxin in the liquid phase for colony formation in vitro.

The effect of PHA+E in vitro

Specific experiments were carried out to study the effect of PHA and endotoxin on colony formation by the leukemic cell population when these substances were added separately to the cultures. The results of such an experiment which is representative of three other experiments have been listed in Table VI. It can be noted that leukemic bone marrow cells without being stimulated in a liquid system did not give rise to colonies in an agar system as listed in Table VI, even when

Table VI: Comparison of Effect of PHA and Endotoxin added Separately and in Combination to the Cultures, on Colony Formation of Marrow Cells from a Relapse (AML (E l))

| | Semi-solid Phase | | | | | | | |
| | Agar Underlayer | | | | Agar + Leuk. Underlayer | | | |
	-*	Endo-toxin	PHA**	(PHA+E***)	-*	Endo-toxin	PHA	(PHA+E***)
No Liquid Phase	0	0	0	0	0	0	0	0
Liquid Phase								
_****	0	0	0	0	0	0	0	0
Endotoxin	0	0	0	0	0	0	0	0
PHA	138*****	145	178	248	124	180	145	205
PHA+E***	155	160	171	228	150	170	217	300

    * Agar underlayer without PHA, endotoxin.
    ** PHA = phytohaemagglutinin; 0.05 ml/ml medium.
    *** E = endotoxin: 10^{-7} g/ml medium.
    **** Liquid phase in which 2×10^6 cells have been cultured for 15 hours in medium without PHA, endotoxin.
    ***** Mean number of colonies from triplicate cultures. Colony number per 10^5 plated cells. The colony incidence in the individual plates do not differ more than 15 % of the mean.

PHA + E were added to the semi-solid phase. When cells were incubated in a liquid system, only PHA could induce colony formation. Addition of endotoxin to the liquid phase had no effect on the untreated colonies generated by PHA, whereas endotoxin added to the semi-solid phase had an amplifying effect on colony formation induced by PHA. Therefore, in the PHA + E in vitro assay as described in the materials and methods, PHA is the essential stimulator for the leukemic cell population.

Analysis of cell type in the in vitro colonies

Evidence of colony formation by the leukemic cell population in the marrow from several leukemics in the PHA + E system was obtained by morphology and chromosome analysis. In several cases (3), May-Grünwald staining of several colonies clearly demonstrated the blastic cell population, predominantly present, whereas the more differentiated cells of the myeloid series were scarce. Since we are aware of the limited value of the May-Grünwald staining procedure as a proof for the leukemic origin of a colony, morphological studies of the colonies were

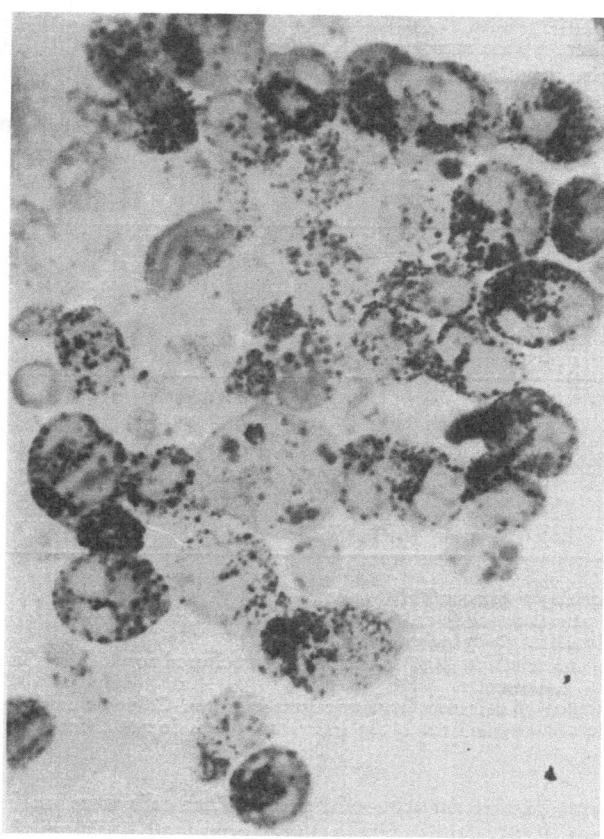

Fig. 2: a. Cross-section of a colony from a seven day marrow culture from patient (El) in AML relapse. Magnification 1700x. The diamino benzidine technique for peroxidase activity clearly shows enzyme activity at the level of granule formation.

performed at the ultrastructural level. Figure 2a is a thick Epon cross-section through a colony grown from an untreated leukemic marrow. The dark granules heavily stained in the cytoplasm of these cells represent the peroxidase positive granules demonstrating the myeloid origin of these cells. Figure 2b represents the typical ultrastructural morphology of one of the colony cells seen in Figure 2a. The cell displays a pocket or bleb on its nuclear surface. This structural abnormality in bone marrow cells has been associated with leukemia and lymphoma by a number of investigators (Achong et al., 1966; Anderson, 1966; Ross et al., 1969). More recently, a correlation between the presence of a high frequency of these nuclear blebs and aneuploidy in acute leukemia has been demonstrated (Ahearn et al, 1974). This particular case (E1) was aneuploid and exhibited a complex chromosome aberration which has been described in several other cases of acute leukemia (45, X, –Y, –C, +D, +E, –G) (Trujillo et al., 1974). This abnormal chromosome pattern could be demonstrated in cells collected from the in vitro colonies of this study and from the liquid cultures incubated with PHA and endotoxin for 15 hours. Twenty-five metaphases were counted of which 19 clearly demonstrated the chromosome abnormality. The remaining six metaphases exhibited a diploid karyotype.

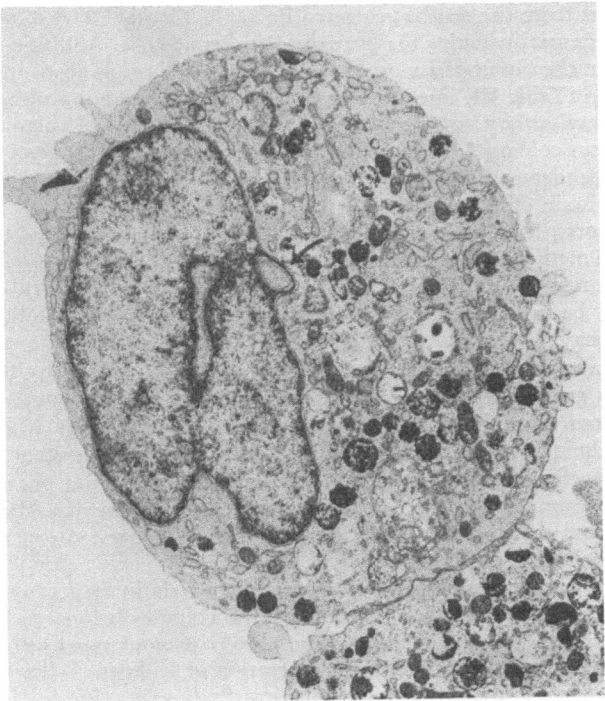

b. Cross-section of a cell from a colony obtained from marrow cultures from patient (E1) suffering from AML relapse. Magnification 300x. The nuclear bleb, indicated by arrow, is clearly visible.

Discussion

It has been clearly demonstrated that leukemic cells can form colonies in vitro in the absence of a feeder layer of leukocytes. This is in contradiction with the data of Moore et al. and Metcalf et al. who observed dependence on CSF* in vitro for leukemic cell proliferation (Moore et al., 1974; Metcalf et al., 1974). An explanation for this discrepancy between our results and the Australian data might be that phytohaemagglutinin stimulates subpopulation(s) of the leukemic cell pool which are different from the leukocyte factor dependent leukemic cells.

In the PHA + E system, aggregates of different sizes are present as can be noted from the results presented in Table IV. This spectrum of aggregate size might be indicative of different sensitivity to the PHA stimulus by the leukemic cell population, reflecting the heterogeneity of the blast cell population. More extensive investigation with respect to the number of clusters (aggregates less than 50 cells) in relation to the number of colonies has to be performed in the future. Just like in the Robinson system, the colony cluster ratio as well as the size of the colonies and the clusters might be of significance for further classification of acute myelogenous leukemia.

It is evident from the results presented in Table VI that PHA in the PHA + E assay is the essential stimulus for growth of leukemic cells. Addition of endotoxin to the PHA in the *liquid*-phase produced no statistically significant increase in colony formation (Table VI, line 4 versus line 5). The combination of endotoxin and PHA in the *semi-solid* phase markedly increased the number of colonies (Table VI, column 3 versus column 4, and column 7 versus column 8). The effect of endotoxin in vivo is dependent on previous incubation of the leukemic cells with PHA. The in vitro endotoxin effect might be an enhancement of leukemic cell sensitivity to PHA. The short period of incubation with PHA in the liquid phase (15 hours, see materials and methods) does not produce cell clumping as was pointed out already in the section results (Table IV). Because of the simplicity, in the future, leukemic cells will only be stimulated by PHA without endotoxin during the liquid phase of the in vitro assay.

PHA was also used as stimulus in an in vitro assay described by Rozenszajn et al. (1974), to grow lymphocyte colonies. As a source of lymphocytes, peripheral leukocytes from normal individuals were used. Although there is similarity between our technique and the assay used by Rozenszajn, in the system employed by the Israeli investigators, PHA was added also to the semi-solid phase, which was obligatory for growing lymphocytes. Moreover, the use of human AB serum in the liquid phase was essential for lymphocyte cultures. In our system, a mixture of horse serum and fetal calf serum was used.

Electronmicroscopic studies and cytogenetic analysis in two cases (El and Fe, Table I), revealed that cells collected from the colonies belong to the leukemic cell population. Nuclear pockets have been clearly demonstrated by Ahearn et al. (1974) to be a consistent ultrastructural alteration of leukemic cell populations associated with aneuploidy. Other morphological findings specific for leukemic cells such as asynchronous nuclear cytoplasmic development, nuclear bodies, and bundles

---

* CSF = colony stimulation factor from leukocytes.

of cytoplasmic fibrils were also found in the cells from the in vitro colonies. These latter findings mark the leukemic cell population in case no abnormal chromosome marker is present in the leukemic cell population. Only a limited number (10) of colonies had been analyzed by electronmicroscopical methods; therefore, these studies do not exclude the possibility that cell types other than leukemic cells proliferate in the PHA + E assay.

Cytogenetic analysis revealed the presence of the aneuploid line in the colonies. The origin of the diploid cells also found in the cultures is still unclear. Possibilities to be considered include the following sources: lymphoid cells, normal immature marrow cells (stem cells?), diploid leukemic elements, etc. This conventional Technique is limited by the fact that only a small number of available metaphases can be recovered. It is possible that the specificity of the PHA stimulation on leukemic cells may be further explored by culturing pure populations of malignant and non-malignant cells using cell separation techniques (Dicke et al., 1973; 1975, in press).

The mode of action of PHA on the leukemic cell population is not known. Colony formation might be a consequence of a humoral factor released by a second cell population stimulated by PHA. Experiments of Aye et al. (1974) support this concept. These investigators observed proliferation of leukemic cells in short term liquid cultures induced by conditioned medium which was prepared from cultures of human peripheral blood cells to which was added PHA. Haematologically normal individuals and patients with acute leukemia were used to prepare these conditioned media. Their data were not conclusive in proving the need of a humoral factor for leukemic cell proliferation due to the fact that residual amounts of PHA were still present in the conditioned medium. Moreover, labelling index and the rate of ^{3}H-TdR incorporation were used as parameters for response of the leukemic cells to the stimulus, which markedly differs from colony formation as measured in our experiments. At the present time, we favor the direct effect of PHA on the leukemic cell population. For the time being, only the linear correlation between the number of leukemic cells plated and the number of colonies per dish as demonstrated in Figure 1 support the above mentioned concept. The value of these results, however, is limited due to the fact that the data were generated from cultures of marrow cells from a single patient. In the future, it will be investigated as to whether this linear relationship is a consistent phenomenon in cultures of marrow from untreated AML and from patient in relapse.

So far, PHA appears to be remarkably specific in stimulating only leukemic cells to form colonies. No effect by PHA was observed on haemopoietic cells in remission. Although the fluctuation of the leukemic sub-populations sensitive to PHA with chemotherapy is not yet understood, it will be of interest to determine whether or not the in vitro phenomenon described in this paper can be used for detection of residual leukemic cells in the remission phase of AML.

References

1. Achong, B. G., and Epstein, M. A. (1966) Fine structure of the Burkitt tumor. Journal of the National Cancer Institute, 36,877.
2. Ahearn, M. J., Trujillo, J. M., Cork, A., Fowler, A. and Hart, J. S. (1974)

The association of nuclear blebs with aneuploidy in human acute leukemia. Cancer Research, 34, 2887.

3. Anderson, D. R. (1966) Ultrastructure of normal and leukemic leukocytes in human peripheral blood. Journal of Ultrastructural Research, 9,24.

4. Aye, M. T., Niho, Y., Till, J. E., and McCulloch, E. A. (1974) Studies of leukemic cell populations in culture. Blood, 44,205.

5. Bull, J. M., Cutteral, J. J., Northrup, J. D., Henderson, E. S., Stashick, E., and Carbone, P. P. (1973) Serial in vitro marrow culture in acute myelocytic leukemia. Blood, 42,679.

6. Chervenick, P. A., and LoBuglio, A. F. (1972) Human blood monocytes. Stimulators of granulocyte and mononuclear colony formation in vitro. Science, 178, 164.

7. Dicke, K. A., van Noord, M. J., Maat, B., Schaefer, U. W. and van Bekkum, D. W. (1973) Identification of cells in primate bone marrow resembling the haemopoietic stem cell in the mouse. Blood, 42,195.

8. Dicke, K. A., Tridente, G., and van Bekkum, D. W. (1969) The selective elimination of immunologically competent cells from bone marrow and lymphocyte cell mixture. III. In vitro test for detection of immunocompetent cells in fractionated mouse spleen cell suspensions and primate bone marrow suspensions. Transplantation, 8,422.

9. Dicke, K. A., van Noord, M. J., Maat, B., Schaefer, U. W. and van Bekkum, D. W. (1973) Attempts at morphological identification of haemopoietic stem cells in primates and rodents. In: Haemopoietic stem cells; CIBA Foundation Symposium. No. 13 (New Series). Amsterdam, Elsevier. Page 47.

10. Golde, D. W. and Cline, M. J. Personal Communication.

11. Greenberg, P. L., Nichols, W. C., and Schrier, S. L. (1971) Granulopoiesis in acute myeloid leukemia in pre-leukemia. New England Journal of Medicine, 284,1225.

12. Gutterman, J. U., Hersh, E. M., Rodriguez, V., McCredie, K. B., Mavligit, G., Reed, R., Burgess, M. A., Gehan, E., Bodey, G. P. and Freireich, E. J. (1974) Chemoimmunotherapy of acute leukemia: prolongation of remission in myeloblastic leukemia with bacillus calmette, Guerin. The Lancet, II, 1405.

13. Hayhoe, G. F. J., Qualino, D., and Doll, R. (1964) The cytology and cytochemistry of acute leukemias. A study of 140 cases. M. R. C. Special Report Series, No. 304, London. Her Majesty's Stationery Office.

14. Iscove, N. N., and Sieber, F. (1975) Erythroid progenitors in mouse bone marrow detected by macroscopic colony formation in culture. Experimental Hematology, 3,32.

15. McCredie, K. B., Hester, J. P., Gutterman, J. U., Gehan, E. A. and Freireich, E. J. (1975) Survival of adults with acute leukemia CI. Proceedings of the AACR, 16,141.

16. Metcalf, D., Moore, M. A. S., Sheridan, J. W., and Spitzer, G. (1974) Responsiveness of human granulocytic leukemic cells to colony stimulating factor. Blood, 43, 847.

17. Metcalf, D. and Moore, M. A. S. (1971) Haemopoietic cells. North Holland Publishing Company. Amsterdam, Holland.

18. Moore, M. A. S., Williams, N., and Metcalf, D. (1973) In vitro colony

formation by normal and leukemic human chemotopoietic cells; interaction between colony forming and colony stimulating cells. Journal of National Cancer Institute, 50,602.

19. Moore, M. A. S., Spitzer, G., Williams, N., and Metcalf, D. (1973) Correlation of agar culture analysis and clinical status in patients with acute myeloid leukemia, haemopoiesis in culture. Second International Workshop. Airlie House, Virginia, page 303.

20. Moore, M. A. S., Spitzer, G., Williams, N., Metcalf, D. and Buckley, J. (1974) Agar culture studies in 127 cases of untreated acute leukemia; the prognostic value of reclassification of leukemia according to in vitro growth characteristics. Blood, 44,1.

21. Pike, B. L. and Robinson, W. A. (1970) Human bone marrow colony growth in agar-gel. Journal of Cellular Physiology, 76,77.

22. Robinson, W. A., Kurnick, J. E., and Pike, B. L. (1971) Colony growth of human leukemic peripheral blood cells in vitro. Blood, 38,500.

23. Robinson, W. A. and Pike, B. L. (1970) Colony growth of human bone marrow in vitro. Symposium on Haematopoietic cellular proliferation. St. Elizabeth's Hospital, Boston. Editor: Frederick Stohlman, Jr. Grune & Stratton, New York.

24. Ross, A., and Harndern, D. (1969) Ultrastructural studies on normal and leukemic human haematopoietic cells. European Journal of Cancer, 5,349.

25. Rozenszajn, L. A., Kalechman, I. and Shohum, D. (1974) Colony proliferation of human stimulated lymphocyte on agar culture; XV. Congress of the International Society of Hematology, page 230.

26. Trujillo, J. M., Cork, A., Hart, J. S., George, S. L. and Freireich, E. J. (1974) Clinical implications of aneuploid cytogenetic profiles in adult acute leukemia. Cancer, 33,824.

27. Van Bekkum, D. W., van Oosterom, P., Dicke, K. A. (In Press) In vitro colony formation of transplantable rat leukemias in comparison with human myeloid leukemia.

Acknowledgements

The criticisms of Dr. Trujillo (M. D. Anderson Hospital and Tumor Institute) is greatly appreciated. Our thanks are also due to Dr. E. Gehan and T. Smith for helping us with the statistical evaluations of the data in this paper. We also acknowledge the excellent technical assistance of Miss M. Lomedico, and of Mr. R. McBee, who prepared the EM pictures.

Clinical Utility of Bone Marrow Culture

Malcolm A. S. Moore
Sloan-Kettering Institute for Cancer Research
New York, USA

Abstract

Standardized culture of bone marrow in soft agar permits the detection of a population of granulocyte-macrophage progenitor cells (CFU-c). A spectrum of qualitative abnormalities serves to distinguish myeloid leukemic CFU-c from normal and remission populations. These abnormalities in maturation and proliferation are diagnostic of a myeloid leukemic state and serve to functionally reclassify acute myeloid leukemia at diagnosis into a number of categories based on in vitro growth pattern. The virtue of this classification is that it permits detection of a substantial number of patients who are refractory to conventional remission induction protocols. The clear distinction between normal and leukemic growth in vitro permits early detection of emerging remission CFU-c during induction therapy and of early onset of relapse in patients who are otherwise in complete remission. In patients with leukemia undergoing allogeneic bone marrow engraftment, marrow culture has proved of value in documenting the reconstitution of the patient and in detecting re-emergence of the original leukemic stem line prior to its detection by cytogenetic and hematological techniques.

Serial studies on patients with chronic myeloid leukemia have allowed early diagnosis of blastic transformation and classification of blastic phase disease on the basis of in vitro growth pattern has revealed a similar spectrum of in vitro abnormalities as seen in AML.

The cloning of normal or leukemic human myeloid progenitor cells (CFU-c) in agar or methylcellulose has permitted analysis of both quantitative and qualitative changes in this cell compartment in leukemia and other myelodysplastic states (1–7). Among these changes are abnormalities in maturation of leukemic cells in vitro (4, 5, 6), defective proliferation as measured by colony size or cluster to colony ratio (5, 6), abnormalities in biophysical characteristics of leukemic CFU-c (4, 5), regulatory defects in responsiveness to positive and negative feedback control mechanisms (8, 9) and the existence of cytogenetic abnormalities in vitro (10,

This research was supported in part by NCI grants CA-08748, CA-17353, CA-17085 and the Gar Reichman Foundation

79

11). Detection of this spectrum of abnormalities has proved of clinical utility in diagnosis of leukemia and preleukemic states (5, 6, 12), in classification of leukemias and myeloproliferative diseases (5, 6), in predicting remission prognosis and response to therapy (5, 13), in predicting onset of remission or relapse in AML (13) and in monitoring the progression of chronic myeloid leukemia or preleukemic disease (4, 14). The present communication serves to illustrate the clinical applications of bone marrow culture in these various areas.

In vitro growth characteristics of untreated Acute Myeloid Leukemia (AML) and its morphological variants

Marrow and, in the majority of cases, peripheral blood cultures, were established from 250 cases of untreated AML and its morphological variants (acute monocytic, myelomonocytic, promyelocytic, stem cell and erythroleukemia). One hundred seventy-four cases represented a random selection of patients presenting at 8 hospitals in Melbourne, Australia, over a period of 3 years and 76 cases presenting at the Memorial Sloan-Kettering Cancer Center over a period of 12

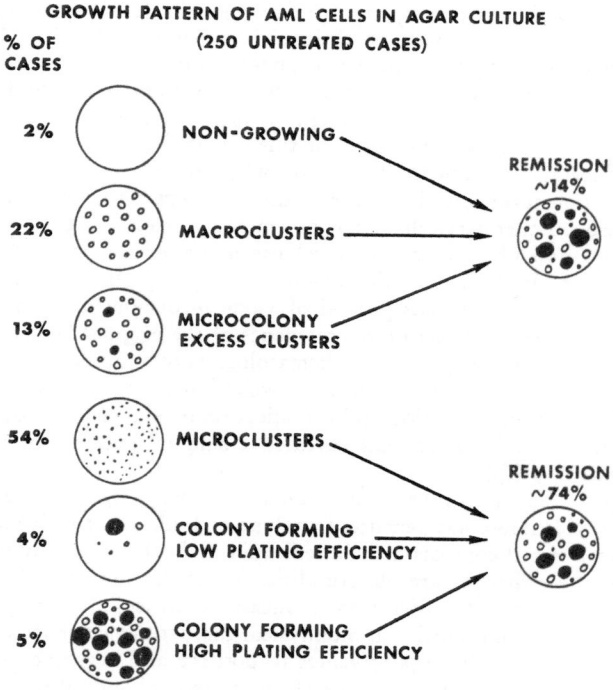

Fig. 1: Schematic representation of the in vitro growth patterns seen in 7 day cultures of marrow cells from 250 patients with untreated AML and its morphological variants. Remission incidence in the non-growing, macrocluster and microcolony category was 14 % and in the remaining categories, 74 %.

months. The clinical and hematological characteristics of these patients have been reported as have the therapeutic protocols and remission criteria (5, 13). All cultures were stimulated by a feeder layer of 1×10^6 normal WBC and were scored at 7 days for the presence of colonies of > 40 cells and clusters of 3–40 cells. For classification of leukemia according to growth in vitro we recognize the following categories of growth pattern (see Fig. 1): (a) non-growing: absence of persisting cells in CSF stimulated cultures with no colony or cluster formation detected in 4 cultures of 2×10^5 marrow cells per plate; (b) microcluster formation: absence of colonies and presence of varying numbers of clusters of 3–20 cells. The great majority of these cases exhibit a pattern of small clusters in marrow culture generally of only 3–10 cells with dispersion and degeneration. Included in this category are examples of extensive persistence of leukemic cells in CSF stimulated cultures without evidence of cluster formation at 7 days. Marrow cultures from these latter patients, when scored prior to 7 days, show cluster formation but with premature dispersion and degeneration of the clusters. The majority of microcluster forming leukemias would be considered as non-growing if scored later than 7 days; (c) macrocluster formation: absence of colonies and presence of varying numbers of clusters approaching the lower limit of colony size, i. e., up to 40 cells. If the cultures are scored later than 7 days, the majority of cases would show evidence of colony formation and merge with category (d); (d) small colonies (microcolonies) with an abnormal cluster to colony ratio: maximum colony size in this group is less than in control cultures and an abnormal excess of aggregates of less than 40 cells is seen (the normal ratio of colonies to clusters is between 2–10); (e) colony forming with a normal cluster to colony ratio at 7 days of culture: we have subdivided this category into cases showing a lower colony incidence than normal and cases with a marked elevation in marrow colony formation invariably associated with a pronounced increase in circulating CFU-c. Both groups share a similar prognosis, however, the former category is mainly comprised of cases where colony growth is non-leukemic, and thus is similar to the pattern seen in acute lymphoblastic leukemia, whereas the latter category merges with the growth patterns seen in chronic myeloid leukemia.

Classification of these patients on the basis of our previously reported correlation between growth pattern and remission rate (5, 6) indicated that 37 % of all these cases fell within a poor prognosis category (Fig. 1). The addition of 76 new cases of AML and their clinical outcome has not significantly altered the correlation we have observed between in vitro growth pattern and remission rate.

Ten patients included in this study had acute undifferentiated or "stem cell" leukemia and classification into myeloblastic or lymphoblastic type was not possible on the basis of morphology, cytochemistry or surface markers. Three of these cases showed a myeloid cluster forming growth pattern in marrow culture, whereas the remainder showed a colony forming pattern with low plating efficiency and normal granulocytic maturation. The indication that colony formation seen in these cases was due to persisting normal CFU-c coexisting with a non-myeloid acute leukemia was supported by cell separation studies. Buoyant density distribution of colony or cluster forming cells was determined by the application of a simplified density "cut" technique in which marrow or blood cells were centrifuged in bovine serum albumin of density 1.062 g/cm^3 and the distribution of CFU-c in the supernatant and pellet fractions determined by subsequent agar culture (4, 5). 56 ± 4 % of cluster forming cells in untreated patients were of density < 1.062 g/cm³ in contrast to the normal distribution of CFU-c (1–10 % < 1.062 g/cm³). This light density distribution of CFU-c was also observed in the microcolony and high cloning efficiency colony forming acute leukemias (96 ± 5 % < 1.062 g/cm³). In contrast, the CFU-c in patients with low cloning efficiency colony forming acute leukemia had a normal density distribution (1.5 ± 1 % < 1.062 g/cm³), as did the CFU-c in untreated acute lymphoblastic leukemia.

Monitoring of relapse-remission status by marrow culture

Unequivocal complete remission was associated with return of a normal growth pattern in marrow culture (Fig. 1), a normal colony incidence and granulocytic maturation and a normal CFU-c buoyant density distribution. The correlation between return of normal colony formation and remission was investigated in a detailed analysis of 57 patients throughout the induction and consolidation phase of therapy (Table 1). patients were selected on the basis of marrow growth characteristics prior to therapy and only examples of non-colony forming AML were studied since appearance of colony formation during remission induction would provide a simple parameter for detection of non-leukemic progenitor cells. Of the 30 patients who showed return of colony formation at some point during induction, 29 achieved complete remission, on average 21 days after first detection of colonies. No examples were observed of a leukemic growth pattern persisting in clinical remission. There was no correlation between the actual number of colonies observed and the time to remission, however, preliminary analysis indicates some correlation between initial colony incidence and duration of remission.

The value of marrow culture in predicting the onset of relapse was investigated in 83 cases of cluster-forming AML where complete remission had been achieved. In this analysis, four patterns of relapse emerged.

Table I: Analysis of Colony Formation During Remission Induction in 57 Patients with Cluster Forming AML

Number of Patients Showing Colony Formation	30/57
Number of Patients Attaining Remission	29/57
Marrow Colony Incidence at Time of First Detection of Colonies (Mean + Range)	27 (1–172)/10⁵
Density Distribution of Colony Forming Cells (% < 1.062 g/cm³)	8.5 ± 0.5
Time to Appearance of Normal Colonies (Days Mean + Range)	41 (5–85)
Time to Complete Clinical Remission (Days Mean + Range)	62 (20–105)

(a) Most frequently observed was a concordance of a clinical diagnosis of relapse with a complete return to a cluster forming leukemic growth pattern.

(b) Loss of colony formation and return to a cluster-forming growth pattern 1–4 weeks prior to clinical and hematological evidence of relapse.

(c) Coexistence of normal and leukemic colony and cluster forming cells for varying periods preceding overt relapse. Discrimination between normal and leukemic cells was possible on the basis of colony size, cell morphology and the dispersion or degeneration of the leukemic clusters. Density gradient separation and cytogenetic analysis of individual colonies and clusters have further confirmed the coexistence of normal and leukemic CFU-c in marrow cultures prior to clinical evidence of relapse.

(d) The fourth category comprised patients who showed evidence of early relapse based on hematological criteria including elevated marrow blast cell incidence (without detectable Auer rods), presence of immature cells in the circulation and, in the case of patients presenting with acute monocytic or myelomonocytic leukemia, abnormal monocytoid cells in marrow and blood with qualitatively normal colony and cluster formation. In this category there exists a clear discrepancy between the interpretation of marrow morphology and the in vitro culture parameters which showed no evidence of leukemic cell proliferation. This paradox was largely resolved by sequential analysis of CFU-c in the marrow of patients in prolonged remission. A striking variation in the incidence of marrow CFU-c was observed in a number of patients which could neither be attributed to technical variation nor in any direct sense, to the maintainance protocol.

Correlated with the periodicity of marrow CFU-c in many patients was a fluctuation in marrow blast cell incidence. A marked increase in CFU-c was frequently associated with or closely followed by an increase in marrow blast count to levels compatible with early relapse. The majority of such cases were treated with intensive reinduction; however, a number were continued on maintainance therapy and, in these cases, both blast cell and CFU-c incidence returned to normal levels in subsequent marrow aspirates and the patients remained in complete remission.

The detection of incipient relapse in patients who presented with leukemia characterized by the formation of microcolonies with an excess of clusters was aided by monitoring the cluster to colony ratio together with morphological analysis of colonies and buoyant density characterization of CFU-c. In the case of colony forming leukemias with a normal cluster to colony ratio, colony morphology and, specifically, CFU-c buoyant density were the main diagnostic parameters capable of distinguishing between relapse and remission status.

Marrow culture parameters in preleukemic disorders

The situation in preleukemic disorders is not unlike that observed in AML remission patients during the time immediately preceding the onset of relapse. We have observed that in such preleukemic states as refractory sideroblastic anemia associated with a variable spectrum of cytopenias or with chronic monocytosis, that a spectrum of qualitative defects can be detected in a proportion of cases. These defects are identical to those seen in overt myeloid leukemia and precede progression to leukemia by 3–18 months. A number of such cases show coexistence of normal and leukemic cell proliferation preceding overt relapse. Clinically identical cases exhibiting no qualitative defects but generally with a depressed incidence of CFU-c in marrow culture did not progress to an acute leukemic phase without first developing qualitative defects in CFU-c maturation or proliferation.

The heterogeneity of AML in relapse is reflected in the spectrum of defects observed in progression from preleukemia to overt leukemia. Prediction of clinical progression of preleukemic disorders must therefore be based on recognition of clonal evolution with progressive derangement in CFU-c proliferation and/or differentiation similar to that observed in the progression from chronic to acute phase in CML (6). Alternatively, the demonstration by cell separation and/or marrow culture of coexisting normal and leukemic populations in "preleukemia" is similar to the situation seen in many cases of early relapse of AML and should be considered not as preleukemia but as early leukemia since the minor leukemic clone progressively expands but retains its characteristic spectrum of qualitative abnormalities.

In vitro characteristics of chronic myeloid leukemia at diagnosis and in blastic transformation

One hundred-three patients with Ph^1 positive CML were studied at various stages of their clinical course; of these 66 were investigated at the time of first diagnosis. With the exception of 8 patients, a characteristic pattern of presentation was seen. The incidence of colony and cluster forming cells in marrow was increased on average 15X normal and circulating CFU-c on average 500X normal. The ratio of clusters to colonies, an important diagnostic parameter when predicting blastic transformation, was consistently within the lower range of normal. CFU-c in CML at all stages of the disease were of an abnormally light buoyant density as determined by continuous density gradient or equilibrium density centrifugation in bovine serum albumin. The abnormal density distribution of CFU-c appears to be a characteristic of the myeloid leukemic state and is only seen in normal hematopoiesis during fetal life (15), suggesting the possibility of an oncofetal transformation associated with leukemogenesis (14).

Analysis of the in vitro characteristics of marrow and blood of 42 patients at the time of clinical diagnosis of blastic transformation revealed in every case defects in proliferation and maturation which served to distinguish this phase from chronic phase disease. A spectrum of different patterns of in vitro growth was seen and the same six categories of proliferative abnormalities were identified as seen in untreated AML (Table 2). Only one patient showed complete absence of colony and cluster formation in marrow and blood culture and the most common pattern was that of macrocluster or microcolony formation with an excess of clusters. These variants accounted for 50 % of the cases studied. The macrocluster variant tended to present with a higher WBC count, higher blast incidence, lower platelet count and after a shorter duration of chronic disease than did the microcolony variant. Both categories showed minimal response to therapy, no remissions were observed and survival in blastic phase was brief. The next most common

Table II: Characteristics of Untreated CML and Blastic Transformation

	No. of Cases	Age (Years)	% Blasts in BM	Marrow/10^5 Colonies	Clusters	Duration of CML (Months)	Blast Phase Survival (Weeks)	Remission Rate
Untreated chronic	58	47	< 5	404	1506	–	–	–
Untreated blastic trans.								
Macrocluster	9	54	50	0	2417	20	7	0/9
Microcolony	12	51	36	22	1043	41	6	0/12
Microcluster	6	39	52	0	136	14	35	3/6
Colony Forming-Blast ProM.	8	52	8	345	1967	13	33	1/8
Colony Forming-Low Plating	6	49	49	4	17	22	27	3/6

variants were cases showing a microcluster growth pattern (14 %) and a colony forming growth pattern with a high plating efficiency and maturation arrest at the blast-promyelocyte stage. Both these categories are associated with a high remission rate in AML. The colony forming cases had higher platelet counts and considerably lower blast counts in marrow and blood than did any other category and generally followed a more subacute course reflected in their longer survival in blasts crisis. The microcluster category of patients were, on average, younger than the other groups and had the longest average survival after diagnosis of blast crisis due to the fact that 50 % achieved complete remission which in two cases was prolonged. The relatively short mean duration of chronic phase disease in the microcluster group may be attributed to the fact that 2/6 cases presented at first diagnosis in blastic crisis with no antecedent history of chronic phase disease. A final category, comprising 14 % of cases was characterized by a low WBC count, high blast count in marrow and blood and a very low incidence of colonies and clusters with normal colony maturation and cluster to colony ratio. As we have previously reported, the blast cells in these patients possessed no discernible myeloblastic features as determined by marrow culture, did not respond to or produce colony stimulating factor and had the buoyant density characteristics of leukemic lymphoblasts rather than myeloblasts (6). A similar growth pattern is seen in acute lymphoblastic leukemia (4) and in the majority of acute undifferentiated leukemias (6). In these latter leukemic states, granulocytic colony formation reflects the persistence of low numbers of normal CFU-c coexisting with a non-myeloid leukemic blast cell population which cannot totally suppress normal granulopoiesis. It appears probable that a similar situation exists in this variant of blastic transformation and that the low incidence of colonies reflect residual chronic phase CFU-c coexisting with an acute leukemic blast population which is either non-myeloid or so undifferentiated that it lacks the capacity to proliferate in response to a regulatory macromolecule (CSF) and is defective in its capacity to specifically suppress chronic phase myelopoiesis. Recognition of this variant of blastic CML may be of particular importance, since we have observed a 50 % remission rate using protocols including vincristine and prednisone.

Of 103 patients who were Ph[1] positive, 8 presented at first diagnosis with abnormalities of in vitro CFU-c proliferation and differentiation characteristic of blastic phase disease. Of these, three were unequivocally in blastic phase at presentation by clinical and hematological criteria. Of the remaining five cases, two died within a week of diagnosis and three progressed to overt blastic transformation within 8–16 weeks.

The number of CML patients who have been sequentially studied using the CFU-c assay is relatively small; however, certain generalizations may be made concerning early detection of acute leukemic clones.

(a) Progressive increase in the cluster to colony ratio in marrow and/or blood cultures may precede by weeks or months clinical or hematological evidence of blastic transformation. During this period, chronic phase CFU-c coexist with emerging acute clones characterized by a microcluster, macrocluster or microcolony growth pattern. The rate of progression may be determined by the relative proportions of the coexisting clones as determined by a changing ratio of clusters to colonies or physical separation and quantitation of CFU-c subpopulations (6, 14). This progression is frequently, but not invariably, associated with cytogenetic evidence of aneuploidy involving additional Ph[1] chromosomes and/or additions or deletions of C, F and G group chromosomes (14).

(b) Progressive increase in the incidence of colony and cluster forming cells in the circulation with a normal cluster to colony ratio and in vitro maturation arrest at the blast-promyelocyte level preceeds a terminal colony forming blast crisis.

(c) A declining incidence of colony and cluster forming cells in marrow and blood with a normocellular to hypercellular marrow and normal to elevated WBC count with an increasing blast cell incidence preceeds clinical evidence of a terminal blast crisis associated with the development of a non-myeloid or undifferentiated acute leukemia. A subnormal incidence of marrow CFU-c with a normal cluster to colony ratio and normal maturation may also be seen in CML patients with myelofibrosis, however, in such cases, circulating CFU-c are increased in number.

Marrow culture studies in allogeneic bone marrow transplantation

The ability of the CFU-c assay to monitor a population of stem cells closely related to the multipotential stem cell compartment, together with its capacity to discriminate between normal and leukemic cell populations, has proved of value in allogeneic marrow transplantation of patients with acute leukemia. The selection of potential transplant recipients is assisted by detection, at first diagnosis, of patients exhibiting a poor prognosis pattern of leukemic CFU-c proliferation. The efficiency of pre-transplant cytoreduction remains a considerable problem in marrow transplantation in leukemia, possibly due to the marked heterogeneity of the disease. We have observed persisting leukemic cell proliferation in AML patients at the time of marrow transplantation and also total absence of detectable leukemic cell proliferation in patients who subsequently relapsed with their original leukemia (16). The regeneration of donor CFU-c following marrow engraftment showed considerable variation, ranging from rapid reconstitution with an overshoot and return to normal incidence, to delayed or absent marrow CFU-c repopulation despite cytogenetic evidence of marrow reconstitution. The number of transplant patient analysed by in vitro culture parameters is, as yet, too small to assign any prognostic significance to the rapidity of regeneration of CFU-c, but from a theoretical standpoint, monitoring reconstitution at the level of a stem cell compartment should provide a more significant parameter than either peripheral WBC counts or analysis of marrow cytogenetic status based on mitosis in predominantly differentiating hematopoietic cells.

The clinical utility of bone marrow culture is illustrated in the case history of marrow transplantation in a patient with acute erythroleukemia (Fig. 2). Seven months prior to transplantation the patient's marrow showed 90 % blast cells and a diagnosis of acute erythroleukemia was made. Despite six courses of cytosine arabinoside and daunomycin, only a transient partial remission was observed. Bone marrow culture 14 days and 10 days prior to transplantation showed a poor prognosis acute leukemic growth pattern of the microcolony type with an excess of poorly differentiated clusters of 3–40 cells and small colonies of 40–60 cells.

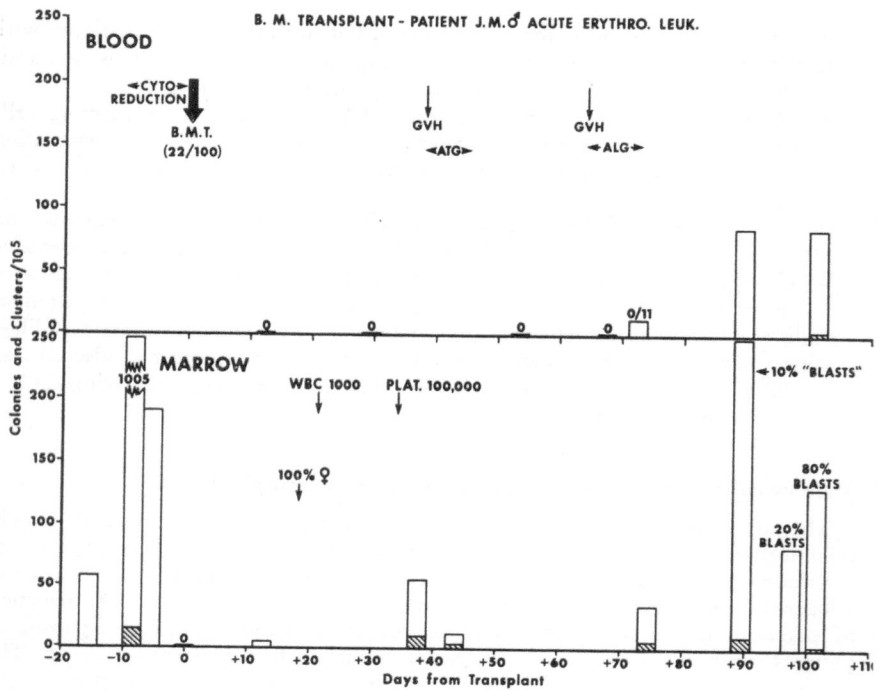

Fig. 2: In vitro culture parameters in the marrow and blood of a patient with acute erythroleukemia before and after a female sibling bone marrow transplant. Note the abnormal ratio of colonies to clusters in the pre-transplant marrow cultures and the return of this leukemic growth pattern in both marrow and blood 70–100 days post-transplantation. Methotrexate was administered at 3, 6, 11 and 18 days post-transplantation and at weekly intervals thereafter.
ATG – Horse anti-human thymocyte globulin
ALG – Goat anti-human lymphoblast gamma globulin

The clusters and small colonies could be further distinguished from normal by their compact nature rather than the dispersed morphology of normal colonies. Following cytoreduction and immunosuppression with daunomycin, cytosine arabinoside, cyclophosphamide and total body irradiation (1,000 rads), the patient received an ABO, HLA and MLC matched female sibling marrow transplant. The donor marrow contained 22 CFU-c per 10^5, indicating minimal dilution with peripheral blood. Engraftment was confirmed by cytogenetic analysis of the marrow on day 18, when 100 % female donor metaphases were observed. Although normal donor colony formation may be detected within 10–12 days following transplantation, this patient showed delayed recovery of marrow colonies which were not seen until 38 days post-transplantation. At no stage of the clinical course did the marrow CFU-c incidence approach or exceed normal levels. A diagnosis of minimal GVH disease in skin, liver and GI tract was made 38 days post-grafting and was reversed with 7 doses of horse anti-human thymocyte globulin (HAHTg). Seventy-two days post-transplantation, peripheral blood cultures which previously had shown no detectable colony and cluster formation, showed a sharp increase in cluster incidence with no detectable colony formation. Bone marrow culture 3 days later showed a mixed population of normal colonies with leukemic clusters and colonies identifiable by their compact nature. At this stage no hematological or cytogenetic evidence of recurrence of leukemia was found. Eighty-nine days post-transplantation both marrow and peripheral blood cultures showed leukemic cell proliferation with a growth pattern and colony formation characteristic of the leukemic clone observed prior to transplantation. No evidence of persisting donor CFU-c was obtained. At this stage the marrow morphology revealed 10 % abnormal proerythroblasts and monocytoid cells; however, an unequivocal-diagnosis of early leukemic relapse was not possible on hematological or clinical grounds. Cytogenetic studies at this time revealed 24/24 normal female donor metaphases. Eight days later, marrow aspiration revealed 20 % blast cells with a persisting leukemic growth pattern and cytogenetic studies showed at least 3 different populations of cells: (1) 24/50 normal female metaphases, (2) 12/50 translocated male metaphases that resembled the original stem line defect and (3) abnormal male cells containing multiple hyperdiploid alterations. The patient expired on day 101 post-transplantation in full hematological relapse with a high circulating blast count and leukemic infiltrations in multiple organs.

It is apparent from studies of this and other patients that marrow culture can detect leukemic relapse following marrow transplantation considerably earlier than conventional diagnostic criteria and at a time when marrow cytogenetic analysis showed no evidence of emerging host leukemic stem lines. More extensive analysis of bone marrow transplantation in patients with AML, aplastic anemia and myeloproliferative disorders will be necessary before the ultimate value of monitoring in vitro culture parameters can be determined, but the preliminary observations suggest that such a venture will not be unrewarding.

References

1. Robinson, W. A., Kurnick, J. E. and Pike, B. L. Blood 38: 500, 1971.
2. Greenberg, P. L., Nichols, W. C. and Schrier, S. L. New Engl. J. Med. 184: 225, 1971.
3. Iscove, N. N., Senn, J. S., Till, J. E. and McCulloch, E. A. Blood 37: 1, 1971.
4. Moore, M. A. S., Williams, N. and Metcalf, D. J. Natl. Cancer Inst. 50: 603, 1973.
5. Moore, M. A. S., Spitzer, G., Williams, N., Metcalf, D. and Buckley, J. Blood 44: 1, 1974.
6. Moore, M. A. S. Blood Cells 1: 149, 1976.
7. Curtis, J. E., Cowan, D. H., Bergsagel, D. E., Hasselback, R. and McCulloch, E. A. CMA Journal 113: 287, 1975.
8. Metcalf, D., Moore, M. A. S., Sheridan, J. W. and Spitzer, G. Blood 43: 47, 1974.
9. Broxmeyer, H. E., Baker, F. and Galbraith, P. G. Blood 47: 389, 1976.
10. Moore, M. A. S. and Metcalf, D. Intl. J. Cancer 11: 143, 1973.

11. Duttera, M. J., Whang-Peng, J., Bull, J. M. C. and Carbone, P. P. Lancet 1: 715, 1972.
12. Moore, M. A. S. and Spitzer, G. In vitro studies in the myeloproliferative disorders. In Lindahl-Kiessling, K., Osoba, D. ed. "Lymphocyte Recognition and Effector Mechanisms" Proc. 8th Leucocyte Culture Conference, Academic Press Inc. 1973 p431.
13. Moore, M. A. S. Blood Cells (In Press) 1976.
14. Moore, M. A. S. Seminars in Hematology (In Press) 1976.
15. Moore, M. A. S. and Williams, N. Cell Tissue Kinet. 6: 461, 1973.
16. Moore, M. A. S., Hansen, J. A., Everson, L. K., O'Reilly, R. and Good, R. A. Trans. Proc. (in Press) 1976.

Proliferative Behavior of Hemopoietic Cells in Preleukemia and Overt Leukemia Observed in One Patient[*]

P. Dörmer

Institute of Hematology of the Gesellschaft für Strahlen- und Umweltforschung, München

Summary

Hemopoietic cell proliferation was studied in a patient suffering from preleukemia characterized by peripheral pancytopenia and hypercellular bone marrow with ineffective erythropoiesis. Two years later when overt acute myelogenous leukemia had developed the study was repeated. The kinetics of proliferation were investigated by a new method which allows evaluation of the rate and time of DNA synthesis in individual morphologically defined cells.

Erythropoiesis was found ineffective to the same degree in both stages of disease. The rate of erythroid cell proliferation, however, was reduced in overt leukemia only. The myeloid system showed a grossly reduced production rate of myeloblasts in preleukemia whilst the same parameter was strongly increased in leukemia. This high production rate of myeloblasts in overt leukemia was interpreted as indication of a far-reaching self-maintenance of the myeloblast pool in this stage of disease. The proliferative activity of the individual myeloblasts was reduced already in preleukemia, and even more so in leukemia. In order to explain the amplification of the myeloblast pool with the onset of overt leukemia a change in the mode of myeloblast divisions is assumed. For this a transition from steady state to some degree of exponential growth gives the most plausible explanation.

A 71 year-old female suffered from severe peripheral pancytopenia with an anemia of 7.9 gm % of hemoglobin, leukopenia of $1,240/mm^3$ and thrombocytopenia of $24,000/mm^3$. The anemia was classified as refractory anemia. The bone marrow was hypercellular with a G:E ratio of 1:2. 69 % of the erythroblasts were ringed sideroblasts according to the Prussian blue reaction. By ferrokinetic examination a highly ineffective erythropoiesis was found with a P.I.T of 3.55 mg Fe/100ml/day whilst the red blood cell lifespan turned out to be normal.

After unsuccessful therapy with vitamins B_6, B_{12} and folic acid the patient received merely occasional transfusions of packed red blood cells. She remained under out-patient control and did not show significant changes for the next 20 months. Then a gradual rise in the white blood cell count with an increasing number of myeloblasts in the blood smear was observed. 2 years after the first examination overt acute myelogenous leukemia (AML) had developed. Retrospectively the phase of pancytopenia was classified as preleukemia.

[*] Study performed under the association contract for hematology between EURATOM and GSF no. 089 721 BIAD. Supported by the Deutsche Forschungsgemeinschaft: SFB 51/ E-3.

In the preleukemic state and at the stage of untreated AML sternal bone marrow was aspirated for the study of cellular proliferation. The suspended cells were incubated in a short-term incubation schedule with ^{14}C-thymidine (^{14}C-TdR) and 5-fluorodeoxyuridine (FUdR). By means of quantitative ^{14}C-autoradiography the duration of DNA synthesis (t_s) was evaluated in individual cells. The method as well as the pertinent principles of cell proliferation kinetics have been discussed in detail elsewhere (2). By Feulgen microphotometry euploid DNA values were obtained for the leukemic myeloblasts.

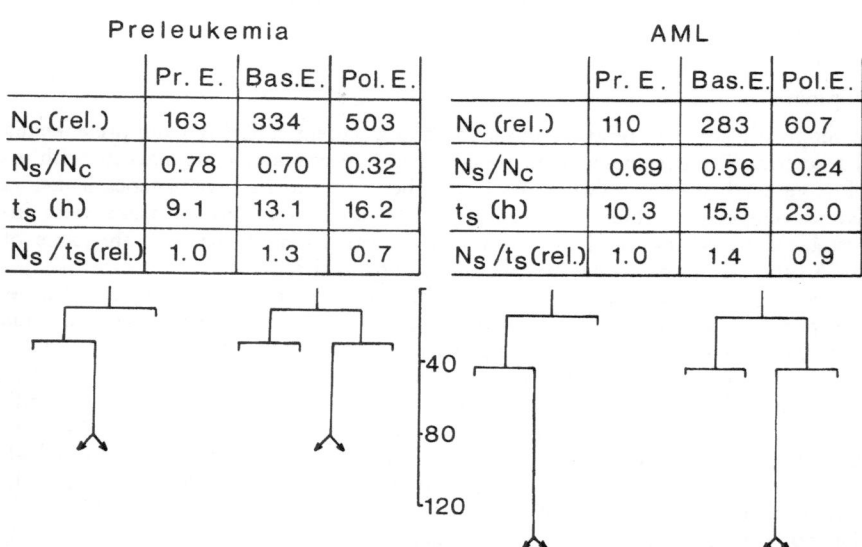

Preleukemia

	Pr. E.	Bas.E.	Pol. E.
N_C (rel.)	163	334	503
N_S/N_C	0.78	0.70	0.32
t_S (h)	9.1	13.1	16.2
N_S/t_S (rel.)	1.0	1.3	0.7

AML

	Pr. E.	Bas.E.	Pol. E.
N_C (rel.)	110	283	607
N_S/N_C	0.69	0.56	0.24
t_S (h)	10.3	15.5	23.0
N_S/t_S (rel.)	1.0	1.4	0.9

Fig. 1: Parameters of cell kinetics and schemes of divisions of erythroid cells in preleukemia (left side) and AML (right side). Between the schemes of divisions a time scale in hours is inserted. Abbreviations: Pr. E. = proerythroblasts; Bas. E. = basophilic erythroblasts; Pol. E. = polychromatic erythroblasts; N_c = relative number of cells in a compartment; N_s/N_c = ^{3}H-TdR labeling index; t_s = DNA synthesis time; N_s/t_s = relative rate of cell production in a compartment.

Fig. 1 contains a compilation of the parameters of erythroid cell proliferation in preleukemia and AML. In preleukemia normal labeling indices (N_s/N_c) as well as normal values of t_s were found for the different morphological cell compartments. These data correspond to the values obtained in a collective of healthy individuals (2). However, the relative production rates (N_s/t_s) show considerable deviation from the normal ratio of 1:2:5 for proerythroblasts:basophilic:polychromatic erythroblasts. The reduction in relative production of more mature erythroblasts most likely is an expression of intramedullary cell death. On the left side of Fig. 1 a scheme of divisions derived from the ratio of production rates illustrates the birth of 3 basophilic erythroblasts from 2 proerythroblasts, and of 2 polychromatic from the 3 basophilic erythroblasts.

92

The scheme of erythropoietic cell division has not changed much in AML (Fig. 1, right side) as is obvious from the ratio of production rates of 1:1.4:0.9. The rate of cell proliferation, however, is reduced as far as conclusions can be drawn using N_s/N_c and t_s only. Similar findings have been reported in other bone marrow infiltrating diseases (2).

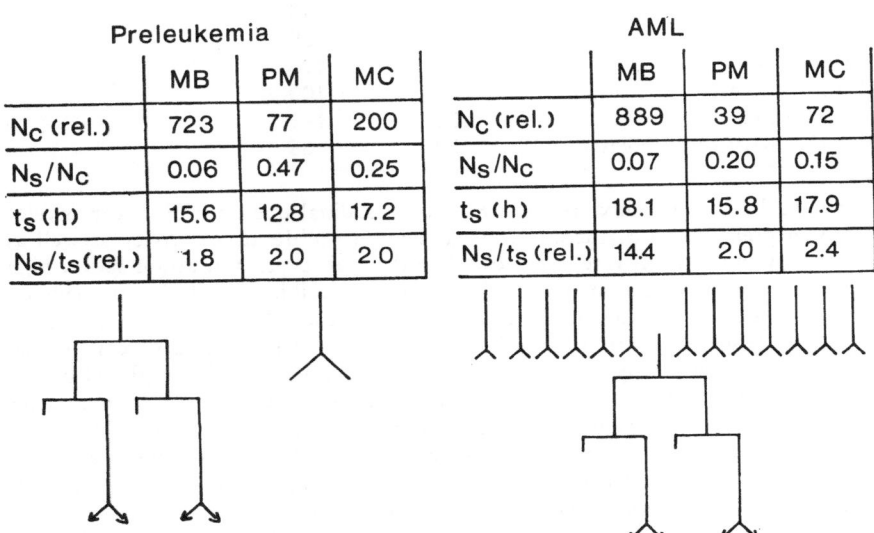

Preleukemia

	MB	PM	MC
N_C (rel.)	723	77	200
N_S/N_C	0.06	0.47	0.25
t_S (h)	15.6	12.8	17.2
N_S/t_S (rel.)	1.8	2.0	2.0

AML

	MB	PM	MC
N_C (rel.)	889	39	72
N_S/N_C	0.07	0.20	0.15
t_S (h)	18.1	15.8	17.9
N_S/t_S (rel.)	14.4	2.0	2.4

Fig. 2: Parameters of cell kinetics and schemes of divisions of myeloid cells in preleukemia (left side) and AML (right side). Abbreviations: MB = myeloblasts; PM = promyelocytes; MC = myelocytes. For the other abbreviations, see legend to Fig. 1.

In the myeloid series (Fig. 2) a prolonged t_s is found already in preleukemic myeloblasts and myelocytes. Normal values for these cells obtained with the same method have been reported by Brinkmann and Dörmer (1). The labeling index of myeloblast in preleukemia is as low as in AML. In this latter stage t_s ist prolonged in all myeloid compartments. From the production rate in AML amounting to 14:2:2 a high degree of self-renewal of the myeloblast compartment can be deduced. In addition, there may be some ineffective myelopoiesis at the stage of myelocytes which is also observed in the preleukemic phase. Possibly the production rates in preleukemia already indicate that half of the myeloblasts do not give rise to promyelocytes after division but remain myeloblasts.

The various parameters of cell proliferation in preleukemia, especially the high percentage of 94 % of myeloblasts in phases other than DNA synthesis, suggest that these cells already constitute a leukemic population. Table 1 shows that the production rate of this population is much lower than that of erythroblasts at the same stage. In normal bone marrow the ratio of production rates of myeloblasts: proerythroblasts is in the order of 1:1 (3). On the other hand, in AML there is a six-fold increase of the myeloblast production rate over that of proerythroblasts.

Table I: Relative Production Rates (Cells Produced per Unit of Time per 100 Proerythroblasts) in Bone Marrow of Preleukemia and AML

	Preleukemia	AML
Myeloblasts	11	640
Promyelocytes	12	89
Myelocytes	12	106
Proerythroblasts	100	100
Basophilic erythroblasts	130	141
Polychromatic erythroblasts	70	88

The findings in this investigation raise one cardinal question: How can myeloblasts in preleukemia characterized by a reduced proliferative activity as well as a very low production rate overgrow the other cell types and attain such a high rate of new cell formation in AML? The most plausible explanation depends on the assumption of a change in the mode of proliferation. By this change is meant a transition from steady state growth of myeloblasts to some kind of exponential expansion. Under steady state conditions a compartment is being replaced by exactly the same number of cells which are leaving it. In exponential growth some of the daughter cells do not leave the compartment and remain mitotable. This increases the production rate of the compartment even if the individual cell looses some of its proliferative activity. In overt AML, finally, the myeloblast compartment has grown to such a size that it can be regarded as mainly self-maintaining. From the present study there is no answer to the question whether at all or to what extent such a compartment is dependent on the influx of stem cells. However, it is most likely that the rate of cell birth in the compartment exceeds by far the rate of influx into it.

Literature

1. Brinkmann, W. and P. Dörmer: Proliferationskinetik der normalen Myelopoese des Menschen, in Stacher, A. and P. Höcker (eds.): Erkrankungen der Myelopoese. München–Wien, Urban & Schwarzenberg 1976.
2. Dörmer, P.: Kinetics of erythropoietic cell proliferation in normal and anemic man. A new approach using quantitative ^{14}C-autoradiography. Progr. Histochem. Cytochem, vol. 6, no. 1, G. Fischer, Stuttgart 1973.
3. Dörmer, P. and W. Brinkmann: A new approach to determine cellcycle parameters in human leukemia, in T. M. Fliedner and S. Perry (eds.): Prognostic factors in human acute leukemia. Oxford, Pergamon Press 1975.

Leukemic Anaplasias Reflecting Physiologic Cytogenesis of Myeloid System

M. R. Parwaresch, H. K. Müller-Hermelink and K. Lennert

Department of clinical and general phatologie
University of Kiel

Cytologcal abnormalities in granulocytes occuring in myeloproliferative diseases prove sometime to be highly revealing in connection with cytogenetical considerations. A good body of techniques have been applied in tracing the developmental line of blood cells. In table 1, a survey of the widely applied methods for the demonstration of the derivation of the granulocytes from their marrow precursors is presented.

Table 1: Survey of methods devised for cytogenetic studies on hemopoetic cells

1. GENERAL MORPHOLOGY
   Size, Form, Granules
2. MORPHOLOGY OF NUCLEI
   Size, Form, Density, Segmentation
3. ULTRASTRUCTURE
4. FUNCTIONAL ACTIVITY
   Phagocytosis, Granule discharge
5. CYTOCHEMICAL PROPERTIES
   Chemical markers
6. DIRECT OBSERVATION
   Derivation in mono-cultures
7. CELL-TRANSFER IN SYNGENEIC ANIMALS
   Radio-labelled
   Enzyme polymorphism
8. MARKER-CHROMOSOMES
9. OBSERVATIONS IN LEUKEMIAS

Revealing informations have been gained on the bases of cytochemical studies. Of special significance proved hydrolytic enzymes as well as dyes with a special affinity to certain cellular structures. These reactions could appropriately be used for the identification of different granulocytic strains. In this context they represent "chemical markers".

Being aware of the differences in the significance of each of these techniques we are going to depict their applicability to the problems of the granulocyte derivation. For the selective visualization of the different granulocytic cell-line the

95

following four techniques have been applied. These methods fulfil the pre-requisites indispensable for cytogenetical considerations: reproducibility, specifity to special cell strain and constancy of the reaction pattern.

1. The naphthol AS-D chloroacetatesterase reaction performed as described by MOLONEY (1960) and LEDER (1964) to visualize promyelocytic azurophil granules and the neutrophilic cell-line (Fig. 1).

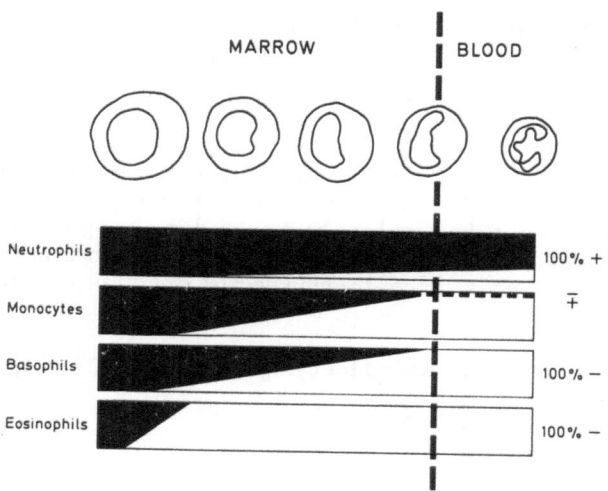

Fig. 1: Naphthol AS-D chlorocetate esterases activity in normal granulopoetic cells from promyelocytes to mature granulocytes.

2. α-naphthylacetatesterase as given by WACHSTEIN and WOLFF (1958) for the staining of blood monocytes (LÖFFLER 1961).
3. Toluidin blue stain for the demonstration of the metachromasia in basophil cell-line following proper fixation of their water soluble granules (PARWA-RESCH and LENNERT 1967).
4. Para – dimethylaminobenzaldehydnitrite (ADAMS 1957) reaction for the selective visualization of eosinophil cell-line (LEDER et al. 1970; LEDER and PAPE 1971). In this reaction structures rich in tryptophane as extracellular fibrin precipitations and RUSSEL bodies reveal also a positive reaction. The separation of these structures however presents no significant difficulties.

Under non neoplastic conditions significant variations in the reaction pattern do not occur. By combination of these methods it is possible to trace back the derivation course of the monocytes (LEDER 1967); basophils (PARWARESCH et al. 1971) and eosinophils (LEDER and PAPE 1971) from the promyelocytes. Promyelocytes, as schematically demonstrated in Fig. 2, gradually develop specific properties of monoytes (activity to α-naphthylacetatesterase reaction) or that of basophils (toluidin blue metachromasia) or that of eosinophils (positive ADAMS reaction). In the same time a progressive reduction of the chloroacetatesterase activity occurs as the specific secondary granules develop. All transitional forms

96

presenting both, properties of promyelocytes and those of individual granulocytes, can easily be detected (fig. 2).

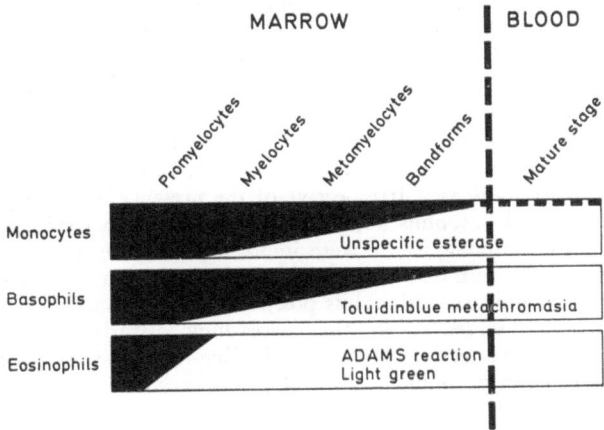

Fig. 2: Demonstration of the granulocyte maturation as observed by the combined application of LEDER's esterase with α-naphthylacetate esterase reaction (monocytic cellline), with toluidin (basophil cell-line) and with light green or ADAMS reaction (eosinophil celline). For further explanation refer to text.

In fig. 3 the reactivity of the individual granulocytes to the four applied methods is demonstrated. In case of naphthol AS-D chloroacetatesterase reaction neutrophils reveal an invariable strong activity. A minor number of monocytes present a fine granular weak reaction. Basophils and eosinophils are invariably

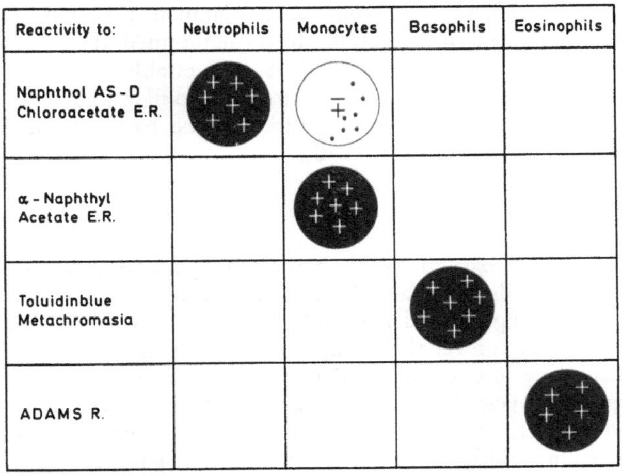

Reactivity to:	Neutrophils	Monocytes	Basophils	Eosinophils
Naphthol AS-D Chloroacetate E.R.	⊕	○		
α-Naphthyl Acetate E.R.		⊕		
Toluidinblue Metachromasia			⊕	
ADAMS R.				⊕

Fig. 3: Reactivity of mature granulocytes and monocytes to the four cytochemical techniques applied.

negative. Monocytes are the only leukocytes presenting a significant activity to α-naphthylacetatesterase reaction. Toluidin blue metachromasia is strictly confined to basophils. The same is valid for eosinophils respecting ADAMS reaction.

In case of myeloproliferative diseases a variety of divergences from the normal reaction pattern have been demonstrated (UNDRITZ 1963; LEDER 1972; PARWARESCH 1975). These deviations have been regarded as neoplastic abnormalities.

There have been reports on basophils (PARWARESCH 1975) and eosinophils positive to chloroacetatesterase reaction (LÖFFLER 1969; LEDER 1970) in cases of myeloproliferative diseases. Irrespective of the presence of this property in the marrow precursors of basophils and eosinophils, theirselves lacking this property as normal mature granulocytes, it were impossible to understand the mechanism and the significance of such an occurance in neoplastic variants. Apparently normal populations of basophils or eosinophils positive to chloroacetatesterase reaction in myeloproliferative diseases reflect the farreaching disturbance of the control mechanisms of the maturation process. This abnormality seen with eosinophils and basophils is strictly confined to myeloproliferative diseases. In fifteen cases of excessive reactive leukocytoses including some leukemoid reactions no single basophil or eosinophil positive to chloroacetatesterase could be detected. It further underscores the exsistence of a single promyelocyte as the common precursors of at least these two granulocyte types and neutrophils. The latter is the only one of the three granulocytes, which retains the azurophil promyelocytic granules up to the mature stage.

A further observation in myeloproliferative diseases is the occurance of granulocytes in bone marrow and peripheral blood which possess specific eosinophil as well as basophil granules. They are positive to chloroacetatesterase and to ADAMS reaction as well as to toluidin blue metachromasia. Coincideing of different properties, specific to individual granulocytes in the same cell is a further and a highly suggestive argument in favour of a common precursor for the three granulocyte types. Recent investigations have maintained further proof for this mode of granulocyte derivation. It could be well established, that monocellular cultures of single promyelocytes give rise to neutrophil granulocytes and monocytes. A fact which has been long expected on the basis of the frequency of myelomonocytic leukemias (LEDER 1970).

Summary

Naphthol AS-D chloroacetatesterase activity in peripheral blood granulocytes is confined to neutrophils which are all positive and to a minor part of monocytes. Its occurance in eosinophils and basophils indicate a myeloproliferative disease. This chemical property can reliably be applied to separate neoplastic from reactive forms of quantitative and qualitative leukocyte alterations. The developmental line of this specific myeloid cellular attribut has been presented to elucidate its diagnostic significance and its validity as proof for existence of a common promyelocyte from which neutrophils, monocytes, basophils and eosinophils originate.

References

Adams, C. W. M.: A p-dimethylaminobenzaldehydnitrite method for the histochemical demonstration of tryptophane and related compounds. J. clin. Path.: *10*, 56–62 (1957).

Leder, L.-D.: Der Nachweis von Naphthol AS-D Chloracetat Esterase und seine Bedeutung für die histologische Diagnostik. Verh. dtsch. Ges. Path.: *48*, 317–320 (1964).

Leder, L.-D.: Die fermentcytochemische Erkennung normaler und neoplastischer Erythropoiesezellen in Schnitt und Ausstrich. Blut: *15*, 289—293 (1967).

Leder, L.-D.: Akute myelo-monocytäre Leukämie mit atypischen Naphthol AS-D Chloracetat Esterase-positiven Eosinophilen. Acta haemat. (Basel): *44*, 52–62 (1970).

Leder, L.-D., H. J. Stutte und B. Pape: Zur selektiven Darstellung von eosinophilen Granulozyten und ihren Vorstufen in Ausstrichen und Schnitten. Klin. Wschr.: *48*, 191–192 (1970).

Leder, L.-D. and B. Pape: Cytological and cytochemical investigations on the origin of human eosinophilic granulocytes. Beitr. Path.: *143*, 241–248 (1971).

Leder, L.-D.: Histochemie und Cytochemie der Leukosen. In: Leukämie. Ed.: R. Gross u. J. van de Loo, Springer Verlag Berlin–Heidelberg–New York (1972).

Löffler, H.: Cytochemischer Nachweis von unspezifischer Esterase in Ausstrichen. Klin. Wschr.: *39*, 1220–1227 (1961).

Löffler, H.: Cytochemische Klassifizierung der akuten Leukosen. In: Chemo- und Immuntherapie der Leukosen und malignen Lymphome (Stacher, A., Hrsg.) Wien: Bohmann-Verlag (1969).

Moloney, W. C., K. McPherson and L. Fliegelman: Esterase activity in leukocytes demonstrated by the use of naphthol AS-D chloroacetate substrate. J. Histochem. Cytochem.: *8*, 200–207 (1960).

Parwaresch, M. R. und K. Lennert: Löslichkeit und Fixierungsmöglichkeiten der Blutbasophilen-Granula des Menschen. Z. Zellforsch.: *83*, 279–287 (1967).

Parwaresch, M. R., L.-D. Leder and K. E. G. Dannenberg: On the origin of human basophilic granulocytes. Acta haemat.: *45*, 273–279 (1971).

Parwaresch, M. R.: Pathologie, Histochemie und Elektronenmikroskopie der basophilen Leukämie. 3. internationale Arbeitstagung über Proliferative Erkrankungen des myeloischen Systems. Wien, 19.–22. März (1975).

Undritz, E.: Die Peroxydasereaktion und ihre praktische Bedeutung. In: Cyto- und Histochemie in der Hämatologie. S. 193—216. 9. Freiburger Symposion (Merker, H. Hrsg.). Berlin–Göttingen–Heidelberg Springer Verlag (1963).

Wachstein, M., and G. Wolf: The histochemical demonstration of esterase activity in human blood and bone marrow smears. J. Histochem. Cytochem.: *6*, 457 (1958).

Membrane Remodeling During Phagocytosis in Chronic Myelogenous Leukemia Cells

Stephen B. Shohet, M. D.
Cancer Research Institute
University of California, San Francisco

Introduction

First, I would like to thank Dr. Neth and the organizers for making this meeting possible. For those of us who have come a long distance, the trip has clearly been educationally profitable and the hospitality of Dr. Neth and his delightful teams of wagon drivers have certainly made this a memorable personal experience as well.

This evening I would like to tell you very briefly the results of some experiments we conducted with chronic myelogenous leukemia cells following phagocytosis. The experiments were initially undertaken in the hope that we could detect some difference in the biochemical behavior of leukemic cells and normal cells which might further our understanding of the former or suggest some therapeutic approaches. At the very beginning, I must tell you that we found no differences between the leukemic and normal cells. However, in both cells we did note some unusual changes in the lipid composition of sub-cellular membrane constituents following phagocytosis of considerable biologic interest. These changes may offer some possibilities for therapeutic manipulation of abnormal phagocytic cells.

Since the lipid composition of biological membranes is a major determinant of their barrier qualities and their permeability characteristics, and since during phagocytosis there is a major architectual rearrangement of membrane constituents in the phagocytic cell, we sought to determine the lipid composition of various permeability barriers within the phagocytic cell both before and after phagocytosis. Although at the time, we were not aware of any therapeutic implications of such potential differences, recent observations of Dr. Tulkens in Brussels suggest that such changes may modulate the effects of some so-called "lysosomotropic" drugs currently utilized in leukemia chemotherapy.

Methods

The basic procedures followed are outlined in Figure 1. In brief, we collected heparin anti-coagulated blood from untreated human patients with chronic myelogenous leukemia. We then separated the CML granulocytes from the red cells and platelets by gravity sedimentation and gentle saline washing. Throughout the isolation procedure, plastic containers and pipettes were used to minimize white cell aggregation. The isolated washed cells were then incubated with an excess of opsonized polystyrene beads so that a large amount of phagocytosis occurred with-

Schema for isolation and lipid analysis of whole cells, Lysosomal Membranes, Plasma Membranes, and Phagosomal Membranes of CML Granulocytes

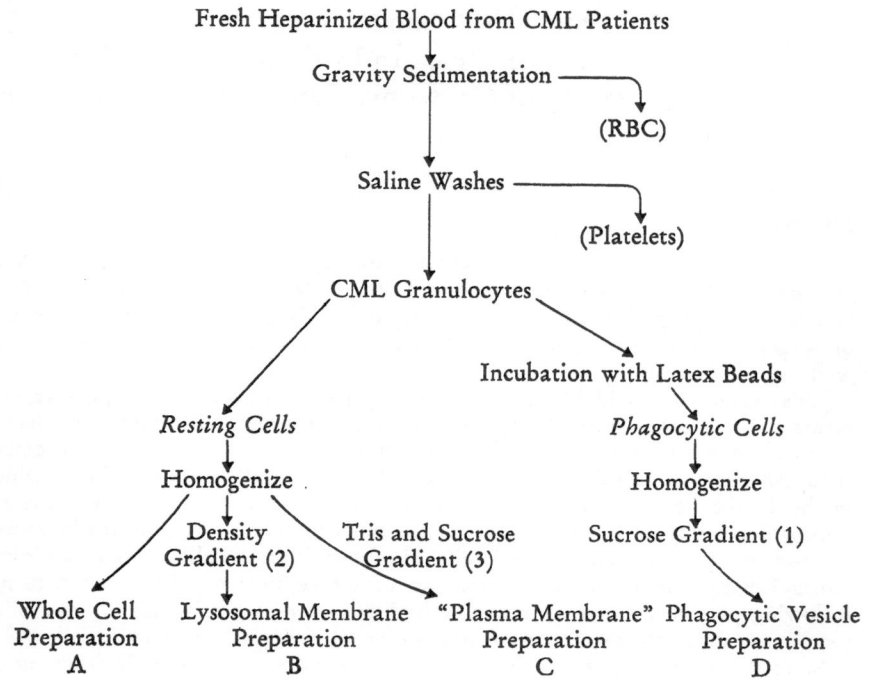

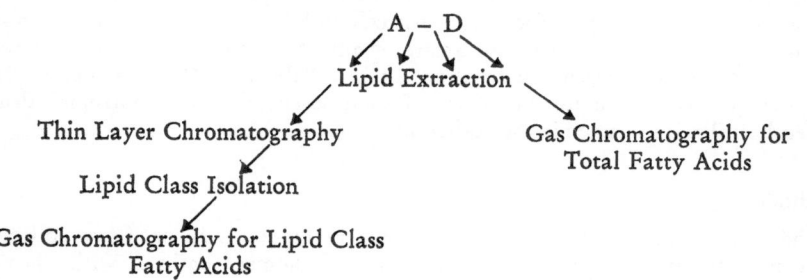

Fig. 1

in approximately 15 minutes. The reaction was stopped by the addition of excess cold saline and the cells were then homogenized in order to liberate the latex beads which were now coated with a phagocytic membrane which was probably derived from a combination of lysosomal membranes and plasma membranes which had fused to form the phagocytic vacuole following particle ingestion. These membranes were then isolated by density centrifugation following the method of Wetzel and Korn (1) while resting cells were similarly homogenized and fractionated to obtain both primary lysosomal membranes and plasma membranes by the methods of Cohn and Hirsch; and Warren, Glick and Nass, respectively (2, 3). The resultant membrane preparations were then extracted for lipid analysis with chloroform and methanol following the method of Folch, Lees, and Sloane Stanley (4) with the modification of adding of one miligram per 100 cc's of Butyrated Hydroxy Toluene as anti-oxidant to all of the solvents. The liquid extracts were then assayed by thin layer chromatography using the method of Skipski, Peterson, and Barclay (5) and by a total lipid phosphorus assay (6). The lipid classes were isolated from the thin-layer plates by elution and analyzed for fatty acids by gas chromatography utilizing methods published elsewhere (7). An "unsaturation index" (U.I.) was calculated for each sample as the sum of the number of double bonds in each fatty acid species multiplied by its mole percentage as determined by the gas chromatography. This index served as a gross estimate of the "fluidity" of the membranes analyzed and also probably reflects their flexibility and permeability.

Results

A summary of the overall results is presented in Table I. Here the "unsaturation index" of the lipids in the whole cells used as starting material is compared to the unsaturation indices of both lysosomes and plasma membranes isolated from those cells prior to phagocytosis, as well as phagocytic vesicles isolated following phagocytosis. Plasma membranes are presented in quotation marks in this table because the product derived by this technique, although the best available, is still subject to some question in terms of purity. In terms of overall unsaturation indices,

Table I: Unsaturation Indices and Representative Fatty Acids of Total Phospholipids in Various Fractions of Chronic Myelogenous Leukemia Granulocytes*

	Whole Cells	Granules	"Plasma Membrane"	Phagocytic Vesicles
U. I.**	110 ± 8	124 ± 4	100 ± 8	65 ± 9
20:4	14 ± 2	17 ± 1	11 ± 2	5 ± 1
16:0	20 ± 3	16 ± 1	28 ± 6	31 ± 6

* Tables I and II modified from Smolen & Shohet (6) with permission of the Journal of Clinical Investigation. ± figures = 1 S. D.
** Unsaturation Index and Sum of Mole % FA Times # Double Bonds/FA.

phatocytic vesicles have a considerably lower unsaturation index than any of the other fractions. This includes particularly both the granule and plasma membrane fractions which are felt to be the precursors of the phagocytic vesicle membranes. When representative polyunsaturated and fully saturated fatty acids are also examined in the same table, it can be seen that there is a consistent reduction in polyunsaturated fatty acid and an increase in saturated fatty acid in the phagocytic vesicles. Similar changes are noted in Table II which presents lipid analyses for the phosphatidylcholine and phospatidylethanolamine lipid sub-classes; again, the data are presented for whole cells prior to phagocytosis and phagocytic vacuoles following phagocytosis. This data may be somewhat more significant than the whole lipid analyses in that the specific lipid sub-classes, which might be expected to enter into metabolic rearrangements following phagocytosis, were particularly analyzed. Again, the phagocytic vesicules have considerably reduced unsaturation indices in both lipid classes in comparison to whole cells, and consistent changes are found when representative fatty acids are examined.

Table II: Unsaturation Indices and Representative Fatty Acids of Separated Phospholipids in Various Fractions of Chronic Myelogenous Leukemia Granulocytes

| | Phosphatidylcholine | | Phosphatidylethanolamine | |
	Whole Cells	Phagocytic Vesicles	Whole Cells	Phagocytic Vesicles
U. I.	70	49	140	122
20:4	35	26	24	98
16:0	33	52	12	43

Discussion

Figure 2 outlines our current understanding of the phagocytic process in terms of the disposition of membrane constituents. Here it can be seen that the phagocytic membrane is composed of elements of both the primary lysosomal membrane and the plasma membrane. Unfortunately, we do not know the percentage of each antecedent constituent and the diagram drawn here is not meant to imply any quantitative accuracy. Nevertheless, it can be seen from Tables I and II that the final lipid composition of the phagocytic vacuole membrane is considerably more saturated than that of either of its parent membranes, so that simple mixing of membrane constituents, in any proportion, can not explain the observed composition of the phagocytic membrane.

Two possible mechanisms for this change in membrane lipid saturation are also outlined in Figure 2. The first is a hydrogen peroxide mediated attack on the unsaturated fatty acid bonds of the lipids making up this membrane. Karnovsky and Sbarra showed long ago that the oxidative burst produced during phagocytosis is related to the generation of hydrogen peroxide within the ingesting granulocyte (8). Many subsequent investigators including most prominately Dr.

MEMBRANE REMODELING TO FORM
'PHAGOSOMES' IN GRANULOCYTES

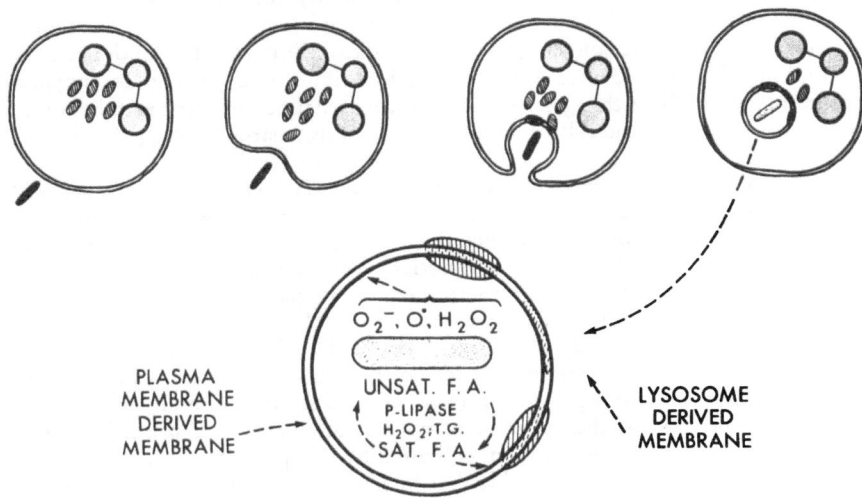

'PHAGOSOME' WITH INJESTED PARTICLE

Fig. 2: A schematic diagram representing changes in lipid membrane constituents of granulocytes during phagocytosis. The plasma membrane invaginates and fuses with lysosomal
membrane elements to form the eventual phagosomal membrane. This new membrane is
thus derived from two parent membranes. However, the final concentration of saturated
fatty acids in the phagosomal membrane is greater than that of either the parent membranes.
It is assumed that either peroxidation of the phagosomal membrane through the action of
hydrogen peroxide or superoxide, or the selective reacylation of that membrane through
the activity of a phospholipase or a reacylation system, is responsible for this remodeling.

Klebanoff (9) have suggested that this hydrogen peroxide may be crucial in
mediating the subsequent killing of the phagocytized bacteria. Hydrogen peroxide
either directly, or indirectly by one of its unstable precursors, superoxide, is well
known to attack double bonds of unsaturated fatty acids; and if liberated in close
proximity to the newly formed phagocytic membrane, might well be responsible
for much of its changed unsaturation index. Alternatively, or perhaps additionally,
a phospholipase-reacylase enzyme cycle has been described in white cells (10)
which, also perhaps under the influence of hydrogen peroxide, may preferentially
attack unsaturated fatty acids on phospholipids replacing them with saturated
fatty acids derived from triglycerides (11, 12).

Whether one or both of these mechanisms is operative, it seems clear that the
permeability of the phagocytic vesicle may be quite different from that of other
membranes within the cell. One might argue that this would be of considerable
importance physiologically in that activated lysosomal products would be retained
in a contained space surrounding the ingested foreign particle. This would facilitate

the rapid destruction of the ingested bacteria on the one hand while protecting the cell from auto-digestion on the other. I should hasten to add that direct measurements of phagocytic vacuole membrane permeability for large enzyme molecules have not been made, and that this line of reasoning is dependent upon assumptions concerning the influence of the unsaturation index. Moreover, it is much more likely that small co-factor permeability would be influenced than gross enzymatic permeability by these changes. Nevertheless, a dynamic compartmentalization of digestive capacity of the cell following phagocytosis is strongly suggested by these experiments.

A possibility of therapeutically exploring these phenomena has been suggested by the recent studies of Dr. Tulkens and this is the reason I wish to bring this data to the attention of this audience this evening. Dr. Tulkens in Dr. DeDuve's laboratory has shown that certain antibiotics permeate lysosomes quite readily and then apparently become trapped there, perhaps in part due to changes in their ionic state induced by the acidic environment (13). Daunomycin and Adriamycin are included within this classification of drugs. Dr. Tulkens also feels that the Daunomycin probably enters the cell by "piggyback endocytosis" a process somewhat analogous to the phagocytosis process we have studied with larger latex granules. It may be that the therapeutic effectiveness of these drugs, which is probably dependent upon nuclear penetration, is limited by this preferential sequestration in the lysosomes. It is not inconceivable that interference with the remodeling process which has been described here, by the addition of an anti-oxidant group to the chemotherapeutic molecules, would reduce lysosomal sequestration and increase the biologic effectiveness of those agents.

References

1. Wetzel, M. G. and Korn, E. D.: Phagocytosis of latex beads by *Acanthamoeba castellanii* (neff). III. Isolation of phagocytic vesicles and their membranes. J. Cell Biol. *43*: 90, 1969.
2. Cohn, Z. A. and Hirsch, J. G.: The isolation and properties of the specific cytoplasmic granules of rabbit polymorphonuclear leukocytes. J. Exp. Med. *112*: 983, 1960.
3. Warren, L., Glick, M. C., and Nass, M. K.: Membranes of animal cells. .I Methods of isolation of the surface membrane. J. Cell. Physiol. *68*: 269, 1966.
4. Folch, J., Lees, M., Jr., and Sloane Stanley, G. H.: A simple method for the isolation and purification of total lipids from animal tissues. J. Biol. Chem. *226*: 497, 1957.
5. Skipski, V. P., Peterson, R. F., and Barclay, M.: Quantitative analysis of phospholipids by thin layer chromatography. Biochem. J. *90*: 374, 1964.
6. Lowry, O. H., Roberts, N. R., Leiner, K. Y., Wu, M. L., and Farr, A. L.: The quantitative histochemistry of brain. I. Chemical methods. J. Biol. Chem. *207*: 1, 1954.
7. Smolen, J. E. and Shohet, S. B.: Remodeling of granulocyte membrane fatty acids during phagocytosis. J. Clin. Invest. *53*: 726, 1974.
8. Karnovsky, M. L. and Sbarra, A. J.: Metabolic changes in leukocytes during phagocytosis studies with C^{14}. Proceedings of the Second United Nations

Geneva Conference on the peaceful uses of atomic energy, New York, 1959, United Nations Press, p. 85.

9. Klebanoff, S. J.: Iodination of bacteria: A bactericidal mechanism. J. Exp. Med. *126*: 1063, 1968.

10. Elsbach, P., Van Den Berg, J. W. O., Van Den Bosch, H., and van Deenen, L. L. M.: Metabolism of phospholipids by polymorphonuclear leukocytes. Biochim. Biophys. Acta *106*:338, 1965.

11. Elsbach, P., and Farrow, S.: Cellular triglyceride as a source of fatty acid for lecithin synthesis during phagocytosis. Biochim. Biophys. Acta *176*: 438, 1969.

12. Shohet, S. B.: Changes in fatty acid metabolism in human leukemic granulocytes during phagocytosis. J. Lab. & Clin. Med. *75*: 659, 1970.

13. Tulkens, P.: Lysosomotropic Drugs: Biological and therapeutical significance. Proceedings of International Conference on Biological Membranes, Crans – Sur-Sierre (Valais) Switzerland, June 15–21, 1975.

Erythroid Cell Differentiation

Bernard G. Forget[1], Jonatham Glass[2], and David Housman[3]

Harvard Medical School, Boston Masschusetts, Institute of
Technilogy, Cambridge

I. Introduction

The study of erythroid cell differentiation is pertinent to the study of human leukemia from two points of view. First, since a common stem cell gives rise to both erythroid and myeloid cells, it is not unexpected that disorders of myeloid cell proliferation and differentiation should be occasionally associated with abnormalities of erythroid cell differentiation. In fact in many cases of human leukemia, there are abnormalities of erythroid cells. Secondly, the study of erythroid cell differentiation can serve as an experimental model for the study of normal and abnormal gene expression, a topic of vital importance to the understanding of the etiology and pathogenesis of human leukemia. The erythoid cell provides a number of advantages as a model system for the study of the control of gene expression. This highly specialized cell devotes approximately 95 % of its protein synthesis to the production of one protein, hemoglobin, and therefore only a limited number of the cell's genes are expressed. In addition, a number of biochemical techniques are currently available for the isolation, characterization and quantitation of globin messenger RNA (mRNA), the necessary intermediary between globin gene expression and globin chain synthesis.

Erythroid cell differentiation can be considered from two points of view: 1) differences between fetal and adult mature red blood cells; and 2) differences between erythroid cells at different stages of morphologic maturation. We will discuss first the abnormalities of red cell differentiation, mainly the emergence of fetal erythropoiesis, which can occur during the course of various human leukemias. Then we will discuss experimental studies on the quantitation of heme synthesis, globin synthesis and globin messenger RNA content in murine erythroid cells at different stages of maturation.

[1] The Divison of Hematology-Oncology of the Department of Medicine, Children's Hospital Medical Center, the Sidney Farber Cancer Center and the Department of Pediatrics, Harvard Medical School, Boston, Mass. 02115.
[2] The Department of Medicine, Beth Israel Hospital and Harvard Medical School, Boston, Mass. 02115.
[3] The Department of Biology and the Center for Cancer Research, Massachusetts Institute of Technology, Cambridge, Mass. 02139.
Abbreviations used:
Hb: hemoglobin; mRNA: messenger RNA.
RNase: ribonuclease.
cDNA: DNA copy of globin mRNA synthesized by RNA dependent DNA polymerase (reverse transcriptase) of avian myeloblastosis virus.

II. Abnormalities of erythroid cells in the human leukemias

1. Abnormal proliferation of erythroid cells.

A number of abnormalities of erythroid cell proliferation and differentiation have been observed in various human leukemias. Some of these abnormalities can be traced to the fact that a common stem cell gives rise to all three types of blood cells: granulocytes, erythroid cells and platelets. In the myeloproliferative disorder, polycythemia vera, which can be considered as a "pre-leukemic" condition, there must be autonomous proliferation of the common progenitor stem cell, because all three cell lines proliferate and accumulate in excess with resulting erythrocytosis, granulocytosis, and thrombocytosis. After many years this condition can revert to myelofibrosis with myeloid metaplasia and/or acute myelogenous leukemia; very rarely Philadelphia chromosome-positive chronic myelogenous leukemia may develop after a long period of myelofibrosis and myeloid metaplasia and prior to acute myeloblastic transformation.

In chronic myelogenous leukemia, the acquired chromosomal marker in the leukemic myeloid cells, the Philadelphia or Ph_1 chromosome is present not only in the granulocytes but also in the erythroid (and megakaryocytic) precursor cells. This finding again points to a lesion in the common progenitor cells as a basis for at least some forms of leukemia.

Since the common stem cell is affected in at least some myeloid leukemias, it is not unexpected that in some forms of myeloid or undifferentiated leukemia, there appears to be an associated frank neoplastic transformation of the erythroid cell line: thus the term erythroleukemia, also referred to as the DiGuglielmo syndrome. In this condition there are bizarre, multinucleated megaloblastic erythroid precursors, clover leaf nuclei, abnormal mitoses with endoreduplication, and bizarre mature red cell morphology; almost invariably there is concomitant or subsequent proliferation of myeloblasts and development of frank acute myeloblastic leukemia.

2. Abnormal hemoglobin synthesis

In certain cases of erythroleukemia and more rarely in other myeloproliferative disorders, an abnormality of hemoglobin synthesis has been detected, termed acquired hemoglobin H (Hb H) disease. Normal hemoglobin consists of two α and two β chains ($\alpha_2\beta_2$), and normally there is equal synthesis and accumulation of α and β chains in erythroid cells. If there is decreased synthesis of α chains relative to β chains, then β chains will accumulate in excess and form tetramers of Hb H (β_4). Hb H is relatively unstable or insoluble: with time it precipitates in the cell, forming inclusion bodies which damage the red cell membrane and lead to premature destruction of the red cell. Studies of globin chain synthesis have been reported in one such case of acquired Hb H disease and these studies directly demonstrated a decrease in α chain synthesis relative to β chain synthesis (1). Other studies have indicated that the defect, in at least the case studied, is a clonal one, and limited to only some but not all of the patient's red cells (?the neoplastic clone) (2).

Hb H disease more commonly occurs as an inherited disorder, a form of α-thalassemia in which there is a genetic defect causing reduction of α chain syn-

110

thesis. In this latter condition, the patient has no increased susceptibility to developing leukemia.

3. Fetal hemoglobin synthesis

During human development there is a change in hemoglobin synthesis from fetal hemoglobin synthesis (Hb F: $\alpha_2\gamma_2$) to adult hemoglobin synthesis (Hb A: $\alpha_2\beta_2$) [Fig. 1]. The phenomenon starts during the third trimester of pregnancy and is

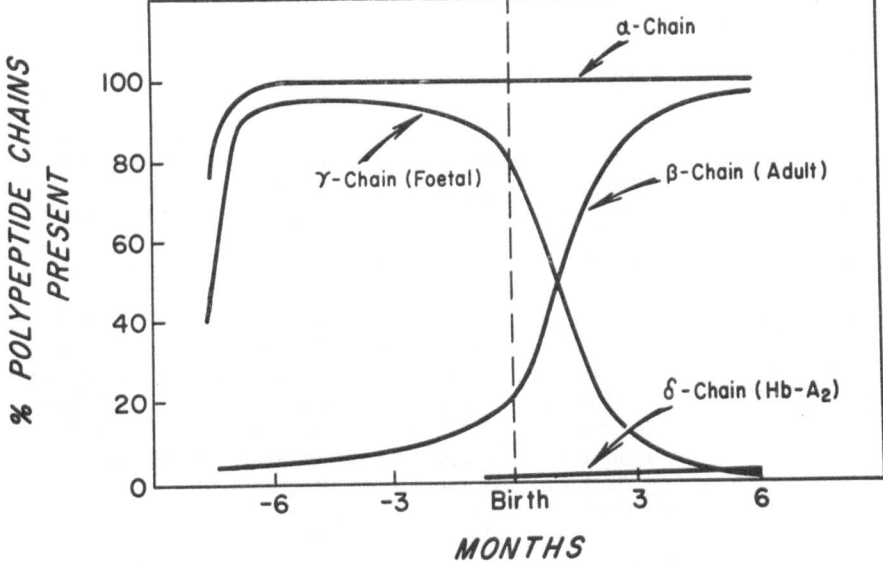

Fig. 1: Diagrammatic representation of the changes in human globin synthesis during prenatal and neonatal development. (Modified from Huehns *et al,* Cold Spring Harbor Symp. Quant. Biol. (1964) *19,* 327).

usually complete by 6 months of age. The process involves the inactivation of the genes for the γ globin chains and the activation of the genes for the β globin chains. The precise mechanism involved and the factors controlling it are unknown. There are two different types of γ chains of Hb F, which are the products of two different genes. The two γ chains differ by only one amino acid residue at position 136 of their amino acid sequence: in one chain it is alanine (the $^A\gamma$ chain), in the other it is glycine (the $^G\gamma$ chain). The relative amounts of $^A\gamma$ and $^G\gamma$ chains produced vary during development: in the fetus and newborn there is more $^G\gamma$ than $^A\gamma$ synthesis, but in the adult the small amount of residual γ chain synthesis consists of more $^A\gamma$ chain synthesis than $^G\gamma$ chain synthesis (Table 1). There are also other differences between fetal and adult red blood cells (Table 1): in fetal cells there is virtual absence of Hb A$_2$ ($\alpha_2\delta_2$) and of the enzyme carbonic anhydrase B, whereas these proteins are easily detected in hemolysates of adult red cells. The fetal and adult red cells also differ by one of their surface antigens: i (fetal) vs I (adult).

Table 1: Features of Fetal Versus Adult Erythroid Cell Differentiation

	Fetal rbc	Adult rbc
Hemoglobin type	Hb F	Hb A
Hemoglobin F subtypes		
gly:ala ratio	3:1	2:3
Membrane antigen	i	I
Carbonic anhydrase B	0	+
Hemoglobin A_2	0	+

In many cases of leukemia there is reactivation of fetal hemoglobin synthesis. This phenomenon is not peculiar to any specific type of leukemia but has been observed in virtually all types of leukemia: erythroleukemia, acute lymphoid leukemia and acute or chronic myeloid leukemia. In most of these cases however, the finding of increased Hb F is variable and the levels observed are usually low (2–15 %). In erythroleukemia elevations of Hb F are more common and the levels can be quite high (up to 60 %) (3).

In one form of leukemia, juvenile chronic myeloid leukemia (CML), striking elevations of Hb F are almost invariable. The Hb F level usually increases as the disease progresses and can attain up to 70 % of the total Hb. This condition is associated with absence of the Ph_1 chromosome and differs in its clinical course from the adult type of chronic myeloid leukemia (3). The fetal Hb in this condition almost invariably is of the true fetal type with respect to its content of ^Gy and ^Ay chains (G/A or gly/ala ratio). As the disease progresses the red cells also gradually acquire other fetal characteristics: increase in i antigen, and diminution of I antigen, Hb A_2 and carbonic anhydrase B. In this condition, there is therefore an apparent total reversion from adult to fetal protein synthesis. In rare cases of erythroleukemia in infants, a similar total reversion to fetal protein synthesis has been observed (4).

In most other cases of leukemia however, the synthesis of Hb F is less striking (2–15 % of total Hb) and when it occurs, the Hb F is heterogeneously distributed among the red cells: it is usually limited to a small proportion or clone of red cells. In these cases there is usually no other evidence of fetal red cell protein synthesis as in juvenile CML. The significance of the phenomenon is uncertain. Reactivation of Hb F synthesis is also seen in a number of other medical conditions, usually associated with some bone marrow stress and hyperplasia. It is possible that these phenomena cause the nonspecific proliferation of usually dormant fetal clones of red cells. On the other hand, the expression of fetal globin genes may be a consequence of the neoplastic process: other neoplastic processes are sometimes associated with the synthesis of other fetal proteins, such as carcinoembryonic antigen (CEA) in colonic carcinoma and α-feto protein in hepatoma. The precise relationship of these events to the malignant process remains to be elucidated.

Another observation has been made which may have relevance to stem cell regeneration and proliferation following chemotherapy for leukemia. Sheridan, *et al* (4) studied hemoglobin synthesis in a number of patients undergoing chemotherapy for acute myelogenous leukemia. In most cases they observed a burst of fetal hemoglobin synthesis at about 90 days after start of therapy usually following a period of marrow hypoplasia which preceded a remission. Peak levels of 13 % were observed. The Hb F was distributed in a distinct cell line and the levels decreased to normal during the period of remission. The G/A ratio of the Hb F produced was usually of the true fetal type rather than of the adult type (4), but other features of fetal protein synthesis were not observed. Similar observations have been made in the early stage of bone marrow regeneration following bone marrow transplantation for aplastic anemia or leukemia (4 a). It is conceivable that stem cells after suppression of growth and during regeneration go through a cycle of producing committed stem cells which proliferate and differentiate as fetal cells. These observations will no doubt serve as the basis for further studies on the mechanisms and control of stem cell growth and proliferation.

III. Hemoglobin synthesis during erythroid cell maturation

1. Introduction

In order to delineate mechanisms involved in the control of gene expression during normal cell development, we studied a model system consisting of erythroid cells at various stages of differentiation. Erythroid precursor cells were isolated from the spleens of anemic mice, then fractionated by velocity sedimentation into relatively pure populations of cells at different morphologic stages of maturation. These cells were then analyzed before and after overnight culture in the presence of erythropoietin for heme synthesis, globin synthesis and globin mRNA content by RNA-DNA hybridization assays using as probes the radioactive DNA copy (cDNA) synthesized from reticulocyte globin mRNA by viral reverse transcriptase. The results demonstrated that heme synthesis is maximal at an earlier stage of maturation than hemoglobin synthesis, indicating a certain degree of asynchronism between heme and globin synthesis during erythroid cell maturation. The least mature cells had a low but substantial level of globin mRNA indicating a greater degree of biochemical differentiation than otherwise suggested by the cells' morphological appearance and very low level of hemoglobin synthesis. After culture overnight with erythropoietin, the globin mRNA content of these cells increased three- to five-fold, to levels found in the more mature erythroid precursor cells. These results indicate that the major control of globin gene expression in this system is probably at the transcriptional level, but some degree of translational control may be operative in the early stages of differentiation.

2. Materials and Methods

Hemolytic anemia was induced in virgin female CD_1 mice (Charles River Breeding Labs), 18–24 grams in weight, by intraperitoneal injections of phenylhydrazine, 30 mg per kg, on days 0, 1 and 3. The spleens were removed on day 4, minced in phosphate buffered saline – 15 % fetal calf serum, forced through stainless steel mesh and filtered through 35 micron Nitex cloth. The more mature erythroid cells were lysed with antibody prepared against adult red cells, according to the method of Borsook et al, (5), and Cantor et al, (6). The cells were then refiltered through Nitex cloth and separated as a function of size by the velocity sedimentation technique (7, 8) in a Staput Cell Separator with an 18 cm diameter bowl. Approximately 7×10^8 cells were loaded in one hour and allowed to settle for 3 hours. After the cone volume was removed, 30 ml fractions were collected and the cells were pelleted at $300 \times g$. Fractions containing similar morphologic classes of cells were combined into larger pools to provide sufficient material for assay of mRNA and for short-term culture.

Replicate aliquots of cells were suspended in modified McCoy's 5A medium containing 15 % fetal calf serum, penicillin (0.1 units/ml), streptomycin (0.1 μg/ ml) and human urinary erythropoietin (0.2 units/ml) at cell concentrations of about 5×10^6 cells/ml. Cells were cultured for 16 hours at 37 °C in a humidified atmosphere with 5 % CO_2. In one experiment cells from fraction I were cultured in the presence of 100 μCi/ml of ^{3}H-uridine, (46.2 Ci/m mole) [New England Nuclear Corp.].

Total cellular RNA was extracted from the various velocity sedimentation cell fractions by SDS-phenol-chloroform-isopropyl alcohol extraction at pH 9.0 (9). The cells labeled with ^{3}H-uridine were washed and lysed by homogenization in 0.1 M Tris, pH 7.5, 0.03 M KCl, 0.002 M $MgCl_2$ containing 1 % Triton X 100 and 50 μg/ml of Dextran 70 (McGraw Laboratories). The nuclei were sedimented at $100 \times g$ and RNA was prepared from the supernatant cytoplasm by SDS-phenol-chloroform extraction. The ethanol precipitated RNA was then fractionated by oligo (dT) cellulose column chromatography (9). The RNA initially bound to the column and subsequently eluted by 10 mM Tris HCl, pH 7.5, was ethanol precipitated in the presence of 50 μg of *E. coli* tRNA. It represented 8 % of the initial total cpm in the cytoplasmic RNA.

Mouse reticulocyte RNA was prepared by detergent-phenol-cresol extraction of membrane-free reticulocyte lysates (10), and fractionated by sucrose gradient centrifugation; the RNA sedimenting between 4S and 18S RNA served as partially purified reticulocyte globin mRNA. Further purification of the globin mRNA was achieved by oligo (dT) cellulose chromatography of the sucrose gradient mRNA fraction. The RNA initially bound and then eluted from the oligo(dT)-cellulose was labeled with ^{125}I by Dr. Wolf Prensky (11).

RNA-dependent DNA polymerase was purified from avian myeloblastosis virus by the method of Verma and Baltimore (12). In some preparations, further purification of the enzyme by phosphocellulose chromatography was omitted. ^{3}H-labeled globin cDNA was synthesized from the sucrose gradient purified reticulocyte globin mRNA as previously described (13, 14). cDNA for DNA excess hybridization was synthesized with the following components: α-^{32}P-TTP 22.5 μCi/ml (116 Ci/mmole); TTP, 0.1 mM; dCTP, dATP, dGTP, 0.5 mM; Tris pH 8.3, 50 mM; Mg acetate, 6 mM; NaCl, 60 mM; dithiothreitol, 8 mM; actinomycin D, 50 μg/ml; globin mRNA, 10 μg/ml; RNA-dependent DNA polymerase, 100 μl/ml; and oligo (dT$_{12-18}$), 2μg/ml. RNA saturation hybridization was then accomplished by incubating a fixed amount of labeled cDNA with varying amounts of total RNA from the different cell fractions for 40 hours at 70 °C, in 0.2 M sodium phosphate, pH 6.8, and 0.5 % SDS (14, 15). Percent hybridization was then determined after digestion of the residual nonhybridized cDNA with the S_1 nuclease of Aspergillus oryzae (14, 15). DNA excess hybridization was performed in 5 μl of 0.2 M sodium phosphate, pH 6.8 and 0.5 % SDS containing 200–400 cpm of either [3]H- or ^{125}I-labeled RNA. Various amounts of ^{32}P-labeled mouse globin cDNA were added to the reaction mixtures which were incubated for 40 hours at 70 °C, in sealed, siliconized, disposable 5 µl micropipettes. After incubation, the reaction mixture was diluted into 2 ml of 2 x SSC (0.3 M NaCl, 0.03 M Na citrate) and incubated for 30 minutes at 37 °C in the presence of 20 µg/ml of boiled pancreatic RNase. Yeast RNA was added to a final concentration of 0.4 mg/ml and TCA added to a final concentration of 10 %. The TCA precipitable radioactivity, collected on Millipore filters was assayed in a Beckman liquid scintillation counter and correction made vor ^{32}P counts.

3. Results

Erythroid precursor cells at different stages of differentiation were obtained from the spleens of mice with phenylhydrazine-induced hemolytic anemia, by immune hemolysis of the more mature cells followed by separation according size by the velocity sedimentation technique. The differential counts of erythroid cells in the three cell fractions examined are listed in Table 2. Fraction I (120 ml)

Table 2: Differential Counts of Erythroid Cells in Velocity Sedimentation Fractions Before and After Culture with Erythropoietin

Velocity Sediment-ation Fraction	Hours in Culture	Erythro-poietin	Pro-normo-blasts	Baso-philic Normo-blasts	Poly-chromat-ophilic Normo-blasts	Ortho-chromat-ophilic Normo-blasts	Enucleat-ed RBCs
			%*	%*	%*	%*	%*
I	0	0	73.3	17.8	7.7	1.0	
	16	+	18.5	35.8	24.3	17.6	5.5
	16	–	1.6	7.0	24.6	48.9	17.9
III	0	0	34.1	30.4	31.3	4.3	
	16	+	1.9	14.6	28.6	34.0	20.3
V	0	0	4.4	25.0	48.7	21.0	
	16	+	0.0	0.9	21.3	56.8	21.3

* Percentage of all erythroid cells. Slides were prepared by cytocentrifugation, stained with benzidine-Wright-Giemsa, and differential cell counts performed on 400 cells using a modification of criteria outlined in Reference no. 5.

contained primarily pronormoblasts 73.3 %), the earliest recognizable erythroid precursor, and basophilic normoblasts (17.8 %). Only 8.7 % of the cells contained demonstrable hemoglobin as evidenced by positive staining with benzidine. The more slowly sedimenting fractions (60 ml each) contained progressively smaller, more mature cells. Fraction III contained approximately equal numbers of pronormoblasts, basophilic normoblasts and polychromatophilic normoblasts, while fraction V consisted primarily of poly- and orthochromatophilic normoblasts. As shown in Table 2, cells from these fractions underwent progressive maturation when cultured for 16 hours in the presence of erythropoietin. Concomitantly, there was a 39–60 % rise in cell number leading to a substantial increase in the absolute numbers of the more mature erythroid cells in each cell population cultured. Cells cultured without erythropoietin differentiated but did not proliferate. Cells from the velocity sedimentation fractions actively synthesized heme and hemoglobin and these functions were also erythropoietin-responsive. The results of heme and globin synthesis by these cells have been reported in detail elsewhere (16). In summary, the results show that, in these cells, heme synthesis is maximal at an earlier stage of differentiation than hemoglobin synthesis indicating a certain degree of asynchronism between heme and hemoglobin synthesis during erythroid cell maturation. These results are summarized in Figure 2. The results of the latter studies

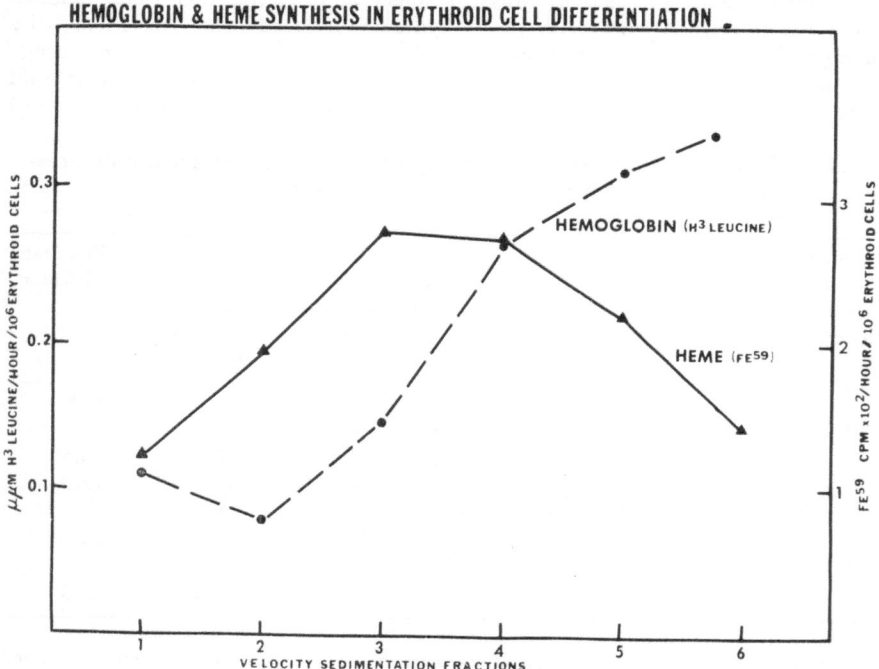

Fig. 2: Relative rates of heme and globin synthesis in the erythroid cells of the various velocity sedimentation cell fractions. The detailed results have been previously published (16) and the figure represents a summary of these results, which indicate a degree of asynchrony between heme and globin synthesis during erythroid cell maturation.

also suggested that erythropoietin is capable of stimulating biochemical differentiation of erythroid precursor cells *in vitro* (16).

Globin mRNA content of the cells was assayed immediately after velocity sedimentation and after culture of replicate samples in the presence of erythropoietin.

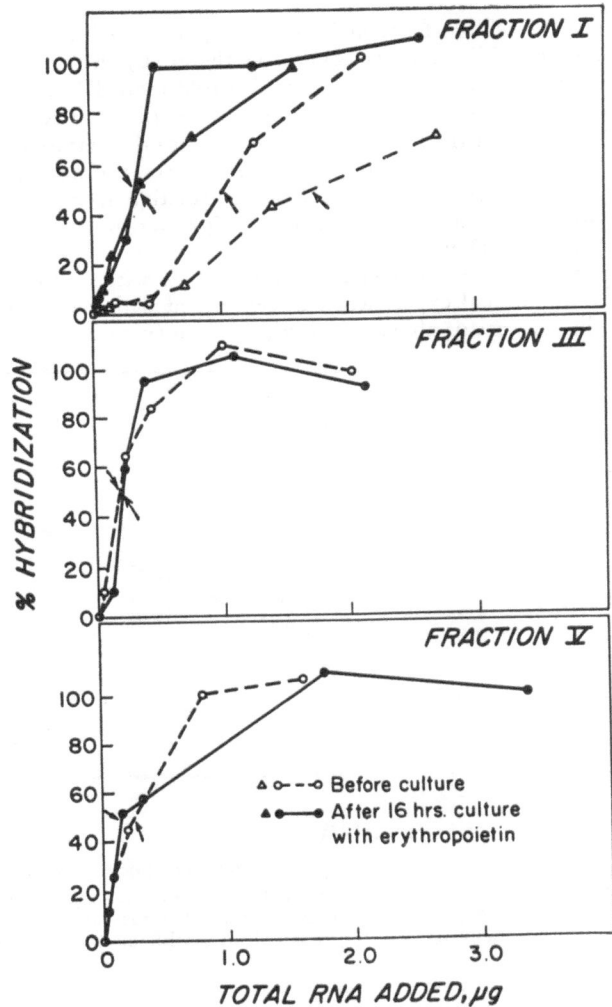

Fig. 3: Hybridization saturation curves using a constant amount of cDNA and increasing amounts of total cellular RNA extracted from velocity sedimentation Fractions I, III, V. Arrows designate 50 % hybridization. The details of the hybridization reaction and its assay are described in Methods. In Fraction I, RNA for the curve (0) was extracted from cells with the differential count listed in Table 2; for the curve (△) the RNA was extracted from a cell population containing only 2.0 % benzidine positive cells (81.5 % pronormoblasts, 16.5 % basophilic normoblasts, 2 % polychromatophilic normoblasts).

Figure 3 shows a series of hybridization-saturation curves using a constant amount of labeled cDNA and increasing amounts of total cellular RNA extracted from the cells in fractions I, III and V. Total cellular RNA varied from about 1.8

A_{260} units per 10^7 cells in fraction I to 1.1 A_{260} units in fraction V. The arrows designate 50 % hybridization. The curve for the most immature cells (fraction I) indicates that 50 % hybridization required 5-fold more RNA than in the more mature fractions III and V; i. e., the proportion of the total RNA that is globin mRNA is 5-fold less in the immature as compared to the mature cells. After overnight incubation of the cells with erythropoietin, the proportion of total RNA that was globin mRNA increased markedly in fraction I; approaching the levels found initially in the more mature fractions. However, no significant change was observed in fractions III and V.

Since globin mRNA levels increased after culture with erythropoietin only in fraction I, an additional experiment was performed with cells from this fraction cultured in the presence or absence of erythropoietin (Figure 4). The 50 % hybrid-

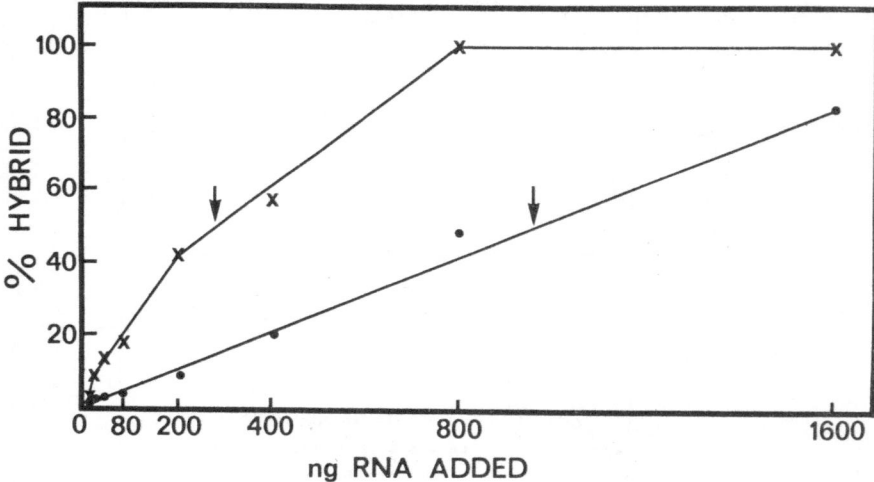

Fig. 4: Hybridization saturation curves using ^{32}p-labeled cDNA and increasing amounts of total cellular RNA from cells of Fraction I cultured in the presence (x) or absence (●) of erythropoietin. Arrows designate 50 % hybridization. The saturation curve for the cells prior to culture was similar to that for cells cultured without erythropoietin and is not presented.

ization values in this experiment indicate that about 3.5 times more globin mRNA was present in the cells cultured with erythropoietin. The level of globin mRNA after culture without erythropoietin was similar to that observed in the same cells prior to culture.

In one experiment the amounts of antiserum and complement used for immune lysis were titered so as to remove nearly all benzidine positive cells (Fig. 3). After velocity sedimentation fraction I contained only 2.0 % benzidine positive polychromatophilic normoblasts. Although the point of 50 % hybridization was achieved with approximately 1.5-fold more added RNA than in previous experiments, the hybridization curve still demonstrated significant levels of globin mRNA.

The quantity of globin mRNA present as a percent of the total cellular RNA was determined by reference to a standard curve for purified mouse globin mRNA hybridized to the same cDNA used in previous studies (14). Levels of mRNA observed in the most immature cells (fraction I) were about 0.008–0.013 % of total cellular RNA and increased to 0.05–0.075 % in more mature precursors (Table 3).

Table 3: Amounts of Globin mRNA in Velocity Sedimentation Fractions Before and After Culture with Erythropoietin

Velocity sedimentation fraction	Hours in culture	Expt. no.:	RNA hybridized to cDNA as % of cell RNA*			
			1	2	3	4
I	0		0.013	0.009	0.012	0.0083
	16		0.05	0.043	–	–
III	0		0.075	–	0.05	–
	16		0.075	–	–	–
V	0		0.075	–	–	–
	16		0.075	–	–	–

* See text for calculation of values.

Similar levels have been observed by Harrison *et al* in studies of fetal erythroid cells (17). On culture with erythropoietin, globin mRNA increased 4–5-fold in fraction I, but remained constant in fraction III and in fraction V. The apparent stability of globin mRNA in the more mature fractions was associated with morphologic maturation to the point that large numbers of orthochromatophilic normoblasts and enucleated RBC's were now present (Table 2).

To demonstrate definitively *de novo* synthesis of globin mRNA, cells from fraction I were cultured in the presence of ^{3}H-uridine and erythropoietin for 16 hours. The poly(A) containing RNA fraction was then isolated by oligo(dT) cellulose chromatography of the total cellular RNA. Approximately 5 % to 8 % of the ^{3}H-labeled RNA was initally bound and subsequently eluted from the oligo(dT) cellulose column. The level of globin mRNA in the poly(A) containing RNA was estimated by hybridization to varying amounts of ^{32}P-labeled mouse globin cDNA. The fraction of ^{3}H-labeled material in hybrid form was determined by resistance of the hybrid to digestion with RNase. Mouse globin mRNA labeled with ^{125}I *in vitro* was also hybridized to mouse globin cDNA to serve as a control. The results are shown in Table 4. At least 65 % of the ^{125}I mRNA could be protected from RNase digestion by the globin cDNA, indicating that the cDNA contains at least 65 % of the sequences of the globin mRNA molecule. Protection of ^{3}H-labeled RNA was about 50 % suggesting that at least 50 % of the stable poly(A) containing cytoplasmic RNA synthesized by erythroid cells of fraction I during the 16 hour incubation period was specifically globin mRNA.

Table 4: DNA Excess Hybridization of Radioactive RNA

RNA added	ng cDNA added	cpm RNA Hybridized	% Hybridization
A) ^{3}H-uridine labeled poly A-containing RNA	0	39.4	–
	0.5	52.7	10
	1.0	60.8	16.5
	2.5	68.9	23
	5	99.2	46.5
	6.6	105.0	51
B) ^{125}I-labeled Mouse Reticulocyte 10S RNA	0	33.3	–
	0.01	44.3	4
	0.025	57.7	7
	0.05	102.5	18
	0.1	192.0	40.5
	0.25	185.5	39
	0.5	244.2	54
	1.0	287.8	65

A fixed amount of radioactive RNA was hybridized to the indicated amounts of cDNA. The quantity of cDNA was calculated on the basis of the specific activity of α-^{32}P-TTP incorporated into the cDNA. The details of the hybridization reaction and its assay are outlined in Methods.

A) Reaction mixtures contained 149 cpm of ^{3}H-labeled RNA derived from the cytoplasm of mouse spleen cells of Fraction I incubated overnight in the presence of erythropoietin and ^{3}H-uridine. Only the poly A-containing RNA (bound to oligo-(dT)-cellulose) was utilized.

B) Reaction mixture contained 418 cpm of ^{125}I-labeled mouse reticulocyte 10S globin mRNA, which had been purified by oligo(dT)-cellulose chromatography prior to iodination. Background was 20 cpm.

4. Discussion

The purpose of this study was to investigate the development of globin mRNA in erythroid cells in an experimental system in which cell differentiation can be readily assessed *in vitro* and which is responsive to erythropoietin. The cell separation methods employed yielded a population of immature cells which contained low levels of globin mRNA but in which the level of globin mRNA increased substantially during the course of incubation with erythropoietin.

The most immature erythroid cell population isolated by the cell separation procedures was comprised primarily of pronormoblasts, the earliest recognizable erythroid cell, whereas the most mature cell population contained predominantly well hemoglobinized precursors. Small amounts of globin mRNA were already detectable in the earliest cell fraction, but levels were higher by a factor of 4–5 in the more mature nucleated erythroid cells. This suggested that the latter must have synthesized significant amounts of globin mRNA as they matured *in vivo*. A similar correlation between globin mRNA levels and progression of erythroid cell maturation has been demonstrated with erythroid cells from the spleens of mice after phenylhydrazine treatment, using a cell-free translation assay (18, 19).

New synthesis of mRNA during erythroid cell maturation was demonstrated more directly in the short-term culture experiments. As the cells in fraction I underwent morphological differentiation *in vitro*, there was a substantial increase in the content of globin mRNA. This change was found only when the cells were cultured in the presence of erythropoietin. Newly synthesized ^{3}H-labeled globin mRNA could also be demonstrated in the ^{3}H-uridine labeled RNA of these cultured cells, using RNA-cDNA hybridization (Table 4). On the other hand, the levels of globin mRNA remained stable with culture of the more mature cell fractions. Erythropoietin has also been shown to increase the globin mRNA content of fetal liver erythroid cells, as measured by both translational (20) and hybridization assays (21).

The precise point in the sequence of erythroid differentiation at which globin mRNA synthesis is initiated is yet to be determined. Terada *et al* have studied this problem by using translation in a cell-free system to assay globin mRNA in primitive erythroid cells from mouse fetal liver (20). These authors found negligible levels of functional globin mRNA in cell populations consisting of about 30 % proerythroblasts, 70 % basophilic erythroblasts and less than 7 % benzidine positive cells. These cells required culture with erythropoietin for at least ten hours before their RNA developed the capacity to direct globin synthesis. Ramirez *et al* (21) using hybridization techniques have found only negligible amounts of globin mRNA in very early fetal erythroid cells, but this level increased 250-fold after culture for 22 hours in the presence of erythropoietin. Using similar cDNA:RNA hybridization assays, we have consistently detected small but significant levels of globin mRNA in the very early erythroid cell population of fraction I.

The low levels of globin mRNA already present in this youngest cell population may have been contributed in part by the nearly 9 % benzidine-positive cells that contaminated this fraction (Table 2). However, substantial hybridization was observed in an experiment in which fraction I contained only 2 % benzidine-positive cells (Fig. 3). Thus, early cells apparently did contain much of the globin mRNA found in the RNA of fraction I cells. This result indicates that there is more biochemical differentiation in these cells than is apparent from the morphology of these otherwise very primitive cells. The erythroid cells were obtained from animals with severe anemia and hence had been subjected to high levels of erythropoietin *in vivo*. As suggested by Harrison *et al* (17), erythropoietin may increase the proportion of pronormoblasts containing globin mRNA.

Other findings which lend support to the presence of globin mRNA in immature erythroid cells have been reported by Harrison *et al* (17, 22). These investigators localized globin mRNA by radioautography after *in situ* hybridization to ^{3}H-labeled cDNA and found a small amount of globin mRNA in the cytoplasm of some pronormoblasts and most basophilic normoblasts from 13.5 day fetal liver in the mouse. The radioautography technique permits localization of mRNA in specific cells, but probably is not as reliable as saturation hybridization to quantitate globin mRNA. The same authors also performed conventional hybridization studies (17), the results of which also indicated that immature fetal erythroid cells contain substantial amounts of globin mRNA. These studies in fetal erythroid cells are therefore very similar to the findings for adult erythroid precursors in the present study. Unexplained are the differences between these results and those which suggest very low levels of globin mRNA in the immature fetal system (20, 21).

The new techniques used in this and other recent studies begin to make it possible to investigate the specific mechanisms controlling the synthesis of globin mRNA. Several groups (23–25) have shown that erythropoietin stimulates the synthesis of several species of RNA in cultures of erythroid precursor cells, but no specific assays were used to identify newly synthesized globin mRNA. In future studies, the use of specific hybridization probes now available for the detection of globin mRNA should lead to a better understanding of the interaction between erythropoietin and the expression of the genes that control globin synthesis.

IV. Summary and Conclusions

We have reviewed erythroid cell differentiation from two points of view: 1) differences between fetal and adult human red cells with particular reference to alterations which can occur in the normal pattern of erythroid cell development during the course of leukemia; 2) beochemical events which occur during erythroid cell maturation, as a model system for the study of the control of gene expression.

During the course of many leukemias there is the synthesis of red cells containing fetal hemoglobin. In most cases this phenomenon is limited to a small population or clone of red cells and probably represents a nonspecific response of the bone marrow to a hematologic stress. However, in juvenile chronic myeloid leukemia and, in rare cases of erythroleukemia, there is a major reversion to fetal erythropoiesis, with progressive increase in fetal hemoglobin levels and synthesis of red cells which contain not only fetal hemoglobin but have a true fetal pattern of protein synthesis affecting proteins other than Hb F, namely Hb A_2, carbonic anhydrase and the membrane antigens i and I. In this case, the fetal erythropoiesis may be a more specific manifestation of the leukemic process and may be related to the phenomenon of fetal protein synthesis (α-fetoprotein of carcinoembryonic antigen) observed in other types of neoplasia.

Further information on the etiology and pathogenesis of abnormal cell proliferation and differentiation in the leukemias can be obtained by the study of experimental systems permitting the investigation of the regulation of gene expression in differentiating mammalian cells. Maturing erythroid cells provide a promsing system for such investigations for many reasons: differentiating erythroid cells can be obtained relatively free of other cell types; a large amount of a well characterized product, hemoglobin, is synthesized; techniques are now available that permit isolation of erythroid precursors at different stages of differentiation (5–8); and finally, highly sensitive methods of measuring globin mRNA levels by DNA-RNA hybridization are currently available (13, 26, 27). We have used such techniques to measure levels of globin mRNA in separated populations of murine erythroid cells at different stages of maturation. These studies demonstrated a correlation between globin mRNA content and degree of morphological maturation. In the least well differentiated cells, however, there appeared to be a disproportionate amount of mRNA for the level of hemoglobin synthesis in these cells. These results suggest the presence of some translational control of globin mRNA in the early stages of erythroid development, although the major control of globin gene expression in this system seems to be at the transcriptional level. Finally, when the immature erythroid cells were cultured in the presence of erythropoietin, *de novo* synthesis of ^{3}H-uridine labeled globin mRNA was demonstrated by the specific RNA-cDNA hybridization assay. These results clearly demonstrate the utility of this model system and these techniques for the study of the interaction between a specific gene and the factors which regulate or modulate its expression.

Acknowledgements

This work was supported by grants from the U.S.P.H.S., Medical Foundation, Inc., Boston, Massachusetts, and National Cancer Institute of Canada. B. Forget is the recipient of a Research Career Development Award from the U.S.P.H.S. J. Glass was supported in part by a fellowship from the Medical Foundation, Inc., Boston. Human urinary erythropoietin (H-4-S4-6SL, 153.0 units/mg) was supplied by the National Institutes of Health. The erythropoietin was collected and concentrated by the Department of Physiology, University of the Northwest, Corrientes, Argentina, and further processed and assayed by the Hematology Research Laboratories, Children's Hospital of Los Angeles, under Research Grant HE-10880. We thank Dr. J. Beard for prividing the avain myeloblastosis virus, and Drs. D. Nathan and S. Robinson for helpful discussions. V. Crickley, L. Lavidor and D. Paci provided skilled technical assistance.

References

1. Hamilton, R. W., Schwartz, E., Atwater, J., and Erslev, A. J. (1971), New Engl. J. Med., *285*, 1217.
2. Pagnier, J., Labie, D., Kaplan, J. C., Junien, C., Najman, A., and Leroux, J. P. (1972), Nouv. Rev. Fr. Hematol., *12*, 317.
3. Weatherall, D. J., Pembrey, M. E., and Pritchard, J. (1974), Clinics in Haematol., *3*, 467.
4. Sheridan, B. L., Weatherall, D. J., Clegg, J. B., Pritchard, J. et al. (1976), Brit. J. Haematol., *32*, 487.
4a. Alter, B. P., Rappeport, J. M., Huisman, T. H. J., and Schroeder, W. A. (1975), Blood 46, 1054.
5. Borsook, H., Ratner, K., and Tattrie, B. (1969), Blood, *34*, 32.
6. Cantor, L., Morris, A., Marks, P., and Rifkind, R. (1972), Proc. Nat. Acad. Sci. (USA), *69*, 1337.
7. Miller, R., and Phillips, R. A. (1969), J. Cell Physiol., *73*, 191.
8. Denton, M. J., and Arnstein, H. R. V. (1973), Brit. J. Haematol., *24*, 7.
9. Aviv, H., and Leder, P. (1972), Proc. Nat. Acad. Sci. (USA), *69*, 1408.
10. Williamson, R., Morrison, M., Lanyon, G., Eason, R., and Paul, J. (1971), Biochemistry, *10*, 3014.
11. Prensky, W., Steffensen, D. M., and Hughes, W. L. (1973), Proc. Nat. Acad. Sci. (USA), *70*, 1860.

12. Verma, I. M., and Baltimore, D. (1973). In Methods in Enzymology, *29*, L. Grossman and K. Moldave, eds. (New York: Academic Press) p. 125.
13. Verma, I. M., Temple, G. F., Fan, H., and Baltimore, D. (1972), Nature New Biology, *235*, 163.
14. Preisler, H. D., Housman, D., Scher, W., and Friend, C. (1973), Proc. Nat. Acad. Sci. (USA), *70*, 2956.
15. Housman, D., Forget, B., Skoultchi, A., and Benz, E. (1973), Proc. Nat. Acad. Sci. (USA), *70*, 1809.
16. Glass, J., Lavidor, L. M., and Robinson, S. H. (1975), J. Cell Biol., *65*, 298.
17. Harrison, P. R., Conkie, D., Affara, N., and Paul, J. (1974), J. Cell Biol., *63*, 402.
18. Cheng, T., Polmar, S. K., and Kazazian, H. H., Jr. (1974), J. Biol. Chem., *249*, 1781.
19. Kazazian, H. H., Cheng, T., Polmar, S. K., and Gunder, G. D. (1974), Ann. N.Y. Acad. Sci., *241*, 170.
20. Terada, M., Cantor, L., Metafora, S., Rifkind, R., Bank, A., and Marks, P. A. (1972), Proc. Nat. Acad. Sci. (USA), *69*, 3575.
21. Ramirez, F., Gambino, R., Maniatis, G. M., Rifkind, R. A., Marks, P. A., and Bank, A. (1975), J. Biol. Chem., *250*, 6054.
22. Harrison, P. R., Conkie, D., and Paul, J. (1973), FEBS Letters, *32*, 109.
23. Gross, M., and Goldwasser, E. (1969), Biochemistry, *8*, 1795.
24. Maniatis, G. M., Rifkind, R. A., Bank, A., and Marks, P. A. (1973), Proc. Nat. Acad. Sci. (USA), *69*, 3575.
25. Nicol, A. G., Conkie, D., Lanyon, W. G., Drewunkiewiez, C. G., Williamson, R., and Paul, J. (1972), Biochim. Biophys. Acta, *277*, 342.
26. Kacian, D. L., Spiegelman, S., Bank, A., Terada, M., Metafora, S., Dow, L., and Marks, P. A. (1972), Nature New Biology, *235*, 167.
27. Ross, J., Aviv, H., Scolnick, E., and Leder, P. (1972), Proc. Nat. Acad. Sci. (USA), *69*, 264.

Molecular Mechanisms in Erythroid Differentiation

John Paul

Beatson Institute for Cancer Research,
132 Hill Street, Glasgow G3 6UD, Scotland.

The most striking molecular event during erythroid differentiation is the accumulation of haemoglobin but this is only one of many overt changes which occur in the maturing erythroid cell. Other proteins accumulate progressively, notably carbonic anhydrase and catalase while yet others, particularly the enzymes of haem synthesis, such as aminolaevulinic acid synthetase, accumulate during early maturation and diminish later (Freshney, R. I. and Paul, J. 1972). Membrane changes also occur. These include the accumulation of spectrin on the inner surface of the membrane, of specific antigens on the outer surface and changes in lectin binding properties. Simultaneously, there is progressive reduction of transcription leading eventually to a complete cessation of RNA synthesis and, indeed, in most mammals, to the extrusion of the nucleus itself. These changes are orchestrated in the orderly manner that we associate with many differentiating systems and, for this reason, erythropoiesis has been regarded as a very good model for investigating normal differentiation in mammals and, hopefully, therefore, for providing information about the mechanisms which are disturbed in leukaemia.

In any experimental situation, it is desirable that one should be able to initiate the process at will and to follow at least some components of it in detail. Erythroid tissues readily respond to increased demand and at least part of this response is mediated through erythropoietin which is produced in the juxtaglomerular cells of the kidney in response to anoxia and promotes the maturation of erythroblasts. It has been possible to purify erythropoietin at least partially and to demonstrate its effects on cultured erythroid tissue *in vitro* (Krantz, S. B., Gallien, Lartigue, O. and Goldwasser, E. 1963; Krantz, S. B. and Goldwasser, E. 1965; Cole, R. J. and Paul, J. 1966). Hence, part of the requirement can be met by using these techniques. Relatively recently, however, an alternative system of considerable power has emerged following the discovery that Friend erythroleukaemic cells of the mouse can be induced to synthesise large amounts of haemoglobin when treated with dimethylsulphoxide although normally they synthesise minimal amounts (Friend, C., Scher, W., Holland, J. G. and Sato, T. 1971; Scher, W., Holland, J. G. and Friend, C. 1971). Experiments with both these systems will be discussed.

In analysing the places in metabolic pathways where the accumulation of a protein can be controlled, the first principle to be appreciated is that accumulation occurs when synthesis exceeds degradation. This applies both to the final product, the protein, and also to intermediates in its synthesis such as messenger RNA. Degradation is unquestionably just as important as synthesis but here are more

125

technical difficulties in studying changes in rates of degradation than in studying changes in patterns of synthesis. Moreover, powerful new tools have been fashioned in recent years to enable us to study the synthesis of specific messenger RNA in cells. Accordingly, this communication will deal mainly with information concerned with the synthesis and accumulation of globin and the nucleic acids involved in its synthesis. However, it is emphasised that our knowledge will be incomplete until we have an equally detailed understanding of degradative processes.

Control of globin synthesis could, theoretically, occur at several levels. There could be an increase in the number of genes for globin chains (gene amplification): the rate at which RNA is transcribed from DNA in chromatin could alter: the processing of newly transcribed RNA into messenger RNA could be subject to control: finally, the efficiency of utilisation of messenger RNA in the translational machinery could be involved. Each of these will be discussed.

Experimental Methods

Globin messenger RNA – The greatest single technical advance in this work has been the isolation of pure messenger RNAs (Williamson, R., Morrison, M., Lanyon, W. G., Eason, R. and Paul, J. 1971). Since a messenger RNA is a direct transcript of a gene, it bears the same absolutely specific relationship to the sense strand of that gene as does a photographic print to its negative. Moreover, it is possible to form hybrid molecules between RNA and DNA and thus it can be used as an absolutely specific probe for globin gene sequences.

Globin messenger RNA was initially isolated from reticulocyte polysomes on the basis of size. More recently, other techniques have become available, especially techniques of affinity chromatography which exploit the existence of a polyadenylate tract at the 3' end of messenger RNA. These methods make it possible to isolate globin messenger RNA in large amounts. That it is a messenger RNA molecule can be proven by using it to programme a cell-free protein synthesising system to make α and β globin chains.

Complementary DNA – The second important technical advance has been the discovery of techniques to prepare DNA copies of messenger RNA with the enzyme reverse transcriptase from RNA tumour viruses (Kacian, D. L. and Spiegelman, S. 1972; Ross, J., Aviv, H., Scolnick, E. and Leder, P. 1972). Since cDNA is an exact transcript of messenger RNA, it is a precise replica of at least part of the sense strand of the globin gene. Consequently, it can be used as an absolutely specific probe both for the nonsense strand of the globin gene and also for globin messenger RNA. Since it is possible to synthesise it at very high specific activity, it is not only an absolutely specific probe but an exquisitely sensitive one.

Results

Is there a change in globin gene number during erythroid differentiation? At least three major possibilities must be entertained. The first is that every cell in an organism has the same number of globin genes. The second is that globin genes are segregated in such a way that most cells have no globin genes whereas erythroid cells do. The third possibility is that all, or most, cells contain globin genes but the number is increased in erythroid tissues, like the ribosomal genes in amphibian oocytes. Within the past two or three years, methods have been devised for measuring the concentration of globin genes in DNA using either messenger RNA or cDNA. The kinetic analysis is very sensitive and has made it possible to determine that, on average, each globin gene occupies about 4×10^{-7} of the genome, i. e. there are 1–2 copies of each globin gene sequence in each genome. These methods are so specific and so sensitive that they have made it possible recently to show that α-thalassaemia is due to a deletion involving the two α genes in the human (Ottolenghi, S., Lanyon, W. G., Paul, J., Williamson, R., Clegg, J., Pritchard, J., Pootrakul, J. and Wong Hock Boon, 1974).

These methods were used to investigate globin gene dosage in different animal tissues (Harrison, P. R., Birnie, G. D., Hell, A., Humphries, S., Young, B. D. and Paul, J. 1974). In particular, we estimated the globin gene concentration in DNA from mouse sperm, from the total mouse embryo and from mouse foetal liver (which is an active erythropoietic tissue). We found that the concentration of globin genes was identical in all three kinds of DNA and corresponded to about one copy of each gene per genome. Hence, the gene segregation and amplification hypotheses can be discarded; all tissues in the mouse seem to have one copy of each globin gene per genome.

Is there evidence for regulation of transcription of the globin gene? It has been shown by a number of workers that it is possible to transcribe mammalian chromatin with bacterial RNA polymerase and that the transcript resembles very closely the nuclear RNA of the cell from which the chromatin was derived. We, therefore, undertook experiments to determine whether we could demonstrate differences between chromatin from erythroid and non-erythroid tissues. Chromatin from mouse foetal liver and from brain was transcribed with *E. coli* RNA polymerase and cDNA was then used to measure the concentration of globin messenger RNA in the transcript (Gilmour, R. S. and Paul, J. 1971; Paul, J., Gilmour, R. S., Affara, N., Birnie, G. D., Harrison, P. R., Hell, A., Humphries, S., Windass, J. and Young, B. 1974). These experiments revealed detectable amounts of newly synthesised globin messenger RNA in the RNA transcribed from mouse foetal liver chromatin but no detectable globin messenger RNA in the RNA transcribed from brain chromatin (Table 1). This, therefore, provided presumptive evidence for transcriptional specificity embodied in the structure of the chromatin itself.

Are there controls at other levels? In the reticulocyte, there is good evidence that

Table I: **Transcription of the globin gene from chromatin by E. coli RNA-dependent RNA polymerase (see Paul et al. 1974, Cold Spring Harbour Symp. Quant. Biol. 28, 885.**

Source of Chromatin	Globin mRNA as fraction of total RNA synthesised $\times 10^7$
Mouse brain	< 3
Mouse fetal liver (erythroid)	25

a control exists at the level of translation. This evidence indicates that there is a high molecular weight diffusible repressor of globin synthesis, the effect of which is inhibited by haemin (Gross, 1974). Hence, haemin can act as an inducer of translation of globin from messenger RNA. Evidence to be cited later indicates that controls at this level may also occur in maturing erythroblasts.

Mode of Action of Erythropoietin – The most primitive erythroid cell to be identified positively in the adult mammal is the colony forming cell (CFC); it can be demonstrated by injecting bone marrow into animals which have received a lethal dose of irradiation, such as to eliminate their own erythroid capacities. If a small enough dose of bone marrow is injected, colonies form in the spleens of the recipient animals and these can give rise either to granulocyte or erythroid cells. There is evidence too that these then give rise to a cell, the erythropoietin-sensitive cell (ESC) which is capable of developing into mature erythroid cells on treatment with erythropoietin. In theory, therefore, erythropoietin could act by influencing the decision of a stem cell to form granuloid or erythroid tissue or to increase, by multiplication, the number of ESC, or again, by stimulating the erythropoietin-sensitive cells to enter into maturation rather than self-maintaining cell divisions or, more specifically, by stimulating the synthesis of globin and other messenger RNAs. There is good experimental evidence against the first and second of these hypotheses, rather good evidence to support the third and mixed evidence concerning the last. Unfortunately, it has not proved possible to culture CFC and ESC continuously. Consequently, most of these deductions are drawn from experiments in whole animals which are sometimes difficult to interpret and experiments with tissue culture material of foetal liver which relate to stages from the proerythroblast onwards. Nevertheless, in short-term cultures, it has proved possible to demonstrate quite striking effects of erythropoietin.

When mouse foetal liver from embryos of 12–14 days gestation is cultured *in vitro*, it retains some capacity to synthesise haemoglobin but this diminishes quite rapidly in the course of 48–72 hours. On the other hand, if erythropoietin is added, then after a lag of about 2 hours, there is increased synthesis of DNA, RNA and haemoglobin at rates which continue to increase for 24 hours and at that time are considerably greater than those of untreated tissue (Figure 1) (Cole, R. J. and Paul, J. 1966; Paul, J. and Hunter, J. 1969; Ortega, J. A. and Dukes, P. P. 1970; Gross, M. and Goldwasser, E. 1969; Gross, M. and Goldwasser, E. 1970; Nicol, A. G., Conkie, D., Lanyon, W. G., Drewienkiewicz, C. E., Williamson, R. and Paul, J. 1972).

Some reports about the response to erythropoietin differ. The increases in messenger RNA and protein synthesis are generally agreed by all workers. Paul and Hunter (1969) originally proposed that while there was an early increase in RNA synthesis, this was followed by an obligatory DNA synthetic step before a specific increase in globin messenger RNA and haemoglobin synthesis occurred. Similar observations have been made by Gross and Goldwasser (1969; 1970) but these have been disputed by Djaldetti, Marks and Rifkind (1972) although this group reported that a rapid decrease in DNA synthesis, which they observed in their cells in culture, was prevented by erythropoietin. Paul. J., Freshney, R. I., Conkie, D. and Burgos, H. (1971) and Harrison, P. R., Conkie, D. and Paul, J. (1973) are of the view that the entire erythropoietin effect in short-term cultures

128

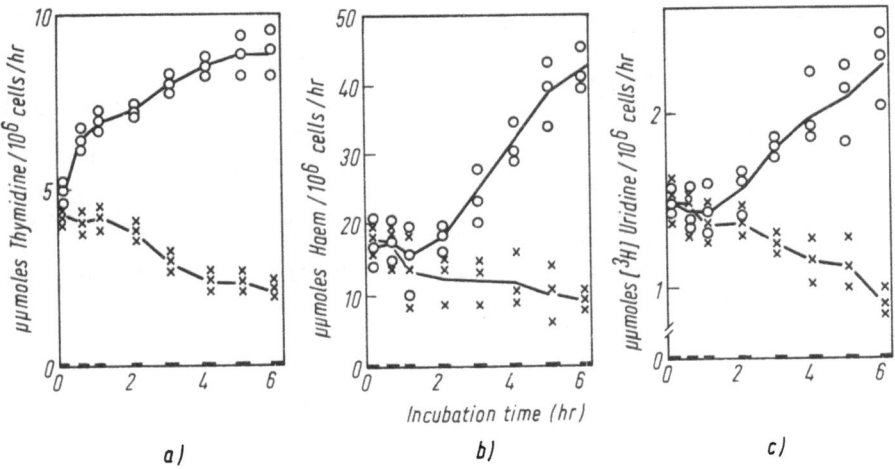

Fig. 1: Rates of synthesis of DNA (a), haemoglobin (b) and RNA (c) in primary mouse foetal liver cultures in the presence or absence of erythropoietin, -x-x-, control; -o-o-o, erythropoietin present from zero time. Labelled precursors were added during the times indicated in the time axis.
(Paul, J. and Hunter, J. A. (1969) P. N. A. S. *42*, 31)

can be explained by increased production of haemoglobin-synthesising cells, achieved by promotion of division of proerythroblasts. They claim that many of the resulting 'G2' cells are unable to divide in tissue culture and form giant cells which are double-sized and contained double the normal amount of haemo-globin. It is certainly agreed that there is no specific increase in the rate of globin synthesis per cell as a result of erythropoietin treatment although there is some disagreement concerning the rate of RNA synthesis.

In this discussion, it is obviously of importance to determine at what stage in erythroid development globin messenger RNA synthesis commences. There is diffi-culty about obtaining sufficient amounts of pure populations of immature eryth-roid cells to permit direct biochemical studies with globin cDNA. Accordingly, Harrison, P. R., Conkie, D., Affara, N. and Paul, J. (1974) applied an *in situ* hybridisation method, developed by Harrison, P. R., Conkie, D., Paul, J. and Jones, K. (1973) which permits the demonstration of the distribution of globin messenger RNA in individual cells. Using this technique, they were able to show that globin messenger RNA makes its appearance during the transition from pro-erythroblast to basophilic erythroblast. This observation is of considerable interest for a number of reasons. For one thing, haemoglobin synthesis is usually not detectable until the next stage in differentiation, the polychromatic erythroblast stage. Hence, the observation provides presumptive evidence for translational control. Secondly, an increase in the number of basophilic erythroblasts at the expense of proerythroblasts is produced by erythropoietin and this also results in the appearance of globin messenger RNA in a few late proerythroblasts. This observation can be considered in the context of other observations by Paul, J.,

Freshney, R. I., Conkie, D. and Burgos, H. (1971) which indicated that erythropoietin was necessary for the completion of cell division in some proerythroblastic cells. It seems possible that erythropoietin is needed to facilitate the maturation divisions which occur in erythrocyte precursors. These may be essential for the transition to occur and to permit activation of globin genes.

The Friend Cell System – Experiments with short-term primary cultures of erythroid tissues have given us some idea of the ways in which globin synthesis may be regulated but unfortunately they leave us with a very incomplete picture of mechanisms. The discovery of the induction of haemoglobin synthesis by dimethylsulphoxide in the Friend system has provided us with a means of studying some of the molecular events (Figure 2).

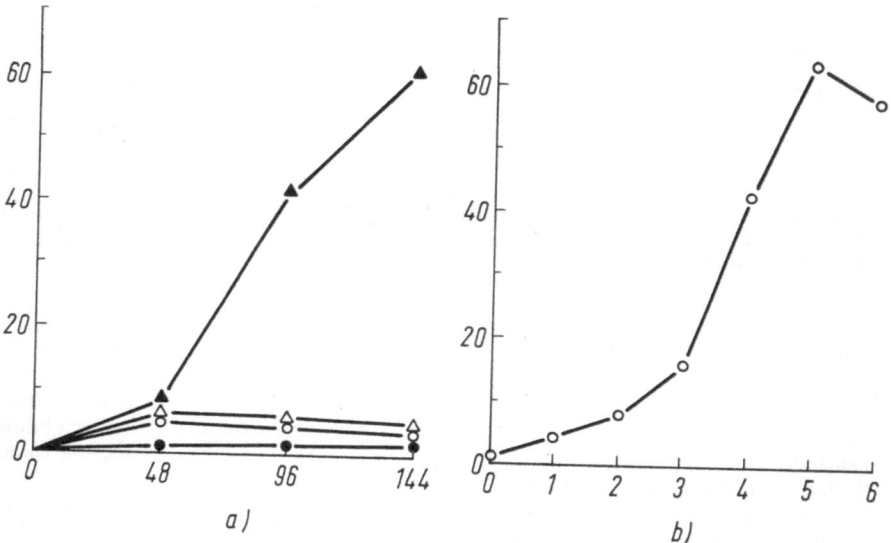

Fig. 2: Induction of haem and benzidine-stained cells following treatment of Friend cells with 2 % DMSO.
1. Abscissa: time (hours; ordinate, pmoles haem/10^6 cells.
FtID+, no DMSO added ($\triangle$–$\triangle$); DMSO added ($\blacktriangle$–$\blacktriangle$).
FwID-, no DMSO added (o-o); DMSO added ($\bullet$–$\bullet$).
2. Abscissa, time (days); ordinate, percentage of cells staining with benzidine.
FtID+.
(From: Paul, J. and Hickey, I. (1974) E. C. R. *87*, 20).

When Friend cells are grown in suspension cultures, they have a doubling time of 12–14 hours and rarely show evidence of haemoglobinisation. Following treatment with dimethylsulphoxide, haemoglobin synthesis occurs at quite a high rate after a lag period of 24–48 hours. The cells rapidly become haemoglobinised until, after about 5 days, upwards of 80 % contain quite large amounts of haemoglobin. Simultaneously, they exhibit many other phenomena characteristic of erythroid differentiation; cell division diminishes and eventually ceases irreversibly; RNA synthesis diminishes and the nucleus becomes condensed and there is some other evidence that other specific molecules accumulate. The accumulation of haemoglobin is accompanied by an accumulation of globin messenger RNA (Ross, J., Ikawa, Y. and Leder, P. 1972; Harrison, P. R., Gilmour, R. S., Affara, N. A., Conkie, D. and Paul, J. 1974; Gilmour, R. S., Harrison, P. R., Windass, J. D., Affara, N. A. and Paul, J. 1974). This may occur slightly ahead of haemoglobin accumulation but for practical purposes, the two events occur almost simultaneously.

At what level does control of haemoglobin synthesis occur? – To determine whether globin messenger RNA synthesis is the controlling step for subsequent processing and translation, we undertook experiments in which cDNA was used to measure the concentration of globin messenger RNA sequences in nuclear, polysomal and cytosol RNA (the cytosol being the non-polysomal cytoplasmic compartment of the cell) (Harrison, P. R., Gilmour, R. S., Affara, N. A., Conkie, D. and Paul, J. 1974; Gilmour, R. S., Harrison, P. R., Windass, J. D., Affara, N. A. and Paul, J. 1974). To our surprise, in the two substrains we first studied, we found evidence for different mechanisms. In one, designated clone M2, we found low levels of messenger RNA in all three cell compartments in uninduced cells but, on induction with demethylsulphoxide, messenger RNA increased both in nucleus and cytoplasm, although the increase in the polysomes was considerably greater than that in the nucleus. This argues for transcriptional control (and possibly translational control) in this cell line. In the other substrain, designated line 707, however, we found that the increase in messenger RNA on induction was confined to the polysomes; there was no evidence of any increase following induction in nuclei of these cells. Hence, the evidence is strongly in favour of post-transcriptional controls. Further support for these conclusions came from experiments in which chromatin was isolated from the two different cells and transcribed with *E. coli* polymerase. It was found that the concentration of globin messenger RNA sequences in transcripts from chromatin from uninduced M2 cells was low and was much higher in transcripts from chromatin from induced M2 cells; in contrast, it was equally high in chromatin from both uninduced and induced 707 cells. Since clone M2 was originally isolated from the 707 cell population, we concluded that the original population had probably contained cells of M2 types in which both transcriptional and post-transcriptional controls and were rather tightly linked. We postulated that during the course of continuous culture, a cell had arisen in which transcriptional control had become relaxed. This cell had eventually extensively overgrown the original cell so that the culture had the characteristics of the variant, but sufficient of the original cells were present that we were able to pick one out by cloning. Whether this speculation is correct or not, these findings immediately suggested a much higher degree of variation among Friend cell clones than we might have expected.

This observation encouraged us to undertake somatic cell genetic studies with a view to elucidating the situation further (Paul, J. and Hickey, I. 1974). It was found that non-inducible variants could be isolated by culturing Friend cells continuously in DMSO. Those cells which differentiated failed to divide further and the population rapidly became overgrown by non-differentiating cells. We therefore attempted to isolate a number of lines of non-inducible cells, to characterise them and to fuse them with other cells. Inadvertently we had already obtained one non-

131

inducible cell line in the laboratory. This cell line, Fw, is therefore of different origin from the other non-inducible variants which will be referred to.

Using standard procedures, lines of cells were now developed which lacked certain of the salvage enzymes of nucleic acid synthesis, namely thymidine kinase (TK) and hypoxanthine-guanine phosphoribosyl transferse (HGPRT). TK⁻ cells and HGPRT⁻ cells will not grow in HAT medium (containing hypoxanthine, aminopterin and thymidine) whereas wild-type cells will. However, if a TK⁻ HGPRT⁺ cell is fused to a TK⁺ HGPRT⁻ cell, the hybrid will survive in HAT medium by complementation. Accordingly, we first prepared stocks of cells which were either TK⁻ or HGPRT⁻ to facilitate the isolation of hybrids. In an early experiment, a hybrid cell was produced by fusing the non-inducible Fw cell line to an inducible Friend cell. The hybrid cell was found to be inducible although to a lesser degree than the parent. This experiment has now been repeated several times and the same result has always been obtained. It would seem, therefore, that in this fusion, inducibility is dominant and exhibits dosage effect.

Other non-inducible variants were produced by mutagenising the two different cell stocks and isolating variants in the presence of DMSO. Many resistant cell lines were isolated in this way but most of them reverted. The selection was, therefore, performed repeatedly until stable resistant cell lines were obtained. One of these was then fused to an inducible line. In this instance, the hybrid was non-inducible. This cross, therefore, provides evidence for transdominant repression.

The nature of the lesion in the Fw cell was further clarified by the finding that, while DMSO would not by itself induce haemoglobin synthesis, addition of haemin to the medium would. In this instance, it would seem that the defect may lie in the haem synthetic pathway.

Further evidence concerning the control steps was obtained by attempting to obtain hybrids between Friend cells and non-erythroid cell lines. In particular, a hybrid was obtained between an inducible Friend cell and a clone (Ly-T) of the L5178Y lymphoma cell. This cell never synthesises haemoglobin although, interestingly enough, very low concentrations of globin messenger RNA can be measured in nuclear RNA. The hybrid cell line proved incapable of synthesising haemoglobin, but it was found to contain quite significant amounts of globin messenger RNA in both nucleus and cytoplasm. Moreover, on treatment with DMSO, the concentration of globin messenger RNA molecules increased although there was little other evidence of erythroid differentiation. When this cell was treated with haemin as well as DMSO, it was then found that it could make haemoglobin. In other words, this hybrid behaved very much like the non-inducible Fw line which had arisen spontaneously from the original Friend cell line. The behaviour of this hybrid accentuates points which have been already made. Clearly, haemin releases a translational block. On the other hand, hybrid cells can make globin messenger RNA and the levels can be induced to higher levels with treatment with DMSO although this has little or no effect on haemoglobin synthesis in the absence of haemin.

Conclusions

Before attempting to draw conclusions from these results, it is necessary to consider the relationship between DMSO stimulation of the Friend cell and erythropoietin induction of mouse foetal liver cells. When mice are inoculated with Friend virus, there immediately ensues an acute condition called Friend disease which is a polycythemia. This occurs in hypertransfused mice which are producing no erythropoietin as well as in normal mice. In this disease, therefore, the normal erythropoietin machinery seems to be by-passed. Moreover, Friend cells are non-responsive to erythropoietin, confirming the suggestion that in these cells the normal process of erythropoietin regulation is in some way by-passed. It seems quite possible that the Friend cell represents a transformed cell closely related to the erythropoietin-sensitive cell.

It is very likely that in normal differentiation, erythropoietin is responsible for an early event, which results in the commitment of ESC to erythroid differentiation. Experiments with cultured foetal liver suggest that the continued presence of erythropoietin accelerates completion of maturation. In the course of normal erythropoiesis, it may be assumed that there is adequate production of haemin but this may be rate-limiting in many Friend cells and the DMSO effect may have to do with increasing haem availability.

The regulation of maturation of erythroid cells clearly involves a series of co-ordinated events, two of which have been considered here. One is the rate of transcription of the globin gene which appears to increase on induction of many inducible Friend cells. The other is the rate of translation for which there is evidence in all varieties of the Friend cell studied. That this may be an important mechanism *in vivo* is also suggested by the fact that globin messenger can be detected in large amounts in basophilic erythroblasts before haemoglobin synthesis is detectable.

Despite their sophistication, one is aware of the deficiencies of some of these methods. In particular, because the measurement of haemoglobin is insensitive, we have to be cautious about drawing hard and fast conclusions about some of these phenomena. Nevertheless, these studies have given us considerable insight into some of the probable mechanisms involved in differentiation and promise quite soon to yield a detailed understanding.

Acknowledgements

Most of the experimental work reported was carried out by my colleagues, G. D. Birnie, R. S. Gilmour, A. Hell, P. R. Harrison, R. Williamson, B. D. Young, N. A. Affara, D. Conkie, S. Humphries, J. Sommerville and J. Windass under grants from M. R. C. and C. R. C.

References

Cole, R. J. and Paul, J. (1966) The effects of erythropoietin on haem synthesis in mouse yolk sac and cultured foetal liver cells. J. Embryol and Exp. Morph. *15*, 245.

Djaldetti, M., Preisler, H., Marks, P. A. and Rifkind, R. A. (1972) Erythropoietin effects on foetal mouse erythroid cells. II. Nucleic acid synthesis and the erythropoietin-sensitive cell. J. Biol. Chem. *247*, 731.

Freshney, R. I. and Paul, J. (1972) The activities of three enzymes of haem synthesis during hepatic erythropoiesis in the mouse embryo. J. Embryol. and Exp. Morph. *26*, 313.

Friend, C., Scher, W., Holland, J. G. and Sato, T. (1971) Haemoglobin synthesis in murine virus-induced leukaemic cells *in vitro*: stimulation of erythroid differentiation by dimethylsulfoxide. Proc. Nat. Acad. Sci. *68*, 378.

Gilmour, R. S., Harrison, P. R., Windass, J. D., Affara, N. A. and Paul, J. (1974) Globin messenger RNA synthesis and processing during haemoglobin induction in Friend cells. I. Evidence for transcriptional control in clone M2. Cell Differ. *3*, 9.

Gilmour, R. S. and Paul, J. (1971) Tissue-specific transcription of the globin gene in isolated chromatin. Proc. Nat. Acad. Sci. *70*, 3440.

Gross, M. (1974) Control of globin synthesis by hemin. Biochim. Biophys. Acta. *340*, 484.

Gross, M. and Goldwasser, E. (1969) On the mechanism of erythropoietin induced differentiation. V. characterisation of the ribonucleic acid formed as a result of erythropoietin action. Biochem. *8*, 1795.

Gross, M. and Goldwasser, E. (1970) On the mechanism of erythropoietin induced differentiation. VII. the relationship between stimulated deoxyribonucleic acid synthesis and ribouncleic acid synthesis. J. Biol. Chem. *245*, 1632.

Harrison, P. R., Birnie, G. D., Hell, A., Humphries, S., Young, B. D. and Paul, J. (1974) Kinetic studies of gene frequency. I. Use of a DNA copy of reticulocyte 9S RNA to estimate globin gene dosage in mouse tissues. J. Mol. Biol. *84*, 539.

Harrison, P. R., Conkie, D. and Paul, J. (1973) Role of cell division and nucleic acid synthesis in erythropoietin-induced maturation of foetal liver cells *in vitro*. Brit. Soc. Dev. Biol. Symp. (eds. M. Balls and F. S. Billet) Cambridge University Press.

Harrison, P. R., Conkie, D., Affara, N. and Paul, J. (1974) *In situ* localisation of globin messenger RNA formation. I. During mouse foetal liver development. J. Cell Biol. *63*, 402.

Harrison, P. R., Conkie, D. and Paul, J. and Jones, K. (1973) Localisation of cellular globin messenger RNA by *in situ* hybridisation to complementary DNA. FEBS Letters *32*, 109.

Harrison, P. R., Gilmour, R. S., Affara, N. A., Conkie, D. and Paul, J. (1974) Globin messenger RNA synthesis and processing during haemoglobin induction in Friend cells. II. Evidence for post-transcriptional control in clone 707. Cell Differ. *3*, 23.

Kacian, D. L. and Spiegelman, S. (1972) *In vitro* synthesis of DNA components of human genes for globins. Nature New Biol. *235*, 167.

Krantz, S. B., Gallien-Lartigue, O. and Goldwasser, E. (1963) The effect of erythropoietin upon heme synthesis by marrow cells *in vitro*. J. Biol. Chem. *238*, 4085.

Krantz, S. B. and Goldwasser, E. (1965) On the mechanism of erythropoietin induced differentiation. IV. Some characteristics of erythropoietin action on haemoglobin synthesis in marrow cell culture. Biochim. Biophys. Acta. *108*, 455.

Mc Culloch, E. A. (1970) Control of haematopoiesis at the cellular level. In: Regulation of Haematopoiesis, ed. A. S. Gordon, volume 1, Chapter 7, p. 132. New York: Appleton-Century-Crofts.

Nicol, A. G., Conkie, D., Lanyon, W. G., Drewienkiewicz, C. E., Williamson, R. and Paul, J. (1972) Characteristics of erythropoietin-induced RNA from foetal mouse liver erythropoietic cell cultures and the effects of FUdR. Biochim. Biophys. Acta. 277, 342.

Ortega, J. A. and Dukes, P. P. (1970) Relationship between erythropoietin effect and reduced DNA synthesis in marrow cell cultures. Biochim. Biophys. Acta. 204, 334.

Ottolenghi, S., Lanyon, W. G., Paul, J., Williamson, R., Clegg, J., Pritchard, J., Pootrakul, J. and Wong Hock Boon (1974) Gene deletion as the cause of α-thalassaemia. Nature, 251, 389.

Paul, J., Freshney, R. I., Conkie, D. and Burgos, H. (1971) Biochemical aspects of foetal erythropoiesis. Proc. of Inter. Conf. on Erythropoiesis. Eds. A. S. Gordon, M. Condorelli and C. Peschle. Il Ponte, Milano. p. 236.

Paul, J., Gilmour, R. S., Affara, N. A., Birnie, G. D, Harrison, P R., Hell, A., Humphries, S., Windass, J. D. and Young, B. D. (1974) Cold Spring Harbour Symp. on Quant. Biology, 28, 885.

Paul, J. and Hickey, I. (1974) Haemoglobin synthesis in inducible uninducible and hybrid Friend cell clones. Exp. Cell Res. 87, 20.

Paul, J. and Hunter, J. A. (1969) Synthesis of macromolecules during induction of haemoglobin synthesis by erythropoietin. J. Mol. Biol. 42, 31.

Ross, J., Aviv, H., Scolnick, E. and Leder, P. (1972b) In vitro synthesis of DNA complementary to purified rabbit globin mRNA. Proc. Nat. Acad. Sci. 69, 264.

Ross, J., Ikawa, Y. and Leder, P. (1972) Globin messenger RNA induction during erythroid differentiation of cultured leukaemia cells. Proc. Nat. Acad. Sci. 69, 3620.

Scher, W., Holland, J. G. and Friend, C. (1971) Haemoglobin synthesis in murine virus-induced leukaemic cells in vitro. I. Partial purification and identification of haemoglobin. Blood 37, 428.

Verma, I., Temple, G. F., Fan, H. and Baltimore, D. (1972) In vitro synthesis of DNA complementary to rabbit reticulocyte 10S RNA. Nature New Biol. 235, 163.

Williamson, R., Morrison, M., Lanyon, W. G., Eason, R. and Paul, J. (1971) Properties of mouse globin messenger RNA and its preparation in milligram quantities. Biochem. 10, 3014.

Analysis by Computer-controlled Cell
Sorter of Friend Virus-transformed Cells
in Different Stages of Differentiation

Donna J. Arndt-Jovin*, Wolfram Ostertag**, Harvey Eisen***,
and Thomas M. Jovin*

  * Abteilung Molekulare Biologie
   Max-Planck-Institut für biophysikalische Chemie
   Postfach 968, D-3400 Goettingen
   Federal Republic of Germany
 ** Abteilung Molekulare Biologie
   Max-Planck-Institut für experimentelle Medizin
   Hermann-Rein-Str. 3, D-3400 Goettingen
   Federal Republic of Germany
*** Département de Biologie Moléculaire
   Université de Genève
   30 Quai de l'École de Médecine
   Geneva, Switzerland

Summary

In most systems involving cellular differentiation and cellular transformation the biological process is non-synchronous and the sample heterogeneous. In order to answer some of the basic questions about the control mechanisms of cellular changes and the order in which they proceed one must have access to homogeneous classes of cells. Friend virus transformed erythroid cells which are stably maintained in tissue culture can be chemically induced to differentiate and are thus very advantageous for *in vitro* studies (1–3).

With such a system the questions which we pose are a) the reversibility of the differentiation process; b) the order of steps in the production of specialized messenger RNA; c) the time of shut-off of undifferentiated messenger production; d) the relationship of viral RNA production to the differentiation process; e) the onset and extent of specific protein synthesis; f) the correlation of DNA metabolism with the timing or course of events. By using a computer-controlled cell separator we can select live cells on the basis of their macromolecular content, membrane properties (using a new parameter, fluorescence emission anisotropy), and size (4, 5, 34). Thus with proper probes as described here, we are able to select cells at different stages in their differentiation and can begin to attack the questions posed above.

Materials and Methods

The Instrument

Systems for separating suspensions of living mammalian cells on the basis of spectroscopic properties present or induced in the cells have been developed in several laboratories (4–7). Our instrument differs from the others in that it is controlled on-line by a computer and thus a) facilitates the use of numerous detectors (up to five) for both light scattering and fluorescence, b) allows the simultaneous separation of cells into four categories to be performed on the basis of complex functions of the measured signals (such as the fluorescence anisotropy shown here) and c) generates, displays and stores frequency distributions of the number of cells having any measured property or the combination of several properties. These features make the instrument ideally suited to the selection of cells from complex biological mixtures.

Figure 1 shows a schematic diagram of the instrument and its general features. The aqueous suspension of cells exits from an inner nozzle 50 microns in diameter and is narrowed into a thin stream by the colaminar flow of the sheath liquid

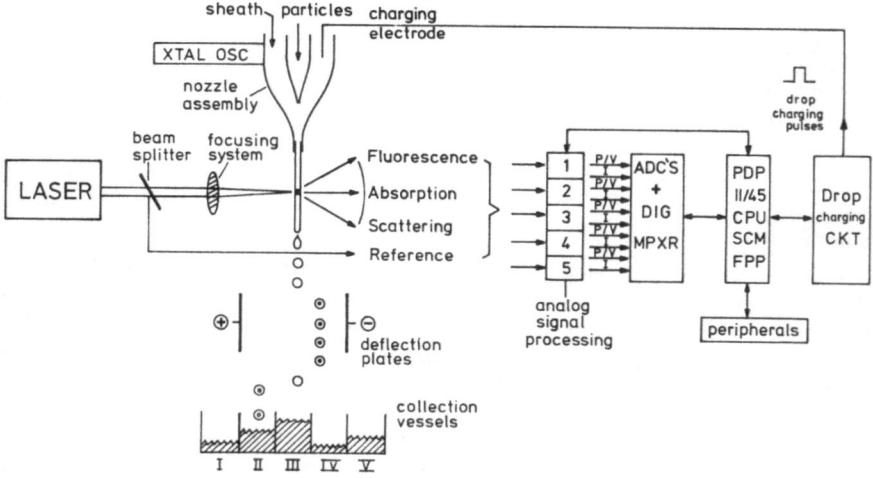

Fig. 1: Schematic diagram of the computer-controlled analyzer-sorter. The flow system leading to the nozzle is omitted. Excitation and detection are represented symbolically; the actual components used are described elsewhere (4, 22). The five independent analog processing modules can accept signals from up to five different detectors, usually a combination of two independent fluorescent detectors and 2 or 3 light scattering detectors and a laser reference signal. The 10 peak or valley (P/V) and integral (I) output signals derived from each cell at the time of intersection with the laser beam are digitized by parallel analog to digital convertors (A2C's) and multiplexed into the central processor (CPU, Digital Equipment Corporation PDP11/45) (taken from reference 4).

138

such that individual cells follow one another. These streams pass through the outer nozzle (also 50 microns in diameter) into air and just below the tip the fluid column intersects a focussed laser beam. As each cell passes through the laser beam a spectroscopic "fingerprint" is registered by the detectors and recorded by the computer. That is, the cells scatter light according to their size, membrane properties, and internal structures. They emit inherent fluorescence if excited in the ultraviolet. More generally, specific fluorescence proportional to the content of macromolecules in the cell or on its surface can be elicited by the use of fluorescent probes. In all cases the magnitudes of the optical signals from an individual cell are measured and converted to a proportional voltage by the various detectors for the light-scattering and fluorescence. These voltages are simultaneously recorded by the computer. Thus each cell is assigned to a particular category by the combination of this information according to freely programable algorithms.

For example, the DNA content of a cell can be determined by the direct proportionality it has to the fluorescence of bound acriflavin after Feulgen treatment or to the fluorescence of bound Hoechst benzimidazole dyes in living cells.[1] The number of antigen binding sites can be determinded by the fluorescent signal from labelled antibody bound to cells and likewise the number of lecitin or hormone binding sites can be measured directly from the fluorescence of labelled hormone or lectin bound to the cells. In addition to determination of content by the absolute fluorescence intensity of the labelled cells one can derive information about the environment of a fluorescent molecule, e. g., the fluidity of the plasma membrane, by measurement of polarized fluorescence emission or anisotropy (5, 34).

Because a crystal oscillator is imposed on the stream the liquid column breaks into droplets at a constant distance from the tip of the nozzle. At the precise moment when the cell reaches the place in the stream where it will be trapped in a droplet the computer gives an electrical charge to the stream, the magnitude and polarity depending upon the category to which the cell has been assigned. Thus the droplet containing the desired cell is given a known charge. The droplets pass through an electrical field established between two metal plates and are deflected according to their charge. Four deflected and the undeflected streams are collected. In addition, the spectroscopic information from each cell is processed by the computer and displayed as the cumulative frequency or number of cells plotted against the size of a particular signal or combination of signals.

Automated cell separators can select living cells sterilely at speeds up to several thousand cells per second with high purity. The fluorescent probes can include, besides those alluded to above: fluorogenic substrates for intracellular enzymes and non-covalent or covalent dyes which equilibrate nonspecifically, e. g. in the cytoplasm as for the purpose of size measurement. Since cells are separated on the basis of an expression of a specific cell function or structure it is a selection related directly to their biological state as opposed to conventional gradient centrifugation or electrophoretic methods which separate on combined gross physical properties often less related to biological function.

---

[1] D. Arndt-Jovin, unpublished results.

The cell system

The Friend virus or spleen focus-forming virus transformed cells are erythroid cells which are arrested in the proerythroblast stage and can be maintained permanently in uncloned or cloned culture (3, 8–10). If aprotonic solvents such as dimethylsulfoxide (DMSO) or dimethoxyethane (2, 3, 11) or short chain fatty acids such as butyric acid (12, 13) are added to the growth medium the cells resume the process of erythroid differentiation which had been blocked by the transformation event. However all cells are not equally responsive to the inducing stimulus (17, 20). During the 2–4 cell divisions required to reach the stage of non-dividing late erythroblast or non-nucleated cell containing 25 % of its soluble cytoplasmic protein as hemoglobin, a number of morphological and biochemical changes in the cells can be observed. Generalized RNA synthesis decreases while mRNA for proteins specific to the differentiated state such as globin increase dramatically (8, 9, 14, 15, 16, 17). The increased production of viral RNA and the activation and release of an endogenous spleen focus-forming virus complex are observed in virus positive cell lines and in some virus negative ones, but no activation of the Friend helper virus takes place (10, 17, 18). These processes are coordinated temporally with the synthesis of globin mRNA (10, 17, 18). In some other virus negative cell lines virus release appears to be inhibited but a 10-fold increase in other endogenous virus-like intracisternal A particles can be observed (10, 17, Krieg *et al.* unpublished observations). The *de novo* synthesis of hemoglobin (3, 19) and the appearance of spectrin in the membrane[2] occur later in differentiation and are characteristic for all the cell lines.

Tissue culture. The isolation and characterization of erythroleukemia cell lines F4N and B8 from DBA/2 mice have been described (3, 8, 10). The lines at a cell density of about 1×10^6 were induced to differentiate by treatment of F4N at 1–1.2 % and B8 at 1.5–2 % DMSO.

Antibody to the H-2 mouse histocompatibility antigens. Antibody was prepared as previously described (5) and used at 1:2 dilution in phosphate buffered saline (PBS). The binding of the antibody to erythroleukemia cells was visualized using fluoresceinated rabbit antimouse IgG as described (5).

Concanavalin A. The methods for the purification and the radioactive and fluorescent labelling of Concanavalin A (Con A) for use in subsequent binding studies to the cells have been described (5).

Labelling of cells with DPH. 1,6-diphenyl-1, 3, 4-hexatriene (DPH) was obtained from Aldrich and a fresh dispersion in PBS was prepared daily as described by Shinitzky and Inbar (29). The methods for labelling cells with DPH and measuring its fluorescence emission anisotropy have been described (5, 34.)

Results

We have investigated various properties of the differentiating Friend cells with the help of the cell separator and correlated them with other biochemical changes as is discussed in more detail elsewhere (5, 21). Table I summarizes the properties

[2] H. Eisen, manuscript in preparation.

TABLE I

MOUSE SPLEENIC CELLS TRANSFORMED WITH FRIEND ERYTHROLEUKEMIA VIRUS
CELLULAR PROPERTIES WHICH CHANGE AFTER DMSO INDUCTION

PROPERTY	CHANGE	BASIS FOR SELECTION IN CELL SEPARATOR
CELL SIZE	DECREASES OVER 2-3 CELL CYCLES	YES, LIGHT SCATTERING
LECTIN BINDING	EARLY: INCREASED AGGLUTINABILITY	NO
	LATE: INCREASED IN NUMBER OF BINDING SITES	YES, FLUORESCENT-LABELLED LECTIN
MEMBRANE VISCOSITY	INCREASES WITH DIFFERENTIATION	YES, ANISOTROPY OF DPH FLUORESCENCE
ANTIGENIC DETERMINANT	H-2 HISTOCOMPATIBILITY ANTIGEN DECREASES	YES, FLUORESCENT ANTIBODY TO THE H-2 LOCUS
SYNTHESIS OF MACROMOLECULES	DNA, CELL CYCLE KINETICS	YES, ACRIFLAVIN-FEULGEN OR HOECHST 33342 STAINING
	SPECIFIC MRNA	NO
	MEMBRANE PROTEIN, SPECTRIN, INCREASES	YES, FLUORESCENT ANTIBODY TO SPECTRIN
	HEMOGLOBIN PRODUCTION	CORRELATES WITH HIGH SPECTRIN CONTENT AND HIGH ANISOTROPY
VIRUS	VIRAL RNA	NO
	VIRUS PRODUCTION	YES, FLUORESCENT ANTIBODY TO VIRAL ANTIGENS

of the cells which change upon induction and how they can be probed by the cell
separator. The following results show representative data for 3 surface phenomena
of the cells.

a) *Lectin binding:* The mobility of the lectin binding sites for Con A on Friend
Virus transformed cells seems to change during the first day of differentiation as
measured by the increased agglutinability of the cells (21) and coincides with a
decrease in membrane permeability 6 hours after addition of DMSO. However,
measurements of the number of binding sites for the lectin assayed both by binding
of ^{125}I-labelled Con A (shown in figure 2) and by fluorescence of bound
fluoresceinated Con A indicate that no net increase in the number of lectin binding
sites occurs until later in differentiation. Although the difference in number of
binding sites is only 2-fold which normally would be difficult to see due to the
rather broad distribution of absolute values for individual cells, some enhancement
of the difference can be achieved by taking advantage of the fact that cells decrease

141

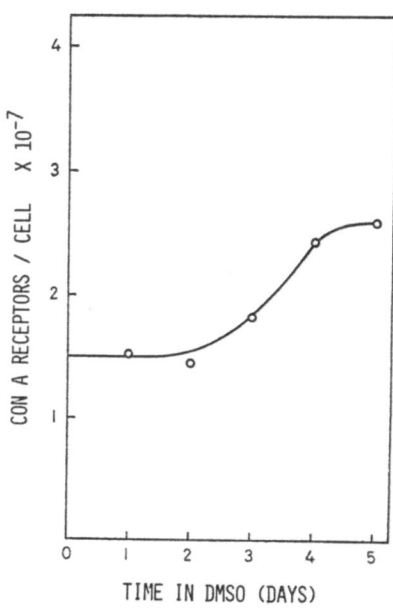

Fig. 2: Increase in Con A receptors per cell for Friend virus transformed cells with time after induction with DMSO. Each point represents the specific binding of ^{125}I-labelled Con A obtained by incubating 10[6] cells in 1 ml PBS from cultures induced in 1 % DMSO for 0–5 days with 150 µg of Con A for 15 minutes and washing through a gradient. Details of labelling and assay procedures have been published (5, 21).

in size as they differentiate. In figure 3 we see such a frequency distribution of the ratio of the fluorescence signal to the light scattering signal (the number of lectin binding sites divided by a function of the cell diameter (22, 23)) for an uninduced and 6-day DMSO unduced population of cells.

b) *H-2 binding sites:* The mature mouse erythrocyte has fewer H-2 histocompatibility antigen sites than the precursor cells as demonstrated by cytotoxicity measurements (24). Thus we can expect and do see a decrease in the number of sites when living cells tagged with fluorescent antibody are measured and sorted in the cell separator. Figure 4 shows a fluorescence micrograph of the antibody complex bound to living uninduced cells and figure 5 the measurement of this antibody binding on individual cells with the cell separator. As expected the mean signal size of the fluorescent cell population decreases with time after induction of the cultures by DMSO.

c) *Membrane fluidity:* The transport of small molecules in induced Friend virus cells is very different from the non-differentiating precursor (8 and unpublished observations). Such effects may reflect changes in the membrane permeability. Additionally, there is considerable evidence in the hemopoietic system for a large increase in the rigidity of the cell membrane between stem cells and erythrocytes. This rigidity can be demonstrated by the fact that lectins and antibodies do not

142

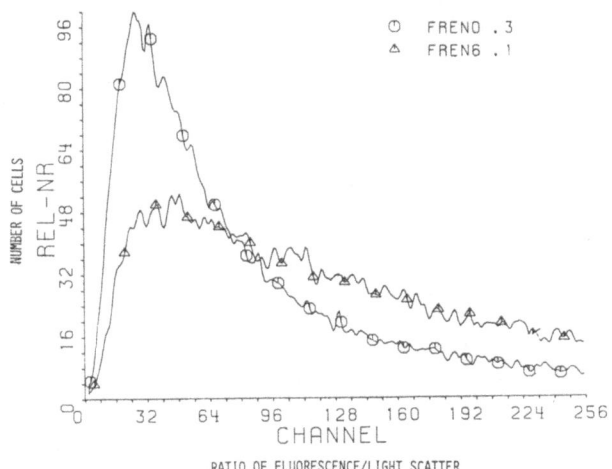

Fig. 3: Change in number of Con A receptors per cell as measured by fluorescence. Fluoresceinated Con A was bound to cells and the ratio of the fluorescence to light scattering signals for each cell monitored in the cell separator (represented by the abscissa). This parameter is larger with increasing number of Con A receptors per cell and/or decreasing cell size. The data are plotted as frequency distributions with relative number of cells for each signal ratio given on the ordinate. A total of 3×10^4 cells from an uninduced culture, -O-, and a 6-day DMSO induced culture, -△-, were measured. The induced culture has a population of resistant cells in a stage of outgrowth as well as differentiating cells.

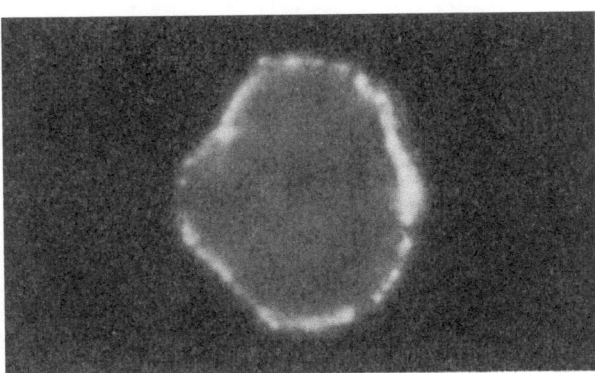

Fig. 4: Immunofluorescence demonstration of H-2 histocompatibility antigen on Friend virus transformed cells. Fluoresceinated rabbit anti-mouse IgG was reacted against anti H-2 mouse IgG bound to uninduced Friend cells. The fluorescence micrograph was taken on a Zeiss epi-illuminated fluorescence microscope, excitation below 480 nm and emission above 530 nm, Kodak Plus X film.

143

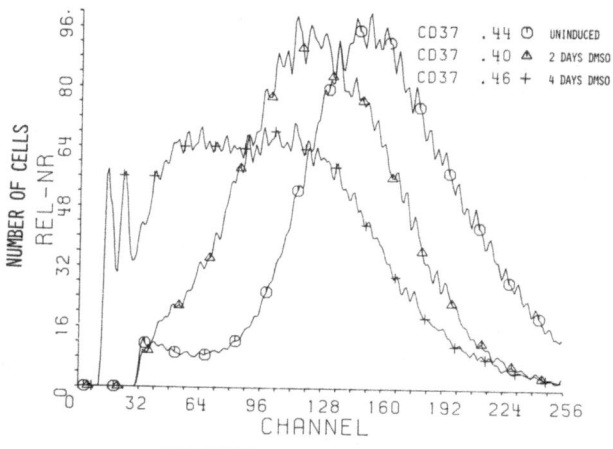

INCREASING H-2 ANTIBODY BINDING

Fig. 5: Measure of the number of H-2 antigen sites in differentiating Friend cells. Indirect fluorescent antibody to H-2 was quantitated in the cell separator for populations of Friend cells with excitation at 488 nm and emission above 530 nm. The data are plotted as frequency distributions with the abscissa indicating increasing antibody binding and the ordinate the number of cells normalized to 10^5. -0-, uninduced cells; -△-, 2 days of 1 % DMSO; -+-, 4 days of 1 % DMSO.

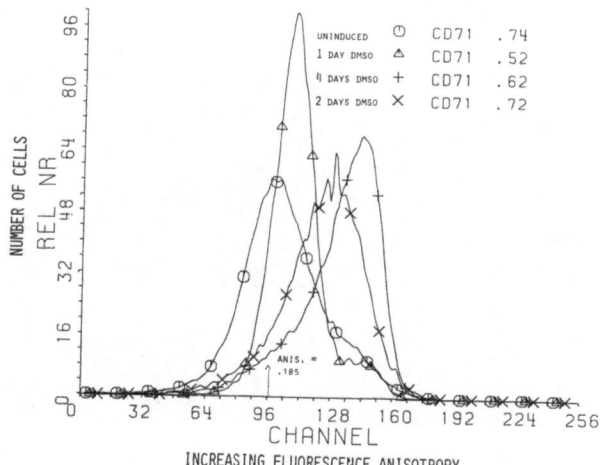

INCREASING FLUORESCENCE ANISOTROPY

Fig. 6: Increase in fluorescence anisotropy with differentiation. The polarized fluorescence of DPH bound to Friend cells was measured in the cell separator and real-time anisotropy functions determined. Frequency distributions for populations of uninduced, -0-; 1 day, 1.2 % DMSO induced, -△-; 2 days induced, -x-; and 4 days induced, -+-, are shown on a single plot. Increasing anisotropy (correlated with increasing membrane viscosity) is plotted on the abscissa and cell number normalized to 10^5 cells on the ordinate.

144

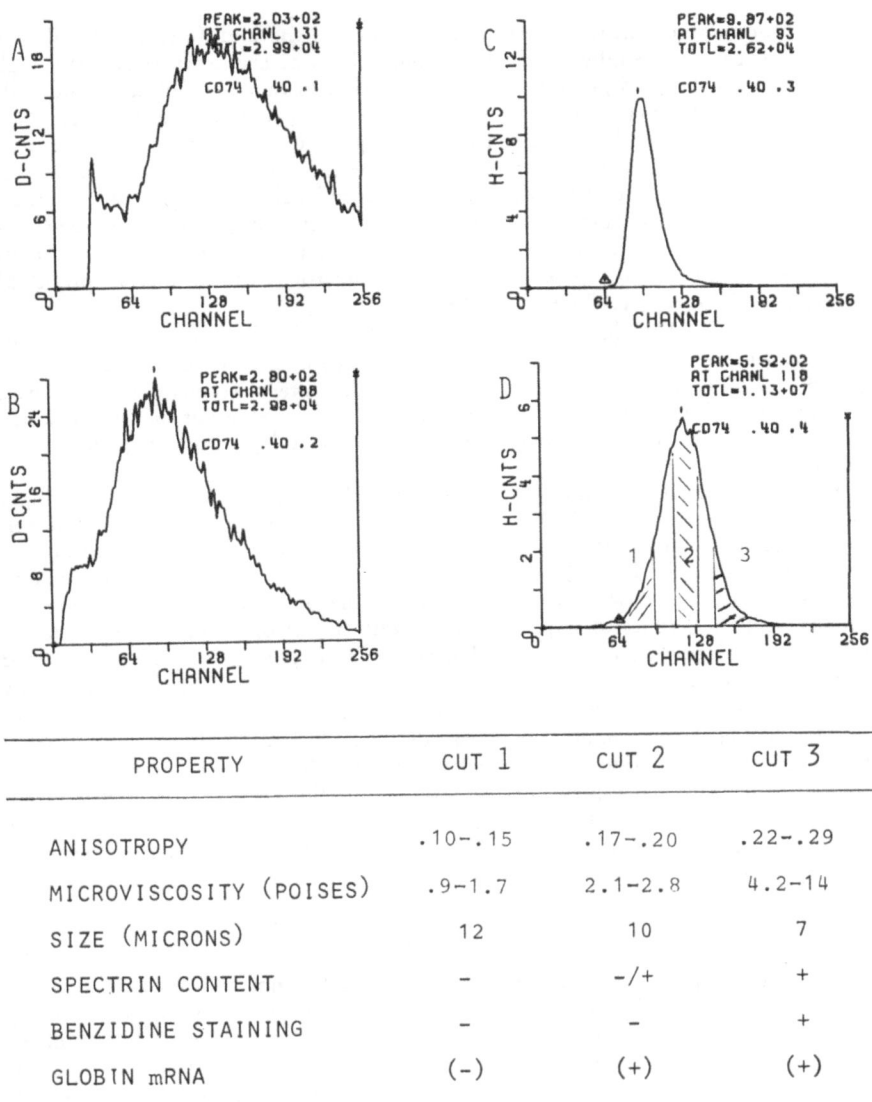

PROPERTY	CUT 1	CUT 2	CUT 3
ANISOTROPY	.10-.15	.17-.20	.22-.29
MICROVISCOSITY (POISES)	.9-1.7	2.1-2.8	4.2-14
SIZE (MICRONS)	12	10	7
SPECTRIN CONTENT	-	-/+	+
BENZIDINE STAINING	-	-	+
GLOBIN mRNA	(-)	(+)	(+)

Fig. 7: Correlation of properties of induced Friend cells sorted on fluorescence anisotropy. The frequency distributions A–D were measured on DPH stained Friend cells after induction in DMSO for 2 days. Plot A is the distribution of the apparent parallel fluorescence intensities; plot B, that of the apparent perpendicular fluorescence intensities; plot C, that of the ratio I_A/I_B; and plot D, that of the fluorescence anisotropy. Cells sorted on the anisotropy according to the indicated cuts can be correlated with other properties as shown in the table.

cap or form large patches in erythrocytes whereas the undifferentiated cells are capable of capping. Studies of the lipid composition of erythrocytes reveal a high cholesterol to phospholipid ratio (25), a condition in model membranes and cells which reduces fluidity (30). Under some conditions, a direct measure of local membrane fluidity can be obtained by measuring the depolarization of fluorescence of a dye situated in the membrane (5, 29, 30, 34). The degree of depolarization is dependent upon the extent to which the excited molecules are displaced from their original orientation during the lifetime of their excited state. The displacement is directly proportional to the hydrodynamic properties of the medium and temperature. Thus the emission polarization (or anisotropy) can be used as probes of membrane viscosity, i. e., fluidity (26–28).

The molecule DPH has been shown to be bound in the hydrocarbon layer of biological membranes and thus functions as a probe of the viscosity of that region (5, 29, 30). The cells continue to grow normally after treatment with the dye. The amount of dye taken up by individual cells is variable but one is concerned primarily with the emission polarization, a function independent of quantity to a first approximation.

Friend virus transformed cells induced with DMSO appear to have increasingly rigid membranes as is shown by the increasing anisotropy of the dye in the cell membranes correlated with time after induction in figure 6. We have been able to demonstrate that the DMSO itself does not appear to alter the dye's emission and one can detect the growth of resistant cells in the population by the appearance at late induction times of a peak of cells with anisotropy like that seen in un-induced populations. In a 2–3 day DMSO induced population there is a broad distribution of cell stages. Separation of the cells on the basis of their anisotropy allows the correlation with other biological properties and the further outgrowth of the homogeneous populations so derived. Figure 7 shows how such a heterogeneous population can be separated and the fractions correlated with cellular functions. The ability to regrow the populations provides us with a means of determining the reversibility of differentiation by assaying for the production of globin messenger in the separated and then regrown cells. These experiments are in progress.

Discussion

The erythroleukemia Friend virus transformed cell is not only a good model for controlled differentiation but may serve to answer some basic questions concerning the role of viruses in leukemias. The fact that one can release these cells from the transformed state and initiate a seemingly normal differentiation provides the means for studying the fate of the transforming virus. Hopefully, such results may suggest means for probing viral etiologies in human leukemias. In addition, the question of reversibility of differentiation although well documented in plants (31) has not been conclusively established for higher animals and is particularly important in any understanding of the mechanism of induction and the mode of treatment for leukemias. As described here with the Friend system, one can select large numbers of cells on the basis of some differentiated function or property with the cell separator and then study the specific mRNA's and specific functional proteins after further culture with and without the inducing agent for differentiation. With this technique it is possible to chronicle the sequence of events leading to reticulocyte-like cells and to compare the process in several cell lines. Once this information is compiled we hope to look at the *in vivo* hemopoietic system with some of these probes to see how comparable the *in vitro* and normal processes are.

The extension of automated cell-separation techniques beyond the quantitation of macromolecular content to obtaining separation on the basis of cellular structure or organization has been described here. We have shown that a complete gradation of differentiating cell stages can be obtained by separating on the basis of the fluorescence emission polarization of a dye, DPH, which appears to bind the plasma membrane and monitor fluidity changes therein.

DPH has been used to monitor the fluidity of membranes of leukemic cells (29) and their lower cholesterol content (32, 33) has been implicated as a factor in their neoplastic behaviour. Our preliminary work on leukemic lymphocytes using the DPH probe with the cell separator indicates that membrane fluidity may be correlated with the nature and state of the disease.

It is probable that the technique of fluorescent anisotropy separation using appropriate fluorescent probes will enable us to look at numerous processes in biological systems which result in changes in cellular permeability or membrane structure, such as response to hormones, infection by virus, other types of differentiation, or transformation.

Thus it would appear that flow systems capable of separating cells on the basis of spectroscopic properties may soon play a larger role in diagnosis of leukemia (e. g. by use of specific fluorescent antibodies, as has been described by Dr. M. Greaves at this symposium), in the recognition of preleukemia states (by perhaps changes in membrane structure or function), and in the early diagnosis of relapse. Flow systems with their rapid screening of statistically significant populations (usually 1000 cells per second) and high sensitivity (laser excitation) should provide a means for large screening programs once enough specific probes are developed.

References

1. Friend, C., Patuleia, M. C., and De Harven, E., *National Cancer Institute Monograph 22:* 505, 1966.
2. Friend, C., Scher, W., Holland, J. G., and Sato, T., *Proc. Nat. Acad. Sci. USA 68:* 378, 1971.
3. Ostertag, W., Melderis, H., Steinheider, G., Kluge, N., and Dube, S. K., *Nature New Biol. 239:* 231, 1972.
4. Arndt-Jovin, D., and Jovin, T. M., *J. Histochem. Cytochem. 22:,* 622, *1974.*
5. Arndt-Jovin, D., Ostertag, W., Eisen, H., Klimek, F., and Jovin, T. M., *J. Histochem. Cytochem.* 24: 332, 1976.
6. Bonner, W. A., Hulett, H. R., Sweet, R. G., and Herzenberg, L. A., *Rev. Sci. Instrum. 43:* 404, 1972.
7. Steinkamp, J. A., Fulwyler, M. J., Coulter, J. R., Hiebert, R. D., Horney, J. L., and Mullaney, P. F., *Rev. Sci. Instrum. 44:* 1301, 1973.

8. Dube, S. K., Gaedicke, G., Kluge, N., Weimann, B. J., Melderis, H., Steinheider, G., Crozier, T., Beckmann, H., and Ostertag, W., in *Differentiation and Control of Malignancy of Tumor Cells*. (Eds. W. Nakahara, T. Ono, T. Sugimura, H. Sugano), University of Tokyo Press, Tokyo, 1974, p. 99.
9. Gaedicke, G., Abedin, Z., Dube, S. K., Kluge, N., Neth, R., Steinheider, G., Weimann, B. J., Ostertag, W., in *Modern Trends in Human Leukemia* (Eds. R. Neth, R. Gallo, S. Spiegelman, F. Stohlman), Grune and Stratton, New York, 1974, p. 278–287.
10. Ostertag, W., Cole, T., Crozier, T., Gaedicke, G., Kind, J., Kluge, N., Krieg, J. C., Roesler, G., Steinheider, G., Weimann, B. J., and Dube, S. K., in *Differentiation and Control of Malignancy of Tumor Cells*. (Eds. W. Nakahara, T. Ono, T. Sugimura, H. Sugano), University of Tokyo Press, Tokyo, 1974, p. 485.
11. Tanaka, M., Levy, J., Terada, M., Breslow, R., Rifkind, R. A., and Marks, P. A., *Proc. Nat. Acad. Sci. USA 72:* 1003, 1975.
12. Leder, A., and Leder, P., *Cell 5:* 319, 1975.
13. Takahashi, E., Yamada, M., Saito, M., Kuboyama, M., and Ogasa, K., *Gann, 66:,* 577, 1975.
14. Gilmour, R. S., Harrison, P. R., Windass, J. D., Affara, N. A., and Paul, J., *Cell Differentiation 3:* 9, 1974.
15. Harrison, P. R., Gilmour, R. S., Affara, N. A., Conkie, D., and Paul, J., *Cell Differentiation 3:* 23, 1974.
16. Ross, J., Ikawa, Y., Leder, P., *Proc. Nat. Acad. Sci. USA 69:* 3620, 1972.
17. Pragnell, I. B., Ostertag, W., Steinheider, G., Takahashi, E., Paul, J., Williamson, R., submitted for publication.
18. Dube, S. K., Pragnell, I. B., Kluge, N., Gaedicke, G., Steinheider, G., and Ostertag, W., *Proc. Nat. Acad. Sci. USA 72:* 1863, 1975.
19. Ross, J., Gielen, J., Packman, S., Ikawa, Y., and Leder, P., *J. Mol. Biol. 87:* 697, 1974.
20. Orkin, S. H., Harosi, F. I., Leder, P., *Proc. Nat. Acad. Sci. USA 72:* 98, 1975.
21. Eisen, H., Ostertag, W., and Arndt-Jovin, D. J., submitted for publication.
22. Jovin, T. M., Morris, S. J., Striker, G., Schultens, H., Digweed, M., and Arndt-Jovin, D., *J. Histochem. Cytochem.* 24: 269, 1976.
23. Arndt-Jovin, D., Jovin, T. M., *FEBS Letters 44:* 247, 1974.
24. Klein, J., *Biology of the Mouse Histocompatibility-2 Complex*. Springer, Heidelberg, 1975, p. 620.
25. Van Deenen, L. L. M., and De Gier, J., in *The Red Blood Cell* (ed. D. M. N. Surgenor), Vol 1, Academic Press, New York and London, 1974, p. 147.
26. Perrin, F., *J. Phys. Radium 7:* 390, 1926.
27. Jablonski, A., *Acta Phys. Polon. 16:* 471, 1957.
28. Jablonski, A., *Bull. Acad. Polon. Sci., Sér sci. math astr. phys. 8:* 259, 1960.
29. Shinitzky, M., and Inbar, M., *J. Mol. Biol. 85:* 603, 1974.
30. Shinitzky, M., and Inbar, M., (in press).
31. Steward, F. C., Mapes, M. O., Kent, A. E., and Holsten, R. D., *Science 143:* 20, 1964.
32. Inbar, M., and Shinitzky, M., *Proc. Nat. Acad. Sci. USA 71:* 2128, 1974.
33. Inbar, M., and Shinitzky, M., *Proc. Nat. Acad. Sci. USA 71:* 4229, 1974.

34. Arndt-Jovin, D. J., and Jovin, T. M., in *Membranes and Neoplasia, Progress in Clinical and Biological Research.* (Ed. F. Fox), Alan Liss, Inc., New York, 1976, in press.

Abbreviations
DMSO = dimethylsulfoxide.
Con A = concanavalin A.
DPH = 1,6-diphenyl-3,4,5-hexatriene.

Hormone Independent in Vitro Erythroid Colony Formation by Mouse Bone Marrow Cells

K. Nooter (1, 2), R. Ghio (3), K. J. v. d. Berg (1) and P. A. J. Bentvelzen (1).

Radiological Institute TNA Rigwigh (ZH), The Netherlands

Introduction

In vitro transformation of normal cells by oncogenic viruses, inducing growth patterns comparable to those of neoplastic cells, has become a powerful tool in the study of these viruses (1, 2). The most used targets for oncogenic viruses are embryonic fibroblasts, but murine leukemia viruses can rarely transform this kind of cell. The obvious targets for this group of viruses seem to be hemopoietic cells. To develop a suitable transformation assay, possibilities to discriminate between normal and leukemic cells on the basis of differences in growth patterns *in vitro* are requied.

Murine erythroid precursor cells (CFU-E) produce within a few days many colonies of hemoglobin-synthesizing cells in vitro in the presence of the hormone erythropoietin (EP) (3, 4). With a longer culture period in the presence of larger amounts of EP, so-called bursts consisting of large, dispersed colonies of erythroid cells appear (3, 5). The burst forming unit (BFU-E) is thought to be a more primitive member of the erythroid series than is the CFU-E.

I. Growth differences between normal and virus-infected B. M. cells

Bone marrow cells from RLV-infected BALB/c mice were compared with cells from uninfected mice with regard to their dependency on EP for the *in vitro* development of erythroid colonies.

BALB/c mice were injected i.p. with RLV and examined twice a week thereafter for the development of the disease. A continuing increase in spleen weight begins at day 5 postinfection; a maximum weight of three grams is reached in the terminal stage at 4–5 weeks after inoculation. The production of *in vitro* erythroid colonies

1. Radiobiological Institute TNO,
   Lange Kleiweg 151,
   Rijswijk (ZH),
   The Netherlands.
2. Part of this investigation was supported by a grant from the Netherlands Organization for Fundamental Medical Research.
3. Riccardo Ghio was on leave of absence from the I.S.M.I., Università Cattedra di Ematologia, Genoa, Italy. He received a fellowship from the Netherlands Organization for the Advancement of Science under the auspices of a treaty between this organization and the Centro Nazionale di Richerche, Italy.

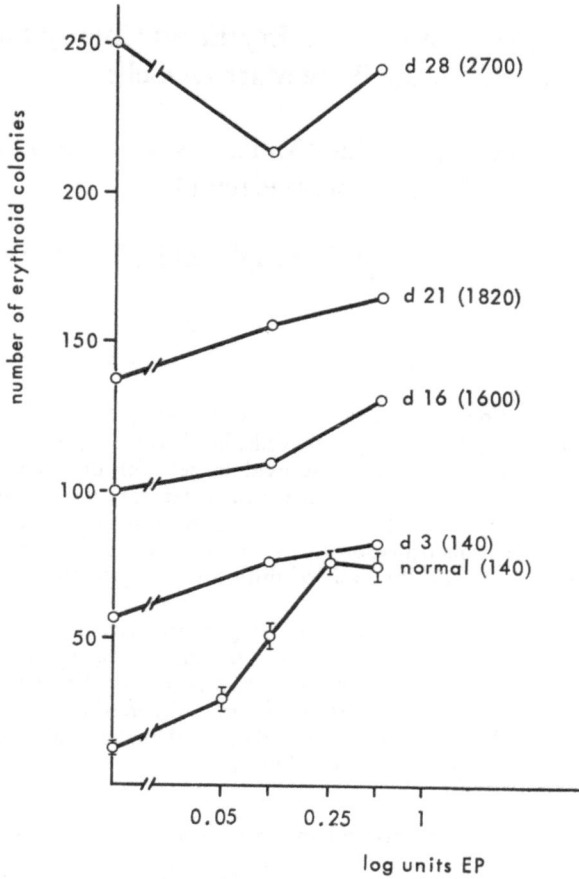

Fig. 1: Erythropoietin dose-response curves of normal and RLV-infected BALB/c mice bone marrow.
Normal curve: mean ± SE of 7 separate experiments. RLV-infected animals: three (d3). sixteen (d16), twenty-one (d21) and twenty-eight (d28) days after infection.
Numbers in parentheses indicate spleen weights.

at several concentrations of EP by normal bone marrow (BM) cells and cells taken from mice at several days after infection with RLV is presented in Fig. 1. A few erythroid colonies are produced by the controls in the absence of exogenous EP (Connaught, Step III), but the addition of the hormone leads to a marked elevation with an optimum at 0.25 I.U. Three days after infection with the virus when clinical signs of the disease are not yet present, a five-fold increase in the number of colonies formed in the absence of exogenous EP is found. During the progression of the disease, a remarkable increase in the number of EP-independent colonies can be observed.

Evidence for the specificity of this spontaneous colony formation is demonstrated by the following experiments: Plating different cell concentrations (1, 2, 5, 10, and 20×10^4) from RLV-infected BM reveals a linear relationship with the number of erythroid colonies formed, both with and without EP in the culture medium. To complete rule out the possibility that the BM cells of RLV-infected mice produce endogenous EP feeder-layer experiments were done with normal and infected BM cells. No significant erythropoietic activity by either normal or RLV-infected BM could be detected which would give rise to erythroid colony formation by normal BM cells.

To exclude the possibility that the observed hormone-independency of BM cells from RLV-infected mice is due only to a high erythropoietic stimulation *in vivo*, we performed the following experiments. Anaemia was induced in BALB/c mice by phenylhydrazine treatment. Two days later the haematocrit and EP responsiveness *in vitro* were determined. The haematocrit values were decreased from 48–50 % to 31–40 %. The maximum number of erythroid colonies per 2×10^5 BM cells increased 3–5 times, but the colony formation was still hormone-dependent. Even after a prolonged phenylhydrazine treatment of 14 days, the erythroid-colony-forming units (CFU-E) were dependent on the addition of EP *in vitro*.

In antoher experiment, RLV-infected mice were hypertransfused with packed red cells at various time intervals after infection. Bone marrow was cultured with 0.25 I.U. EP and in medium containing no EP. Both infected and uninfected mice showed a drastic decrease in the number of colonies in the presence of EP. However, the colony formation was still completely EP-independent in the infected animals, while the BM cells of the controls needed the hormone.

Not only the CFU-E but also the BFU-E seems to have become hormone independent as large bursts of erythroid cells after 10 days of cultures are found by BM cells from mice which have been infected with RLV 15 days earlier (Table 1).

Table I: **Number of EP-independent BFU-E in bone of marrow of RLV-infected BALB/c mice 15 days after injection**

	number of bursts after 10 days of culture	
Treatment animals	+ EP*	− EP
−	17	2
RLV	21	8

* The amount of EP added to the cultures is 1 I. U.

II. Enhancement of erythroblasts by CFA

Complete Freund's adjuvant (CFA) strongly enhances the erythroblastosis induced by Rauscher murine leukemia virus (RLV) (6, 7). On the basis of this fact, it was concluded that the pluripotent hemopoietic stem cell would be involved in the development of splenomegaly (6). On the other hand, the course of the disease can be influenced by manipulation of the erythroid compartment (8, 11) suggesting that an erythroipoietic-sensitive cell would be the target for the transforming activity of the virus.

The *in vitro* techniques mentioned above were used to determine the mechanism by which CFA enhances RLV-induced erythroblastosis.

BALB/c mice were injected with crude cell-free RLV preparation and the same day with CFA(0.2 ml. i.p.).

The number of CFU-E per 10^5 normal bone marrow cells as determined in methylcellulose cultures with erythropoietin greatly increases after administration of CFA (fig. 2). A peak is reached at 5 days after inoculation; after which a plateau level is maintained.

The number of CFU-E producing erythroid colonies in the absence of erythropoietin increases steadily after RLV-infection (fig. 3). The administration of CFA also has an enhancing effect on the number of EP-independent CFU-E, but this effect becomes noticeable only when bone marrow is taken 10 days or later after infection. The most likely explanation for the strong increase induced by the treatment with CFA is the recruitment of new target cells for virus released by previously infected cells.

Rather unexpected was the marked increase in CFU-E after CFA administration. This is certainly not due to the slight anemia induced by CFA, because that is preceded by the rise in CFU-E. Furthermore, a drop of less than 10 % in the hematocrit does not induce a 6-fold increase in CFU-E (12). The adjuvant, like other antigens, is known to stimulate the proliferation of pluripotent hemopoietic stem cells as has been described for a variety of other antigen (133). There is probably no competition at the stem cell level for differentiation into a a specific

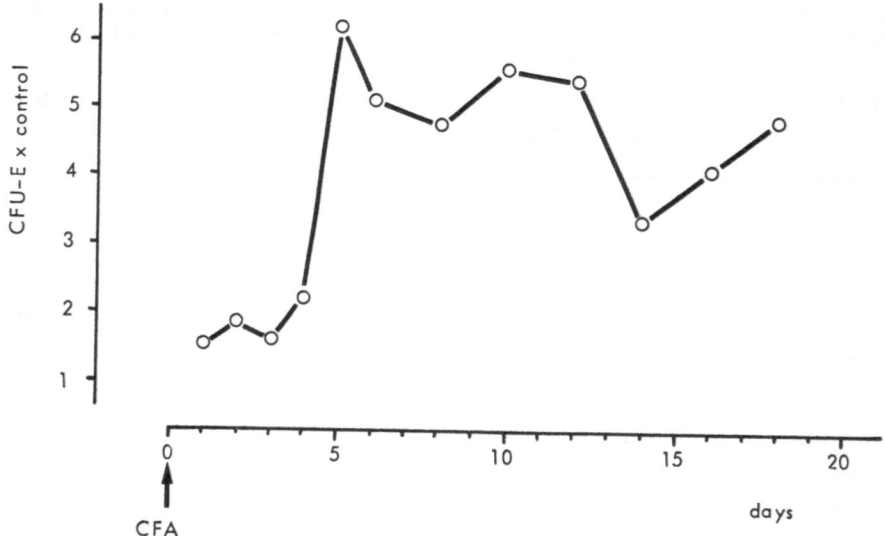

Fig. 2: Increase in the number of CFU-E in bone marrow of BALB-c mice induced by CFA, expressed proportional to control bone marrow of untreated animals.

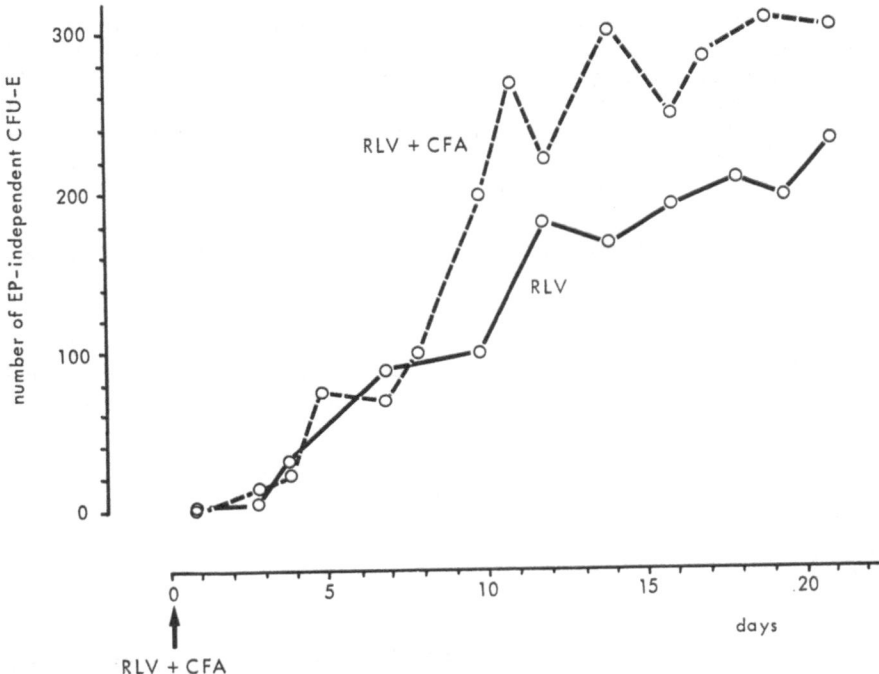

Fig. 3: Number of EP-independent CFU-E in bone marrow of BALB/c mice treated with only RLV or RLV + CFA.

hematologic series which would promote proliferation of myeloid progenitor cells over that of erythropoietic-sensitive cells. The very marked increase in CFU-E does not lead to polycythemia. There is even a slight decrease in the hematocrit. The number of erythroblasts in the bone marrow also declines after administration of CFA (14). There seems to be an maturation block *in vivo* beyond the stage of CFU-E.

III. Transformation in vitro

A subsequent step in our study was the induction of such hormone-indepency by incubation *in vitro* of normal BM cells with RLV. In table 2 is presented the number of erythroid colonies produced at various intervals after plating for bone marrow incubated with 10^7 XC-PFU of purified RLV isolated from leukemic spleen. As controls, the results of bone marrow kept for 4 hours under the same conditions in the absence of RLV are given. An additional control is the addition of EP to the culture medium. Already 2 days after plating no sign of EP-dependency can be observed in the RLV-infected cells, while the addition of EP to the normal bone marrow cultures leads to a marked elevation in colony production. A very high number of EP-independent colonies is noticed at day 5 after plating of RLV-incubated cells. The numbers of erythroid colonies produced 5 days after plating in the absence of EP and after incubation with various dilutions of RLV are presented in table 3. The results suggest a linear dose-response relationship. An endpoint seems to be reached at the dilution of 3200x, which corresponds with 10^4 PFU in the reverse XC test. Transformation could be prevented by incubation with specific antiserum. Mammary tumor virus or a myeloid leukemia virus did not induce this physiologic transformation.

Table II: In vitro induction by RLV of E.P.-independency of erythroid colony formation

Days after plating	Incubated with RLV number of erythroid colonies[1]		Incubated without RLV number of erythroid colonies[1]	
	presence of EP[2]	absence of EP	presence of EP[2]	absence of EP
2	166	207	290	82
5	1404	1342	174	54
7	1306	1211	201	43

[1] per 2 x 10^5 B. M. cells.
[2] 0.5 I. U. per dish.

Table III: Dose-response relationship of EP-independent colony-formation after incubation with R.L.V.

Dilution of RLV stock suspension	Number of EP-independent colonies 5 days after plating[1]
10	538
100	481
200	374
400	220
800	96
1600	58
3200	24
6400	15
12800	19

[1] per 2 x 10^5 B. M. cells.

The influence of EP on *in vitro* transformation was investigated by incubating bone marrow with RLV in the presence of EP for 16 hours. Thereafter, the cells were plated in the same way as described above. A slight inhibitory effect of the hormone on *in vitro* transformation can be observed in both experiments (table 4).

Possibly during the 16 hour incubation period the hormone induces maturation of the target cells beyond a stage where transformation can still take place. The hormone cannot compensate for this by the production of new target cells from more primitive hemopoietic cells under the employed *in vitro* conditions.

Table IV: Influence of incubation with EP on in vitro transformation by RLV

Incubation		Number of EP-independent colonies at day 5[1]	
1 mg RLV	1 IU EP	Experiment 1	Experiment 2
−	−	32	76
−	+	15	53
+	−	686	939
+	+	483	632

[1] per 2 x 10⁵ B. M. cells.

IV. Transfection

Hill and Hillova (15) were the first to carry out "transfection" experiments using proviral DNA of Rous sarcoma virus. Their results gave clear evidence that DNA from RNA virus-infected cells can carry virus-specific information responsible for the transformation.

In the present study, we used spontaneous erythroid colony formation by mouse bone marrow cells as a criterion for transformation. DNA was isolated by standard procedures from spleen cells of BALB/c mice which had been infected with RLV. The DNA solution was buffered with Hepesphosphate and treated with a high calcium concentration according to Graham and Van der Eb (16). A 0.5 ml sample of DNA suspension was then incubated with BALB/c mouse bone marrow cells for 4 hr and after washing the cells were plated in methyl-cellulose in the absence of erythropoietin.

After 5 days the number of erythroid colonies were counted. From table 5 it can be seen that DNA prepared from RLV-infected spleen cells has a transforming capacity. The control experiments show that the observed phenomenon is specific. Experiments with the reversed XC-test (17) showed that virus reproduction also

Table V: Transfection of mouse bone marrow cells with proviral DNA

Additions	Number of EP-independent colonies at day 5[1]
RLV-spleen-DNA 50 ug	744
rat-spleen-DNA 50 ug	22
RLV-spleen-DNA[2] 50 ug + DNA-se	16
High calcium buffer only	20

[1] per 2 x 10⁵ B. M. cells.
[2] incubated for 60 min. at 37 °C with 50 ug/ml of DNA-se before addition of calcium.

takes place after incubation of bone marrow cells with DNA from RLV-infected cells. The procedure utilized here to isolate DNA may give a range of molecular weights between 20 x 10⁶ and 200 x 10⁶ daltons. More detailed studies will be undertaken to determine the minimal size of the DNA fragments which can lead to virus reproduction and to transformation of haemopoietic cells.

V. Concluding remarks

B.M. cells of RLV-infected BALB/c mice can proliferate in methylcellulose in the absence of E.P., while normal B.M. cells cannot (12). Not only the CFU-E but also the more primitive BFU-E shows hormone-independency (18). This phenomenon is in favour of the view that the Rauscher virus induced erythroblastosis is a true neoplasia although transplantation experiments failed so far.

The experiments in which transformation *in vitro* of B.M. cells by RLV is established (19) show that the CFU-E can serve as a target for the virus.

Treatment of normal mice with CFA leads to a rapid increase in CFU-E in the bone marrow (18). Splenomegaly of RLV-infected mice is enhanced by CFA-treatment probably due to an increase in targets. Transfection with proviral DNA also can transform the CFU-E of BALB-c mice. This approach allows *in vitro* studies on the resistence of mouse strains to RLV *in vitro*.

The studies are of interest for the human disease in two aspects. *In vitro* transformation assays are needed to study the oncogenic potential of putative human leukemia viruses. Furthermore the studies have yielded some new insight in the pathogenesis of virally induced erythroblastosis. This might serve as a model for e.g. acute myeloid leukemia in man.

References

1. Macpherson, I. The characteristics of animal cells transformed in vitro. Adv. Cancer Res. *13*, 169–209 (1970).
2. Pontén, J. Spontaneous and virus induced transformation in cell culture. Virology Monogr. *8*, Springer Verlag, New York (1971).
3. Iscove, F. N. and Sieber, F. Erythroid progenitor in mouse bone marrow detected by macroscopic colony formation in culture. Exp. Hematol. *3*, 32–43 (1975).
4. Stephenson, J. R., Axelrad, A. A., McLeod, D. L. et al. Induction of colonies of hemoglobin-synthesizing cells by erythropoietin in vitro. Proc. Nat. Acad. Sci. USA *68*, 1542–1546 (1971).
5. Axelrad, A. A., McLeod, D. L., Shreeve, M. M. et al. Properties of cells that produce erythrocytic colonies in vitro. In hemopoiesis in culture. (Robinson, W. A., ed.). DHEW publication No (NIH) 74–205 (1974), pp. 226–234.
6. Siegel, B. V., and Morton, J. I. Immunologic stimuli in relation to leukemogenesis. I. Potentiation of Rauscher viral leukemia by Freund's adjuvants. J. Nat. Cancer Inst. *48*, 1681–1686 (1972).
7. Brommer, E. J. and Bentvelzen, P. A. J. Interactions between differentiation and leukaemogenesis in Rauscher murine leukaemia. Bibl. Haemat. *39*, 929–934 (1973).

8. Dunn, T. B., Malmgren, R. A. and Carney, P. C. et al. PTU and transfusion modification of the effects of Rauscher virus in BALB/c mice. J. Nat. Cancer Inst. *36*, 1003–1025 (1966).
9. Pluznik, D. H., Sachs, L. and Resnitzky, P. The mechanism of leukemogenesis by the Rauscher leukemia virus. Nat. Cancer Inst. Monogr. *22*, 3–14 (1966).
10. Brommer, E. J. The role of the stem cell in Rauscher murine leukaemia TNO, The Hague, (1973).
11. Seidel, H. J. Die Blutzellbildung bei der Rauscher-Leukämie (Mäusestamm BALB/c) und ihre Beeinflussung durch Hypertransfusion. Z.Schr. Krebsforsch. *77*, 155–165 (1972).
12. Nooter, K. and Ghio, R. Hormone-independent in vitro erythroid colony formation by bone marrow cells from Rauscher virus-infected mice. J. Nat. Cancer Inst. *55*, 59–64 (1975).
13. Boggs, D. R., Marsh, J. C. and Chervenick, P. A. et al. Factors influencing hematopoietic spleen colony formation in irradiated mice. J. Exp. Med. *126*, 851–870 (1967).
14. McNeill, T. A. Antigenic stimulation of bone marrow colony forming cells. Immunology *18*, 61–72 (1970).
15. Hill, M. and Hillowa, J. Virus recovering in chicken cells tested with Rous sarcoma cell DNA. Nature New Biology *237*, 35–39 (1972).
16. Graham, F. L. and Van der Eb, A. J. A new technique for the assay of infectivity of human adeno virus 5 DNA. Virology *52*, 456–467 (1973).
17. Niwa, O., Declève, A. and Liberman, M. et al. Adaptation of plague assay methods to the in vitro quantitation of radiation leukemia virus. J. Virol. *12*, 68–73 (1973).
18. Nooter, K. and Bentvelzen, P. A. J. In vitro studies on the enhancement of Rauscher virus-induced erythroblastosis by complete Freund's adjuvant in BALB/c mice. J. Nat. Cancer Inst. In press. (1976).
19. Nooter, K. and Bentvelzen, P. A. J. In vitro transformation of murine erythroid cells by Rauscher leukemia virus. Cancer letters, 155–160 (1976).

In Vitro and Preliminary in Vivo Studies of Compounds which Induce the Differentiation of Friend Leukemia Cells*

H. D. Preisler, M. D.

Roswell Park Memorial Institute
Department of Medicine A
Buffalo, New York 14263

The progeny of normal hematopoietic stem cells ultimately become mature functional cells through a process involving both cell replication and differentiation. The proliferative aspect is limited and in fact as full maturation is approached the cells lose their proliferative potentital. Built into the process of differentiation is an inherent limitation of the life span of the maturing cells. In essence, acute myelogenous leukemia (AML) results from a disruption of the normal maturation process. Leukemic stem cells proliferate without normal constraints and their progeny for the most part remain at the stem cell level. This latter phenomenon results in the cells retaining their proliferative potential and endows the cells with a life span which is longer than that of normal cells. The resulting increasing mass of leukemic cells, through an as yet undefined process, interferes with the proliferation and maturation of normal myeloid elements ultimately causing the pancytopenia which is directly responsible for the morbidity and mortality which accompanies AML.

Current approaches to the therapy of AML are directed towards the destruction of the leukemic cells by the administration of cytotoxic chemotherapy. Unfortunately the chemotherapeutic agents are also toxic for normal hematopoietic stem cells and one of the major side effects of this form of therapy is pancytopenia – with attendant morbidity and mortality.

A variety of studies have demonstrated that malignant cells possess the potential to differentiate and that differentiation is frequently associated with a decrease in or a loss of malignant potential (1–4). These observations suggest that it may be possible to treat cancer (including AML) by inducing the differentiation of the malignant cells. Such an approach, even if only moderately effective, might result in the production of mature granulocytes which could alleviate the granulocytopenia associated with the disease.

Friend Leukemia as a Model System

The Friend leukemia is a viral induced murine leukemia (5). The disease is characterized by the proliferation of blast cells with the spleen being the major site of leukemic cell proliferation. Some of the progeny of leukemic cells prolife-

* This research was supported by U. S. P. H. S. grant CA-5834.

rating in the spleen undergo erythroid differentiation while the same leukemic cells growing subcutaneously produce tumors which are devoid of differentiating erythroid cells (6). These tumors have been classifield as "reticulum cell sarcomas" (7).

Several investigators have established long-term suspension culture cell lines from the leukemic mice (8–10). These leukemic cells grow in suspension culture as morphologically undifferentiated blast cells. A small proportion of the tissue culture cells (usually < 1 %) spontaneously differentiate along the erythroid pathway. It was found that the addition of either dimethylsulfoxide (DMSO) (11) or dimethylformamide (DMF) (12) to the culture media of these cells induced a substantial proportion of the leukemic cells to differentiate along the erythroid pathway. These observations led to the conclusion that the Friend leukemia cells growing in suspension culture represented a class of committed erythroid precursor cells whose normal maturation had been prevented by their neoplastic transformation.

Recent studies in our laboratory have made the question of the nature (multipotential stem cell vs. erythroid progenitor) of the Friend cells growing in culture more complex than had previously been appreciated. We have found that when these tissue culture cells (line 745A) are innoculated subcutaneously into mice, the majority of tumor cells growing at the site of innoculation contain chloroacetate esterase (CAE) and some of the cells are peroxidase positive as well (13). Both enzymes are felt to be characteristic of granulocytic cells and have not been reported to be present in cells of the erythroid series nor in reticulum cell sarcomas. Some of the tumor cells appear morphologically to be undergoing abortive granulocytic maturation. The tissue culture cells themselves are all chloroacetate esterase positive (14). It should be noted that Friend virus infection of mice is associated with a significant increase in granulocyte colony forming units (15). It is not known if this increase is due to neoplastic transformation of granulocytic progenitor cells or if it is merely reactive proliferation of normal progenitor cells.

Thus the question as to the nature of the Friend leukemia cell is more complicated than had hitherto been realized. Are they erythroid progenitors whose maturation has been arrested by the leukemic state and whose genomic regulation has been so distorted by malignant change that it programs for the synthesis of enzymes which are normally not present in erythroid cells? Or are they granulocytic (CAE positive) stem cells which in the in vitro environment have a greater potential for erythroid rather than granuloid differentiation? One interesting aspect of this problem is the fact that while DMSO-induced erythroid differentiation in vitro appears to be associated with a decrease in the degree of CAE positivity of the cells, the majority of cells remain CAE positive and in fact we have found cells which are simultaneously strongly positive for both CAE and heme (benzidine stain). At present wo do not know if the CAE present in cells which are synthesizing heme is being actively synthesized or if CAE synthesis ceases with the onset of erythroid differentiation and we are detecting residual enzyme. In any event, it is clear that the cells which are induced to differentiate along the erythroid pathway are the cells which had previously synthesized an enzyme believed to be characteristic of granulocytic differentiation. Hence if CAE positivity denotes granulocytic differentiation then either the cell can simultaneously differentiate along two different pathways or alternatively the cell must dediffer-

162

entiate from the granulocytic pathway and then differentiate along the erythroid pathway. At the present time assigning the Friend cell to a particular cell series appears to be essentially a problem of semantics.

The ability to induce erythroid differentiation in vitro and the ability of the tissue culture cells to produce leukemia when inoculated intravenously into DBA 2/J mice suggested that this system could serve as a prototype for determining if agents which induce leukemic cell differentiation in vitro could function as chemotherapeutic agents in vivo.

Cryoprotective Agents as Inducers of Differentiation

Our initial studies demonstrated that both DMSO and DMF were too toxic to permit chemotherapeutic trials in mice. Since both inducers were aproteic polar solvents which were cryoprotective agents as well, we studied the ability of other cryoprotective agents to induce the differentiation of Friend leukemia cells in vitro. These studies ultimately led to the recognition of other inducing agents which were more potent and less toxic than DMSO or DMF (16, 17).

Table I

Inducer	$^0/_0$ B + cells*
Tetramethylurea	70
Dimethylacetamide	70
N-methylacetamide	55
Pyridine N oxide	55
Dimethyl sulfoxide	55
Dimethyl formamide	30
Acetamide	16
Dimethylurea	13
Pyridazine	10
Diethylene glycol	7
Control	0.3

* $^0/_0$ of benzidine positive cell after 5 days of culture in the presence of the inducing agent.

Table I lists some of the compounds which we tested and their effects on the proportion of differentiated cells in Friend leukemia cell cultures. Fig. 1 demonstrates that the compounds exhibited various physical structures ranging from linear molecules to aromatic molecules. The agents are all small, polar, freely diffusible compounds. Nash has conducted extensive studies of the physical properties of cryoprotective compounds and has found that the cryoprotective potential of a compound correlates with the ability of the compound to donate free electron pairs (to function as a Lewis base) (18, 19). This same property also correlates with the relative ability of compounds within a family (such as tetramethylurea, dimethylurea, and urea) to induce differentiation (17). While compounds vary widely in their inducing potency, it appears that once begun the biology of the

163

process of differentiation is the same regardless of the agent used to induce differentiation (17).

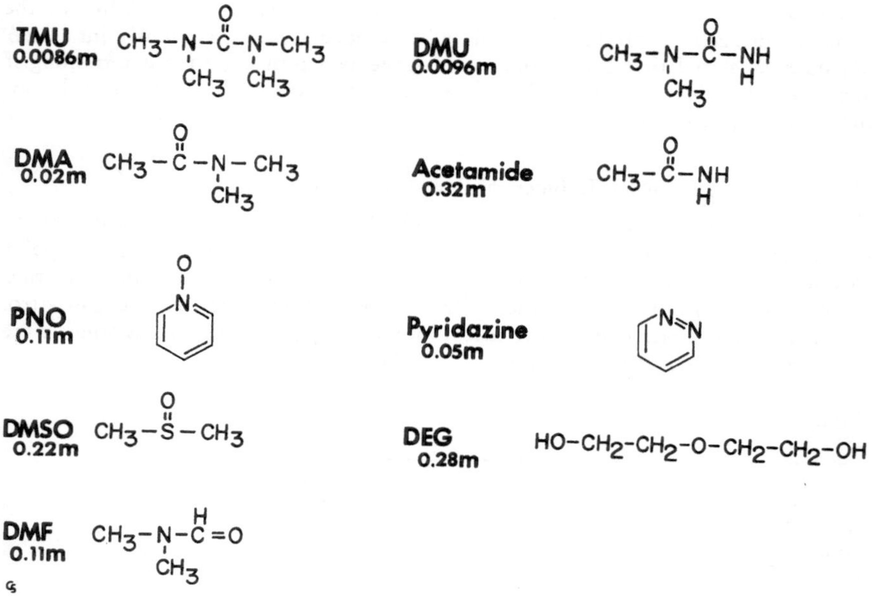

TMU 0.0086m $CH_3-N-\overset{\overset{\displaystyle O}{\|}}{C}-N-CH_3$ with CH_3 and CH_3

DMU 0.0096m $CH_3-N-\overset{\overset{\displaystyle O}{\|}}{C}-\overset{H}{N}$ with CH_3

DMA 0.02m $CH_3-\overset{\overset{\displaystyle O}{\|}}{C}-N-CH_3$ with CH_3

Acetamide 0.32m $CH_3-\overset{\overset{\displaystyle O}{\|}}{C}-\overset{H}{N}$

PNO 0.11m (pyridine N-oxide structure)

Pyridazine 0.05m (pyridazine ring structure, N=N)

DMSO 0.22m $CH_3-\overset{\overset{\displaystyle O}{\|}}{S}-CH_3$

DEG 0.28m $HO-CH_2-CH_2-O-CH_2-CH_2-OH$

DMF 0.11m $CH_3-\overset{H}{N}-\overset{H}{C}=O$ with CH_3

G

Fig. 1: Physical structure of the inducing agents listed in Table I. Numbers under names of compounds indicate optional inducing concentrations.

This research was supported by U.S.P.H.S. grant CA-5834.

Despite the obvious similarities between the inducing agents and the general similarities in the process of induced differentiation, it should be recognized that not all of the effects of the inducing agents are identical or necessarily related to differentiation per se. For example, when line 745A cells are cultured in the presence of DMSO there is an 80 % decline in the acid soluble ATP pool size by the end of 5 days of culture. This significant fall in ATP pool size is not seen when cells are cultured in the presence of tetramethylurea, a more potent inducer of differentiation than DMSO (20). In this case there is only a 20–25 % decline in pool size. Furthermore BUdR-inhibition of DMSO-induced differentiation does not prevent the decline in ATP pool size. Thus a biological or biochemical phenomenon which accompanies chemical-induced differentiation is not necessarily part of or even related to the process of differentiation.

The situation is further complicated by our observations that cells may be resistant to the inducing effects of one compound and yet be induced to differentiate by a different compound. We have conducted studies with a cell line which is not induced to differentiate by DMSO (cell line 745D). This cell line is responsive, albeit to a low degree, to pyridine N-oxide, N-methylacetamide and DMF (17).

Furthermore, this cell line responds to a significant extent (greater than 20 % of cells induced to differentiate) to butyric acid (14), a compound demonstrated by Leder & Leder to be an effective inducer of differentiation in their Friend leukemia cell line (21). Despite the fact that butyric acid is a much better inducer of 745D differentiation than is DMSO, the former is a less potent inducer of 745A differentiation. From these observations it is apparent that caution must be exercised in interpreting and generalizing from experimental studies since: 1) equally potent inducers of differentiation may exert differing biological and biochemical effects 2) different cell lines may have differing sensitivities to the various inducers of differentiation.

Mechanism of Action of Inducing Agents

The differentiation of FLC in vitro is accompanied by the accumulation of globin mRNA (22, 23). Bromodeoxyuridine (BUdR) which interferes with globin mRNA accumulation inhibits DMSO-induced differentiation (24). Accumulation of globin mRNA during differentiation has been noted in most studies. Therefore any stimulus which induces the differentiation of these cells appears to ultimately act through the process of transcription. There may be however an exception to this statement (25). Paul et. al. have presented evidence for translational control of differentiation of a Friend leukemia line.

Our initial studies of the effects of BUdR on DMSO-induced differentiation led us to postulate the presence of a repressor of differentiation in the leukemic cells with DMSO-induced differentiation resulting either in a decreased affinity of repressor for operon or in a decrease in the level of intracellular inhibitor (24). The recognition of the fact that the inducers were small molecules whose inducing potency appeared to be related to their ability to donate lone pair electrons permitted a broadening of this concept with the actual physical interaction involved in transcription being related to: 1) disruption of water structure with secondary alterations in hydrophobic bonding of regulatory molecules to DNA (such as histones) 2) interaction between inducers and acidic nucleoproteins, or 3) perhaps direct disruption of the internal hydrogen bonding within the DNA helix permitting transcription of the resultant single stranded DNA sequences (16). In support of this possible mode of action are the reports of DMSO stimulates DNA transcription in vitro (26) and the studies of the effects of BUdR and DMSO on chromatin structure (27).

On the other hand, the ability of inducers to cryoprotect erythrocytes suggested that these compounds have significant effects on the cell membrane. Using differential scanning calorimetry (DSC) we have found that the inducing-cryoprotective agents increase the melting temperature of artificial acidic phospholipid vesicles, a finding we interpret as indicative of a decrease in the fluidity of the vesicle membranes. Compounds, such as topical anesthetics, which increase the fluidity of phospholipid membranes in vitro, interfere with the effects of the inducers on the phospholipid vesicles and also inhibit the induction of differentiation of Friend leukemia cells in suspension culture (28). In fact, to date, using DSC and the artificial phospholipid vesicle system we have been able not only to account for our previous observations (such as apparent synergistic induction of differentiation by the combination of DMSO and DMF and the only additive effects of DMSO and PNO) but also have been able to prospectively predict the effects of agents and combinations on the differentiation of FLC 745A in vitro. These observations suggest that the initial event during the induction of differentiation by cryoprotective agents may occur at the cell surface with transcription being a necessary but secondary phenomenon mediated perhaps by communication between the cell membrane and nucleus.

It is clear that at this time it is not possible to state whether the chemical agents induce differentiation by directly stimulating transcription of those DNA sequences which code for erythroid differentiation or by interacting with the cell membrane and thus indirectly inducing differentiation. It is possible that the same physical properties (low molecular weight, Lewis bascity, etc.) which produce the effects on acidic phospholipid vesicles and provide cryoprotection to erythocytes are also responsible for directly altering the transcription of DNA. To complicate matters further, as noted above, some Friend leukemia cell lines are responsive to some agents and more or less responsive to others. In at least one cell line butyric acid has been found to interfere with DMSO-induced differentiation (21). Conversely, but leading to a similar potential conclusion, the combination of some inducing agents appear to be "synergistic" while others are "additive" (16). Hence it is possible that there is more than one mechanism by which chemical agents induce the differentiation of FLC in vitro or alternatively the various cell lines may differ in the way in which they metabolize the inducers (exclude, activate, or deactivate the compounds) or differ in the composition of their cell membranes and hence while differences in membrane composition result in different inducer sensitivities the acutal changes in the cell membranes produced by the agents may be identical (for example all may decrease membrane fluidity).

Whatever their mechanism of action in vitro, the recognition of a wide variety of inducing agents has made possible the in vivo testing of their possible chemotherapeutic efficacy.

In Vivo Chemotherapy

Our initial studies have employed the intravenous innoculation of FLC lines 745A into syngeneic DBA 2/J mice followed 1 week later by the daily administration of N-methylacetamide. This therapy significantly and consistently inhibited the proliferation of FLC in the spleens of the treated mice and to a somewhat lesser degree the proliferation of leukemic cells in the bone marrows of the mice (29). Survival of the mice has not been consistently prolonged, perhaps a result of the hepatoxicity of the compound. In any event we are now in the position to determine whether the studies of leukemic cell differentiation in vitro are applicable to the treatment of leukemia in vivo.

Future Perspective

The induction of leukemic cell differentiation in vivo may provide a mode of therapy which is significantly different from that currently employed. It now appears feasible to test this proposition in vivo in mice.

References

1. Pierce, G. B. and Wallace, C. (1971) Cancer Res. 31: 127–134.
2. Prasad, K. N. (1972) Cytobios 6: 163–166.
3. De Cosse, J. J., Gossens, C. L., Kuzma, J. F. and Unsworth, B. R. (1973) Science 181: 1057–1058.
4. Ichikawa, Y. (1969) J. Cell. Physiol. 74: 223–234.
5. Friend, C. (1957) J. Exp. Med. 105: 307–318.
6. Friend, C., Preisler, H. D., and Scher, W. (1974) Curr. Top. Develop. Biol. 8: 81–101.
7. Buffet, R. F. and Furth, J. (1959) Cancer Res. 19, 1063–1069.
8. Friend, C., Patuleia, M. C. and Harven, (1966) Natl. Cancer Inst. Monogr. 22: 505–522.
9. Ostertag, W., Melderis, H., Steinheider, G., Kluge, N. and Dube, S. (1972) Nature (New Biol) 239: 231–234.
10. Ikawa, Y., Furusawa, M. and Sugano, H. (1973) in: Unifying Concepts of Leukemia. Bibl. Haemat. No 39, 955–967.
11. Friend, C., Scher, W., Holland, J. G. and Sato, T. (1971) Proc. Nat. Acad. Sci. (USA) 68: 378–382.
12. Scher, W., Preisler, H. D. and Friend, C. (1973) J. Cell Physiol. 81: 63–70.
13. Preisler, H. D., Bjornsson, S., Mori, M. and Barcos, M. (1975). Cell Diff. 4:213–283.
14. Preisler, H. D., Shiraishi, Y., Mori, M., and Sandberg., A. A. Submitted to Cell Diff.
15. Golde, D. W., Faille, A., Sullivan, A., and Friend, C. (1975) in: Proc. Amer. Assoc. Cancer Res. 16:13.
16. Preisler, H. D. and Lyman, G. (1975) Cell Differ. 4: 179–185.
17. Preisler, H. D., Christoff, G. and Taylor, E. (1976). Blood. 47:363–368.
18. Nash, T. (1962) J. Gen. Physiol. 46: 167–175.
19. Nash, T. in: Meryman, H. T. (ed): Cryobiology. New York, Academic Press 1966, Chapter 5, 179–211.
20. Preisler, H. D. and Rustum, Y. (1975) Life Sciences. 17:1287–1290.
21. Leder, A. and Leder, P. (1975) Science. 5:319–322.
22. Ross, J., Ikawa, Y. and Leder, P. (1972) Proc. Nat. Acad. Sci. (USA) 69: 3620–3623.
23. Preisler, H. D., Scher, W. and Friend, C. (1974) Differ, 1: 27–37.
24. Preisler, H. D., Housman, D., Scher, W., and Friend, C. (1973) Proc. Nat. Acad. Sci. (USA) 70: 2956–2959.
25. Harrison, P. R., Gilmour, R. S., Affara, N. A., Conkie, C. and Paul, J. (1974) Cell Differ. 3: 23–30.
26. Travers, A. (1974) Eur. J. Biochem 47: 435–441.
27. Lapeyre, J. and Bekhor, I. (1974) J. Mol. Bio. 89: 137–162.
28. Lyman, G., Preisler, H. D. and Papauadjopoulous, D. submitted to Nature.
29. Preisler, H. D., Bjornsson, S., Mori, M. and Lyman, G. Presented at the American Society of Hematology Meetings, Dallas (1975).

Target Cells for Transformation with Avian Leukosis Viruses

T. Graf, B. Royer-Pokora and H. Beug

Max-Planck-Institut für Virusforschung, Tübingen

Introduction

Leukemia is a widespread disorder of the hemopoietic system of vertebrates which has been particularly well analyzed in chickens, mice and recently also in cats (for review see 1). It seems now safe to assume that the majority of the different ypes of leukemias found in animals are caused by infection with or activation of C-type leukemia viruses (1). In fact, it has been known since 1908 that leukemia can be induced by a filterable agent, i.e., a virus (2). With the availability of modern biochemical technology and quantitative biological assays, leukosis-sarcoma viruses have since then been thoroughly analyzed in their structure, mechanism of replication and genetics (1). Little is known, however, about the mechanism of virus-induced leukemogenesis.

The existence of highly oncogenic chicken virus trains which specifically induce certain types of acute leukemias such as myeloblastosis or erythroblastosis stimulated us to attempt to define the corresponding target cells. An important prerequisite for these studies was the availability of in vitro transformation assays. While such assays had been developed for two strains causing myeloid leukemia (avian myeloblastosis) (AMV) (3, 4) and avian myelocytomatosis strain MC29 (5, 6) no in vitro transformation system was known for viruses causing leukemias of other types of hemopoietic cells.

Here some of the features of a newly developed in vitro transformation assay with avian erythroblastosis virus will be described. In addition, data will be discussed which suggest that the target cells for leukemogenesis with chicken erythroid and myeloid leukosis viruses are not pluripotent stem cells but are committed to differentiate along the erythropoietic and granulopoietic series respectively.

In vitro transformation of hemopoietic cells with avian erythroblastosis virus

Avian erythroblastosis virus (AEV) is known to cause the corresponding disease at an incidence of over 50 % in young and adult birds within only a few weeks after infection (for ref. see 7). The picture of a blood smear of a diseased bird is shown in Fig. 1.

Two strains, AEV-R and AEV-ES4, were studied and similar results were obtained with both. They will therefore collectively be referred to as AEV. Infection of freshly prepared bone marrow cell cultures with AEV resulted in the appearance of foci of small refractile, round, rapidly growing cells (Fig. 2). The details of the assay as well as the origin of the virus strains, the methods used for their assay and propagation, and the preparation and culture of bone marrow cells will be described in another communication (8). Here it may suffice to mention

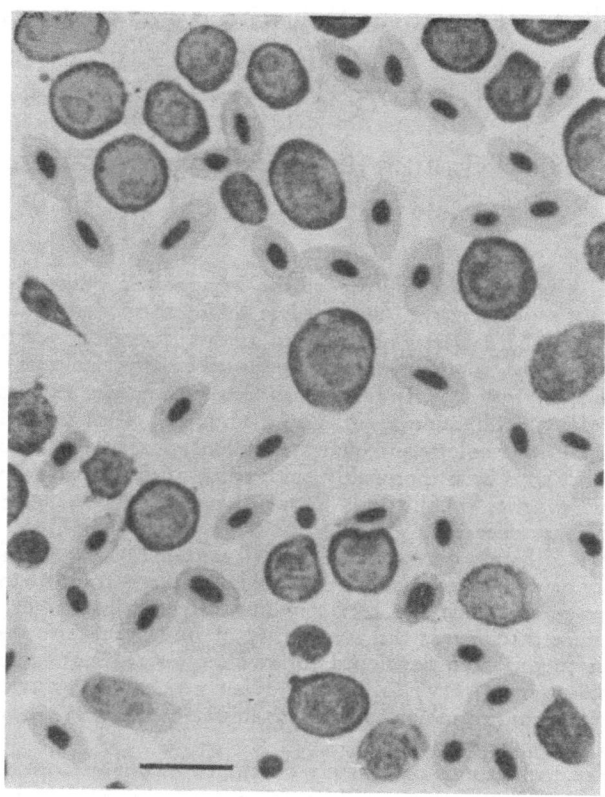

Fig. 1: Smear (stained with Wright-Giemsa) of peripheral blood from a chicken infected with AEV. Note that the chicken erythrocytes are nucleated. Bar represents 20 μ.

that the culture medium contained calf serum and chicken serum and that the addition of 1 %/o DMSO greatly improved the assay. The *in vitro* transformed cells were indistinguishable in their staining properties from leukemic erythroblasts induced *in vivo* and maintained in culture (Fig. 3).

To determine the proliferative capacity of the *in vitro* transformed cells, 22 randomly selected 7-day-old single foci were isolated and propagated separately. The cells from each culture were then counted and passaged at appropriate intervals. After two weeks of growth (the best cultures duplicating every 15–20 hours), most of the cultures started to accumulate degenerated cell forms and slowed down in their rate of growth. By 4 weeks no more increase in cell number was obtained and the experiment was terminated. From the total number of cells obtained with each clone (the values ranged from $4 \cdot 10^5$ to $7 \cdot 10^8$) the number of population doublings was calculated. As can be seen from Fig. 4, the *in vitro* transformed cells studied were capable of dividing in average for 18–29 generations. These values are

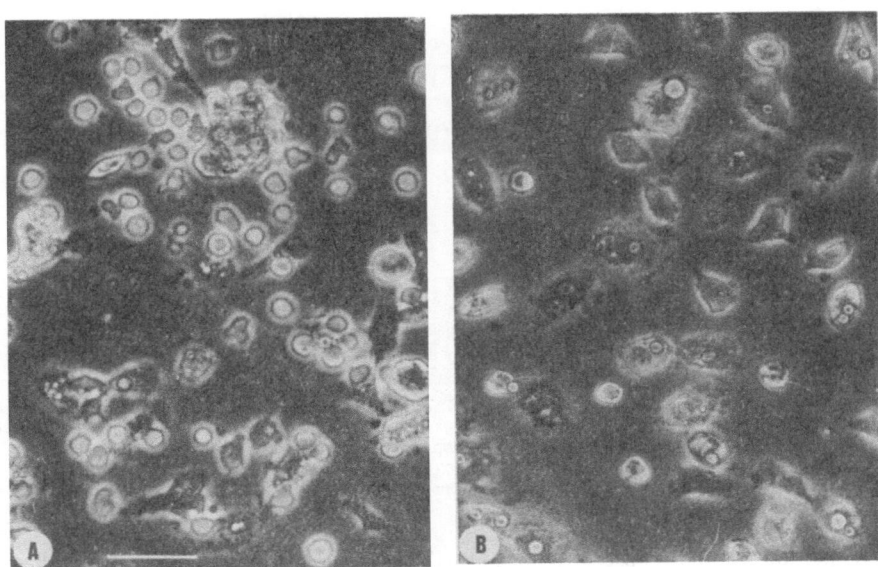

Fig. 2: Phase micrographs of chicken bone marrow cells. (A) Focus of cells transformed *in vitro* 5 days after infection with AEV. (B) Uninfected bone marrow culture. Bar represents 40 μ.

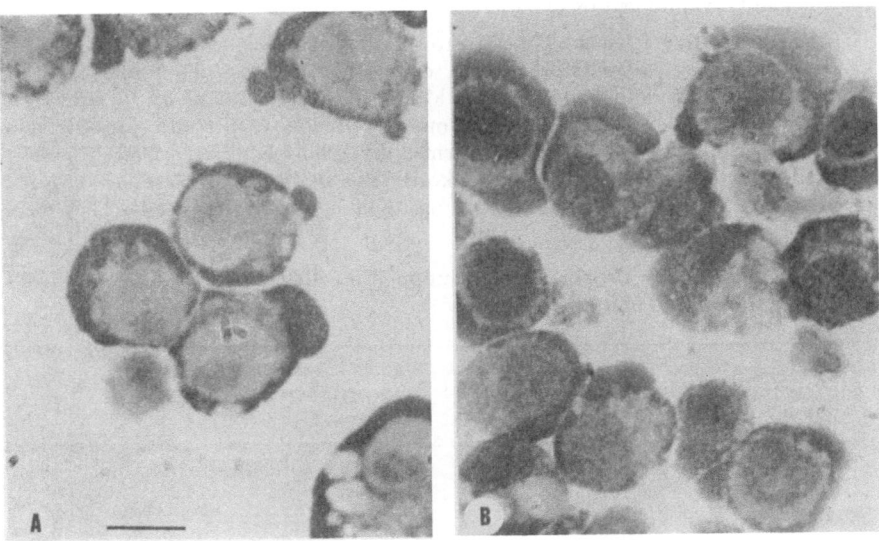

Fig. 3: Smears (stained with Wright-Giemsa) of erythroblasts transformed *in vitro* (A), and transformed *in vivo* and maintained in culture for 10 days (B). Bar represents 10 μ.

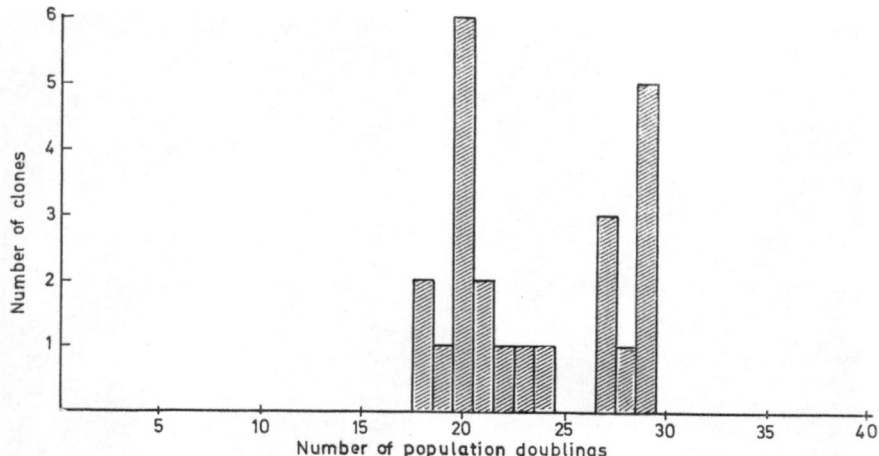

Fig. 4: Frequency distribution of the number of population doublings obtained with 22 clones of *in vitro* transformed erythroblasts.

comparable to those observed for normal or sarcoma virus-transformed chicken fibroblasts (9).

Comparative properties of bone marrow cells transformed in vitro by erythroblastosis and myeloid leukosis viruses

To further characterize the bone marrow cells transformed *in vitro* by AEV as erythroblasts, they were compared in a series of properties to bone marrow cells transformed by myeloid leukosis virus MC29. A fuller account of these experiments will be given elsewhere. A summary of the results are presented in Table 1. As can be seen, *in vitro* transformed erythroblasts differed from hemopoietic cells transformed by a myeloid leukosis virus in that they were negative for the following properties characteristic of granulopoietic (myeloid) cells: They were

Table I: Comparative properties of hemopoietic cells transformed by erythroid and myeloid leukosis viruses

Bone marrow cells transformed *in vitro* by	
Avian erythroblastosis virus (AEV-R)	Avian myelocytomatosis virus (MC29)
Erythroblast-like morphology	Macrophage-like morphology
Non adherent	Adherent
No phagocytic activity	Phagocytic activity
Colony formation in semisolid media not CSF dependent	Colony formation in semisolid agar is CSF dependent

172

not adherent, did not phagocytize bacteria, and were not dependent on colony stimulating factor (CSF) for colony formation in semisolid agar. Other more specific markers of erythroid differentiation could not yet be determined. Like the *in vivo* induced leukemic erythroblasts, *in vitro* transformed erythroblasts were hemoglobin negative (as determined by benzidine staining) and could not be induced to synthesize hemoglobin by the addition of DMSO, as it is possible with mouse erythroid cells transformed by Friend leukemia virus (10). Neither could the effect of erythropoietin on the growth of these cells be evaluated since avian erythropoietin was not available and mammalian erythropoietin has been found to be inactive in birds (11).

Models explaining the transformation specificity of avian leukosis viruses

Two basic models will be discussed to account for our findings. In accordance with current notions about normal hemopoiesis it is assumed that all differentiated hemopoietic cells arise from pluripotent stem cells by a series of maturation steps (12). In the drawings of the models in Fig. 5 only the erythropoietic and granulopoietic (or myeloid) series of differentiation were included. The terms "transformation of hemopoietic cells" or "leukotransformation" are defined as the process by which certain hemopoietic cells are morphologically altered and induced to proliferate by infection with a leukosis virus.

Model 1. Transformation of specific committed progenitor cells. Avian erythroblastosis virus (AEV) transforms *erythroid* cells at an early stage of maturation whereas avian myeloblastosis virus (AMV) and myelocytomatosis virus (MC29) transform immature *myeloid* cells. The target cells for the latter two viruses differ

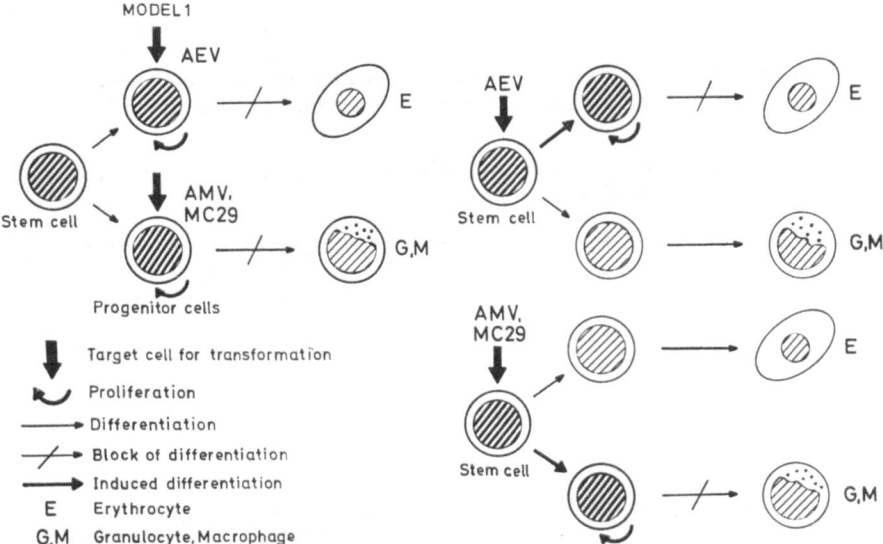

Fig. 5: Two basic models concerning the involvement of hemopoietic cells in leukemogenesis.

in their degree of maturation. Experimental observations indicate that concomitantly with leukotransformation normal differentiation is arrested. The model also allows room for the possibility that leukosis viruses induce a limited maturation or dedifferentiation of their target cells. A testable prediction arising from this model is that the target cells for erythroid and myeloid virus strains can be physically separated or selectively eliminated prior to infection.

Model 2. Involvement of stem cells. In this case, AEV induces pluripotent stem cells to differentiate into transformed erythroblasts. Conversely, AMV and MC29 viruses induce the formation of transformed myeloid cells of different stages of maturation. A similar specificity could also be achieved if it is assumed that these viruses are capable of selectively blocking the differentiation of hemopoietic cells belonging to series other than those transformed. As in model 1, once the cells are transformed they do not usually differentiate anymore. If this model is correct it should not be possible to separate or selectively eliminate target cells for erythroid and myeloid leukosis viruses.

Preliminary data supporting model 1

Most of freshly seeded chicken bone marrow cells die within a few days of incubation and a population of adherent cells survive. Cultures of these cells consist in their majority of macrophage-like cells (13). They can be passaged by trypsinization and maintained with a net increase in cell number for several months (unpublished observations). To determine the incidence of target cells for transformation in freshly prepared cultures of bone marrow and in cultures of adherent cells at different passages, they were infected with AEV and MC29 viruses and the number of foci obtained with each virus scored. As can be seen from Table 2, AEV-induced erythroblast foci were only obtained in freshly prepared cultures and not in the cultures passaged up to 3 times. This suggests that the target cells for AEV are non adherent cells or that they have been otherwise eliminated during the transfer procedure. In contrast, MC29 induced foci in all cultures. The much

Table II: **Incidence of bone marrow cells transformed by avian erythroid and myeloid leukosis viruses**[a]

	Fresh cultures	Passaged cultures (number of passages)		
		1	2	3
Avian erythroblastosis virus (AEV)	55[b]	0	0	0
Avian myelocytomatosis virus (MC29)	160	15.000	5.400	4.400

a) Cultures were prepared from a 4-week-old chicken and passaged at 5-day intervals.
b) Average number of transformed foci. Duplicate cultures in 35 mm dishes were seeded with 10^3, 10^4, 10^5 and 10^6 cells and infected with 10^4–10^5 transforming units of virus per dish.

higher efficiency of transformation with this virus in cultures which had been transferred at least once can be explained by a selection of a population of myeloid cells particularly susceptible to transformation with myeloid leukosis virus. These results demonstrate that the target cells for AEV can be selectively eliminated and are therefore probably not identical to the target cells for MC29. Cell separation experiments devised to further test this interpretation are currently being performed.

Concluding Remarks

Chromosomal studies of human leukemic cells strongly suggest that chronic myeloid leukemia (CML) and possibly also acute myeloid leukemia (AML) are stem cell diseases (for review see 14). The data presented show that other mechanisms probably exist in a model animal system. A diversity of target cells as suggested for chicken leukosis viruses, however, does not rule out the possibility that stem cells are also affected.

In drawing parallels to C-type virus induced leukemogenesis in animals it is assumed that human leukemia is induced by similar agents. Recently, evidence has accumulated demonstrating the presence of C-type viruses or some of their components in human leukemic cells (see articles by Spiegelman, Gallo, Todaro, Bentvelzen and Till in this volume). It is not clear, however, whether these viruses are cause or consequence of the disease. And, even if the former is assumed, it remains to be determined whether they are endogenous agents that become activated, as postulated by the oncogene theory (15), or whether they represent infectious viruses as suggested by the work of Spiegelman, Gallo and their coworkers (16, 17). It appears as if both of these possible mechanisms of virus-induced leukemogenesis are realized in animals (1).

Studies performed with another highly oncogenic strain, the murine leukemia virus FLV, indicate that transformation of *committed* hemopoietic cells is a mechanism not restricted to avian viruses (18). It is, however, questionable whether the so-called lymphoid leukosis viruses, the C-type virus strains found most frequently under natural conditions in the chicken and which possess an extensive period of latency (19), also act on committed hemopoietic cells as proposed here for highly oncogenic strains. So far, because of the lack of *in vitro* transformation assays, the mechanism of leukemogenesis by these "weakly" oncogenic viruses has not been well analyzed.

The isolation of infectious human leukemia viruses might allow studying the question of whether or not all leukemias are stem cell disorders by an approach such as described here in a model system. Besides its academic interest the answer to this question may have implications for the therapy of the disease.

References

1. Tooze, J. (Ed.), The Molecular Biology of Tumour Viruses. Cold Spring Harbor Laboratory, 1973.
2. Ellermann, V., and Bang, O., *Centr. Bakteriol. Parasitenk., Abt. I, Orig. 46:* 595, 1908.

3. Beaudreau, G. S., Becker, C., Bonar, R. A., Wallbank, A. M., Beard, D., and Beard, J. W., *J. Nat. Cancer Inst. 24:* 395, 1960.
4. Baluda, M. A., Moscovici, C., and Goetz, I. E., *J. Nat. Cancer Inst. Monograph 17:* 449 (1964).
5. Langlois, A. J., Fritz, R. B., Heine, U., Beard, D., Bolognesi, D. P., and Beard, J. W., *Cancer Res. 29:* 2056, 1969.
6. Graf, T., *Virology, 54:* 398, 1973.
7. Beard, J. W., *Adv. in Cancer Res. 7:* 1, 1963.
8. Graf, T., Z. Naturforsch. *30c* 847, 1975.
9. Pontén, J., *Int. J. Cancer 6:* 323, 1970.
10. Friend, C., Scher, W., Holland, J. G., and Sato, T., *Proc. Nat. Acad. Sci. U.S. 68:* 378, 1971.
11. Rosse, W. F., and Waldmann, T., *Blood, 27:* 654, 1966.
12. Metcalf, D., and Moore, M. A. S., Haemopoietic cells. North Holland Publishing Co., Amsterdam, London, 1971.
13. Moscovici, C., and Moscovici, M. G., *In:* Methods in Cell Physiology Vol. 7. D. M. Prescott (Ed.) (Academic Press, New York and London) pp. 313–328, 1973.
14. Sandberg, A. S., and Hossfeld, D. K., *Ann. Rev. Med. 21:* 379, 1970.
15. Huebner, R. J., and Todaro, G. J., *Proc. Nat. Acad. Sci. U.S. 64:* 1087, 1969.
16. Baxt, W., Yates, J. W., Wallace, H. J., Holland, J. F. and Spiegelman, S., *Proc. Nat. Acad. Sci. U.S. 70:* 2629, 1973.
17. R. E. Gallagher, and R. C. Gallo, *Science 187:* 350, 1975.
18. Tambourin, P. E., and Wendling, F., *Nature 256:* 321, 1975.
19. Purchase, H. G., and Burmester, B. R. *In:* Diseases of Poultry, Hofstad, M. S. et al. (Eds.) Sixth edition (The Iowa State University Press) pp. 502–571, 1972.

Fusion Experiments with Human Tumour Cells

J. F. Watkins

Dept. of Medical Microbiology
The Welsh National School of Medicine
Cardiff, Wales

This paper reports some results of experiments in which cells from human tumours have been fused with mouse cells by Sendai virus inactivated by ultraviolet irradiation (1, 2, 3). The reasons for wanting to perform these experiments are as follows:

1. If malignant change in human tumour cells is determined by the product of a specific gene locus, it may be possible, by hybridisation with mouse cells, to generate a mouse tumour containing only one human chromosome, since human chromosomes are usually lost from mouse x human hybrid cells.
2. If the human tumour cells contain an oncogenic virus, one or more of the following phenomena may occur as a result of fusion:
   a) Maintenance of part of the tumour cell genome as part of the genome of a continuously growing hybrid line may lead to spontaneous induction of virus.
   b) If the virus is xenotropic the hybrid environment may be permissive, allowing full expression of the virus genome.
   c) A mouse tumor may be produced in which all human chromosomes have been lost, but malignancy is maintained by translocation of an integrated human viral genome to the mouse genome.
3. Because of possible rearrangement of antigenic determinants on the surface of hybrid cells, such cells may have applications in attempts at immunotherapy.

Tumour material is obtained within a few hours of surgical removal. The tissue is coarsely minced and incubated in pronase for one to two hours. The cell suspension is centrifuged and resuspended in culture medium. The suspension consists of clumps of tumour cells mixed with single cells many of which are dead. The clumps at first attach loosely or not at all to the plastic surface of the culture bottle, whereas fibroblasts attach readily. In this way some separation of tumour cells and fibroblasts can be achieved. Depending on the conditions the clumps often start to flatten within a few days, and then appear as colonies of up to a few hundred cells, within which small numbers of cells are seen in mitosis. After a month or two the colonies are not much larger than their original size and they gradually degenerate. This pattern of events has occurred in material from carcinoma of colon, rectum, stomach, bladder, thyroid, parathyroid, and breast. Fusion experiments are carried out either immediately after pronase treatment or after a day or two in culture, before the clumps have attached to the bottle. A suspension of tumour clumps is mixed with mouse cells and inactivated Sendai virus; the agglutinated cells are incubated in plastic bottles for periods up to several months, and examined repeatedly for evidence of hybrid cell formation.

Thirteen tumours (carcinoma of bladder, parathyroid, breast, colon, and vulva, and glioma and melanoma) have been fused with primary kidney cells from inbred CBA mice. During periods of incubation of up to six months, with one possible exception, there was no evidence of hybrid cells growing more rapidly than the mouse kidney cells, although from time to time single hybrid metaphases were seen. CBA mice injected with stamples of the cultures have so far not developed tumours. The reason for this failure may be technical, or it may be more fundamental. In a fusion experiment in which melanoma cells were fused with CBA kidney cells the heterokaryons did not follow the expected course. The nuclei remained separate, with no evidence of synchronous mitosis, for up to nine days.

In one of the above experiments, eleven weeks after fusion of cells from a carcinoma of the colon, a single rapidly growing colony of transformed appearance was noticed. This colony, which has grown up into a line disignated 33FA1, has some interesting characteristics. It shows mixed haemadsorption with a rabbit antiserum against human fibroblasts; this antiserum does not react with primary CBA mouse kidney cells. A rabbit antiserum raised against 33FA1 reacts with human fibroblasts as well as CBA mouse kidney cells. The cells are subtetraploid, with 60 to 80 telocentric and acrocentric chromosomes. Chromosomal examinations of the line are still in progress. So far it looks as though a D-group chromosome, and possibly a G-group chromosome may be present. The cells have been examined by Professor Bodmer for the presence of β_2-microglobulin, the gene for which he and his colleagues have assigned to chromosome 15 (Goodfellow, et al. (1975). Nature, 254:267). No evidence of β_2 microglobulin was found. If a human D-group chromosome is present, therefore, it will probably be 13 or 14.

The cells of this line were carrying a virus which could be labelled with tritiated uridine and which banded on sucrose density gradient equilibrium centrifugation at a density of 1.23, which is the same density as Sendai virus. However, electron microscopy of phosphotungstate stained preparations of the virus, showed particles of diameter 85nm to 150nm, which is smaller than paramyxoviruses (150–300nm). Haemadsorption tests on the cells have been repeatedly negative, and after two successive passages of the virus in the allantoic cavity of hens' eggs no haemagglutinating activity could be detected. A rabbit antiserum prepared against the cells, and their carried virus, did not inhibit haemagglutination by Sendai virus. The virus is cytopathogenic for primary CBA mouse kidney cells. Electron microscopy of sections of detached cells in the 33FA1 cultures showed particles of the same size as those visualised by phosphotungstate staining. Similar particles have now been seen after repeated electron microscopic examination of the original tumour. We are continuing investigations on this virus to determine whether it is, after all, Sendai virus, or a defective variant of Sendai virus, which has persisted since the initial fusion. It could also be a virus from the gut, fortuitously present in the tumour, or a mouse virus contaminating the CBA mouse kidney cells. Whatever the virus proves to be, this line at least illustrates some of the problems of interpretation which can arise as a result of this experimental approach.

Primary mouse kidney cells, like most human tumour cells, divide slowly in culture, so perhaps it is not surprising that a hybrid between them should divide slowly. Some fusion experiments were therefore done with 3T3 cells (mouse fibroblasts). Many hybrid metaphase spreads, in company with 3T3 cell metaphase spreads, were seen in a fusion experiment with thyroid carcinoma cells, but it proved impossible to separate a hybrid clone from the background of 3T3 cells. 10^7 cells of the whole culture were injected into nude mice by Dr. Stiles, in Dr. Sato's laboratory. So far, after two months, no tumours have developed. A visible tumour in nude mice contains about 10^8 cells. If a single malignant cell was present in the original inoculum it must therefore have a generation time, if it is dividing at all, of more than two or three days.

In order to overcome some of the technical problems referred to above, CBA mouse kidney cells were transformed with SV40 virus. One of the transformed clones was mutagenised, and a mutant clone selected which was resistant to thioguanine. This mutant does not incorporate hypoxanthine, and therefore dies in medium containing azaserine and hypoxanthine in which wild-type cells grow readily. Two fusion experiments using this clone, one with cells from carcinoma of the rectum, the other with a primary culture of melanoma cells, have both produced hybrid colonies within a few weeks. Recent fusion cultures made with carcinoma of the colon and carcinoma of the breast also contain actively growing cells with some morphological characteristics of hybrid cells. The fact that SV40 virus is present in the hybrid cells may create further problems of interpretation as the work develops. These problems may not be too great, as the SV40-transformed CBA mouse kidney cells have so far failed to produce tumours in CBA mice.

It is therefore possible to make hybrid lines from human tumour primary suspensions fused with a continuous mouse line. The question of whether a particular hybrid is derived from tumour cells, or from normal cells associated with the tumour is difficult to answer. The only guidance can come from the properties of the hybrid in vitro and in vivo. For example, if the original tumour is producing a hormone, then hormone production by the hybrid would be evidence favouring the view that the human parental cell was a tumour cell, especially if the tumour material was derived from a metastatic deposit. Malignancy of a hybrid line in nude mice would also be consistent with a tumour cell parent. Chromosomal abnormalities in the original tumour would also help interpretation. These problems do not arise, of course, in the rare cases where a hybrid can be made by fusion of a cell line derived from the human tumor, provided that, as with melanoma cultures, the line has undoubtedly developed from malignant cells.

Summary

Some preliminary results are reported of etperiments aimed at establishing hybrid cell systems for the study of the somatic cell genetics of human tomour cells.

References

1. H. Harris and J. F. Watkins, Hybrid cells derived from mouse and man: artificial heterokaryons of mammalian cells from different species. Nature, 1965, 205: 640.
2. J. F. Watkins, Cell fusion for virus studies and the production of hybrid cell

lines, in 'Methods in Virology', volume V, ed. Koprowski & Maramorosch, Academic Press, New York, 1971, pp. 1–31.

3. J. F. Watkins, Cell fusion in the study of tumour cells, International Review of Experimental Pathology, volume 10, Academic Press, New York. 1971. pp. 115–139.

Effect of Cytochalasin B on Malingant Cells

Françoise Kelly

Département de Biologie Moléculaire
Institut Pasteur
Paris, France.

Introduction

By contrast to their untransformed parents, mouse cells transformed by SV40 are killed by cytochalasin B (Kelly and Sambrook, 1973), a drug which prevents cytoplasmic division and inhibits movement in animal cells (Carter, 1967). When exposed to cytochalasin B, normal cells become binucleated but further division is blocked and upon removal of the drug, the binucleated cells undergo cellular division and retain their viability even after a prolonged treatment. In transformed cells, nuclear division and cellular division are no longer coupled precesses. When cytoplasmic division is blocked by cytochalasin B, most cells become multinucleated and do no recover after removal of the drug.

We have used the ability of cytochalasin B to discriminate normal from transformed cells as a basis for selecting drug resistant variants from the SVT2 line of SV40-transformed mouse cells. These cells which had regained a normal response to the drug have been shown to have an altered expression of virus specific functions and contain less integrated viral DNA sequences than the parental cells. (Kelly and Sambrook, 1974)

The cytochalasin B resistant variants were shown to have unexpected growth properties *in vivo*: by contrast to their transformed parents, they failed to give rise to tumors when injected into mice of the same Balb/c strain, although they were tumorigenic in immunodeficient 'nude' mice. Normal mice, previously injected with the cytochalasin B resistant cells did not develop tumors when challenged later with the transformed parent cells. These results suggested that the variant cells were capable of eliciting an immune rejection response and therefore might be useful in an approach to cancer immunotherapy (Sato *et al*, submitted for publication).

We report in this paper that Lewis lung carcinoma cells respond to cytochalasin B in a manner similar to that of SV40-transformed cells and are efficiently killed by the drug.

Effect of cytochalasin B on lewis lung carcinoma cells

Cells from the Lewis lung carcinoma have been examined for their susceptibility to cytochalasin B. They were compared to a differentiated cell line, PDC1, which has been derived from the mouse teratocarcinoma and shown to have normal growth properties (Boon et al, 1974). Cells growing in culture were treated with cytochalasin B at a concentration of 2 and 5 μg.ml $^{-1}$. After 4 days, the medium was replaced with medium to allow the spreading of the cells and examination of the nuclei. Most PCD1 were binucleated, whereas most Lewis lung carcinoma cells had more than 2 nuclei per cell with often as many as 8 to 12 nuclei per cell. The viability of the cells was determined by plating efficiency. As shown in table I the viability of the Lewis lung carcinoma cells is markedly reduced by a 4 days exposure to the drug. At both concentrations used, only 1 in 10^4 cells appeared capable of forming a colony. PCD1 cells were only little affected by the same treatment.

Table I: Efficiency of plating of Lewis Lung Carcinoma and PCDl Cells

Incubation in cytochalasin B		
(ug. ml^{-1})	LLC	PCD1
0	55	100
2	0.0001	25
5	0.0001	20

Table I: LLC cells were derived from a lung metastasis of the Lewis Lung Carcinoma, after two passages in culture and were obtained from Dr. R. Fauve. PCD1 cells were obtained from Dr. T. Boon.
Cells were grown in plastic Petri dishes in Dulbecco's modified Eagle medium containing 10 % fetal calf serum, at 37° and 12 % CO_2. Cells were seeded at a density of 10^4 cells/cm^2 and cytochalasin B dissolved in DMSO was added 12 h. later at the concentration indicated. After 4 days the medium was removed and cells were allowed to spread in fresh medium. They were resuspended 6 h. later and plated at various dilutions. The efficiency of plating is expressed in % of cells forming colonies after two weeks.

We are presently investigating the effect of cytochalasin B on the *in vivo* growth of the Lewis lung carcinoma cells injected into syngeneic C57B1/6 mice. Preliminary results indicate that the appearance of local tumor and metastasis is retarded when animals are injected with the drug.

Discussion

When treated in culture with cytochalasin B, cells from the Lewis lung carcinoma become multinucleated and their viability is drastically reduced, a behaviour previously reported for SV40-transformed mouse cells (Kelly and Sambrook 1973). Other studies on cells from different species transformed by various DNA tumor viruses (Wright and Hayflick, 1972; Hirano and Kurimura, 1974), and studies on cytochalasin B resistant variants of SV40-transformed mouse cells (Kelly and Sambrook, 1974) have suggested that the response to cytochalasin B is a consequence of the expression in transformed cells of a specific viral function. It is of interest that cells from the Lewis lung carcinoma, a spontaneous tumor of the mouse, exhibit a similar response to the drug.

Because of its ability to discriminate between normal and transformed cells, cytochalasin B is a potential chemotherapeutic agent. In addition to its direct killing effect on malignant cells, the drug may also be useful through the selection of variant cells capable of eliciting an immune rejection reaction of the tumor cells.

We are investigating these possibilities on the Lewis lung carcinoma. We have shown that the cells are very efficiently killed *in vitro* by cytochalasin B and preliminary experiments indicate that the drug may also be active *in vivo*. Further studies are needed to determine optimal conditions of action *in vivo* and whether or not cytochalasin B acts directly on the tumor cells in a manner similar to that observed in culture. We have recently isolated a cytochalasin B resistant cell line from the lung carcinoma cells (unpublished results). If these cells indeed present the property described for the resistant variants of SV40-transformed mouse cells to immunise animals against the parental tumor cells, they will provide a useful tool in an approach to immunotherapy.

References

Boon, T., Buckingham, M. E., Dexter, D. L., Jakob, H. et F. Jacob. 1974. Terato-carcinome de la souris: isolement et propriétés de deux lignées de myoblastes. Ann. Microbiol. (Inst. Pasteur), *125 B*: 13.

Carter, S. B. 1967. Effect of cytochalasin B on mammalian cells. Nature. *213:* 261.

Hirano, A. and T. Kurimura. 1974. Virally transformed cells and cytochalasin B. I. The effect of cytochalasin B on cytokinesis, karyokinesis and DNA synthesis in cells. Exp. Cell. Res. *89:* 111.

Kelly, F., and J. Sambrook. 1973. Differential effect of cytochalasin B on normal and transformed cells. Nature, *242:* 217.

Kelly, F. and J. Sambrook. 1974. Variants of Simian virus 40-transformed mouse cells that are resistant to cytochalasin B. Cold Spring Harbor Symp. Quant. Biol. *39:* 345.

Sato, G., Desmond, W., Kelly, F. and P. Roberts. Studies of growth behaviour of tumor cells in culture and in animal hosts. Submitted for publication.

Wright, W. E. and L. Hayflick. 1972. Formation of anucleate and multinucleate cells in normal and SV40 transformed WI-38 by cytochalasin B. Exp. Cell. Res. *74:* 187.

Growth Regulation and Suppression of Metastasis In the Congenitally Athymic Nude Mouse

Charles D. Stiles, Penelope E. Roberts,
Milton H. Saier Jr. and Gordon Sato

Department of Biology
John Muir College
University of California, San Diego
La Jolla, California 92037, U.S.A.

Introduction

The physiologically relevant site for studies on growth regulation is within intact modulated circuits which have evolved for maintenance of tissue and organ animal hosts. Animal cells in culture are disconnected from complex hormonally homeostasis (Furth, 1967). Paradoxically the most detailed information on growth control has been generated from studies on animal fibroblasts and lymphocytes grown *in vitro*. In the tissue culture environment, the growth of cloned populations of animal cells, in defined or semidefined media may be easily quantitated.

By studying the growth of established and cloned cell lines in heterologous animal hosts, the tactical advantages of tissue culture technology can be exploited in a biologically relevant framework. Heterologous cells can be recovered from animal hosts, identified and quantitated by virtue of their differential morphology, antigenic composition and karyotype. Clearly, however such studies can only be conducted in an immunologically tolerant host.

The congenitally athymic nude mouse does not display the cell mediated immune response and never rejects heterologous skin grafts (For review, see Rygaard, 1973). We have examined the capacity of nude mice to support and control the growth of a variety of heterologous tissue culture cell lines. This paper will deal with the results of these studies which demonstrate (1) that a variety of epithelioid and fibroblastic cell lines which grow forever *in vitro* do not grow tumors in nude mice; (2) that the failure of cell lines to grow tumors in nude mice is an authentic growth regulatory response; (3) that the growth behavior of cells in tissue culture is not a reliable indicator of tumorigenic potential; and (4) that the capacity of tumor cells to grow in suspension, invade surrounding tissues and develop secondary metastases possibly requires a thymus dependent function.

Table I

Category	Cell line or strain	Tissue of origin	Transforming agent	No. tumors formed / No. mice injected
I. Embryonic Cell Strains	Balb / c	mouse embryo	none	0/8
	HFL-Johnson	human fetal lung	none	0/13
	HFL 2	human fetal lung	none	0/4
II. Established Lines of Neoplastic Origin	RPMI 2650	human carcinoma	spontaneous	8/9
	C6	rat glioma	N-nitro-somethylurea	10/10
	B-16	mouse melanoma	spontaneous	20/20
	HeLa	human carcinoma	spontaneous	15/15
	BRL-4143	human melanoma	spontaneous	5/16
III. Established Lines from Normal Tissue	Balb / c 3T3	mouse embryo	none	0/12
	MDCK	dog kidney	none	0/16
	BRL	rat liver	none	0/20
	31A	rat ovary	none	0/12
	3T6	mouse embryo	none	7/7
IV. Lines Transformed *in vitro*	SVT2	mouse embryo	SV_{40}	10/10
	56-1	mouse embryo	SV_{40}	10/10
	T	mouse embryo	SV_{40}	10/10
	XIII	mouse embryo	SV_{40}	10/10
	VA2-8-aza-G^r	human fetal lung	SV_{40}	0/12
	RBSV3	human skin	SV_{40}	0/12
	RBSV-1A	human fetal lung	SV_{40}	0/10
	LNSV	human skin	SV_{40}	0/6
	PY 3T3	mouse embryo	polyoma	5/5
	A-9	mouse muscle	methyl-cholanthrine	10/10
	WI-L2	human spleen	spontaneous	2/5

Table 1: Tumorigenicity of heterologous cells in athymic nude mice. The tumorigenic potential of the various cell lines was examined by injecting from 10^6 to 2×10^6 viable cells subcutaneously into the scapular region. All cell lines were tested in both male and female mice. Cell lines were classed as tumorigenic when nodules grew progressively to greater than 5 mm in diameter at the site of injection. Most tumorigenic cell lines produced tumors from 7 to 21 days post inoculation. Mice injected with RPMI 2650 developed tumors in 20 to 60 days. Before cell lines were classed as nontumorigenic, the test animals were observed for at least four months and a second series of nude mice was challenged with a larger cell inoculum (5×10^6 to 10^7 cells).

Results

Tumorigenicity of Heterologous Cells in Nude Mice

Table 1 summarizes the tumorigenic potential of heterologous cell lines in athymic nude mice. Embryonic cell strains never grew tumors in nude mice. All established cell lines of neoplastic origin were tumorigenic. Established cell lines derived from explants of nonneoplastic animal tissue were generally not tumorigenic. Every line of SV40 transformed mouse cells tested was tumorigenic. Curiously, none of 5 lines of SV40 transformed human cells produced tumors even though each of 3 human lines derived from authentic neoplasms and a line of human lymphocytes from a non-leukemic patient were tumorigenic. Dr. James Robb at the University of California, San Diego School of Medicine kindly screened the SV40 transformed human lines for the presence of viral T antigen by immunofluorescence and found all of them to be T-antigen positive.

Basis of Growth Suppression in Nude Mice

A variety of control experiments indicated that the failure of particular cell lines to grow tumors in nude mice was not a trivial result but rather indicated an authentic response to host mediated growth regulatory signals.

Attempts to "vaccinate" nude mice against human tumor cells (Hela) by repeated inoculation of normal human lung fibroblasts in Freund's adjuvant were unsuccessful. Mice which had been inoculated with human fetal lung cells in Freund's adjuvant were bled and the serum was tested for the presence of cytotoxic antibodies directed either against fetal lung cells or against Hela cells. No evidence of cytotoxic antibodies directed against either cell type was found. These experiments indicate that the failure of human fetal lung cells to grow tumors in nude mice is not due to rejection by either the cell mediated or humoral immune response.

Fate of Nontumorigenic Cells in Nude Mice

The hairless condition of these athymic animal hosts facilitates observation of nontumorigenic cells which are injected subcutaneously. An inoculum of 10^6 cells is visable as a light colored subcutaneous mass from one to two mm in diameter twenty four hours after injection. The persistance of these masses is variable from cell line to cell line. Most nontumorigenic cells appear to survive no longer than 10 days beneath the skin of nude mice; however, an Inoculum of 10^6 dog kidney epithelial cells (MDCK) is still detectable in some animals at two months post-injection. One subcutaneous mass measuring 1.6 mm in diameter was removed from a mouse which had been injected with 10^7 MDCK cells two months previously. The tissue was plated into culture and cells with the MDCK epithelioid morphology were observed growing amid mouse fibroblasts. A clone of the epithelioid cells was isolated and metaphase chromosomes were stained with Geimsa. A modal chromosome number of 76 and the presence of a large metacentric X chromosome (fig. 1) identified the cells as MDCK. Thus cell lines which do not induce progressively growing tumors can persist for long periods of time in nude mice and be recovered in a viable state.

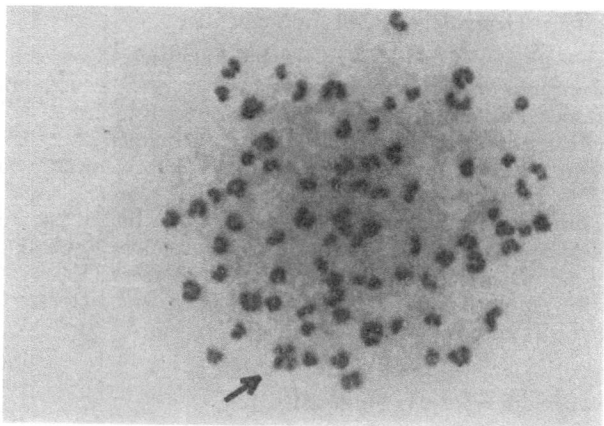

Fig. 1: Metaphase cell recovered from a nude mouse injected two months previously with MDCK dog kidney cells. The arrow indicates the large metacentric X chromosome which characterizes the canine karyotype.

* In each experiment, one C57 mouse died prior to three weeks and could not be autopsied

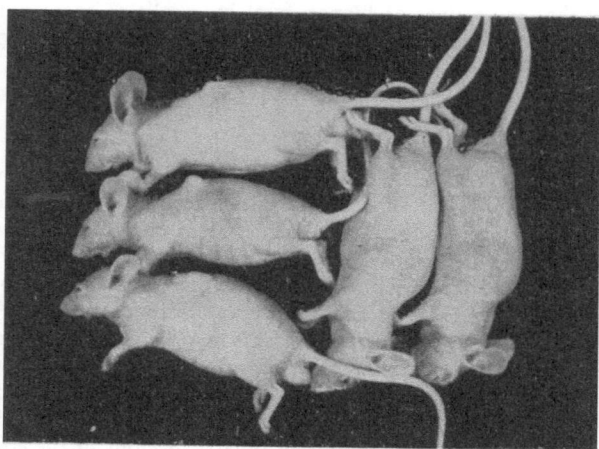

Fig. 2: The three mice on the left received 10⁶ MDCK cells subcuntaneously along the midline of the back one day after birth. The two mice on the right received 2 x 10⁶ MDCK cells subcutaneously on the right flank as adults. The mice on the left were photographed 30 days after injection and the mice on the right were photographed 60 days after injection.

188

Growth Response of Nontumorigenic Cells in Nude Mice

MDCK cells did not induce tumors when injected into nude mice. Previous experiments indicated that nude mice do not reject heterologous cells immunologically and it was shown that MDCK cells surived for long periods in nude mice with no net growth. To determine whether the MDCK line could respond to host growth regulatory signals, 10^6 cells were injected subcutaneously into 1 day old nude mice. At birth the nude mouse weighs approximately 1 gram and over the next 30 days, mass increases to about 20 grams. Figure 2 demonstrates that in rapidly growing mice inocula of 10^6 MDCK cells formed nodules measuring 0.5cm in diameter whereas twice as many cells injected into adult animals failed to grow. MDCK nodules formed in neonatal animals did not continue to grow once the animals attained adult mass. Thus the failure of MDCK cells to grow tumors in nude mice does not seem to be caused by rejection or any intrinsic deficiency on the part of the host. Rather these cells seem responsive to host mediated growth regulatory signals.

Relationship of Growth Behavior in vitro to Tumorigenicity

The observation that 5 human cell lines infected with, and morphologically transformed by SV40 virus were not tumorigenic suggested that many of those characteristics which serve to define the transformed state *in vitro* are only

Table II

	Cell Line	Growth in 1 % fetal calf serum	Saturation density greater than 10^5 cells/cm²	Growth in methocel suspension	Growth on confluent mouse cell monolayers
Tumor-igenic Cell Lines	3T6	+	+	−	+
	RPMI-2650	+	+	+	+
	Hela	+	+	+	+
	BRL-4143	+	−	+	+
	C-6	+	+	+	+
	B-16	−	+	+	+
	SVT2	+	+	−	+
	PY3T3	+	+	+	+
	A-9	+	+	+	+
Non-tumor-igenic Cell Lines	3T3	−	−	−	−
	MDCK	+	+	+	+
	31A	−	+	−	+
	BRL	+	+	−	+
	VA2-8-azaGr	−	+	+	+
	LNSV	−	+	−	+

Table2: Correlation of growth behavior *in vitro* with tumorigenicity in nude mice.

189

coincidentally related to malignant potential in animals. The serum growth requirement, the ability to grow on top of stationary phase mouse monolayer cultures, the ability to grow in methocel suspension and the cell saturation density were determined for various cell lines. The correlation of these *in vitro* growth parameters with tumorigenicity in athymic nude mice is summarized in table 2. As can be seen, there is no absolute correlation between any *in vitro* growth parameter and tumorigenic potential in immunologically tolerant hosts. In fact with the exception of secondary mouse embryo fibroblasts and 3T3 cells, every nontumorigenic cell line displayed one or more of those cell growth characteristics *in vitro* which have come to be associated with the transformed state.

Suppression of Metastasis in the Nude Mouse

In the course of testing various cell lines for tumorigenicity we were struck with the complete absence of tumor metastasis in these athymic hosts. Despite the diverse origin of the nine tumor producing lines depicted in table 1 and the large number of animals tested, tumor growth was always restricted to the region where cells were inoculated. To investigate this phenomenon in more detail, the malignant potential of a highly metastatic subclone of the B-16 mouse melanoma was tested in nude mice. B-16 melanoma clone #2 cells were derived by inoculating tumor cells subcutaneously into C57 black mice and culturing the metastatic nodules which arose in occasional animals. The parental B-16 line seldom metastasized in C57 black mice whereas within 3 weeks the B-16 clone #2 cells metastasized to the lungs, lymph nodes and spleen of sixty percent of the animals tested (table 3 and

Table III

B-16	C57 Mouse			Nude Mouse		
Cell Clone	# mice injected	mean tumor mass at autopsy	# mice with metastatic nodules	# mice injected	mean tumor mass at autopsy	# mice with metastatic nodules
B-16 #2	9	1.0 ± 1.0 g	6	10	1.6 ± 1.2 g	1
B-16 #2s	10	2.0 ± 0.85 g	8	10	3.7 ± 0.5 g	0

Table 3: Suppression of metastasis in nude mice. Two highly invasive subclones of the B-16 mouse melanoma were injected subcutaneously into the scapular region of C57 black mice or into nude mice. Each mouse received 10^6 cells and all mice developed tumors. At three weeks postinjection the animals were sacrificed. Tumors were weighed and the animals were examined for black melanoma nodules in the lungs, lymph nodes and spleens.

fig. 3). In athymic nude mice, B-16 clone #2 cells induce large pigmented tumors (table 3) but, with one exception in 20 challenges, none of the nude mice showed secondary tumor metastasis at autopsy (table 3).

One clue to the mechanism whereby metastasis is suppressed in athymic nude mice may be found in the growth behavior of human lymphocytes in these animal

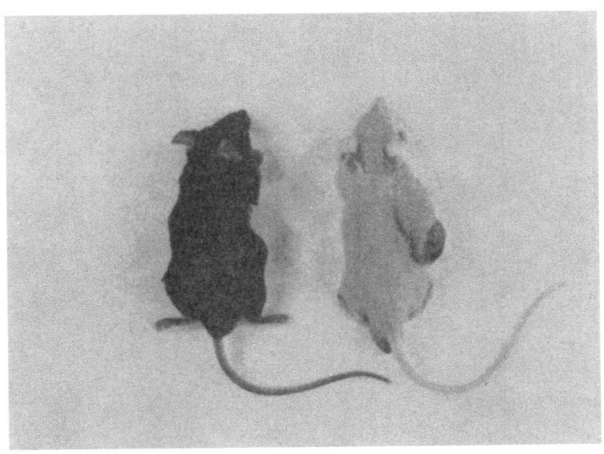

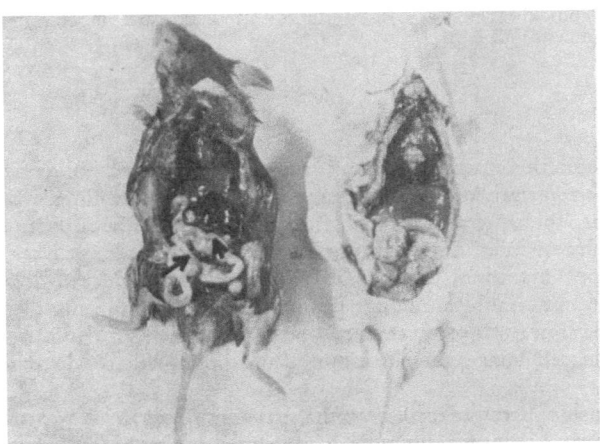

Fig. 3: Top; C57 mouse on left and nude mouse on right, 3 weeks following injection of 10^6 B-16 clone # 2_8 cells. Arrows indicate large pigmented tumors growing at site of injection in animals. Bottom; Same animals as above after dissection. Arrows indicate metastatic melanoma nodules in C57 mouse. No metastasis was detectable in the nude mouse.

hosts. The WI-L2 cell line was derived from spleen cells of a patient free from malignant disease but bearing antibodies to Epstein Barr virus. In culture the cells grow entirely in suspension showing no tendency to adhere to coated plastic tissue culture dishes. WI-L2 cells are tumorigenic in nude mice but the tumors formed are solid lymphosarcomas (fig. 4). No ascites formation was noted in 4 nude mice injected intraperitonially with two million cells per mouse.

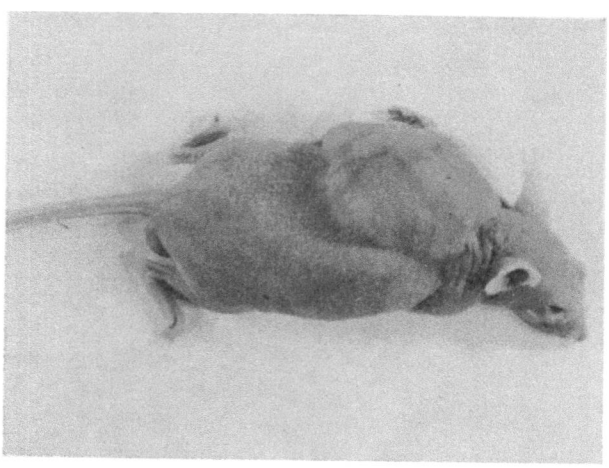

Fig. 4: Nude mouse bearing large solid tumor 2 months after inoculation with 2 x 10⁶ human lymphoid cells (WI-L2).

Discussion

The purpose of this research was to assess the capacity of nude mice to support and control the growth of heterologous tissue culture cell lines. We found that many cell lines which grow forever in tissue culture did not form tumors in nude mice. The failure of individual cell lines to grow tumors did not have an apparent immunologic or nutritional basis. Cells from a nontumorigenic dog kidney line were recovered in a viable state after prolonged incubation in nude mice. We conclude that the failure to grow tumors in nude mice is not a trivial result. Rather, nontumorigenic cell lines may be responsive to host mediated growth regulatory signals.

The relationship between cell growth behavior *in vitro* to growth control in animals has long been of interest to cancer biologists. Many laboratories have sought to determine whether growth behavior *in vitro* correlates with tumorigenicity in animal hosts; the published conclusions are at variance. Aaronson and Todaro (1963) concluded that the ability to grow to high saturation density correlated best with tumorigenicity. Weiss *et al.* (1973) suggested that loss of contact inhibition of growth and of locomotion was the best indicator of tumorigenic potential. Di Mayorca *et al.* (1973) and Freedman and Shin (1974) have concluded that loss of anchorage requirement is essential to tumorigenicity. The congenitally athymic nude mouse would seem to be the most useful animal host for correlative studies between growth behavior *in vitro* and tumorigenicity; in the immunologically tolerant nude mouse, a cellular growth response in the host cannot be masked by a host immune response to the cells. We have found that under uniform culture conditions, none of those *in vitro* growth parameters which serve to define "transformation" in tissue culture correlate with tumorigenicity in nude mice. These experiments indicate that the most reliable and physiologically meaningful assay for malignant transformation may be cell tumorigenicity in nude mice.

The pathologic consequences of malignant transformation are more a reflection of tumor cell invasiveness than of tumor growth potential (Kark, W. 1966). The mechanisms whereby malignant tumor cells migrate through surrounding tissue, penetrate the blood vascular and lymphatic systems and lodge at distal sites to form secondary tumors are difficult to study in tissue culture. Growth of malignant tumors in heterologous animal hosts, wherein the origin of distal metastasis may be determined unambiguously, may provide insight into these problems. Giovionella (1973) reported the occurrence of metastasis from a human melanoma in athymic nude mice. On the other hand, this laboratory and others (Freedman and Shin, 1974) have not observed metastasis in nude mice, although more than 50 human and animal cell lines have been studied. A direct test of metastatic potential in nude mice using mouse melanoma cells of proven invasive capabilities confirmed that metastasis is suppressed in athymic nude mice (table 4 and fig. 2). These observation corroborate the finds of Fidler (1974) who, in a series of experiments using B-16 melanoma cells with properties similar to those described here, found that low numbers of lymphocytes from tumor bearing animals actually promoted metastasis in thymectomized -X- irradiated C57 mice.

The incongruous growth behavior of human lymphocytes, which formed solid tumors in nude mice while growing as suspension cells in tissue culture may provide a clue to the supression of metastasis. Freedman and Shin (1974) reported a similar modification of growth behavior for Erlich Ascites cells which grew only as solid tumors in nude mice. These results suggest that a thymus dependent function is required in order for cells to grow in suspension in animal hosts.

The experiments described in this communication demonstrate that the growth behavior of cells in tissue culture is in many respects not indicative of their behavior in animals. It is likely that growth of normal animal tissues is regulated by hormone like agents and cellular interactions which have yet to be described *in vitro*. Observations on the growth of heterologous tissue culture cell lines in immunologically tolerant nude mice may assist in the reconstruction of these growth regulatory interactions *in vitro*.

Acknowledgements

This research was supported by Special Grant #741 from the California Division of the American Cancer Society, a grant from the University of California Cancer Research Coordinating Committee and NIH grant #15503-02. M.H.S. is supported by Career Development Award CA001138-01. C.D.S. is supported by a postdoctoral fellowship award from the USPHS #DE03366.

Bibliography

Aaronson, S. A. and Todaro, G. J. 1968. Basis for Acquisition of Malignant Potential by Mouse Cells Cultivated *in vitro*. Science, 162: 1024–1026.

Di Mayorca, G., Greenblatt, M., Frauthen, T., Loller, A., and Giordano, R. 1973. Malignant Transformation of BHK_{21}, Clone 13 Cells *in vitro* by Nitrosamines – A Conditional State. Proc. Nat. Acad. Sci. U.S.A., 70: 46–49.

Freedman, V. H. and Shin, S. 1974. Cellular Tumorigenicity in Nude Mice: Correlation with Growth in Semi-Solid Medium. Cell, *3*: 355–359.

Fidler, I. J., 1974. Immune Stimulation-Inhibition of Experimental Cancer Metastasis. Cancer Res., *34*: 491–498.

Furth, J. 1967. Pioitary Cybernetics and Neoplasia. Harvey Lectures, *63:* 47–72.

Giovannella, B. C., Yim, S. O., A. C. Morgan, J. S. Stehlin and L. J. Williams, Jr. 1973. Brief Communication: Metastases of Human Melanoma Transplanted in "nude" Mice. J. Nat. Cancer Inst., *48*: 1531–1533.

Karl, W. 1966. A Synopsis of Cancer. Williams and Wilkinson Co.

Rygaard, J. 1973. Thymus and Self. F.A.D.L. Copenhagen (C) 1973 Jørgen Rygaard, Copenhagen, Henmark.

Weiss, R. A., Vesely, P. and Sindelarova, J. 1973. Growth Regulation and Tumor Formation of Normal and Neoplastic Rats Cells. INT. J. Cancer, *11*: 77–89.

Cell-Mediated Immunity to Leukemia Associated Antigens in Experimental Models and in Man

Ronald B. Herberman

Laboratory of Immundiagnosis
National Cancer Institute
Bethesda, Maryland USA 20014

Cell-mediated immune reactions against leukemia associated antigens have been detected in experimental animal models and in patients with acute leukemia. The occurrence of specific cellular immune reactivity has important implications for the diagnosis and therapy of human acute leukemia. As summarized in Table 1,

Table I: Application of Assays of Cell-Mediated Immunity to Diagnosis and Therapy

---

1. Initial diagnosis
   a. Specificity: Are antigens leukemia assqciated?
   b. Reactivity: Is reactivity found only with leukemia patients?
2. Monitoring of patients during clinical course
   a. Correlation with clinical status
   b. Indication of prognosis or response to therapy
3. Therapy
   a. Antigens: Can they induce transplantation protection?
   b. Proximity of reactive cells to tumor cells
   c. Augmentation of specific immune reactivity

---

assays of cellular immunity could be applied to the initial detection and diagnosis of leukemia, to the monitoring of patients during and after therapy, and to the planning of rational immunotherapeutic trials. For initial diagnosis, the specificity of the detected antigens and the distribution of reactivity among patients with leukemia and other individuals need to be carefully defined. For immunologic monitoring of leukemia patients, only assays which correlate with extent of disease or with responsiveness to therapy would be useful. Techniques which can measure leukemia associated transplantation antigens would be very useful for selection of materials for specific immunotherapy. In addition, such assays could be used to detect relevant responses to immunotherapeutic manipulations, and to subsequently design optimal schedules of immunotherapy. However, before such practical clinical applications can be realized, additional information in several areas needs to be accumulated. For all of these objectives, standardization of reagents will be very important. There appears to be considerable heterogeneity in the antigens on leukemia cells and in the quantitative expression of each of these antigens (1). Some of the variability in results and some of the negative reactions could be ascribed to the use of poorly antigenic leukemic cells. Selection of large supplies of highly antigenic cells and extracts, with known specificities, and provision for long term preservation of antigenicity will help to ensure adequate sensitivity of the assays. Preservation of highly reactive lymphocytes, and reduction in day-to-day variability in the assays, will also be major steps in the standardization of the assays. Although progress in these areas is being made in clinical studies, there are a number of logistical problems. The use of leukemia models in syngeneic animal systems should be helpful to work out approaches might could then be applied to studies of leukemia patients. In this paper, I will review some of the information which has been obtained in animal systems, and try to relate this to the clinical objectives.

Specificity of Cell-Mediated Immunity in Experimental Mogels

Tumors induced by oncogenic viruses have been shown to have cell surface antigens specific for the particular virus and also antigens common to other types of tumors and to fetal cells (2, 3). We have shown, by quantitative absorption tests, that syngeneic mice and rats may respond to tumor cell inoculation by formation of antibodies with differing specificities. It is equally important to determine the nature of the antigens detected in assays of cell-mediated immunity. However, it is considerably more difficult to define the specificity of cellular reactions and few extensive studies have been done. Recently, an inhibition assay was developed which permits definition of the specificity of the ^{51}Cr release cytotoxicity assay for cell-mediated immunity (4). Unlabelled cells were added to the mixture of lymphocytes and labelled target cells. If the added cells had the same antigens as those on the target cells, competitive inhibition of lysis was seen. In studies of the Gross virus-induced leukemia (C58NT)D in W/Fu rats, the detected antigenic specificity was found to be quite distinct from any of those detected by humoral antibodies. The antigen was only found on rat cells and not on mouse cells transformed by Gross or other leukemia viruses (4). The antigen appears to be related to expression of rat endogenous type C virus (Table 2) and has been designated REV-SA-1 (5). We have also used this inhibition assay to study the specificity of the cell-mediated reactivity induced in mice by murine sarcoma virus (MSV). MSV induces local tumors in mice, which then usually

Table II: Specificity of Cell-Mediated Immunity in Experimental Models

1. Immunity to Gross virus-induced leukemia, (C58NT)D: antigens associated with rat endogenous type C viruses (REV-SA-1).
2. Murine sarcoma virus (MSV) induced immunity: antigens associated with mouse endogenous type C viruses (MEV-SA-1), present on leukemia cells but also on variety of other cells.
3. Immunity to Friend virus-induced leukemia, FBL-3:
   a. F and FMR antigens
   b. MEV-SA-1

regress. Many laboratories have studied the cell-mediated immune response in this system, and since positive reactions were seen with some leukemic cells, the detected antigens have been presumed to be related to FMR leukemia antigens (6–8). However, we have found that cytotoxic lymphocytes of immune C57BL/6 mice react against an antigenic specificity distinct from any of the expected specificities (9). This antigen has been designated MEV-SA-1 (Table 2) since it appears to be related to expression of mouse endogenous type C virus. The most direct evidence for the association of this antigen to endogenous virus has come from studies involving infection of a mouse cell line SC-1 and a rabbit cell line SIRC with viruses from antigen positive cells (10). Some of the infected cells rapidly became antigen positive (Table 3). Recent studies, with an ^{125}IUdR release cytotoxicity assay, of

Table III: Inhibition of MSV-Induced Cytotoxicity by MEV*-Infected Cells

Cell Line	Infected with virus from:	Inhibition of cytotoxicity
SIRC	none	−
	BALB/3T3 clones	
	S16 C1-2	+
	S2 C1-3	+
	S3	+
	EL-4 ascites	+
	E♂ G2	−
SC-1	MCDV-12 ascites	+
	none	−
	EL-4 ascites	+
	E♂ G2	−
	MCDV-12 ascites	−

* Mouse endogenous type C virus.

cell-mediated immunity against a Friend virus-induced leukemia FBL-3 have indicated reactivity against the FMR serologic specificity and also against MEV-SA-1 (11, 12).

Nature of Effector Cells in Experimental Models

A further complexity in the analysis of cell-mediated immunity is that different types of effector cells can be involved, even within the same tumor system (Table 4). These different subpopulations of cells can develop reactivity with disparate kinetics, and can be directed against different specificities. In each of the three animal model systems mentioned above, thymus derived lymphocytes (T cells) appear to be responsible for the reactivity in isotopic release cytotoxicity assays, of animals immunized by tumor cells or by virus (13–16). In addition, immune reactivity in a microcytotoxicity assay (16) and in a lymphocyte proliferation assay (17) in our MSV system, and the lymphoproliferative response of immune

Table IV: Nature of reactive cells in experimental models

1. T cells: responsible for specific immune reactivity (cytotoxicity and lymphocyte proliferation) induced by MSV, FBL-3, (C58NT)D.
2. Macrophages: responsible for nonspecific growth inhibiton induced by MSV and by other tumors.
3. N cells: responsible for specific natural immunity against mouse and rat leukemias.

cells against (C58NT)D (18) are dependent on T cells. Effector cells have also been detected in the MSV tumor system by a growth inhibition assay, in which cytostasis is measured by inhibition of uptake of ^{3}H-thymidine (19). Macrophages appear to be responsible for these effects, and in contrast to the specificity of the immune T cells, growth inhibitory activity appears to be nonspecific, with marked effects on a variety of leukemia cells and other tumor cells (19, 20). In addition to the T cells and macrophage effector cells in immune animals, the lymphocytes of many normal mice and rats have been shown to have specific cytotoxic reactivity against leukemia cells (21, 22). The natural cytotoxic reactivity of mice was not dependent on T cells, being unaffected by treatment with anti-$\ominus$ serum plus complement, and with high levels being found in athymic, nude mice (Table 5; 23). Treatment of reactive mouse cells by procedures known to deplete or in-

Table V: Effects of various treatments on MSV immune and BALB/c nude spleen cell cytotoxicity against RBL-5 target cells

Treatment of spleen cells	MSV immune		BALB/c nude	
	Untreated	Treated	Untreated	Treated
Anti-$\ominus$ + C	32*	4	38	25
Carbonyl iron/magnet	21	22	15	15
Nylon column	27	23	15	38
Carrageenan (200μg)	45	45	12	12
EA monolayer	24	31	28	21
EAC monolayer	24	28	28	34
Anti-γ globulin (1:20)	48	40	23	22

* % cytotoxicity.

activate macrophages, complement receptor bearing cells, or immunoglobulin receptor bearing cells also had no effect on cytotoxicity. Similarly, the natural rat effector cells had no identifiable surface marker (Table 6; 22). The subpopulation of lymphocytes responsible for the natural cytotoxicity has been tentatively designated N cells (23). The natural cytotoxicity appears to be directed against antigens associated with endogenous type C viruses of the particular species, but some differences have been noted between these specificities and those detected by immune T cells (22, 23). The finding of cytotoxic reactivity against some tumor

Table VI: Effects of various treatments on (C58NT)D immune and normal spleen cell cytotoxicity against (C58NT)D target cells

Treatment	Immune		Normal	
	Untreated	Treated	Untreated	Treated
Anti-T (NIH) + C	68*	3	13	12
Anti-T (Scripps) + C	32	3	12	11
Carbonyl Iron/magnet	11	24	6	8
Nylon column	24	41	8	10
EA monolayer	9	9	4	3
EAC monolayer	9	13	4	5
EAC column	46	53	4	5

* % cytotoxicity.

associated antigens in normal animals has important implications for the use of cell-mediated dytotoxicity assays for diagnosis of cancer. On the one hand, the wide distribution of reactivity, not only in tumor immune animals, but also in many normal individuals, would seem to eliminate the diagnostic usefulness of these assays. However, since different subpopulations of effector cells are involred, methods could be worked out to distinguish the nature of the reaction seen with a particular individual.

Correlation of Cell-Mediated Immunity in Experimental Models with Tumor Growth

In order to evaluate the usefulness of assays of cell-mediated immunity for monitoring of individuals with leukemia, it is important to determine the relationship of reactivity to course of disease. In each of our three animal model systems, it has been possible to induce progressive tumor growth (such animals are designated progressors) or transient tumor growth followed by complete regression (such animals are designated regressors). In both regressors and progressors, the T cell cytotoxic responses were transient, with peak levels soon after inoculation (8, 12, 24). However, the responses of progressors in each of these systems were considerably lower than those seen in regressors (Table 7). In the growth inhibition assay, more reactivity has been seen in progressors than in regressors. The activity appeared to be correlated with presence of large tumors, and it persisted in the progressors (19, 20). In the lymphocyte proliferation response to (C58NT)D, the difference between regressors and progressors was particularly striking. Reactivity has been detected in regressors at 15 days or more after tumor cell inoculation. In contrast, no reactivity was seen with lymphocytes from progressors (25). This lack of detectable direct reactivity was found not to be due to an absence of lymphocytes capable of response, but rather to the presence of suppressor cells. After removal of these suppressor cells, positive proliferative responses could then be observed.

In addition to these *in vitro* studies of correlation with *in vivo* host resistance

Table VII: Correlation of cell-mediated immunity with tumor growth

	Regressors	Progressors
Cytolysis		
MSV	peak at 14 days; then rapid decline to low levels	similar time course, but low levels
FBL-3	biphasic response	similar time course, but much lower levels
(C58NT) D	peak at 10 days; then rapid decline to low levels	similar time course, but low levels
Growth inhibition	transient activity at peak of tumor growth	persistent activity
Lymphocyte proliferation		
(C58NT) D	detectable after 15–20 days	not detectable, except after removal of suppressor cells
Adoptive transfer of immunity		
MSV	good protection against	weak protection against cell
FBL-3	tumor cell challenge	challenge

to tumor growth, we have also performed some systemic adoptive transfer experiments in the MSV and FBL-3 systems, with lymphocytes from regressors and progressors (15). Cells from regressors conferred considerably better protection against challenge with leukemia cells than did cells from progressors.

Secondary Cytotoxic Responses in Experimental Model Systems

One of the major apparent discrepancies between the results of *in vitro* cytotoxicity assays and *in vivo* events in our model systems was the short duration of strong cytotoxic reactivity after tumor or virus inoculation. This was in contrast to the very long-lasting resistance of previously inoculated animals to rechallenge with leukemia cells. This raised serious questions about the *in vivo* relevance of the cytotoxic reactions. Recently, a series of experiments has been performed which resolves this problem. When immune animals were rechallenged with tumor cells,

Table VIII: In vivo generation of secondary cytotoxic response to tumor cells

Tumor system	% Cytotoxicity*	
	no challenge	challenge with tumor cells
MSV	−0.2	34.1
FBL-3	3.5	33.0
(C58NT) D	2.3	47.2

* Immune animals were challenged intraperitoneally with tumor cells and 3–5 days later, peritoneal exudate cells were tested for cytotoxicity against labelled target cells. In the MSV system, RBL-5 ascites tumor cells were used for challenge and as target cells.

strong cytotoxic reactivity rapidly developed but tended to be restricted to the region of challenge (Table 8; 26–28). Similar results have also been obtained *in vitro*, by incubation of immune lymphocytes with tumor cells for 5–9 days (Table 9; 29–31). These data clearly indicate that immune animals have memory cells for cytotoxicity, but re-exposure to antigen is needed for generation of reactivity. Since the *in vivo* transplantation protection experiments involve such re-exposure to tumor cells, the data from the secondary response experiments are quite concordant with the persistence of *in vivo* resistance to challenge.

Table IX: In vitro generation of secondary cytotoxic response to tumor cells

| Tumor system | % Cytotoxicity* | |
	immune cells alone	immune cells + tumor cells**
MSV	9.1	33.5
FBL-3	3.0	69.1
(C58NT) D	6.1	66.7

* At end of 5–9 days in culture, effector cells tested against ^{51}Cr labelled target cells, at ratio of 50:1, or in FBL-3 system, against $^{125}IUdR$ labelled cells, at 15:1 ratio. In MSV system, RBL-5 ascites tumor cells were used as target.
** Immune spleen cells were obtained 30–40 day after virus or tumor cell inoculation. Incubation performed with mitomycin C treated tumor cells.

Standardization of Assays of Cell-Mediated Immunity

For reliable practical applications of the assays of cell-mediated immunity, standardization of reagents and reduction in day-to-day variability of the assays is quite important. We have focused on the ^{51}Cr release cytotoxicity, and have been able to cryopreserve functional effector cells and tumor target cells (32, 33). Cryopreserved tumor cells have also been quite useful in the cytotoxicity inhibition assays. These cyropreserved cells have yielded very reproducible results over a long period of time, and have reduced the number of variables in the assays. In addition, they have allowed us to include internal standards in assays, so that we can accurately compare experimental results among different experiments. Cryopreserved tumor cells have also been effective for stimulation of lymphocyte proliferation and for *in vitro* generation of secondary cytotoxic responses.

Cell-Mediated Immunity to Human Leukemia Associated Antigens

Cell-mediated immune reactions have also been detected against human leukemia associated antigens. My laboratory has primarily used skin tests for delayed hypersensitivity and ^{51}Cr release cytotoxicity assays for these studies. Some of the characteristics of the observed reactions are summarized in Table 10. The initial delayed hypersensitivity studies were performed with membrane extracts of autologous leukemic and remission leukocytes. Positive reactions were obtained with leukemic extracts and not with the extracts of remission cells (34). Although these data indicate an association of the antigens with leukemia, it was not possible

Table X: Characteristics of cell-mediated immunity in human leukemias

Assay	Specificity	Clinical Correlation
Skin tests		
autologous cells	leukemia associated	higher incidence of reactivity in remission than in relapse
allogeneic cells	leukemia (same type) associated	higher incidence of reactivity in remission than in relapse
Raji	broader specificity: mainly ALL* and Burkitt's lymphoma	higher incidence of reactivity in remission than in relapse
HKLY 28	broad specificity: mainly NPC** and ALL	higher incidence of reactivity in remission and with localized tumor
51CR release cytotoxicity		
autologous cells	leukemia associated	?
allogeneic cells	antigens on blast cells and remission cells of leukemia patients; considerable normal reactivity	?
tissue culture lines	high incidence of normal reactivity	depressed during chemotherapy

* Acute hymphocytic leukemias.
** Nasopharygeal carcinom.

to evaluate the distribution of a particular antigen. Therefore, a series of experiments were performed with extracts of allogeneic cells (35). Extracts of allogeneic acute leukemia cells produced positive reactions in about one third of patients with the same type of leukemia, but were unreactive in patients with the dissimilar type of leukemia. Extracts of allogeneic remission cells or of normal leukocytes gave negative results. Therefore, the skin tests with the blast extracts detected reactions to antigens common to acute leukemia (ALL) and to distinct common acute myelogeous leukemia (AML) antigens. However, these antigens did not appear to be equally represented in all extracts. Some preparations gave positive reactions in more than half of the appropriate leukemia patients, whereas others were poorly or non-reactive. Partly as an attempt to obtain large amounts of standard test materials, extracts have been prepared from human lymphoid tissue culture cell lines, derived from leukemia, other tumors, or from normal keukocytes (36). Extracts of some of these lines have given positive skin reactions in patients. A summary of data with some of these extracts is given in Table 11. The Raji line, derived from a patient with Burkitt's lymphoma, has given reactions in 40 %/o of American patients with ALL, several patients with AML, and over 60 %/o of patients with Burkitt's lymphoma (37). Only a small proportion of French ALL patients (38, 39) and none of the Canadian ALL patients reacted to Raji (40). This could

Table XI: Delayed skin reactions to extracts of lymphoid cell lines

Patients	Tests positive/total tests (%o +) Tumor derived cell lines			
	RAJI	MOLT	HKLY 28	F-265
ALL* (U.S.)	26/65 (40)	6/17 (35)		1/54 (2)
ALL (French-Oldham)	4/49 (8)			0/49 (0)
ALL (French-Levine)	1/12 (8)		1/10 (10)	0/10 (0)
ALL (Canada)				
before therapy	0/14 (0)	0/14 (0)	0/14 (0)	0/14 (0)
remission	0/22 (0)	0/22 (0)	7/22 (32)	0/22 (0)
Burkitt's lymphoma	29/47 (62)			2/47 (4)
NPC**	10/34 (29)		24/36 (67)	6/35 (17)
Other carcinomas	10/72 (14)		12/59 (20)	1/69 (2)

* Acute lymphocytic leukemia.
** Nasopharyngeal carcinoma.

be partially ascribed to differences between lots of antigen, even from the same cell line; however, American ALL patients reacted well to the same lot as that used in the study in France. The extract from HKLY28, a lymphoid cell line derived from a patient with nasopharyngeal carcinoma (NPC), gave a different pattern of reactivity. Patients with NPC had a high incidence of reactivity (38), Canadian ALL patients also reacted (40), but only 1 of 10 French ALL patients reacted (39). It is clear from these data that the antigens detected on the cultured cells have considerably broader specificity than the blast cell extracts. However, the reactions showed some clear specificity, since patients with carcinomas other than NPC had a low incidence of reactivity. The HKLY28 cell line produces Epstein-Barr virus (EBV) and Raji contains the EBV genome. The skin reactive antigens on these cells could be related to EBV. However, the F-265 cell line has a similar expression of EBV genome as Raji, yet elicited very few reactions. Furthermore, the MOLT cell line, derived from a patient with ALL and lacking the EBV genome, produced almost as high an incidence of reactions in American ALL patients as did Raji.

In the skin tests with membrane extracts of either blast cells or of cell lines, reactivity has correlated with clinical status (Tabele 10). Patients with ALL or Burkitt's lymphoma in remission had a significantly higher incidence of reactivity than did patients in relapse (35, 37, 38). Patients with positive skin tests have also tended to have a better prognosis. Similarly, NPC patients with localized disease have had a higher incidence of reactions to HKLYL8 than those with more advanced disease (41).

The main limitation in the skin test studies has been the inability, for ethical reasons, to test the extracts in control individuals, with benign or no disease. *In vitro* studies of cytotoxicity, using the ^{51}Cr release assay against cryopreserved leukemic target cells, have allowed a more extensive study of reactivity in controls as well as in patients (Table 10). Testing of autologous reactivity of leukemia patients showed reactions against leukemia associated antigens, with no reactions against remission target cells (42). In allogeneic testing, a broader pattern of reactivity was seen. Positive results were obtained against remission lymphocytes of leukemia patients, as well as against blast cells (43, 44). A considerable number of normal individuals reacted against the target cells from leukemia patients, but hey did not react against their own lymphocytes or against allogeneic normal lymphocytes. Reactivity of normal individuals, higher than that of leukemia patients, was also seen against lymphoid tissue culture target cells, including the F-265 line (45). As noted in Table 10, cytotoxic reactivity of the leukemia patients has not correlated well with clinical status. Patients with bone marrow relapse, as well as those in complete remission, gave positive reactions (42).

Major Areas for Further Study of Human Leukemia

Considerably more work will be needed before the assays of cell-mediated immunity can be used for practical clinical problems. Table 12 outlines some of the major problems which need to be addressed. From the tests performed thus far, it

Table XII: Major areas in human leukemia to be investigated

1. Preparation of large, standardized batches of antigenic materials.
2. Better characterization of antigens.
3. Nature of effector cells in patients and in controls.
4. Conditions for augmentation of cell-mediated immunity to leukemia associated antigens.

appears that the antigens on human leukemia cells, similar to those on experimental leukemias, are heterogeneous and quite complex. In order to sort these antigens out, it will be important to work with large, standardized batches of cells or extracts. Cells obtained by the cell separator machines or from tissue culture lines should be quite useful in this regard. Further characterization of the antigens, both by fractionation studies and also by further specificity testing (e.g. by the cytotoxicity inhibition assay), is needed. It will be of interest to determine whether any of the antigenic specificities detected by the cellular immunity assays are the same as those described by others at this Workshop, using serologic techniques.

It will also be of interest to determine the nature of the effector cells in the cytotoxicity reactions. It has recently been suggested that cytotoxicity by effector cells from patients is mediated by T cells, whereas the natural cytotoxicity is mediated by complement receptor bearing cells (46, 47). This would be analogous to the differences seen in the experimental tumor models. However, our preliminary studies have indicated that both T cells and non-T cells of normal individuals can be cytotoxic against the lymphoid cell lines (48). Further studies will be needed to resolve this issue, and determine whether the cytotoxicity assay can be used for diagnosis of leukemia or for monitoring of patients.

The assays of cell-mediated immunity should be helpful to determine conditions for immunotherapy. If the antigens detected are relevant to host resistance, as some appear to be in the experimental model systems, then procedures which augment reactivity would be expected to have a beneficial *in vivo* effect. Better schedules of therapy, and selection of antigenic materials for inoculation, could be determined by appropriate immunologic testing.

References

1. Char, D. H., Lepourhiet, A., Leventhal, B. G., and Herberman, R. B.; Int. J. Cancer 12: 409, 1973.
2. Herberman, R. B.; J. Natl. Cancer Inst. 48: 265, 1972.
3. Ting, C. C., Ortaldo, J. R., and Herberman, R. B.; J. Natl. Cancer Inst. 52: 815, 1974.
4. Ortiz de Landazuri, M., and Herberman, R. B.; Nature New Biol. 238: 18, 1972.
5. Nunn, M. E., Djeu, J. Y., Glaser, M., Lavrin, D. H., and Herbermann, R. B.; J. Natl. Cancer Inst. 56: 393, 1976.
6. Lamon, E. W., Skurzak, H. M., and Klein, E.; Int. J. Cancer 10: 581, 1972.
7. Leclerc, J. C., Gomard, E., and Levy, J. P.; Int. J. Cancer 10: 589, 1972.
8. Lavrin, D. H., Herberman, R. B., Nunn, M., and Soares, N.; J. Natl. Cancer Inst. 51: 1497, 1973.
9. Herberman, R. B., Aoki, T., Nunn, M., Lavrin, D. H., Soares, N., Gazdar, A., Holden, H., and Chang, K. S. S.; J. Natl. Cancer Inst. 53: 1103, 1974.
10. Aoki, T., Herberman, R. B., Hartley, J. W., Liu, M., Walling, M. J., and Nunn, M.; submitted for publication.
11. Ting, C. C., Shiu, G., Rodrigues, D., and Herberman, R. B.; Cancer Res. 34: 1684, 1974.
12. Ting, C. C., Rodrigues, D., Bushar, G. S., and Herberman, R. B.; J. Immunol., in press, 1975.
13. Herberman, R. B., Nunn, M. E., Lavrin, D. H., and Asofsky, R.; J. Natl. Cancer Inst. 51: 1509, 1973.
14. Djeu, J. Y., Glaser, M., Kirchner, H., Huang, K. Y., and Herberman, R. B.; Cellular Immunol. 12: 164, 1974.
15. Herberman, R. B., Ting, C. C., Holden, H. T., Glaser, M., and Lavrin, D.; Proceedings XI International Cancer Congress, Excerpta Medica, Vol. 1: 258, 1975.
16. Fossati, G., Holden, H., and Herberman, R. B.; Cancer Res. 35: 2600, 1975.
17. Kirchner, H., Glaser, M., Holden, H. T., and Herberman, R. B.; Int. J. Cancer, in press, 1976.
18. Glaser, M., Herberman, R. B., Kirchner, H., and Djeu, J. Y.; Cancer Res. 34: 2165, 1974.
19. Kirchner, H., Muchmore, A. V., Chused, T., Holden, H. T., and Herberman, R. B.; J. Immunol. 114: 206, 1975.
20. Kirchner, H., Holden, H. T., and Herberman, R. B.; J. Natl. Cancer Inst., 59: 971, 1975.
21. Herberman, R. B., Nunn, M. E., and Lavrin, D. H.; Int. J. Cancer, in press, 1975.
22. Nunn, M. E., Djeu, J. Y., Glaser, M., Lavrin, D. H., and Herberman, R. B.; J. Natl. Cancer Inst., 56: 393, 1976.

23. Herberman, R. B., Nunn, M. E., Holden, H. T., and Lavrin, D. H.; Int. J. Cancer, 16: 230, 1975.
24. Oren, M. E., Herberman, R. B., and Canty, T. G.; J. Natl. Cancer Inst. 46: 621, 1971.
25. Glaser, M., Kirchner, H., and Herberman, R. B.; Int. J. Cancer, 16: 384, 1975.
26. Holden, H. T., Kirchner, H., and Herberman, R. B.; J. Immunol. 115: 327, 1975.
27. Ting, C. C., Kirchner, H., Rodrigues, D., Park, J. Y., and Herberman, R. B.; J. Immunol., 116: 244, 1976.
28. Glaser, M., and Herberman, R. B.; J. Natl. Cancer Inst., in press, 1976.
29. Glaser, M.; unpublished observations.
30. Ting, C. C., and Bonnard, G. D.; J. Immunol., in press, 1976.
31. Glaser, M., Bonnard, G. D., and Herberman, R. B.; J. Immunol. 116: 430, 1976.
32. Holden, H. T., Oldham, R. K., Ortaldo, J. R., and Herberman, R. B.; J. Natl. Cancer Inst., in press, 1976.
33. Ortaldo, J. R., Oldham, R. K., Holden, H. T., and Herberman, R. B.; Cell. Immunol., in press, 1976.
34. Oren, M. E., and Herberman, R. B.; Clin. Exper. Immunol. 9: 45, 1971.
35. Char, D. H., Lepourhiet, A., Leventhal, B. G., and Herberman, R. B.; Int. J. Cancer 12: 409, 1973.
36. Herberman, R. B., McCoy, J. L., and Levine, P. H.; Cancer Res. 34: 1222, 1974.
37. Nkrumah, F.; unpublished observations.
38. Herberman, R. B., Char, D., Oldman, R., Levine, P., Leventhal, B. G., McCoy, J. L., Ho, H. C., and Chau, J. C. W.; In Comparative Leukemia Research 1973, Leukemogenesis, (ed. Ito, Y. and Dutcher, R. M.), p. 649, Tokyo Press, Tokyo, 1975.
39. Levine, P., H., de The, G. B., Brugere, J., Schwaab, G., Mourali N., Herberman, R. B., Ambrozioni, J. C., and Revol, P.; Int. J. Cancer, in press, 1976.
40. Lee, S.; unpublished observations.
41. Ho, H. C., and Chau, J. W.; unpublished observations.
42. Leventhal, B. G., Halterman, R. H., Rosenberg, E. B., and Herberman, R. B.; Cancer Res. 32: 1820, 1972.
43. Rosenberg, E. B., Herberman, R. B., Levine, P. H., Halterman, R. H., McCoy, J. L., and Wunderlich, J. R.; Int. J. Cancer 9: 648, 1972.
44. Herberman, R. B., Rosenberg, E. G., Halterman, R. H., McCoy, J. L., and Leventhal, B. G.; Natl. Cancer Inst. Monogr. 35: 259, 1972.
45. Rosenberg, E. B., McCoy, J. L., Green, S. S., Donnelly, F. C., Siwarski, D. F., Levine, P. H., and Herberman, R. B.; J. Natl. Cancer Inst. 52: 345, 1974.
46. Svedmyr, E., and Jondal, M.; Proc. Nat. Acad. Sci. USA 72: 1622, 1975.
47. Jondal, M.,Svedmyr, E., Klein, E., and Singh, S.; Nature 255: 405, 1975.
48. Dean, J. H., Silva, J. S., McCoy, J. L., Leward, C. M., Cannon, G. B., and Herberman, R. B.; J. Immunol., 115: 1449, 1975.

Surface Features of Cells in Human Lymphoproliferative Disorders. An Immunoelectron Microscopy Study.

M. F. Gourdin, F. Reyes, J. L. Lejonc, P. Mannoni and B. Dreyfus

Unite de Recherches sur les Anémies. INSERM. U. 91 and
C. D. T. S. du Val de Marne. CHU Henri Mondor.
94010 CRETEIL FRANCE

Summary

Peroxidase conjugated antibodies were applied to cell suspensions in order to detect surface associated immunoglobulins. Cell suspensions were fixed prior to incubation with reagents, a procedure avoiding membrane alterations induced by antibodies to surface component. By immunoelectron microscopy an identification of B lymphocytes could be made with simultaneous observation of their surface architecture.

Basic findings were that normal circulating human B lymphocytes had a villous surface. This relationship was not confirmed however by examinating samples from various B and T cell proliferations establishing that surface morphology is not sufficient to categorize cells in disease.

Specimens from hairy cell leukemia were also examined. Despite salient surface characteristics as revealed by the present method, the categorization of cells remains unclear.

Introduction

The recognition of T and B lymphocytes by their surface properties is well documented and has led to numerous studies in humans. Among several available assays the detection of surface immunoglobulins is essential for the chraracterization of B cells (1). Immunoelectron microscopy (I.E.M.) gives the possibility of studying the surface architecture and structure of cells with simultaneous detection of membrane components.

This work was supported by grants from I. N. S. E. R. M.

We are grateful to Mr. REBOUL for photographic assistance and Mrs. M. SEGEAR for secretarial work.

CORRESPONDANCE:
F. REYES
Unité de Recherches sur les Anémies. INSERM U. 91
Hôpital Henri Mondor.
94010 CRETELL FRANCE

Therefore this technic has been largely applied to lymphoid cells. Until recently however no striking differences of the surface morphology were reported between immunoglobulin-bearing (B) lymphocytes and the others, when antibodies conjugated with various markers were applied to live lymphocytes (for review see (2)). Recent data have shown that a clear distinction can be made between B cells and the others on the basis of surface morphology, when normal human blood lymphocytes are reacted with conjugated anti-immunoglobulin reagents as fixed cell suspension (2, 3). These observations have confirmed by immunologic identification previous observations by scanning electron microscopy (S.E.M.) of Polliack and co-workers (4).

In this paper basic findings on normal human B lymphocytes will be recalled and cells from various proliferative disorders described.

Material and Methods

1. *Samples.* The following samples were examined: blood buffy coat from eight normal individuals, ten untreated patients with chronic lymphocytic leukemia (C.L.L.), two with Waldenström macroglobulinemia, four with "prolymphocytic leukemia", two with Sezary syndrom and four with hairy cell leukemia. Splenectomy was performed in two patients of the "prolymphocytic" type. Blood leukocytes were prepared by simple sedimentation at room temperature without other separation procedure and washed in Hank's. Spleen were teased in Hank's with fine forceps, cell clumps discarded and cell suspension obtained after several centrifugations and washings.

2. *Preparation of specimens for I.E.M.* This was carried out as detailled elsewhere (2). Briefly, extensively washed cell suspensions were first glutaraldehyde-fixed. They were then reacted with peroxidase conjugated anti-immunoglobulin reagents, post-fixed with glutaraldehyde and reacted with diaminobenzidine for peroxidase detection. Cell pellets were further post-fixed with osmium and processed for embedding by usual procedures.

3. *Reagents.* Anti-immunoglobulin antibodies were raised in rabbits and sheep, and purified by immunoadsorption (5). They were rendered monospecific for μ, γ, α and $\varkappa$, λ chains (2). Anti-human IgD serum was purchased from C.D.T.S., Bois-Guillaume, Rouen, France; after further absorption on insolubilized whole human serum with a high IgM content, anti-δ antibodies were purified by elution from insolubilized IgD myeloma serum. Anti-F_{ab} antibodies were used as polyvalent anti-immunoglobulin reagent; they were prepared by similar adsorption procedures as previously detailled (6).

4. *Controls.* The specificity of surface labeling was checked by appropriate cellular and serological controls (2).

Results

1. *Normal lymphocytes*

A specific surface staining was found in about 15 % of blood lymphocytes after reacting suspensions with the anti-F_{ab} reagent. IgM-bearing cells were largely predominant over IgG or IgA-bearing lymphocytes, which were uncommon in

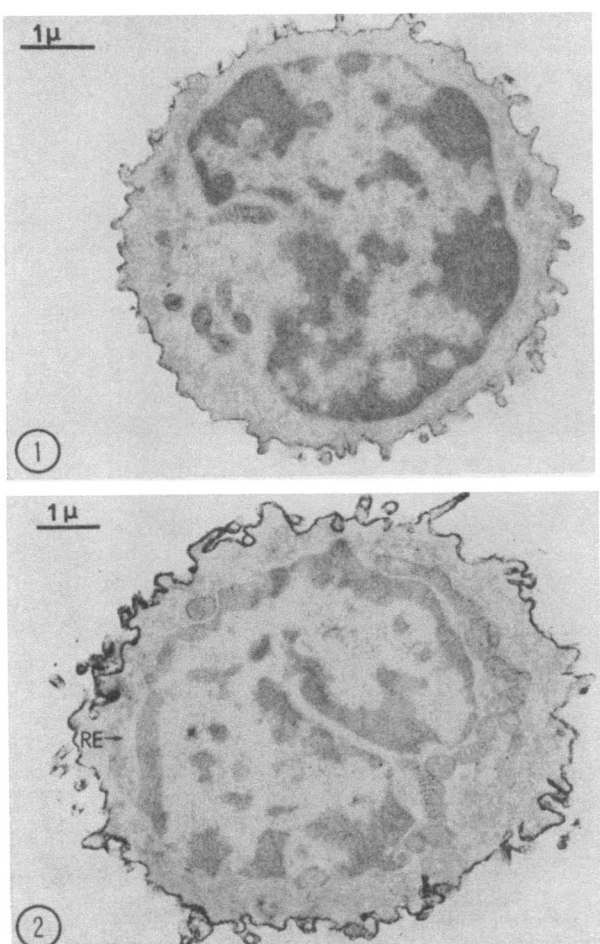

Fig. 1, 2: Normal human blood B lymphocytes. Villous cells are labeled by peroxidase conjugated anti-Fab. Surface immunoglobulins are revealed by a black reaction product due to the cytochemical detection of peroxidase. Variations of the number and length of microvilli, and of surface staining intensity can be appreciated by comparing these two figures. Short strands of endoplasmic reticulum are appearant. (RE →). Fig. 1 x 13350, Fig. 2 x 11700.

sections. Anti-δ reagent was applied to two samples and IgD-bearing lymphocytes found in sections although less numerous than IgM-bearing cells.

In every sample however the labeling pattern was similar, whatever the s.Ig class detected, in that the surface staining was continuous and diffuse all around the cell. No periodicity or patchy pattern was observed on labeled cells. This did not preclude some variations of the staining intensity in a given sample; IgD

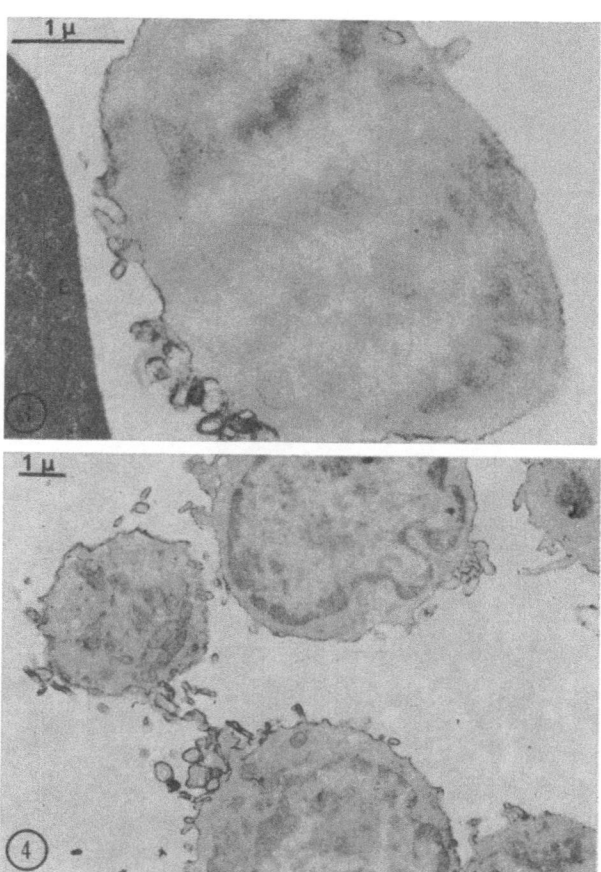

Fig. 3, 4: These are two examples of polar concentration of microvilli in B lymphocytes from C.L.L., with surface Ig Mϰ. Cells are labeled by conjugated anti-μ. E is an erythrocyte. Fig. 3 x 21150, Fig. 4 x 9450.

positive cells for instance were moderately stained when compared to IgM-bearing lymphocytes.

Whatever the class of detected s.Ig, labeled B lymphocytes had a characteristic appearance because of the presence of numerous microvilli (Fig. 1, 2). Non labeled cells had a general smooth surface with sometimes only rare short and spaced microvilli. A few cells were also found which had an intermediate amount of microvilli and a weak surface labeling, therefore considered as B lymphocytes.

2. Lympho-proliferative disorders.

In C.L.L. samples most cells confirmed the relationship between the presence of detectable s.Ig and a villous surface, as previously reported (2). Lymphocytes

210

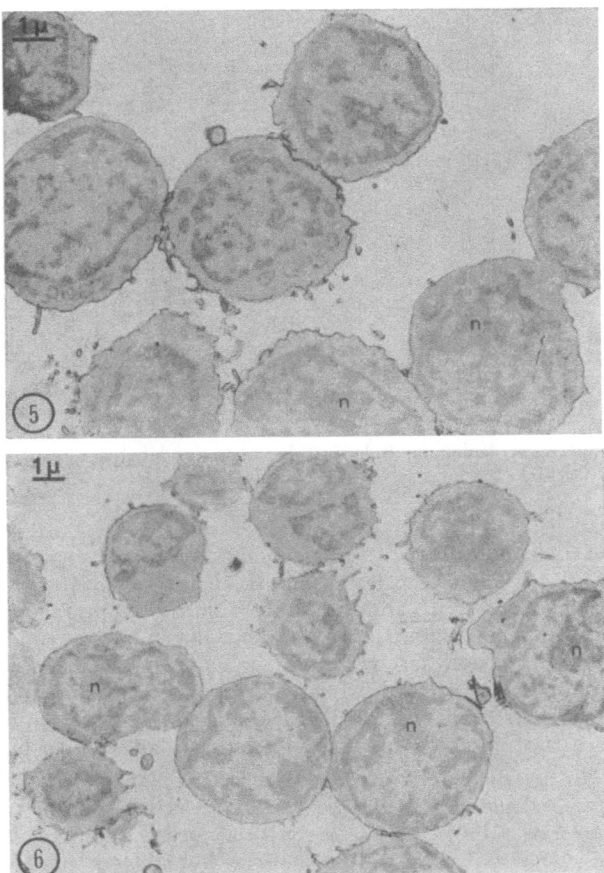

Fig. 5, 6: Sample from prolymphocytic leukemia with surface Ig M λ. Cells are labeled by anti-μ in Fig. 5, by anti-λ in Fig. 6. Moderately villous and smooth cells can be seen. Nuclei contain coarse chromation. n =nucleolus.
Fig. 5 x 7900, Fig. 6 x 6190.

were identified as B cells by polyvalent anti-Fab reagent and their monoclonal distribution of s.Ig shown by monospecific anti-heavy and light chains reagents (IgM ϰ in 5 cases, IgM λ in 2, IgG ϰ in 1). Among cells classified as mature small lymphocytes on the basis of their ultrastructural appearance, variations of the number of microvilli could be seen paralleled by variations of the staining intensity; therefore in some samples the surface morphology ranged from moderately villous to "hairy" cells. In addition cells were found in some sections exhibiting a polar concentration of labeled microvilli with a remaining smooth surface (Fig. 3, 4).

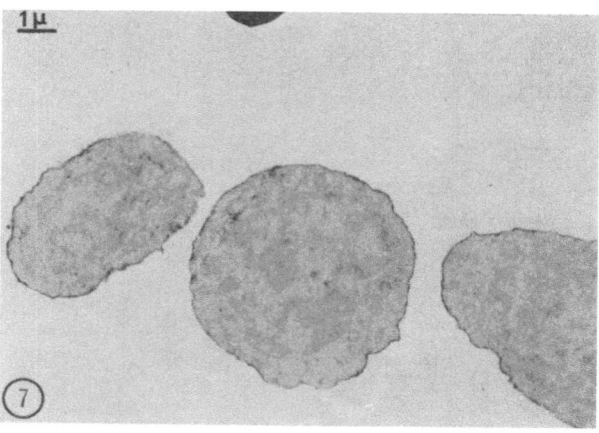

Fig. 7: Prolymphocytic leukemia. Spleen B lymphocytes labeled by anti-µ and with a smooth surface. x 7400.

In some C.L.L. samples careful survey disclosed a minor population of larger cells, either with prominent nucleolus but condensed chromatin, or with large nucleolus and dispersed chromatin (i.e. with "blastic" appearance). These cells were shown to bear the same s.Ig class as remaining mature lymphocytes; they had however a rather smooth surface with rare microvilli.

The presence of smooth labeled B lymphocytes was still more obvious in blood samples from patients with "prolymphocytic leukemia". These cases were diagnosed on the basis of clinical and cytological criteria as reported by Galton and co-workers (7). Specimens contained variable proportions of small villous B lymphocytes and a minor population of "blastic" smooth B cells. The predominant cell type was in fact a large lymphocyte with a nuclear structure similar to that of small lymphocytes – i.e. coarse chromatin – but a large compact nucleolus; cytoplasm also contained some short strands of endoplasmic reticulum. Most of these large cells had few microvilli and their general shape was smooth, although specifically stained by corresponding monospecific anti-immunoglobulin antibodies (Fig. 5, 6). These smooth large B cells were also the predominant feature of splenic suspensions in these patients (Fig. 7).

Blood leukocytes were obtained from two patients with Wäldenström macro-globulinemia. In one patient all lymphocytes were labeled by anti-µ and anti-ϰ reagents; in the other IgM ϰ B cells were only part of circulating lymphocytes (30 %). In both cases a villous surface characterized the mature lymphocytes, as in C.L.L. (Fig. 8, 9). In addition some "intermediate" lymphoid cells were present with some development of endoplasmic reticulum; they were weakly labeled and had a rather smooth surface, but also exhibited a faint specific reaction in the perinuclear space and endoplasmic reticulum lamellae (Fig. 8).

In blood specimens from Sezary syndrom, large abnormal lymphocytes with a typical convoluted nucleus were found. They were regularly free of labeling by

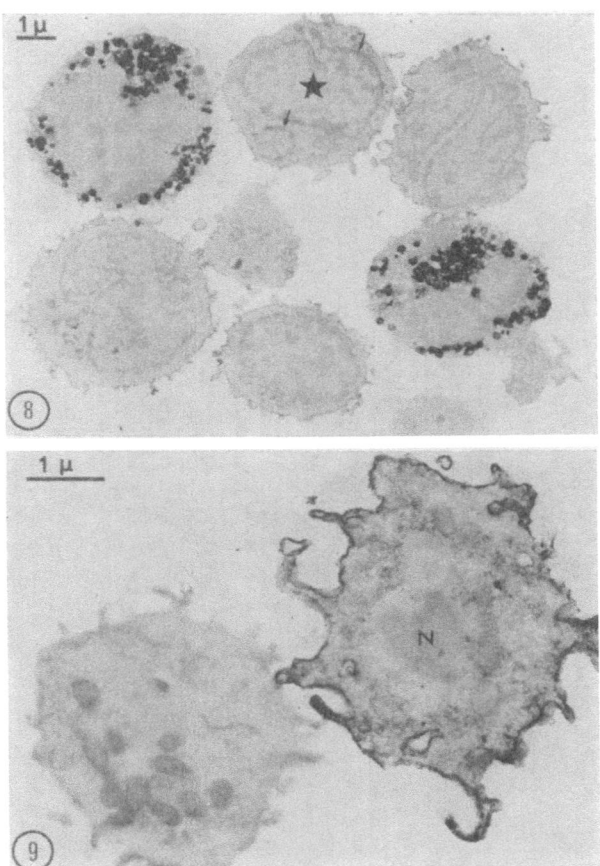

Fig. 8: Blood leukocytes from Waldenström macroglobulinemia. This micrograph shows two polymorphs with endogenous peroxidase in granules; their membrane is not labeled. Three villous B lymphocytes as revealed by anti-μ can be seen. In addition a smooth lymphoid cell (✳) with weak surface labeling also exhibits specific staining in perinuclear space and endoplasmic reticulum (→). x 7250.
Fig. 9: Tangential section of two villous lymphocytes in another sample from macroglobulinemia. One cell with long microvilli is heavily labeled by anti-μ reagent. N is the nucleus. x 14850.

anti-immunoglobulin reagents although segments of their membrane could exhibit numerous microvilli, the remaining surface being smooth (Fig. 10, 11).

3. Hairy cell leukemia

Blood buffy coat was obtained in four cases diagnosed by current clinical and morphological criteria (8, 9). In our experimental conditions these abnormal nononuclear cells exhibited three main characteristics (Fig. 12): 1) they had a very

213

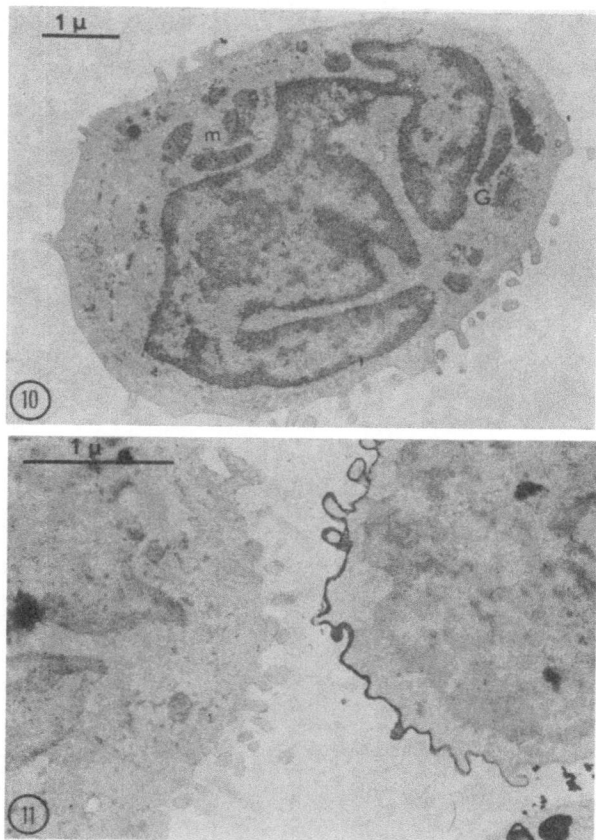

Fig. 10: Sezary syndrom. A typical abnormal cell with convoluted nucleus is seen. Cytoplasm contains lysosomes and numerous lucent vesicles; G is the Golgi apparatus, m are mitochondria. This cell has segments of villous and smooth membrane, without any detectable labeling by anti-Fab. x 15000.

Fig. 11: Sezary syndrom. Part of facing Sezary cell and B lymphocytes. Note that microvilli of Sezary cell are not labeled. Lower right: part of a polymorph with peroxidase containing granules. x 30000.

irregular surface, covered by numerous long microvilli and finger-like projections; 2) they had a high density of associated s.Ig., as revealed by anti-Fab reagent; 3) they lacked detectable endogeneous peroxidase in either endoplasmic reticulum or granules.

However, these cells failed to exhibit a monoclonal pattern of s.Ig. since both x and λ light chains were detected in every sample. Moreover cells strongly reacted with anti-γ antibodies but not with anti-μ, anti-δ, or anti-α antibodies.

214

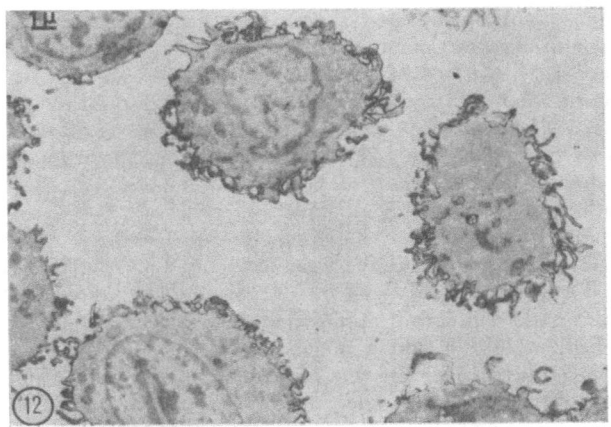

Fig. 12: Blood sample from hairy cell leukemia. These large mononuclear cells have a very irregular surface, covered by long villous processes. There is a high density of surface immunoglobulins as revealed by the diffuse black reaction product outlining the cell surface. No endogeneous peroxidase is detectable. These cells have been labeled with anti-γ reagent. x 5450.

Discussion

The present findings establish a clear duality based on the surface morphology of normal human blood lymphocytes, when first glutaraldehyde-fixed and then identified by peroxidase-conjugated anti-immunoglobin reagents. The distinction between normal villous B cells and smooth (presumed) T cells is not absolute since a minor population of intermediate forms can be found, most of them being however recognized as B cells (2, 3). Thus previous S.E.M. observations by Polliack and co-workers (4) are confirmed by I.E.M.

It is worth noting that until recently no major morphological distinction had emerged from previous I.E.M. studies using various markers; the reasons for this have been discussed already (2). We will only emphasize that when incubation with anti-immunoglobulin reagents is carried out on cells in a living state, B lymphocytes are rendered smooth as a result of a redistribution phenomenon which involves an invagination of surface microvilli (10). Similar observations of smoothing of the surface by antibody-induced redistribution have been made on cells from hairy cell leukemia (unpublished observations).

Such data illustrate the possible induction of morphological cell alterations by factors related to experimental procedures. Another example is the surface alteration of lymphoid cells when involved in rosetting with erythrocytes (11). Therefore the appreciation of the surface morphology of B and T cells after identification by rosetting procedures seems questionable and may explain conflicting reports (12, 13, 14).

However the villous nature of B lymphocytes as found in normal human blood – and recently in mouse lymphoid organs (15) – is still controverted by recent reports in human (16) and mouse (17, 18). It is difficult to know to what extent preparative conditions are similar in published reports, either at the level of cell collection for S.E.M. (16) or of separation procedures such as density gradient centrifugation or column filtration. At this point we can only reiterate that when observed after a simple procedure involving spontaneous sedimentation, washing and fixation of normal human blood buffy coat, lymphocytes can be separated into two predominant populations of villous and smooth cells, the former being associated with the presence of s.Ig.

The functional implications of B lymphocytes microvilli is not clearly determined however. This peculiar surface architecture may be related to some physical properties of B cells as revealed in vitro (for more detailled discussion see (2)).

On the other hand a practical application of this peculiar surface architecture would be its utilization as a simple morphological marker, detectable by scanning or conventional transmission electron microscopy, for the classification of cells from lymphoproliferative states. The present study which was undertaken to test the reliability of such a marker clearly shows that it is not the case.

In C.L.L. and macroglobulinemia, known as monoclonal B cell disorders (1) the villous nature of lymphocytes was confirmed. However samples also contained some smooth cells belonging to the same proliferative process as revealed by simultaneous immunologic identification; they were larger cells with a distinct nucleo-cytoplasmic features. The presence of smooth large B cells was further confirmed by examinating prolymphocytic leukemia samples in which this cell type was predominant over villous small lymphocytes, although they were part of the same proliferative process. A smooth surface also characterized those cells present in blood specimens from macroglobulinemia which were termed "intermediate" because of their developing endoplasmic reticulum; they were also shown to be of B deviration by the simultaneous detection of immunoglobulins both at the surface and in secretory apparatus.

These observations therefore demonstrate that B cells involved in the same proliferative process may have a different surface morphology. Similar conclusions were recently suggested by S.E.M. examination of C.L.L. samples (19, 20). These villous and smooth patterns may represent different stages in the maturation process of B cells. This view suggested by the present findings, is further supported by the surface pattern of B immunoblasts, as found in some lymphomas (to be published). It is also corroborated by the finding of smooth precursor B cells, as recently reported in chicken bursal cells (15).

Examination of abnormal Sezary cells also disclosed an exception to the general relationship between microvilli and s.Ig, as found in normal blood lymphocytes. Sezary cells have been shown to have membrane properties common to T lymphocytes (21, 22). In this study they were found to lack detectable s.Ig including at the level of their segment of villous membrane.

Taken all together our observations of B and T cell disorders emphasize that surface morphology alone is not a suitable criterion for classifying cells of lymphoproliferative disorders. Immunologic identification is in fact essential for that purpose.

The lymphocytic or monocytic nature of abnormal cells found in hairy cell leukemia keeps on being the subject of controversial reports (for review see (23,

24, 25)), despite the use of various sophisticated methods. In this study cells lack detectable endogeneous peroxidase, an essential cytochemical feature of normal marrow and blood monocytes (26). Their peculiar surface morphology can be compared to that of some very villous, "hairy", B lymphocytes, but also to the ruffled membrane of monocytes (25). Despite the presence of great amounts of s.Ig. their lymphocytic nature is not ascertained. In the present experiment we failed to demonstrate surface IgM or IgD; such B cell markers were recently reported to be present in hairy cell leukemia (27). On the other hand surface polyclonal IgG were regularly detected in our study, a result suggesting that s.Ig were adsorbed cytophilic immunoglobulins rather than an actual cell product; the presence of receptors for the Fc portion of IgG has been previously demonstrated in hairy cell leukemia, favoring its monocytic origin (24). Culture experiments are actually in progress in order to clarify this problem. However, as recently pointed out by King and his colleagues, the identification of these malignant cells is "plagued by the universal problem of categorizing abnormal cells on the basis of assays usually reserved for identifying normal cells". (28).

References

1. Seligmann, M., J. L. Preud'homme, and J. C. Brouet. 1973. B and T cell markers in human proliferative blood diseases and primary immunodeficiencies, with special reference to membrane bound immunoglobulin. Transplant. Rev. *16*: 85.
2. Reyes, F., J. L. Lejonc, M. F. Gourdin, P. Mannoni, and B. Dreyfus. 1975. The surface morphology of human B lymphocytes as revealed by immunoelectron microscopy. J. Exp. Med. *141*: 392.
3. Reyes, F., J. L. Lejonc, M. F. Gourdin, P. Mannoni, and B. Dreyfus. 1974. Démonstration de la présence d'immunoglobulines de membranes sur les villosités des lymphocytes humains. C. R. Acad. Sci. Paris, Série D. *278*: 2373.
4. Polliack, A., N. Lampen, B. D. Clarshson, E. de Harven, Z. Bentwich, and H. G. Kunkel. 1973. Identification of human B and T lymphocytes by scanning electron microscopy. J. Exp. Med. *138*: 607.
5. Avrameas, S., and T. Ternynck. 1969. The cross-linking of proteins with glutaraldehyde and its use for the preparation of immunoadsorbents. Immunochemistry. *6*: 53.
6. Sapin, C., A. Massez, A. Contet, and P. Druet. 1975. Isolation of normal human Ig A, Ig M and Ig G fragments by polyacrylamide beads immunoadsorbents. J. Immunol. Methods. *9*: 27.
7. Galton, D. A. G., J. M. Goldman, E. Wiltshaw, D. Catovsky, K. Henry, and G. J. Goldenberg. 1974. Prolymphocytic leukaemia. Brit. J. Haemat. *27*: 7.
8. Flandrin, G., M. T. Daniel, M. Fourcade, and N. Chelloul. 1973. Leucémies à "Tricholeucocyte: (Hairy cell Leukaemia)". Nouv. Rev. Fr. Hémat. *13*: 609.
9. Catovsky, D., J. E. Petit, D. A. G. Galton, A. J. D. Spiers, and C. V. Harrison. 1974. Leukaemic reticuloendotheliosis ("Hairy cell Leukaemia"): a distinct clinico-pathological entity. Brit. J. Haemat. *26:* 9.
10. Gourdin, M. F., F. Reyes, J. L. Lejonc, J. Breton-Gorius, P. Mannoni, and

B. Dreyfus. 1976. Ultrastructural studies of human erythrocyte and lymphocyte series with peroxidase conjugated antibodies. In "Proceedings of the 1ˢᵗ International Symposium on Immunoenzymatics Technics". North Holland publ. in press.

11. Reyes, F., A. Le Go, F. Delrieu, and J. F. Bach. 1974. Ultrastructure of cell binding immunoglobulin-coated erythrocytes in rheumatoid arthritis. Clin. Exp. Immunol. *17*: 533.

12. Lin, P. S., A. G. Cooper, and H. H. Wortis. 1973. Scanning electron microscopy of human T-cell and B-cell rosettes. N. Engl. J. Med. *289*: 548.

13. Kay, M. M., B. Belohradsky, K. Yee, J. Vogel, D. Butcher, J. Wybran, and H. H. Fudenberg. 1974. Cellular interactions: scanning electron microscopy of human thymus-derived rosette-forming lymphocytes. Clin. Immunol. Immunopath. 2: 301.

14. Polliack, A., S. M. Fu, S. D. Douglas, Z. Bentwich, N. Lampen, and E. de Harven. 1974. Scanning electron microscopy of human lymphocyte-sheep erythrocyte rosettes. J. Exp. Med. *140*: 146.

15. Polliack, A., U. Hämmerling, N. Lampen, and E. de Harven. 1975. Surface morphology of murine B and T lymphocytes: a comparative study by scanning electron microscopy. Eur. J. Immunol. *5*: 32.

16. Alexander, E. L., and B. Wetzel. 1975. Human lymphocytes: similarity of B and T cell surface morphology. Science *188*: 732.

17. Linthicum, D. S., S. Sell, R. M. Wagner, and P. Trefts. 1974. Scanning electron microscopy of mouse B and T lymphocytes. Nature *252*: 173.

18. Baur, P. S., G. B. Thurman, and A. L. Goldstein. 1975. Reappraisal of lymphocyte classification by means of surface morphology. J. Immunol. *115*: 1375.

19. Polliack, A., and E. de Harven. 1975. Surface features of normal and leukemic lymphocytes as seen by scanning electron microscopy. Clin. Immunol. Immunopath. *3*: 412.

20. Catovsky, D., B. Frisch, and S. Van Noorden. 1975. B, T and "null" cell leukaemias. Electron cytochemistry and surface morphology. Blood cells *1*: 115.

21. Brouet, J. C., G. Flandrin, and M. Seligmann. 1973. Indications for the thymus derived nature of the proliferating cells in six patients with Sézary's syndrome. N. Eng. J. Med. *289*: 341.

22. Zucker-Franklin, D., J. W. Melton, and F. Quagliata. 1974. Ultrastructural, immunologic, and functional studies on Sézary cells: a neoplastic variant of thymus-derived (T) lymphocytes. Proc. Natl. Acad. Sci. U.S.A. *71*: 1877.

23. Daniel, M. Th., and G. Flandrin. 1974. Fine structure of abnormal cells in hairy cell (tricholeukocytic) leukemia, with special reference to their in vitro phagocytic capacity. Lab. Invest. *30*: 1.

24. Jaffe, E. S., E. M. Shevach, M. M. Frank, and I. Green. 1974. Leukemic reticuloendotheliosis: presence of a receptor cytophilic antibody. Amer. J. Med. *57*: 108.

25. Golomb, H. M., R. Braylan, and A. Polliack. 1975. Hairy cell leukemia: a scanning electron microscopic study of eight cases. Brit. J. Haemat. *29*: 455.

26. Breton-Gorius, J., and F. Reyes. 1976. Ultrastructure of human bone marrow cell maturation. International Review of Cytology. Academic Press. In press.

27. Fu, S. M., J. Winchester, K. R. Rai, and H. G. Kunkel. 1974. Hairy cell leukemia: proliferation of a cell with phagocytic and B-lymphocyte properties. Scand. J. Ummunol. *3*: 847.
28. King, G. W., P. E. Hurtubise, A. L. Sagone, A. Lo Buglio, and E. N. Metz. 1975. Leukemic reticuloendotheliosis. A study of origin of the malignant cell. Amer. J. Med. *59*: 411.

Immunological Characterization of Blast Cells in Patients with Acute Lymphoblastic Leukemia. Evaluation of its Clinical Significance.

J. C. Brouet and A. Chevalier

Laboratory of Immunochemistry and Immunopathology, U 108, INSERM, Research Institute on Blood Diseases, Hôpital Saint-Louis, Paris, France.

Summary

A panel of lymphocyte surface markers was used to identify blast cells from 111 patients with acute lymphoblastic leukemia (ALL). Three groups of patients were found. 1) 14 patients with B derived ALL. Only three patients had a common ALL; in the other cases the blastic proliferation was featured by Burkitt's tumor cells or supervened in patients affected with chronic lymphocytic leukemia (CLL). 2) The blast cells from 28 % of the patients with common ALL had T cell properties. 3) The cells from the largest group of patients did not bear B or T cell markers but were featured by the presence of a leukemia-associated antigen revealed by a rabbit antiserum to CLL B cells. Studies with another antiserum to CLL B cells as well as with an antiserum to foetal thymocytes revealed also leukemia-associated antigens but these antigenic determinants were present on all acute leukemia cells which had been tested and were therefore of no help to classify various leukemias. A number of clinical and hematological findings were more frequent in the group of patients with T cell ALL: high white blood cell counts, tumoral disease, thymic enlargement, meningeal involvement, strong acid phosphatase activity in blast cells. However no difference in the survival curve is yet apparent at 30 months.

Introduction

Rwo main immunological approaches were used in the recent years to characterize the blast cells in various leukemias and specially acute lymphoblastic leukemias (ALL). The expression at the surface of ALL blast cells of membrane markers which are considered specific for T or B lymphoid cell lines may help to elucidate the cellular origin of the neoplastic cells. Such studies showed that a minor group of ALL was B cell derived (1, 2) that nearly 30 % of ALL had T cell features (1, 3–8) whereas the majority of ALL blast cells did not possess B or T cell markers. On the other hand the identification at the surface of leukemic cells of some antigenic determinants which are leukemia associated or leukemia specific has been developed (9–14, 18) and there is much evidence now that there is a complexity of serologically detectable antigenic determinants on leukemic cells.

These two approaches to the characterization of leukemic cells are not inconsistent with each other. They may both be helpful to classify various leukemias on objective criteria and hopefully will have some therapeutic or prognostic implications. This report deals with the immunological characterization of blast cells in 111 patients with ALL and with a search for possible correlations between the nature of the leukemic cells and clinical, morphological and cytochemical data as well as with the evolution and prognosis of the disease.

Methods and their critical Evaluation

The methods used for the detection of B or T cell membrane markers have been described elsewhere (15, 16).

Three different antisera to B CLL cells and an antiserum to foetal thymocytes were raised in rabbits and tested for their reactivity with various normal and leukemic cells. Rabbits were immunized with 20 to 40. 10^6 cells intravenously, boosted with the same number of cells 14 days later and bled 7 days following each immunization. After heat inactivation, serial absorptions were performed with human liver (x3), human AB erythrocytes (x 3), normal human serum and immunoglobulin (Ig) chains coupled to Sepharose 4B. The anti CLL sera were further absorbed with peripheral T cells (serum 1 and 2) or with peripheral T cells and thymocytes (serum 3). The antiserum to foetal thymocytes was absorbed on CLL B cells. Absorptions were usually carried out with a 3 to 1 serum to packed cells ratio for 60 minutes at + 4 °C. The reactivity of these antisera was assessed by either cytotoxicity or indirect immunofluorescence on 1) normal blood and tonsil lymphocytes. 2) T lymphocytes obtained after nylon filtration of blood or tonsil lymphocytes, 3) B lymphocytes from CLL patients, 4) T lymphocytes from T derived CLL, 5) T or B lymphoid cultured cell lines, 6) thymocytes, 7) phytohemagglutinin transformed lymphocytes, 8) blast cells from various acute leukemias (T derived ALL, non T non B ALL, acute myeloblastic leukemia (AML)).

The interpretation of the results of such investigations requires much caution since they are exposed to a number of pitfalls. Among lymphocyte surface markers, membrane bound Ig detected by immunofluorescence constitute the most reliable marker of B cells and may represent a clonal marker of B cell proliferations when monospecific antisera to the various Ig chains are used. But the mere presence of immunoglobulins at the surface of a cell does not necessarily mean that they are produced by that cell. Erroneous interpretations may result from the attachment of circulating immune complexes or IgG aggregates to any cell carrying receptors for C3 or Fc, from an anti-IgG activity of membrane bound IgM (17) or from the presence of antibodies directed to lymphocyte surface determinants (16). In vitro experiments may therefore be required to ensure that surface immunoglobulins are synthesized by the cells under study (17). Most heteroantisera to B or T cells are only relatively specific. When they can be used only in cytotoxicity tests and not in immunofluorescence, they do not allow direct checking for other markers and direct examination of the positive cells.

Current studies have shown that the delineation between B and T lymphocyte markers is less clear cut than previously appraised and that cell subpopulations characterized by different surface markers exist within these two broad categories. Is should be stressed that a classification of cells in terms of B or T origin which may be relatively safe for normal lymphocytes may not be valid when extrapolated to undifferentiated or neoplastic cells. Such cells may express membrane antigens only at certain stages of the cell cycle or experience surface changes which prevent their identification.

Reactive antigenic determinants on leukemic cells may represent viral coded determinants, foetal, stem cell or even derepressed normal antigens. The precise nature and significance of leukemic associated antigens remains largely unknown. Some antisera appear truly leukemia specific since they react only with leukemic cells, usually of various cellular types (10–14); other antisera reveal leukemic associated antigens which may also be found on a population of normal cells (14, 18, 19).

Results

Lymphocyte membrane markers in 111 patients with ALL

B derived ALL

A monoclonal B cell proliferation was found in 14 patients. The cells bore a homogeneous surface IgM in all cases but one where IgG ϰ molecules were detected. These blast cells also bound IgG aggregates but lacked T cell markers in all cases studied.

Most of these patients were not affected with a common ALL. In 3 cases the blastic proleferation supervened in patients previously affected with common CLL. In one of these patients the finding of an identical anti-IgG antibody activity of the surface Ig on both small lymphocytes and blast cells ascertained that the two cell populations derived from the same clone (20). In 8 cases the blast cells possessed all the cytological features of Burkitt's tumor cells (2). Only 3 patients with a monoclonal B cell process belonged to the group of unselected patients with common ALL. In 2 of these cases the blast cells showed some unusual cytological features similar to that of cells from lymphosarcoma.

T derived ALL

Blast cells from 28 patients out of 100 cases of common ALL (i.e. patients with Burkitt's tumor cells or with ALL supervening on CLL excluded) had T cell surface characteristics (Table I). In 26 of these 28 patients the blast cells formed spontaneous rosettes. In 10 cases only the percentage of rosetting blasts was higher than 60 %; in the remaining 16 patients the percentage of rosette forming blast cells was lower (10 to 60 %). The cells from 18 patients were studied with an antiserum to peripheral T cells. In 17 cases including the 2 patients whose blast cells did not form rosettes, the cells were killed by this antiserum.

Non T non B ALL (Table I)

In 59 patients, all blast cells were devoid of surface Ig and did not bind IgG aggregates. In the remaining 10 patients a small percentage (less than 15 %) of cells were stained by antisera to γ, ϰ, λ and sometimes μ chains. The staining pattern was unusual with an irregular or grossly spotted aspect. These cells did not bind IgG aggregates. In the 2 cases where trypsinization experiments were per-

Table I: B and T membrane markers on blast cells in common ALL.

	N° studied	N° positive
Surface Ig	100	3 μ x
		μ λ
		μ λ
Fc receptor	70	0
Spontaneous rosette formation	100	26 (only 8 with > 80 % of RFC)
Killing by anti-T serum	50	17

formed, no evidence in favor of an actual Ig synthesis by the cells in vitro was obtained.

In 63 cases the blast cells did not form rosettes with sheep erythrocytes. Small cells (presumably the residual T lymphocytes present in the suspension) accounted for most of all of the few rosette-forming cells. However in the last 6 patients, it was difficult to exclude the possibility that a small percentage of the blasts were rosetting cells. These 6 patients could not be studied with other T cells markers. In the 32 patients who were studied with an antiserum to peripheral T cells, the blast cells were unreactive. By contrast in most cases the cells were killed by an anti-CLL serum which recognized leukemia associated antigens (see infra).

Correlations between lymphocyte membrane markers on blast cells and clinical and hematological data

All patients with a B derived ALL experienced a very poor prognosis. Patients with Burkitt's tumor cells did not respond to chemotherapy or relapsed after a short remission. Among the patients with B derived "common" ALL one 5-year old child died from hematological relapse after five years survival whereas two male adults had no remission under chemotherapy.

Among patients with T ALL or non T non B ALL, there was no difference in the sex and age distribution. The cytological subclassification of ALL did not differentiate the two groups. Cytochemical studies showed that a strong positivity for acid phosphatase was more often found in blast cells from T derived ALL ($p = 0.01$). PAS positivity or beta-glucuronidase activity were not different in the two groups of patients.

Initial anemia or thrombocytopenia were equally found in both groups of patients. An initial high white blood cell count was more often associated with T ALL ($p = 0.05$). A tumoral presentation occurred in 36 patients; 17 of these patients were affected with a T ALL ($p = 0.05$). 15 patients had a mediastinal involvement. Seven of those 8 patients who had a predominantly antero-superior mediastinal enlargement and hence presumably a thymic enlargement were affected with T ALL.

The actuarial survival curve shows no difference between the group of patients with T ALL and non T non B ALL at 30 months. Hematological relapses were found equally in both groups of patients. 5 patients experienced a meningeal involvement in the group of T ALL whereas a single patient had a meningeal relapse in the non T non B group (p = 0.02).

Reactivity of ALLblast cells with antisera to CLL B cell or foestal-thymoctes

The reactivity of anti-B CLL cells sera 1 and 2 on normal and leukemic cells is shown on Table II. These antisera reacted with B cells from normal or leukemic individuals and from various B cell lines. They gave negative reactions with peripheral T cells, on T derived cultured lines, T derived CLL and PHA transformed cells. However they did react with thymocytes. Among patients with leukemias they did not react with AML cells or T derived ALL blasts (with a single exception) but were positive on blast cells from non T non B ALL cases. The reactivity with the latter cells was abolished by absorption with thymocytes and vice versa. The results of this cross-absorption experiments and the presence of at least one determinant on thymocytes showed that these leukemia associated antigens shared by CLL, non T non B ALL and thymocytes are distinct from B cell antigens.

Table II: Reactivity of leukemic and normal cells with rabbit antisera to CLL B cells (sera 1 and 2)

Absorption	B cells	Peripheral T cells	Thymocytes	T ALL	Non T non B ALL	AML
A						
RBC						
Liver	+	−	+	−	+	−
Ig						
Peripheral T cells						
B						
Abs. A						
+	+	−	−	−	−	−
Thymocytes						
C						
Abs. A +						
Non T non B	+	−	−	−	−	−
All cells						

Another serum raised in rabbits to CLL B cells had a different pattern of reactivity (Table III). It was absorbed on peripheral T cells and thymocytes. It contained antibodies to B cells and gave negative results on peripheral T cells or thymocytes. However it was reactive with PHA transformed T lymphocytes. This reactivity was only transient and disappeared in late cultures. This serum stained AML and ALL blast cells; the latter reactivity disappeared after absorption with AML cells and it is most likely that this antiserum contained antibodies to cell cycle antigens.

Table III: Reactivity of leukemic and normal cells with a rabbit antiserum to CLL B cells (serum 3)

Absorption	B cells	Peripheral T cells	Thymocytes	Non T non B ALL	AML	PHA transformed T cells 3rd day	8th day
RBC Liver Ig Peripheral T cells Thymocytes	+	–	–	+	+	+	–
Idem + AML cells	+	–	–	–	–	–	–

A rabbit antiserum to foetal thymocytes, reacted after suitable absorptions with T cells and blast cells from ALL or AML (Table IV). Absorption of this antiserum with AML cells abolished the reactivity with non T non B ALL blast cells but not with T ALL and T cell antibodies were not removed by this absorption.

Table IV: Reactivity of leukemic and normal cells with a rabbit antiserum to foetal thymocytes

Absorption	B cells	Peripheral T cells	Thymocytes	T ALL	non T non B ALL	AML
RBC Liver Ig B CLL cells	–	+	+	+	+	+
Idem + AML cells	–	+	+	+	–	–

Discussion

The study of the expression of B or T membrane markers on blast cells in ALL allowed the distinction between three groups of patients. A minor group is characterized by B derived blast cells. In our experience these B ALL cells bore homogeneous surface Ig and thus are presumably of monoclonal origin. Patients with B ALL belonged mostly to two specific antities namely ALL supervening on CLL and ALL featured by Burkitt's tumor cells. It is striking that in 2 out of 3 patients with a "common" B ALL, the cells had unusual cytologic features suggestive of poorly differentiated lymphocytic lymphoma, a disease which is usually of B cell origin in adults. These findings suggest that most if not all patients with B type ALL may in fact be affected with a lymphoma with leukemic presentation.

Less than a third of common ALL are featured by T derived blast cells. This study and other reports (4–8) demonstrated that such patients often had leukemias with high risk factors, such as high WBC, tumoral presentation and often a thymic mass. It is thus likely that the survival of patients with T ALL will be poorer than that of patients with non T non B ALL, although at present no difference is apparent at 30 months. It will be important to look for the survival of patients with T ALL or non T non B ALL which will be matched for initial clinical parameters in order to determine whether the T nature of the blast cells is by itself of poor prognostic value.

In the largest group of patients with ALL the blast cells did not possess any of the current B or T lymphocyte membrane markers. The question of the true cellular origin of non T non B ALL remains presently unsettled. The involvement of lymphoid stem cells devoid of mature B or T lymphocyte markers or the occurrence of surface changes due to the malignant process may explain the lack of detectable T cell markers. The finding of a specific thymic enzyme in blast cells from 11 out of 13 ALL patients (21) would support this hypothesis and it seems unlikely that these non T non B cells do not involve the lymphoid differentiation pathway at all. In this context, it is of great interest that blast cells from non T non B ALL were characterized in this study by a positive finding, i.e. a leukemia ssociated antigens as discussed below.

The proposed immunologic classifcation of ALL in three main groups appears to be valid. Hopefully the classification will not remain purely academic but will prove to be of some practical value. If confirmed by the study of a large number of patients, the results obtained in this report give some hope that a battery of less sophisticated methods such as for instance myeloperoxidase and acid phosphatase staining, E rosette formation and binding of IgG aggregates will improve in any case the accuracy and reproducibility of the classification of acute leukemias.

The study of leukemic cells with rabbit antisera to feotal thymocytes or CLL B cells pointed to the presence of distinct leukemia associated antigens. The former antiserum reacted with blast cells from different cellular origin (i.e. AML or ALL cells). A wide pattern of reactivity among leukemic cells was also found by Mohnakumar and Metzgar using a primate antiserum to thymocytes (19). The results obtained with antisera to thymic cells must therefore be carefully interpreted when evaluating the possible T origin of leukemic cells.

Another approach to leukemic surface antigens was evaluated in this study using antisera to CLL B cells. Two antisera reacted, after suitable absorptions, with thymocytes (and not peripheral T cells), CLL and non T non B ALL cells whereas negative results were obtained with T ALL or AML blasts. It is of interest that such a distinction between non T non B ALL cells and T derived blasts was also achieved by Greaves et al. using a rabbit antiserum to non T ALL cells (14). Since their antiserum did not react with CLL cells it is likely that at least two different sets of leukemia related antigenic determinants are expressed on non T non B ALL cells.

In contrast previous studies performed with antisera to B cell line extracts or B CLL cells yielded different results. The antigenic systems involved in such studies were found on all ALL and CLL cells tested when monkey antisera were used (10) whereas rabbit antisera reacted with all acute leukemias (12, 13, 22). In the present report one out of three rabbit antisera to CLL cells had such a broad reactivity; it contained presumably antibodies to cell cycle dependent antigens since normal lymphocytes were transiently positive when stimulated by PHA.

The purification and characterization of leukemia associated antigens (23, 24) are clearly warranted to evaluate the potential use of such antisera in the management of patients with acute leukemia.

We are grateful to Dr. H. R. Toben who provided some antisera used in this study. This work was supported in part by INSERM (grant ATP 1.73.16.17) and DGRST (Grant 75.7.0786).

References

1. Brouet, J. C., Toben, H. R., Chevalier, A., Seligmann, M. *Ann. Immunol. Paris, 125C,* 691, 1974.
2. Flandrin, G., Brouet, J. C., Daniel, M.T., Preud'homme, J. L. *Blood, 45,* 183, 1975.
3. Belpomme, D., Dautcher, D., Du Rusquec, E., Grandjon, D., Huchet, R., Pouillart, P., Schwarzenberg, L., Amiel, J. L., Mathe, G. *Biomedicine, 20,* 109, 1974.
4. Sen, L., Borella, L. *New Engl. J. Med., 292,* 828, 1975.
5. Brown, G., Greaves, M. F., Lister, T. A., Rapson, N., Papamichael, M. *Lancet, 11,* 753, 1974.
6. Catovsky, D., Goldman, J. M., Okos, A., Frisch, B., Galton, D. A. G. *Brit. Med. J., 2,* 643, 1974.
7. Chin, A. H., Saiki, J. H., Trujillo, J. M., Williams, R. C. *Clin. Immunol. Immunopath., 1,* 499, 1973.
8. Kersey, J. H., Sabad, A., Gajl-Peczalska, K. J., Hallgren, H. M., Yunis, E. J., Nesbit, M. E. *Science, 182,* 1355, 1973.
9. Bias, W. B., Santos, G. W., Burke, P. J., Mullins, G. M., Humphrey, R. L. *Science, 178,* 304, 1972.
10. Metzgar, R. S., Mohanakumar, T., Miller, D. S. *Science, 178,* 986, 1972.
11. Baker, M. A., Ramachandar, C., Taub, R. N. *J. Clin. Invest., 54,* 1273, 1974.
12. Mann, D. L., Rogentine, G. N., Halterman, R., Leventhal, B. *Science, 174,* 1136, 1971.
13. Billing, R., Terasaki, P. I. *J. Nat. Cancer Inst., 53,* 1639, 1974.
14. Greaves, M. F., Brown, G., Rapson, R., Lister, A. *Clin. Immunol. Immunopath., 4,* 67, 1975.
15. Seligmann, M., Preud'homme, J. L., Brouet, J. C. *Transpl. Rev., 16,* 85, 1973.
16. Preud'homme, J. L., Seligmann, M. *Blood, 40,* 777, 1972.
17. Preud'homme, J. L., Seligmann, M. *Proc. Nat. Acad. Sci., 69,* 2132, 1972.
18. Brouet, J. C., Preud'homme, J. L., Seligmann, M. *Blood Cells, 1,* 81, 1975.
19. Mohanakumar, T., Metzgar, R. S. *Cellul. Immunol., 12,* 30, 1974.
20. Brouet, J. C., Preud'homme, J. L., Seligmann, M., Bernard, J. *Brit. Med. J., 4,* 23, 1973.
21. McCaffrey, R., Harrison, T. A., Parkman, R. B. S., Baltimore, D. *New Engl. J. Med., 292,* 775, 1975.
22. Mohanakumar, T., Metzgar, R. S., Miller, D. S. *J. Nat. Cancer Inst., 52,* 1435, 1974.
23. Metzgar, R. S., Mohanakumar, T., Greeen, R. W., Miller, D. S. Bolognesi, D. P. *J. Nat. Cancer Inst., 52,* 1445, 1974.
24. Billing, G., Terasaki, P. I. *J. Nat. Cancer Inst., 53,* 1645, 1974.

Immunological Membrane Markers of Hodgkin's Cells

Marshall E. Kadin, M. D. [1, 2, 3]
Sondra Gold, Ph. D. [3]
Eileen M. Garratty, A. I. M. L. S. [3]
Daniel P. Stites, M. D. [1, 2]

From the Departments of Medicine[1] and Laboratory Medicine[2],
the Division of Hematology and the Cancer Research Institute[3]
University of California, San Francisco, CA 94143, U. S. A.

Summary

Reed-Sternberg and other Hodgkin's giant cells derived from involved spleens and lymph nodes of patients with Hodgkin's disease were examined for surface markers of T and B cells and macrophages. Attachment and phagocytosis of untreated (E) or sensitized (EA and EAC) sheep red blood cells and yeast by Reed-Sternberg cells did not occur. IgG frequently detected at the membrane of Reed-Sternberg cells was partially removed by incubation and washing at 37 °C. Fluorescence with a specific anti-T cell serum was not seen on Reed-Sternberg and other Hodgkin's giant cells. These studies indicate that Reed-Sternberg and other Hodgkin's giant cells lack most detectable normal human lymphoid cell markers, but do exhibit membrane bound immunoglobulin possibly of exogenous origin.

Introduction

Morphological criteria alone are inadequate for the recognition of the Hodgkin's cell. These criteria lack specificity since Reed-Sternberg cells may be observed in a number of other disorders including infectious mononucleosis (1), and they do not permit identification of the perhaps more proliferative precursors of the Reed-Sternberg cell (2). It would be attractive to find a membrane marker or combination of markers to characterize these cells. Therefore, we have examined isolated viable Hodgkin's cells for the presence of membrane markers typical for normal histiocytes and lymphocytes.

Initial studies in our laboratory (3) and by Braylan et al (4) indicated that the cytologically malignant giant cells in Hodgkin's tissues lack normal T cell markers. We have extended these observations and further examined these cells for receptors for sheep erythrocytes sensitized with IgG, or IgM and complement which are surface markers for histiocytes and B lymphocytes. We have also studied their capacity for the phagocytosis of opsonized yeast and latex particles. Finally, we have looked for surface immunoglobulins and are currently investigating the possible exogenous origin of the surface IgG which we have detected.

Methods

All of the experiments were performed with cells sterily isolated from Hodgkin's lesions of nine involved lymph nodes and six spleens by careful mincing in RPMI 1640 culture medium. Erythrocytes were lysed in 0.83 % NH_4Cl and the resulting cell suspension washed 3 times in media. Cells were then resuspended in media containing 10 % fetal calf serum at 5×10^6 cells/ml for the rosetting and phagocytosis studies. The cell viability as determined by trypan blue dye exclusion was at least 90 %.

Rosetting and phagocytosis studies

T lymphocytes were detected by the spontaneous formation of rosettes with washed sheep red blood cells (SRBC) using the method of Jondal et al (5). Briefly, 0.25 ml cells from tissue suspensions were incubated with 0.25 ml washed SRBC (1 % in Hank's balanced salt solution – 10 % FCS) at 37° for 5 minutes. The cells were then centrifuged at 1000 rpm for 10 minutes at room temperature and stored overnight at 4°. Tubes were inverted gently, cells were added to trypan blue, and 200 viable cells were counted with the hemocytometer. A rosette was defined as a cell having 3 or more SRBC bound to its surface. Cytocentrifuge preparations were also made and stained with Wright-Giemsa.

Fc and complement receptors were detected by the method of Shevach et al (6). Fresh SRBC (E) were washed and sensitized either with 7S (IgG) rabbit anti-SRBC (7S EA) or with 19S (IgM) rabbit anti-SRBC (19S EA). The anti-SRBC reagents are from Cordis Laboratories, Miami, Florida. For complement receptor detection, the 19S EA was further incubated with fresh mouse complement diluted 1:20 with gelatin-veronal buffer. 0.25 ml of the appropriate reagent – 7S EA (for Fc receptor), 19S EA (for non-specific binding), 19S EAC (for C_3 receptor) was mixed with 0.25 ml tissue cell suspension and put on a rotator at 37° for 30 minutes. Hemocytometer counts were made as for the T-rosettes, with the additional observation of any phagocytic cells. Cytocentrifuge preparations were also made and were the best means of observing phagocytosis.

Normal peripheral blood lymphocytes did not demonstrate Fc receptors with the 7S EA reagent; normal and malignant histiocytes did rosette and phagocytose 7S EA. Normal peripheral blood lymphocytes (10–25 %) and most monocytes rosetted with 19S EAC as did the majority of CLL cells. Monocytes and histiocytes also phagocytosed the 19S EAC reagent. T-rosettes were formed by 50–70 % of peripheral blood lymphocytes and by 99 % of normal thymocytes.

Phagocytosis was studied further in two cases by prolonging incubation with 7S EA or 19S EAC to 150 minutes. At the end of the incubation period aliquots were taken and on one portion the percentage of rosetted and phagocytic cells were counted. Cytocentrifuge preparations were also made. The other portion of the incubation mixture was treated with NH_4Cl to lyse the SRBC in order to differentiate between ingested and external SRBC's since ingested SRBC's are not lysed by NH_4Cl. Rosetting and phagocytosis was assessed by hemocytometer counts and cytocentrifuge preparations. Opsonized Baker's yeast was also used as a phagocytic stimulant at a ratio of 100 yeast particles to one white cell. This mixture was incubated on a rotator at 37° for one hour and cytocentrifuge preparations made to assess the degree of phagocytosis.

Immunofluorescence

In four cases cells from tumor tissues were examined by indirect immunofluorescence with an antiserum specific for human T-cells. This antiserum was prepared by immunizing rabbits with pooled fetal thymocytes and rendered specific for T-cells by repeated absorptions with chronic lymphocytic leukemia cells (B-cells) and pooled human RBC. The antiserum was heat inactivated for 30 minutes at 56° and stored at –40 °C until used. The antiserum detected 95–100 % of thymocytes, 70 ± 5 % of human peripheral blood lymphocytes, malignant cells from mycosis fungoides, and Sternberg sarcoma cells. It did not detect CLL B-cells. All tests were done by indirect immunofluorescence with a goat-anti-rabbit Fc (IgG) reagent conjugated to fluorescein. Cells were incubated at 4 °C with the anti-T serum appropriately diluted in 1 % BSA-PBS with 2.5 x 10⁻⁵ molar sodium azide for 30 minutes. They were then washed, and incubated for an additional 30 minutes at 4° with the goat-anti-rabbit Fc conjugate.

Direct immunofluorescence was performed with fluorescein-conjugated anti-IgG serum (Behring Diagnostics, Somerville, NJ) for surface IgG. Staining with anti-IgG was done at 4 °C on cells which had been preincubated in 1 % BSA-PBS at either 37 °C or 4 °C for 30 minutes. Preincubation at 37° was performed to elute absorbed antibodies (7). Cells were washed at 37 °C or 4 °C respectively and examined unfixed by epifluorescence and phase microscopy in order to distinguish cellular morphology. Cells exhibiting diffuse cytoplasmic fluorescence were interpreted as dead.

Latex particles were added to cell suspensions at the beginning of the incubation period in an attempt to facilitate the distinction of Hodgkin's cells from histiocytes, monocytes, and reticulum cells. This proved to be of limited value because in many instances the latex particles seemed to adhere to the irregular surface of the Hodgkin's giant cells. Furthermore, these cells had prominent cytoplasmic granulations not readily distinguished from the latex particles. The Hodgkin's giant cells were best differentiated from histiocytes and reticulum cells by their much larger, more irregular nuclei and prominent, often huge, nucleoli. Hodgkin's giant cells with multiple separate nuclei or distinct nuclear lobulations, each with individual nucleoli, were judged to be Reed-Sternberg cells. Both Reed-Sternberg and mononuclear Hodgkin's cells exhibited long spike-like and foot-shaped projections. Multiple small lymphocytes frequently were attached to the surface of these Hodgkin's giant cells. Fluorescence was therefore judged only on those cells with adequate free cell membrane and those without attached lymphocytes. In the anti-T serum preparations an additional difficulty encountered was a tendency towards leukagglutination. We did not attempt to judge fluorescence of clumped cells.

Results

Cell suspensions derived from involved lymph nodes and spleens of patients with Hodgkin's disease contained Reed-Sternberg and mononuclear Hodgkin's giant cells, frequently with adherent small lymphocytes. The majority of the lymphocytes were identified as T-cells by their linear membrane fluorescence with specific anti-T cell serum and their capacity to form spontaneous rosettes with non-sensitized SRBC (E rosettes) (Fig. 1). By contrast, the Hodgkin's giant cells never formed E rosettes (Fig. 2) and showed no linear membrane fluorescence with the anti-T cell serum. Fluorescence at the interface of a Hodgkin's cell and an

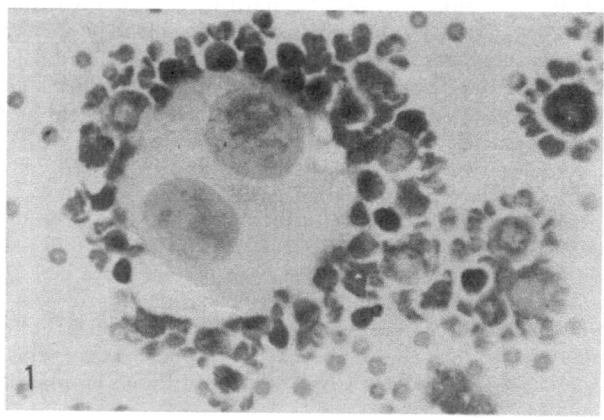

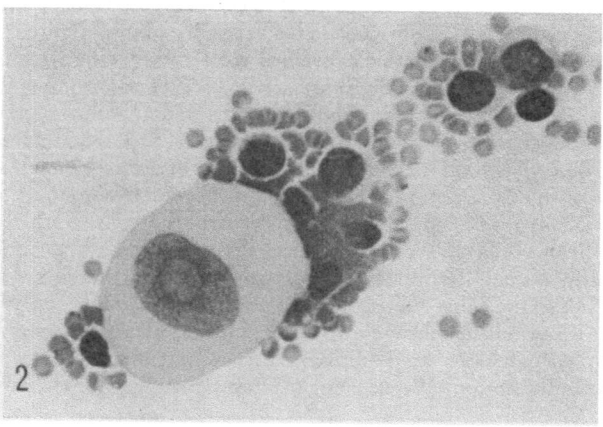

Fig. 1: A large binucleate Reed-Sternberg cell surrounded by small lymphocytes identified as T-cells by their rosetting with untreated sheep erythrocytes (E).

Fig. 2: A mononucleate Hodgkin's giant cell is partially surrounded by rosetted T-lymphocytes but has no T-cell marker (E) attached to its membrane.

adherent lymphocyte was disregarded since it was assumed to be a property of the lymphocyte.

When the large Hodgkin's cells were examined for Fc and complement receptors no rosettes were formed. Normal B-lymphocytes and histiocytes did rosette, and histiocytes frequently showed phagocytosis. In some cytocentrifuge preparations, a few large Hodgkin's cells appeared to contain one or more erythrocytes and large vacuoles, possibly with digested erythrocyte material. Since we considered that this might be an artifact caused by the impingement of erythrocytes on the much larger Hodgkin's cells in the cytocentrifuge, phagocytosis was further examined by lysis of non-ingested erythrocytes prior to cytocentrifugation. Figure 3 shows that no erythrocytes were found in Hodgkin's cells after such treatment whereas erythrocytes phagocytosed by macrophages were not lysed. Hodgkin's cells were also unable to phagocytose heat-killed Baker's yeast.

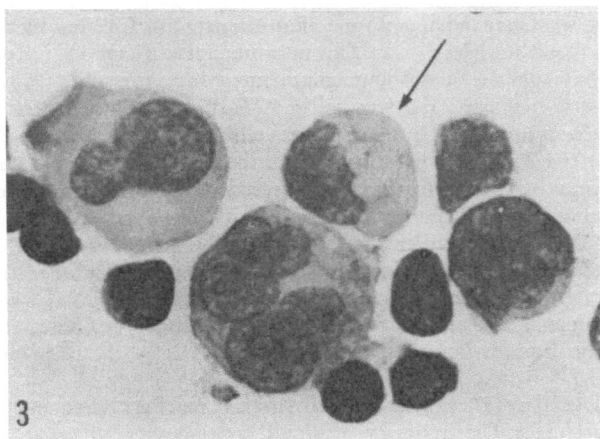

Fig. 3: The splenic macrophage (arrow) has phagocytosed several complement-coated sheep erythrocytes (EAC) while the adjacent Hodgkin's cells from a case of nodular sclerosis have not phagocytosed this reagent.

Examination of surface immunoglobulins by direct immunofluorescence revealed speckled membrane fluorescence with anti-IgG on 54 % of large Hodgkin's cells but not on the surrounding T-lymphocytes. To determine whether this surface IgG might be absorbed antibody, which could be eluted at 37 °C, immunofluorescence studies were also carried out following incubation and washing of the cells at 37 °C (7). Following this treatment the proportion of Hodgkin's cells staining was reduced to 26 % and the degree of residual fluorescence on stained cells was moderately diminished.

Discussion

The derivation of the Reed-Sternberg cell cannot be determined solely on morphological grounds. Various morphological observations have suggested its relationship to either a macrophage (8, 9, 10) or transformed lymphocyte (1, 11, 12). We have therefore sought to characterize these giant Hodgkin's cells in terms of immunological markers. Except for IgG which could be partially eluted at 37 °C, we found no markers of normal lymphocytes or macrophages on these cells. Reed-Sternberg cells showed no avidity for sensitized erythrocytes or opsonized yeast and therefore could not qualify as "professional" phagocytes (13). Their ability to ingest smaller latex particles could not be accurately determined with the light microscope and awaits ultrastructural studies.

In these studies, the complement receptor, frequently detected on benign and malignant B cells (14, 15) was not observed on Hodgkin's cells. As shown earlier by Leech (16), we observed membrane fluorescence for IgG on Hodgkin's giant cells including Reed-Sternberg cells. This may suggest a B-cell origin for these cells; B cells may have surface Ig without complement receptors (15). However, when the cells were pre-incubated and washed in 1 % BSA at 37 °C, there was a 50 % reduction in the number of stained giant cells and the degree of fluorescence, indicating that the IgG may be absorbed antibody which may be eluted (7, 17). The situation may be similar to that encountered by Preud'homme and Seligmann in some examples of CLL where absorbed IgG removed by trypsin was not regenerated (18). Further evidence for the possible exogenous origin of the SIgG on Reed-Sternberg cells may be inferred from the work of Taylor (19). He clearly demonstrated that cytoplasmic immunoglobulins within individual Reed-Sternberg cells are sometimes not restricted to a single light chain type. Since this implies a polyclonal origin for this immunoglobulin, its synthesis by the Reed-Sternberg cell is unlikely (20).

As reported earlier (3), normal T cell surface markers were not detected on Hodgkin's giant cells. The majority of small lymphocytes adherent to the Reed-Sternberg cells rosetted with nonsensitized sheep red blood cells and showed membrane fluorescence with antithymocyte serum. *In vivo* ultrastructural observations indicate that this close apposition of the small T-lymphocytes is correlated with significant cytotoxic changes in the large neoplastic cells (21).

If the Reed-Sternberg cell were derived from a T-cell, the detection of T cell surface markers may be prevented by the presence of a blocking antibody. Cytotoxic IgG antibodies have been demonstrated in the serum and on the peripheral blood lymphocytes of patients with Hodgkin's disease (22), where they may be produced in large part by the spleen (23). Such antibodies can inhibit formation of E rosettes, PHA responsiveness, and allograft rejection by normal T cells (24–26). If directed against an antigen shared by the peripheral blood T cells and Reed-Sternberg cells these antibodies could account for the impaired cellular immunity found in early stages of Hodgkin's disease and our present inability to detect normal T cell surface markers on the Reed-Sternberg cell.

234

Acknowledgements

We wish to thank Doctors Stephen B. Shohet, George Brecher and Louis K. Diamond for their thoughtful advice and support.

This investigation was supported by U.S.P.H.S. Research Grants CA 15182 and HD03939 from the National Cancer Institute and the National Institute for Child Health and Human Development. Dr. Stites is the recipient of a Senior Fellowship (D-237) from the American Cancer Society-California Division.

References

1. Lukes, R. J., Tindle, B. H., and Parker, J. W. (1969) Lancet 2, 1003.
2. Peckham, M. J. and Cooper, E. H. (1969) Cancer 24, 135.
3. Kadin, M. E., Newcom, S. R., Gold, S. B., and Stites, D. .P (1974) Lancet 2, 167.
4. Braylan, R. C., Jaffe, E. S., and Berard, C. W. (1974) Lancet 2, 1328.
5. Jondal, M., Holm, G., and Wigzell, H. (1972) J. Exp. Med. 136, 207.
6. Shevach, E. M., Jaffe, E. S., and Green, I. (1973) Transplant. Rev. 16, 3.
7. Lobo, P. I., Westervelt, F. B., and Horwitz, D. A. (1975) J. Immunol. 114, 116.
8. Rappaport, H. (1966) Tumors of the Hematopoietic System. Section III Fascicle 8.
9. Kay, M. M. B. and Kadin, M. E. (1975) Lancet I, 748.
10. Carr, I. (1975) Lancet I, 926.
11. Tindle, B. H., Parker, J. W., and Lukes, R. J. (1972) Am. J. Clin. Path. 48, 607.
12. Dorfman, R. F., Rice, D. F., Mitchell, A. D., Kempson, R. L., and Levine, G. (1973) Natl. Cancer Inst. Monogr. 37, 221.
13. Rabinovitch, M. (1968) Seminars in Hematology 5, 134.
14. Pincus, S., Bianco, C., and Nussenzweig, V. (1972) Blood 40, 303.
15. Ross, G. D., Rabellino, E. M., Polley, M. J., and Grey, H. M. (1973) J. Clin. Invest. 52, 377.
16. Leech, J. (1973) Lancet 2, 265.
17. Phillips, T. M. and Lewis, M. G. (1971) Rev. Europ. Études Clin. et Biol. 16, 1052.
18. Preud'homme, J. L. and Seligmann, M. (1972) Blood 40, 777.
19. Taylor, C. R. (1974) Lancet 2, 802.
20. Spriggs, A. I. (1971) Lancet 1, 857.
21. Archibald, R. B. and Frenster, J. H. (1973) Natl. Cancer Inst. Monogr. 36, 239.
22. Grifoni, V., Giaco, G. S., Manconi, P. E., and Tognella, S. (1972) Lancet 1, 848.
23. Longmire, R. L., McMillan, R., Yelenosky, R., Armstrong, S., Lang, J. E., and Craddock, C. G. (1973) NEJM 289, 763.
24. Bach, J. F., Dormont, J., Dardenne, M., and Balner, H. (1969) Transplantation 8, 265.

25. Wortis, H. H., Cooper, A. G., and Brown, M. C. (1973) Nature New Biol. 243, 110.
26. Kaplan, H. S., Bobrove, A. M., Fuks, Z., Strober, S., (1974) NEJM 290, 971.

Abbreviations used

FCS	=	Fetal calf serum
BSA-PBS	=	bovine serum albumin-phosphate buffered saline
CLL	=	chronic lymphocytic leukemia
SIgG	=	surface-bound immunoglobulin G

Human Leukemia-Lymphoma Associated Antigen Detected by Heteroantisera

Ronald Billing, Ph. D., Bahman Rafizadeh, M. D.,
Andrzej Zebrowski, M. D. Gary Hartmann, M. D.
and Paul I. Terasaki, Ph. D.

Department of Surgery, School of Medicine
University of California
Los Angeles, California 90024

The identification of tumor-specific antigens on leukemia cells would facilitate the diagnosis and possibly the treatment of the disease. To detect such antigens, one widely used approach has been to raise antibodies in animals against leukemia cells or leukemia cell extracts. Although many variations of this approach have been used previously, in most cases the antisera produced have not been unequivocally shown to be leukemia specific. The more recent tests used to determine the specificity of the antisera have been more discriminating and some progress has been made. The tests used must be sensitive, capable of screening a large variety of cells, and able to detect small subfractions of positive cells. In our studies these critera were applied to the two main tests used to determine antiserum specificity. Complement-dependent microcytotoxicity was used to screen large numbers of normal and leukemic cells, and the immunofluorescent staining technique was used to detect small subpopulations of positive cells. The latter technique was essential for locating positive cells in heterogeneous populations such as bone marrow samples or peripheral blood lymphocyte preparations.

The heterogeneity of the antisera produced is dependent on the nature of the immunogen used and the type of animal which is immunized. In the past, a variety of different antigenic sources and animals has been used (1–9). In our studies whole leukemia cells produced very heterogeneous antisera whereas soluble membrane extracts produced more specific reagents. Animals either tolerant to normal cell antigens (1, 2, 8), or nonhuman primates (9) that are phylogenetically closer to man, have been immunized so that the response produced against normal antigens is lowered. However, when these animals were immunized with whole leukemia cells, the antisera that was produced still required absorption with normal tissue to show leukemic specificity.

Our approach has been to immunize rabbits with papain-solubilized extracts of purified cell membranes from human lymphomas (10, 11). The antisera produced were tested without prior absorption by the methods described above. Complement-dependent microcytotoxicity indicated that the antisera had specificity for leukemia cells from about 75 % of patients having all subclasses of leukemia. The

Table I: Cytotoxic titers of rabbit antisera against normal human lymphocytes and leukemia cells

Rabbit Number	Normal Lymphocytes[a]	Leukemia Cells
63	1	128
64	4	1024
66	0	512
68	0	1024
69	8	512
70	8	2048
71	0	10000
74	0	512
75	0	512
77	8	4000
78	0	1500
79	0	400
80	0	256
P413[b]	0	512

[a] Average titer against cells from 100 different donors.
[b] IgG fraction from antisera 68.

more discriminating fluorescein test revealed a small percentage of normal peripheral lymphocytes and normal bone marrow cells that were also positive.

Table 1 shows the complement-dependent cytotoxicity titers of antisera obtained from 13 different rabbits immunized with papain digests of cell membrane from human histiocytic lymphoma. The titers against normal lymphocytes were low (1:8 or less) while titers against leukemia cells were high, ranging from 1:128 to 1:10,000. This strongly indicates that the antigen being detected is present on leukemia cells but is not present on the majority of normal lymphocytes. However, the cytotoxicity test using total lymphocytes as targets is unable to detect a small subfraction of normal lymphocytes such as B cells which might also be positive. The specificity of the antisera for several different types of normal white cells and leukemic cells is presented in Table 2. Peripheral blood leukemia cells from patients with high white cell counts were positive whereas lymphocytes, granulocytes, and bone marrow from normal healthy donors were negative. However, not all leukemia cells were positive; 70–75 % of ALL, AML, and CML and 100 % (7/7) CLL were positive. Thirteen out of fifteen cultured lymphoblastoid cell lines were positive, the lines Molt 4 and 6410/EBV were negative. Normal lymphocytes from remission patients and phytohemagglutinin blast cells were negative.

The antisera would also kill leukemia cells when normal human lymphocyte effector cells were used in place of complement. In lymphocyte-dependent antibody lympholysis (LDA) the titer of the rabbit antiserum, 78008, was very high (10^6) against leukemia cells and cultured lymphoblastoid lines 6410 and RAJI

Table II: Cytotoxicity of rabbit antisera against various types of normal and leukemia cells

Cell type	Clinical Status	Cytotoxicity	
		No. positive[1] No. tested[2]	Average titer
PWBC[3]	AML relapse	30/40	1 = 512
PWBC	CML relapse	9/13	1 = 512
PWBC	ALL relapse	28/41	1 = 512
PWBC	CLL relapse	7/7	1 = 512
Lymphocytes	Normal	0/500	–
Granulocytes	Normal	0/56	–
Bone Marrow	Normal	0/2	–
PHA lymphoblasts	Normal	0/4	–
C L B[4]		13/15	1 = 64
PBWC	Leukemia[5]-remission	0/13	–

[1] More than 80 % cells killed.
[2] Number of different patients tested.
[3] Peripheral white blood cells.
[4] Cultured lymphoblastoid lines.
[5] 8 ALL, 4 AML, 1 CML.

whereas the LDA titer against normal peripheral blood lymphocytes was undetectable (Table 3). The control serà taken from the same rabbit prior to immunization (78000) was negative against leukemia cells. The LDA titers were found to be over 1000-fold higher then the complement-dependent microcytotoxicity titers. This large difference in titer between normal cells and leukemia cells further suggests that the antigen is not found on the majority of normal peripheral blood lymphocytes.

Neither the complement-dependent cytotoxicity test nor the LDA test are, however, capable of detecting minor subpopulations of positive target cells. In order to detect such positive cells in bone marrow or peripheral blood an immunofluorescent staining technique was used. The target cells were first incubated for

Table III: LDA and complement-dependent antibody titers of rabbit antileukemia sera

TARGET	78008		78000	
	LDA	Compl.	LDA	Compl.
6410	10[6]	64	N	N
RAJI	10[6]	64	N	N
Leukemia cells	10[6]	512	N	N
Normal Human Lymphocytes	N	N	N	N
N = negative				

30 min with the rabbit antisera at a dilution of 1:200. After washing, the cells were then treated with fluorescein-conjugated goat antirabbit IgG and examined microscopically for fluorescence. Positive leukemia cells and certain cultured lymphoblastoid lines gave a very bright continuous membrane fluorescence which can be seen in Fig. 1.

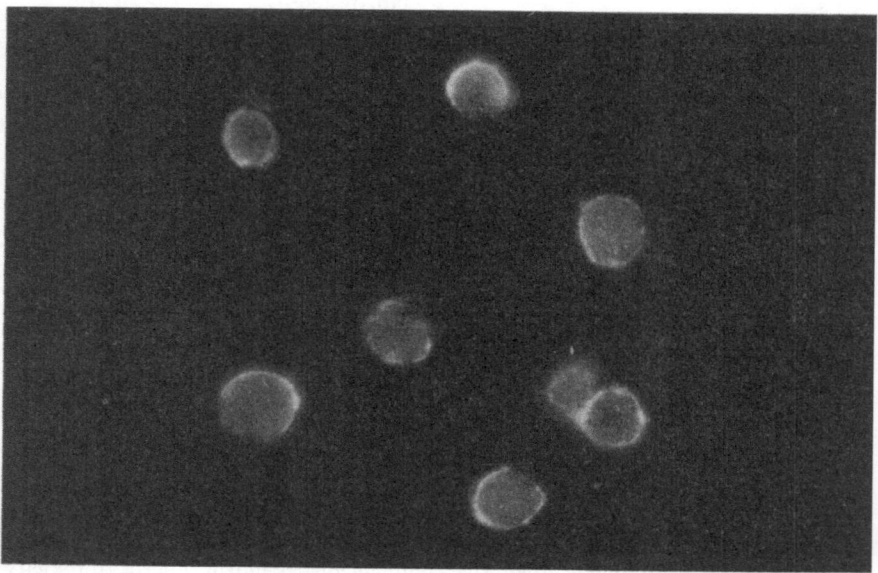

Fig. 1: Immunofluorescence staining of leukemia cells.

Whereas in the microcytotoxicity and LDA tests the rabbit antisera were negative against normal peripheral lymphocytes, the fluorescence test showed the presence of 6–15 % positive cells among peripheral lymphocytes from 40 healthy donors. Bone marrow cells from normal healthy donors had 0–2 % fluorescein-positive cells. This positivity of normal lymphocytes did not appear to be due to non-specific binding to B cells through the Fc receptors because F (ab)₂ fragments of the rabbit antibody gave similar results. Therefore, the leukemia-associated (LA) antigen appears also to be found on a subpopulation of normal peripheral lymphocytes. Preliminary results indicate that the positive peripheral blood lymphocyte is a B cell.

Bone marrow samples from children with leukemia were examined before and after chemotherapy. The numbers of fluorescein-positive cells were found to correspond to the stage of the disease as determined by morphological examination (Table 4). In newly diagnosed cases, the number of fluorescein-positive cells in the bone marrow was high (over 80 %). After chemotherapy the numbers of positive cells decreased to 0–2 % which was in general agreement with the number of blast cells found at this time by morphological examination. In relapse cases the increase

Table IV: Bone marrow samples tested for LA by fluorescein technique

Patient	Treatment	Diagnosis	% Blasts (Morphology)	% LA Positive (Fluorescen)
G. E.	Untreated	ALL New Case	87	90
	Chemotherapy	ALL Remission	1	Neg.
P. R.	Untreated	ALL New Case	93	70
	Chemotherapy	ALL Remission	0	2
S. J.	Untreated	ALL New Case	97	80
	Chemotherapy	ALL Remission	0	1
A. E.	Chemotherapy	ALL Remission	0	10
S. J.	Chemotherapy	ALL Partial Relapse	8	30
R. M.	Chemotherapy	ALL Relapse	72	60

of fluorescein-positive cells was again commensurate with the increased numbers of blast cells.

Although the immunofluorescence test was able to detect small numbers of positive leukemia cells its potential for early diagnosis of relapse remains to be determined. Before this can be achieved, the 0–2 % positive cells present in normal bone marrow must be eliminated. At the present time a more practical use of the test might be to distinguish between different clinical forms of leukemia. A preliminary study in children indicated that negative cases which constitute 25 % of the ALL cases studied appear to have a more virulent form of the disease which is characteristic of T cell leukemia. If this result can be substantiated, then the presence or absence of this cell marker may aid diagnosis and therapy of not only acute lymphocytic leukemia but also acute and chronic myeloid leukemia.

Acknowledgements

We thank Ms. Patricia Peterson, Ms. Angela Gillet, and Mr. Maj Safani from UCLA and Betsy Manchester at Children's Hospital for their skilled technical assistance. This work was supported in part by NIH grants AI 12366-01 and CA 01137.

References

1. Garb, S., Stein A. A., Sims G: The Production of Antihuman Leukemic Serum in Rabbits. J. Immunol 88: 142–152, 1962.
2. Hyde, R. M., Garb, S., Bennett, A. J.: Demonstration by Immunoelectrophoresis of Antigen in Human Myelogenous Leukemia. J. Natl Cancer Inst. 38: 909–919, 1967.
3. Viza, D., Davies, D. A., Harris R.: Solubilization and Partial Purification of Human Leukemic Specific Antigens. Nature (Lond) 227: 1249–1251, 1970.
4. Mann, D., Rogentine, G. N., Halterman, R., Levanthal, B.: Detection of Antigen Associated with Acute Leukemia. Science 174: 1136–1137, 1971.

5. Halterman, R. H., Levanthal, B. G., Mann, D. L.: An Acute-Leukemia Antigen: Correlation with Clinical Status. N Engl J Med 287: 1272–1274, 1972.
6. Bentwich, Z., Weiss, D. W., Sultizeanu, D., Kedar, E., Izak, B., Cohen, I., Eyal, O.: Antigenic Changes on the Surface of Lymphocytes from Patients with Chronic Lymphocyte Leukemia. Cancer Res 32: 1375–1383, 1972.
7. Harris, R.: Leukemia Antigens and Immunity in Man. Nature (Lond) 241: 95–100, 1973.
8. Baker, M. A., Ramachander, K., Taub, R. N.: Specificity of Heteroantisera to Human Acute Leukemia-Associated Antigens. J Clin Invest 54: 1273–1278, 1974.
9. Mohanakumar, T., Metzgar, R. S., Miller, D. S.: Human Leukemia Cell Antigens: Serological Characterization with Xenoantisera. J Natl Cancer Inst 52: 1435–1444, 1974.
10. Billing, R., Terasaki, P. I.: Human Leukemia Antigen. I. Production and Characterization of Antisera. J Natl Cancer Inst 53: 1635–1638, 1974.
11. Billing, R., Terasaki, P. I.: Human Leukemia Antigen II. Purification. J Natl Cancer Inst 53: 1639–1643, 1974.

Analysis of Human Leukaemic Cells Using Cell Surface Binding Probes and the Fluorescence Activated Cell Sorter

M. Greaves, D. Capellaro, G. Brown
T. Revesz and G. Janossy
ICRF Tumour Immunology Unit,
Department of Zoology,
University College London

T. A. Lister
ICRF Medical Oncology Unit,
St. Bartholomew's Hospital, London

M. Beard
Department of Haematology,
St. Bartholomew's Hospital, London

N. Rapson
Department of Haematology,
Institute of Child Health, London
and
D. Catovsky
MRC Leukaemia Unit,
Royal Postgraduate Medical School, London

Abbreviations used

AUL	: Acute Undifferentiated Leukaemia
ALL	: Acute Lymphoblastic Leukaemia
AML	: Acute Myeloblastic Leukaemia
AMML	: Acute Myelo-Monocytic Leukaemia
AMonL	: Acute Monocytic Leukaemia
CML	: Chronic Myeloid Leukaemia
CLL	: Chronic Lymphocytic Leukaemia
Ph[1]	: Philadelphia chromosome

PHA	: Phytohaemagglutinin
T	: Thymus-derived lymphocyte
B	: 'Bursa equivalent' derived lymphocyte
FACS	: Fluorescence Activated Cell Sorter
G_{M1}	: Monosialoganglioside (a charged glycolipid of known structure)
SmIg	: Surface membrane immunoglobulin

This paper is dedicated to our colleague Professor G. Hamilton- Fairley who was tragically and savagely killed by a terrorist bomb in London on October 23, 1975.

Summary

Cell surface binding fluorescent ligands have been used to distinguish between different types of leukaemic cells and between leukaemic cells and their presumed normal counterparts or progenitors. Binding of these probes was evaluated using the Fluorescence Activated Cell Sorter (FACS) which provides both rapid, objective and quantitative recording of fluorescent signals from individual cells plus physical separation of cells of particular interest. Binding sites for cholera toxin (monosialoganglioside G_{M1}) were found to be normally expressed in chronic leukaemias but greatly diminished or absent in acute leukaemias irrespective of their morphological type. Antibodies specific for the common form of acute lymphoblastic leukaemia (ALL, non-T, non-B) have been produced in rabbits. After extensive absorption and testing these were shown to define a cell surface antigen of non-T, non-B type ALLs. The antigen is absent from other leukaemias with two interesting exceptions – the majority of acute undifferentiated leukaemias express the antigen as do a proportion of chronic granulocytic leukaemias in blast crisis relapse.

The anti-ALL antibodies can therefore be used to distinguish different leukaemias and, more significantly, can identify the existence of relatively rare leukaemic cells in the blood of untreated patients and the marrow of treated patients considered to be in remission.

Introduction

Human leukaemia is a monoclonal proliferative disease (1). The leukaemias as a group are recognised as being heterogeneous, reflecting in part the cellular heterogeneity of the haemopoeitic system itself and the potential range of 'target' cells for the malignant process. The cellular diversity of disease is not surprisingly associated with a great variation in prognosis. In view of the corresponding range of therapeutic protocols available, it is clearly of great importance to establish the correct diagnosis.

Acute leukaemias still pose a considerable problem of classification. Whilst it is relatively easy to subdivide this group into myeloid and non-myeloid types, subgroupings are difficult if not impossible by morphological and histochemical criteria. Cell surface markers now provide a new and potentially more discriminating set of probes for cellular identity in leukaemia.

244

The philosophy and technology behind this approach has been reviewed recently (2). Cell surface phenotyping can be regarded as a form of molecular morphology with the capacity to reveal the existence of 'silent' structures on cell surfaces which can thereby serve as convenient identity tags.

Lymphoid malignancies have been extensively analysed for cell surface differentiation antigens and receptors which are characteristic of different populations or subsets of normal lymphocytes (2–4) or monocytes (5). This has led to a greater appreciation of the likely target cells involved in leukaemic processes. For example, chronic lymphocytic leukaemia is, with few exceptions, a B lymphocyte neoplasm (6) as is nodular or follicular lymphoma (7). In contrast, virtually every cutaneous lymphoma (e.g. Sezary syndrome, mycosis fungoides) appears to involve T lymphocyte derivatives (8). Acute Lymphoblastic Leukaemias appear by surface marker criteria to involve at least three separate cell types (2, 3) 70–75 $^0/0$ are non-T, non-B-like, 20–25 $^0/0$ are T cell-like, and rare cases (1–3 $^0/0$) are B cell-like (cf. Burkitt's Lymphoma – ref. 9). There is suggestive evidence that those with a T cell surface phenotype have a poorer prognosis (10, 11). They usually present with higher white cell counts in the blood and in our experience are predominantly males (14 out of 15 cases). We have recently explored the potential use of two additional cell surface markers which may be particularly revealing.

We have used the binding of cholera toxin to its natural 'receptor' – Monosialoganglioside G_{M1} (12) as a probe for defective cell membrane glycolipid in leukaemias. The rationale of this approach is based upon the extensive evidence that transformation of animal cells by viruses or carcinogens is usually associated with pronounced simplification of membrane glycolipids including gangliosides (13). Our results suggest that cholera toxin may provide an extremely useful indicator of acute leukaemic cells.

The second type of marker system employs an antiserum specific for a particular type of leukaemia. There is a long and somewhat tortuous history of attempts to produce such reagents and it is only very recently that some success has been achieved (14, 15, reviewed in 2). We have raised antisera in rabbits to the non-T, non-B or common form of ALL. After extensive absorption the sera can be used to identify ALL cells.

Three key features of this analysis are (1) the availability of chemically homogenous markers with well defined specificity; (2) fluorescent labelling of probes of marker antibodies to permit identification of individual cells; (3) evaluation of reactivity using the Fluorescence Activated Cell Sorter or FACS (2). All the fluorescence reactions on living cells we carry out can, in fact, be reasonably well analysed by conventional methods (e. g. ultra-violet microscopy with plume or incident illumination). However, the FACS provides a rapid objective and quantitative evaluation of cell surface binding reactions. In addition, fluorescent and non-fluorescent cells can be physically separated for further independent analysis.

Full experimental details of the development and application of these probes are published elsewhere (2, 4, 5, 16, 17). In this paper an up to date summary of results is provided.

Materials and Methods

Patients:

Leukaemia patients studied were attending clinics at St. Bartholomew's Hospital, London, the Hospital for Sick Children, London, or the Hammersmith Hospital, London. Diagnosis of their leukaemia was by standard clinical and haematological criteria (i.e. morphology and staining with Sudan Black and periodic acid Schiff). Blood and bone marrow samples, and in cases of central nervous system relapse, cerebro-spinal fluid, were taken. In some cases (particularly untreated AMLs) circulating white cells were removed using an IBM cell separator.

Preparation of cell suspensions:

In high count leukaemias the buffy coat was taken for study. In other cases heparinised blood or marrow were separated on ficoll-isopaque density gradient (18). Control, non-leukaemic cell suspensions were obtained from blood, tonsils, and bone marrow (ribs removed during thoracic surgery) and treated similarly.

Analysis and separation of fluorescent cells using the Fluorescence Activated Cell Sorter:

The Fluorescence Activated Cell Sorter (FACS)[1] is a recently developed and potentially extremely important automatic electronic device currently in operation in five or six laboratories, including our own (2). This machine has the dual capacity to rapidly and accurately analyse cells in suspension, in terms of size and fluorescence, and also to separate cells that are of particular interest. The principles involved in these two procedures are simple and have been described in detail previously (19, 20).

Figure 1 shows a simplified diagram which illustrates the general principles. The cells are contained in saline and emerge essentially in single file from an ultrasonically vibrated nozzle which eventually breaks up into regularly spaced droplets forming a stream of 50 μ diameter. The beam from an argon-ion laser intersects the cell stream just below the nozzle. As individual cells pass through the beam they scatter some of the light, and, if labelled, they also fluoresce. The two types of signals from cells are detected separately (using microscope objectives), amplified and converted into voltage pulses, the size of which is proportional to the input signal. After pulse height analysis these data are displayed in the form of a histogram; the ordinates representing the number of events (i.e. cells) recorded against pulse height (i. e. cell fluorescence intensity or size) – see following sections. Cells having particular characteristics of interest can be both enumerated and physically separated from the remainder. Separation is achieved by imparting a charge to the droplet stream. By 'informing' the FACS of the characteristics of the cells to be separated (e.g. fluorescent versus non-fluorescent, small cells versus large cells) and by finely controlled timing, droplets containing cells of interest charged and deflected into collection tubes, as they fall between charged plates (see Fig. 1). The time taken to accurately enumerate and separate various cell populations is determined by the flow rate. This will vary depending upon the particular experiment, but is

[1] Manufactured by Becton Dickinson Limited, Mountain View, California. Similar instruments are also currently under manufacture by other companies.

obviously geared to the rarity of the particular cells one is interested in. In general for analytical purposes, we screen lymphocyte preparations at 10^3–4×10^3 cells/second and red cell suspensions at up to 10^4 second, an analysis of 40,000 lymphocytes in the presence of red cells taking only a few seconds. For separation of relatively minor cell populations (see below) and for high purity, a lower sample flow rate of 1–3×10^3/second is usually employed. The FACS has the great advantage of being able to analyse very large numbers of cells at high speed and to efficiently separate reasonable numbers for functional analysis. Separations can be performed under sterile conditions with minimal loss of cell viability and function. There are no theoretical limits to the soluble fluorescent probes employed (e.g. lectins, antibodies, toxins, etc.). In general, cell surface reactive probes have been used; however, intracellular fluorescein diacetate can be used to distinguish live from dead cells (only the former give cytoplasmic fluorescence) and acriflavine and mithramycin dyes which bind to nucleic acids have been used to map cell cycle positions. As the sensors in the sorter measures only total energy, its function is independent of the cellular distribution of fluorescence (i.e. intracellular versus cell surface, random, diffuse versus concentrated or localised).

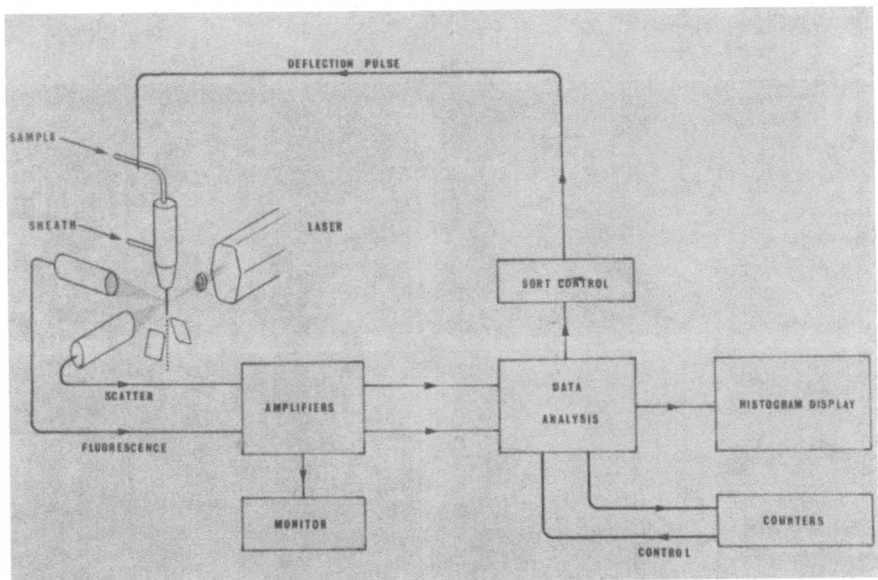

Fig. 1: The Fluorescence Activated Cell Sorter. Simplified block diagram.
Legend: See text for explanation.

Reagents:

Cholera toxin (choleragen) and horse anti-toxin were gifts from Dr A. Finkelstein. The former is now distributed through Schwartz-Mann Antisera to All was produced in rabbits as previously published (16). In brief, rabbits received two intravenous injections of viable ALL cells pre-coated in vitro with antibodies produced in rabbits against normal lymphocyte antigens. Following heat inactivation of complement components the sera were absorbed with red cells, liver homogenate, tonsil lymphocytes, AML cells and normal bone marrow cells. Absorptions were checked for efficiency and completeness using the Fluorescence Activated Cell Sorter (17).

Immunofluorescent labelling of cells:

Cells were labelled on their surfaces by indirect immunofluorescent methods. Binding of cholera toxin was detected by sequential treatment of cells with appropriate concentrations of cholera toxin, horse anti-toxin, followed by fluoresceinated rabbit anti-horse IgG. Binding of anti-ALL was similarly detected by adding sequentially rabbit anti-ALL followed by fluoresceinated goat anti-rabbit IgG. In standard tests 10^6 cells were used (in 100 µl). The first ligand was added at room temperature and subsequent steps performed at 4 °C in the presence of 0.2 % sodium azide.

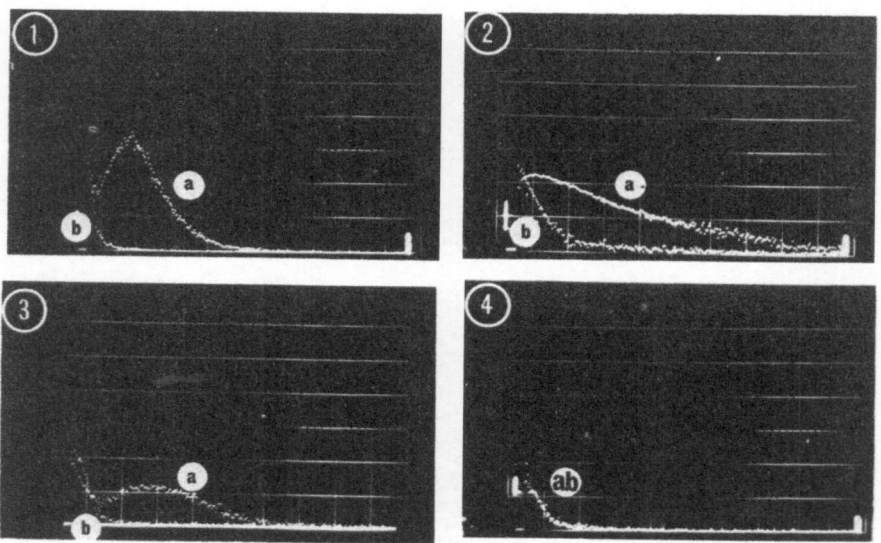

Fig. 2: Fluorescence Activated Cell Sorter (FACS) analysis of cholera toxin binding.
Legend: Vertical axis: relative cell number. Horizontal axis: relative fluorescence intensity.
1. Thymus cells (4 yr donor, cardiac surgery) (a) cholera toxin, (b) control (see methods).
2. Tonsil lymphocytes (a) cholera toxin (b) cholera toxin pre-incubated with G_{M1}.
3. Chronic lymphocytic leukaemia cells (a) cholera toxin, (b) control.
4. Acute lymphoblastic leukaemia cells (a) cholera toxin, (b) superimposed control.
Taken from ref. 21.

Results and Discussion

1. Binding sites for cholera toxin

A variety of human leukaemias have been analysed for cell surface cholera toxin binding sites (21). Results to date (Autumn, 1975) are given in Table 1 and Fig. 2. Irrespective of morphological type all chronic leukaemias have cholera toxin receptors whereas acute leukaemias have few if any. Philadelphia chromosome positive CML, like CLL, has an apparently normal expression of G_{M1}. CML usually progresses to a terminal phase characterised by blast crisis relapse. This is generally regarded as an acute transformation of the Ph^1 positive malignant clone (22). As indicated in Table 1 blast crisis relapse cases of CML in contrast to CML itself lacked cholera toxin receptors. This observation re-inforces the argument that this test discriminates between acute and chronic phase cells. The exact proportion of G_{M1} negative cells in blast crisis relapse was quite variable and each patient had a mixed population of blast cells and granulocytic cells. This point can be clearly illustrated by cell sorting experiments. The FACS was used to identify and separate

Table I: Cholera toxin staining of human leukaemia cells

Leukemia type	Cholera toxin labelling		
	+	±	−
ALL – untreated (or relapse)			
1. Non-T, non-B*			12
2. T**			3
3. B (Burkitt-like)***			2
ALL – in remission	2		
AML – untreated	1	4	9
AML – in remission	3		
CLL	11		
CML (Ph^1+)	16		
CML in blast crisis (Ph^1+)			20
Others:			
Sezary syndrome		1	
Prolymphocyte leukaemia	3	1	2
Hairy cell leukaemia			2

+ 75–100 % cells strongly positive.
± 15–75 % of cells weakly positive.
− < 15 % of cells weakly positive.
   * E rosette: neg, SmIg: neg, anti-ALL: pos.
  ** E rosette: pos, SmIg: neg, anti-ALL: neg.
*** E rosette: neg, SmIg: pos, anti-ALL: neg.
Taken from ref. 21.

$G_{M_1}+$ and $G_{M_1}-$ cells in a case of blast crisis of CML (Fig. 3). The separated fractions were re-run in the FACS for analysis and also smeared onto slides and stained. The results showed that G_{M_1} negative cells were exclusively undifferentiated blast cells whereas the positive cells were granulocytic. These data suggest that acute blastic transformation in CML might be detected at an early stage by the appearance of G_{M_1} negative cells. Negative acute leukaemias can be converted into positive cholera toxin binders by two simple manoeuvres (Fig. 4): (i) insertion of purified G_{M_1} ganglioside (the receptor for cholera toxin – ref. 12) into the cell membrane of the leukaemic cells. (ii) Treatment of cells with neuraminidase which cleaves off sialic acid residues from more complex gangliosides converting them into monosialoganglioside G_{M_1} in which the single sialic acid residue is sialidase resistant.

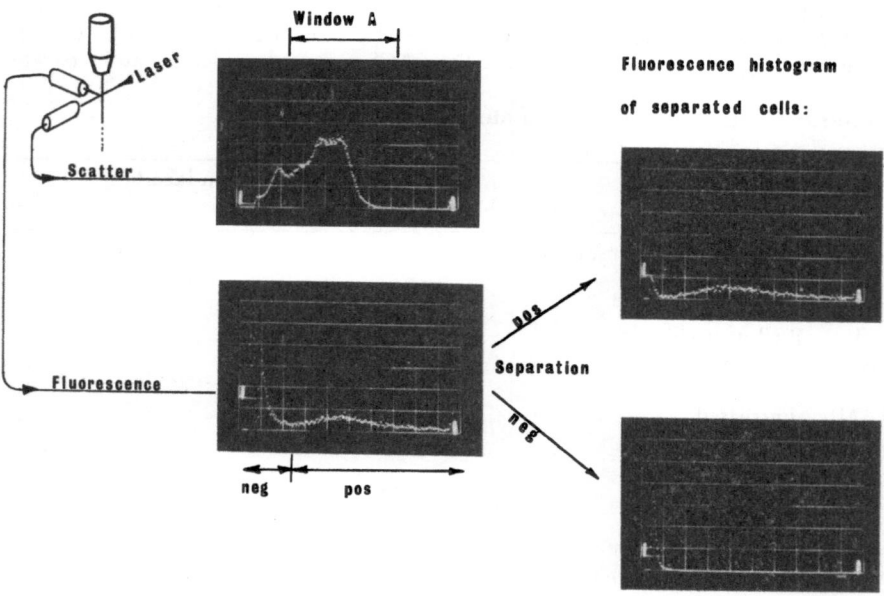

Fig. 3: Separation of positive and negative cholera toxin binding cells from a blood sample of a CML patient in blast crisis relapse.
Legend: see Methods section for technique taken from ref. 23.

We take these observations to imply that there is no defect at the level of G_{M_1} insertion in the membrane and that the ganglioside deficiency in acute leukaemia may be more pronounced in G_{M_1} than other more complex gangliosides. The latter observation contrasts with what is seen when the same experiments are carried out with the transformed BHK (hamster kidney) cell line which has been shown by chemical criteria to be defective in all gangliosides (24 and D. Critchley, personal communication). Here neuraminidase treatment is without effect (Fig. 4).

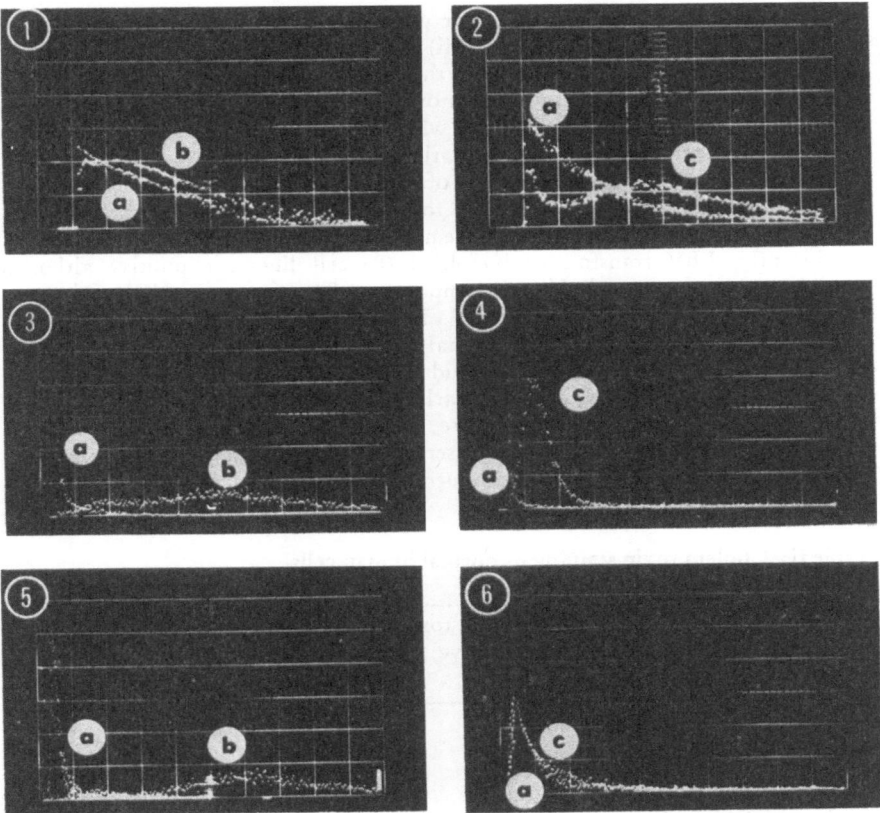

Fig. 4: Reconstitution of G_{M1} receptors for cholera toxin.
Legend: FACS analysis, axes as in Fig. 2.
(1) and (2) tonsil cells, (3) and (4) acute leukaemic cells, (5) and (6) Transformed Hamster BHK fibroblasts.
(a) cholera toxin binding, (b) cholera toxin binding after G_{M1} insertion into cells (see methods), (c) cholera toxin binding after treating cells with neuraminidase.
Taken from Ref. 21.

Although the G_{M1} deficit in acute leukaemia may be fairly selective, preliminary chemical analyses of these same cells suggest that a general reduction of charged glycolipids may exist (B. Murray and M. Greaves, unpublished observations). These observations are consistent with the view that a simplification of glycolipids occurs in transformed cells. The primary locus for the effect may be at the level of glycosyl transferase enzyme activity (13, 25).

Precisely what a deficiency in cholera toxin receptors can tell us about the acute leukaemia cell is unclear. Three general interpretations can be considered: (i) the deficiency is a primary or indirect consequence of the malignant process itself; (ii) the variable expression of cholera toxin binding sites (probably G_{M1} molecules) in leukaemia reflects cell cycle position or general growth/proliferative status independent of the neoplastic condition; (iii) the expression of cholera toxin binding sites on leukaemic cells simply reflects the status of these same structures on the normal cellular counterpart or progenitor, i.e. acute leukaemias are a malignant derivative of a (undifferentiated?) cell which itself has no receptor for the toxin. We cannot as yet determine which of these three, if any, is correct. However, several clues are available. A number of normal proliferating and non-proliferating cell types have also been tested for cholera toxin receptors and the only negative cells so far identified are members of the erythroid series (Table 2). Significantly, EBV transformed lymphoid (B) cell lines are positive although possibly less so than non-dividing B lymphocytes. Thymocytes and T lymphocytes are also positive which implies that T-ALLs may differ from their normal cellular counterparts or progenitors. The normal function of G_{M1} is inknown. Indirect evidence suggests this and other glycolipids might play an important role in growth control (13) but this remains to be clearly established. G_{M1} negative human and murine leukaemias and lymphomas are available (De Cicco and Greaves, unpublished observation), and the easy insertion of G_{M1} into such cells suggests that it may be possible to determine the influence of G_{M1} molecules on cell growth and malignancy.

Table II: Cholera toxin staining of normal human cells

Cell type	Cholera toxin labelling	
	% Positive	Intensity of staining
Red blood cells	0	−
Polymorphs	98	+++
Monocytes	95	+++
Peripheral lymphocytes	92	++
Thymocytes	99	++
Spleen cells	96	++
Tonsil cells	95	++
Bone marrow	85	++→+++
Cord blood		
Polymorphs	99	+++
Lymphocytes	92	++
Normoblasts	0	−
PHA lymphoblasts	95	++
B-lymphoblasts	78–95	+/++
B-lymphoid cell lines (11)		

Taken from ref. 21.

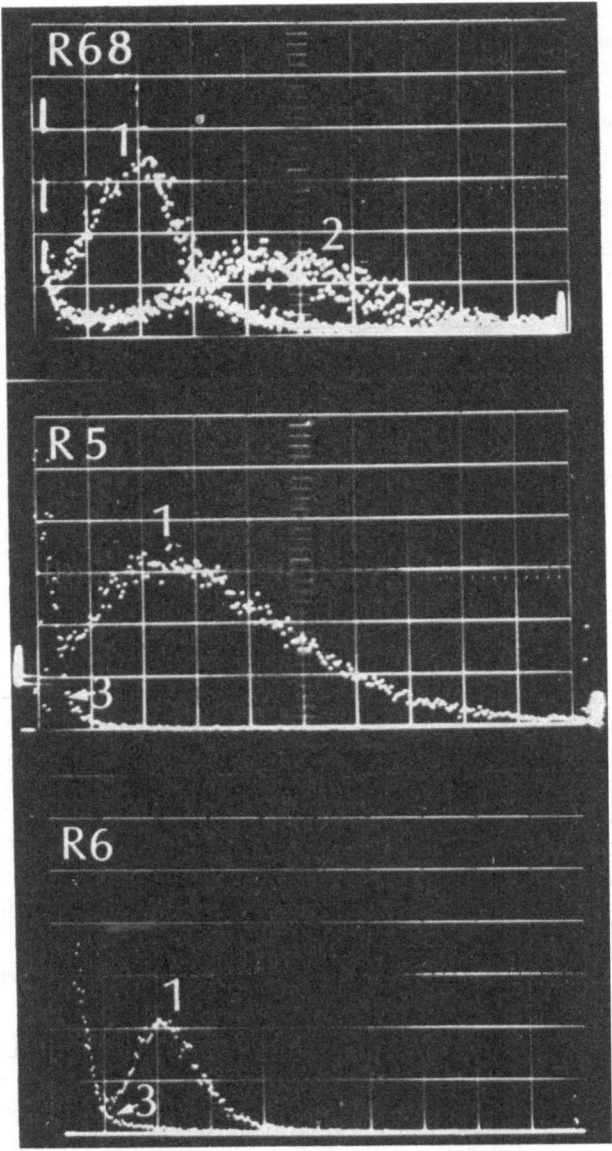

Fig. 5: FACS analysis of the binding of anti-ALL sera to non-T, non-B All cells.
Legend: Ordinate: relative cell number.
Abscissa: relative fluorescence intensity.
R68, R.5 and R.6 – three different rabbit sera.
1. Fully absorbed sera (red cells, liver, lymphocytes, bone marrow, AML).
2. Absorbed red cells, liver, lymphocytes only.
3. Controls: normal rabbit serum or anti-ALL absorbed with ALL cells.
Taken from ref. 17.

2. *Antisera to common (non-T, non-B) ALL*

After absorption with red cells, liver, lyphocytes, AML and bone marrow, antisera to ALL are specific for ALL as judged by indirect immunofluorescence and absorption tests (16, 17). Table 3 lists non-leukaemic cells which have been shown to be negative. The antigen(s) being detected would appear *not* to be a cryptic, cell cycle or foetal (phase specific) determinant.

Table III: Possible antigenic specificities defined by antisera to ALL

Potential Antigen	Cells tested	Cross reactive with anti-ALL?[1]
1. 'Normal' antigen	thymus*, tonsil*, appendix, blood w. b. c., spleen, bone marrow*, liver*	No[2]
2. 'Cryptic' normal lymphocyte antigen	Tonsil lymphocytes treated with trypsin[3], pronase[4] or neurominidase[5]	No
3. Lymphocyte antigens expressed during mitosis	Mitogen activated tonsil T and B lymphocytes[6]. Lymphoblastoid cell lines[7]. Lymphoblasts from blood of patients with infectious mononucleosis	No
4. 'Foetal' antigens	Spleen 13–22 wk, Thymus 15–22 wk, liver (9–22 wk)*	No

[1] All cells tested by indirect immunofluorescence with anti-ALL. Cell types marked with asterisk * were also tested for their capacity to absorb out anti-ALL antibodies.
[2] No reactivity = less than 0.5 % positive cells recorded which is the "background" recorded with normal control sera, or alternatively, in absorption experiments, reflects no shift in the FACS profile on anti-ALL against ALL cells.
[3] Trypsin (Sigma 12,000 BAEE units/mg. 2X crystallised) 50 µg/10⁶ cells/1 ml/30 min/ 37 °C.
[4] Pronase (BDH 45,000 PuK units per g) 50 µg/10⁶ cells/1 ml/30 min/37 °C.
[5] Neurominidase (vibrio cholera Calbiochem. Grade B) 0.5 u/10⁶ cells/1 ml/30 min/37 °C.
[6] Tonsil T lymphocytes cultured with phytohaemagglutinin or Concanavalin A or spleen B lymphocytes cultured with pokeweed mitogen.
[7] Derived from normal adult blood or from blood of patients with infectious mononucleosis, Burkitt's lymphoma or ALL.

Figures 5 and 6 illustrate reactivity of leukaemic cells with anti-ALL as analysed by the FACS. In Table 4 the pattern of reactivity in leukaemias is presented. Virtually every common ALL reacts whereas all T and B ALLs do not. Other types of leukaemias do not react, with two interesting exceptions – AUL and CML in blast crisis. Six out of eight AUL patients and nine out of 19 patients with CML blast crisis had a high proportion of cells reacting with the anti-ALL serum. Blast cells in CML acute crisis can be predominantly 'lymphoid' or 'myeloid' by morphological and cytochemical criteria (22). ALL antigen positive cells were only found in the 'lymphoid' crisis, although not in all such cases. In all cases studied, however, the blast crisis involved Ph[1] positive cells (23). In one particularly interesting case an ALL antigen negative 'lymphoid' blast crisis in blood was followed by CNS relapse which was ALL positive (i.e. the cells in cerebro-spinal fluid). In the same sample, all metaphases were Ph[1] positive. These results provide direct evidence for earlier suggestions that CML can enter an ALL-like phase (26, 27) and parallels recent findings using terminal deoxynucleotidyl transferase enzyme as a marker for ALL (28, see also Sabin and McCaffrey in this symposium).

Table IV: Reactivity of different leukaemias with anti-ALL serum[1]

Diagnosis:	Common, non-T non-B, ALL	ALL T-type ALL	B-type ALL	AUL	AML	AMML	CML	CML-BC[3]	CLL[4]
Proportion of positive cases:	47/50[2]	0/14	0/3	7/9	1/48	0/10	0/10	9/19	0/12

[1] The sera were raised against lymphoblasts from children with typical non-T, non-B type ALL.
[2] Pooled data from adults and children.
[3] Chronic Myeloid Leukaemia in Blast crisis relapse (see ref. 23). All nine positive cases had a 'lymphoid' morphology. All 19 cases were Ph[1] chromosome positive.
[4] All leukaemias were diagnosed (using marrow or blood cells) by standard morphological and histochemical methods (including Romanowsky, Sudan Black, periodic-acid Schiff and Acid phosphatase staining).

The most likely interpretations of these findings are that: 1. ALL of both children and adults can involve three different cell types and therefore probably derives from three different progenitors – T lymphocyte related cells (probably thymocytes), B lymphocyte related cells, and in the majority of cases, a non-T, non-B cell which could be either a lymphoid precursor (28) and/or a pluripotential stem cell. 2. Common ALL, most AUL cases and a proportion of CML blast crises involve the same cell type. Important corollaries of this are that (i) CML is, in at least some cases, a malignancy induced in a pluripotential stem cell rather than a myeloid stem cell. A similar suggestion was made previously based on the results referred to above with terminal transferase enzyme (29). (ii) the ALL antigen(s) can be expressed in diseases involving a common target cell but a different aetiology (e.g. Ph[1] positive or negative). This might lead one to suspect that the ALL antigen would be found on the normal counterpart or progenitor of the 'ALL' spectrum of diseases. If this is the case then we can say that this cell has a frequency in formal bone marrow of less than 0.1 %. This in turn implies either a derivation of ALL from a very rare cell (e.g. a pluripotential stem cell) or that the ALL antigen(s) is only expressed on transformed derivatives.

The nature of ALL antigen has recently been investigated (30). It is glycoprotein as judged by sensitivity to pronase and interaction with lentil lectin. It does not

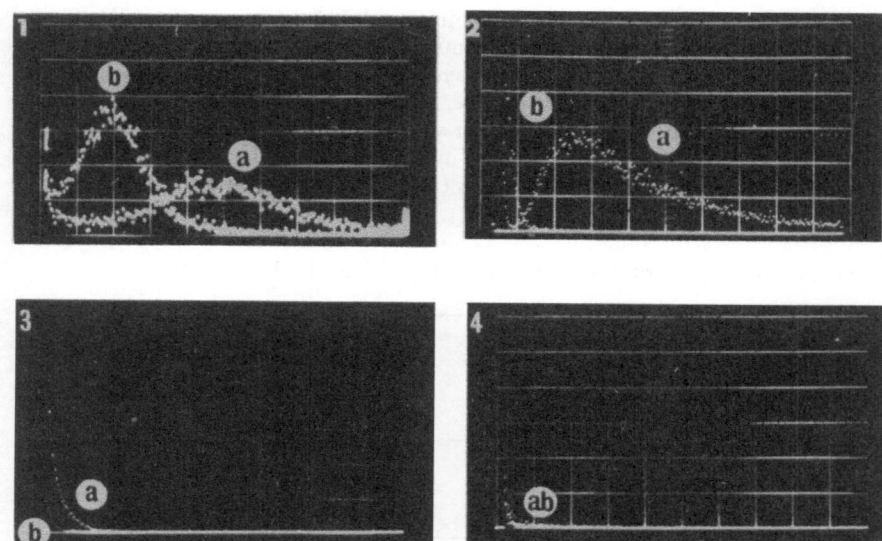

Fig. 6: FACS analysis of the binding of anti-ALL sera to different leukaemias.
Legend: Ordinate: relative cell number.
Abscissa: relative fluorescence intensity.
1. Untreated non-T, non-B ALL (Blood) as in Fig. 5.
2. Non-T, non-B ALL (CNS relapse) cerebro-spinal fluid.
3. Untreated AML (Blood, IBM separated).
4. Untreated T-like ALL (Blood).
(a) Anti-ALL, (b) Control (as in Fig. 5).
Note small difference between (a) and (b) in 3 can be removed by a further single absorption with AML, cells (17).

appear to cross-react immunologically with a variety of C-type RNA oncorna-viruses including murine Moloney and Gross viruses, Feline leukaemia virus, Simian Sarcoma virus and the recently isolated human leukaemia (AML) virus, HuLV-23-1 (31).

Selective binding of anti-ALL sera can be demonstrated in a quantitative manner by the iodinated anti-globulin binding method (Sutherland and Greaves, unpublished observations). This result also raises the possibility of developing a sentitive radioimmune assay for cell-free leukaemic antigens in patients' serum and cerebro-spinal fluid.

The precise selectivity and sensitivity of the anti-ALL probe suggests that it should be possible to use it to detect rare leukaemia cells in situations where they would appear to be absent by standard haematological tests. We have been able to do this in two situations so far. A proportion of untreated ALL patients present with a typical lymphoblastic bone marrow but with no obvious leukaemic cells in the peripheral blood picture. Five of such patients (included in Table 4) we studied, had no leukaemic blasts by routine haematological assessment, but we

256

found 1 to 5 %/o leukaemic cells in the blood of all five, using anti-ALL sera. This result suggests that anti-ALL antibodies could be used to detect early emergence of the leukaemic clone into the circulation. One would obviously like to detect early expansion of the malignant cell in the marrow itself. One approach to this problem is to study the marrow of patients prospectively through treatment, in order to assay for residual disease and/or early signs of relapse. Such trials are in progress and, meanwhile, spot checks on individual patients indicate that rare leukaemic cells may indeed be present in the bone marrow of patients considered to be in complete remission (17).

The availability of antisera to leukaemia specific or leukaemia associated antigens raises the possibility of therapeutic applications. Our antisera are not directly cytotoxic (in the presence of complement) and we are currently exploring their potential use as selective 'bullets' in antibody dependent cell induced killing systems (cf. ref. 32) and as carriers of cytotoxic drugs (cf. ref. 33). It is also possible that the leukaemic antigen(s) itself, once isolated, could be rendered highly immunogenic and re-introduced to the patient.

In conclusion, we suggest that fluorescent cell surface binding probes provide a new incisive tool for characterising or 'phenotyping' leukaemic cells. Table 5 is a summary of all the membrane markers we have studied and the current distribution of reactivity among different leukaemias. Of these various test systems anti-leukaemia antibodies in combination with analytical efficiency of the Fluorescence Activated Cell Sorter provide a particularly exciting approach for accurate

Table V: Cell surface phenotype of human leukaemic cells tested at University College (1972–1975)

Membrane markers	Refs.	Common or non-T, non B type	T-type	B-type	AUL	AML	AMML	A. Mon. L	CML	CML-BC	CLL
A. LYMPHOCYTE MARKERS											
i. Anti-lymphocyte serum[1]		▨	▨	▨							▨
ii. T-markers. Anti-T serum[2] E rosettes	(4,2)		▨								
iii. B-markers. Anti-Ig serum Anti-CLL (B) serum	(4,2, 34)			▨							▨
B. MYELOID MARKERS											
i. Anti-monocyte serum	(5,2)							▨			
ii. Anti-granulocyte serum[3]	-					▨	▨	▨	▨		
C. LEUKAEMIA MARKER Anti-ALL serum	(16, 17,30)	▨			▨	▨				▨	▨
D. CHOLERA TOXIN	(21,2)								▨	▨	▨

[1] Rabbit anti-thymus serum absorbed with normal blood granulocytes and AML cells (Brown & Greaves unpublished observations).
[2] Antisera to thymus or brain (4, 2).
[3] Kindly provided by Dr. A. B. de la Riviere. This rabbit serum was raised as previously described by Engelfriet et al. (35).
Shaded areas represent proportion of positive cases.

and sensitive diagnosis of disease and monitoring the response of patients to therapy.

Acknowledgements

This work was supported by the Imperial Cancer Research Fund and the International Agency for Research in Cancer (Fellowship to T.R.). We are most grateful to our many colleagues who participated in these studies by providing patient material and haematological data. We also thank Dr Finkelstein for supplying cholera toxin and anti-toxin reagents and Dr R. K. Murray (University of Toronto) and Dr D. Critchley (ICRF) for gifts of gangliosides and for collaboration in some of the experiments.

References

1. Fialkow, P. (1974) The origin and development of human tumours studied with cell markers. New Engl. J. Med., *270*, 26.
2. Greaves, M. F. (1975) Clinical applications of cell surface markers. Progr. Haematol. I, 255.
3. Seligmann, M. (1975) Membrane cell markers in human leukaemias and lymphomas. Brit. J. Haematol., *31* (suppl.), p. 1.
4. Brown, G., Greaves, M. F., Lister, T. A., Rapson, N. and Papamichael, M. (1974) Expression of human T and B lymphocyte cell surface markers on leukaemia cells. Lancet, *ii*, 753.
5. Baker, M. A., Falk, R., Falk, J. and Greaves, M. F. (1975) Detection of a monocyte specific antigen on human acute leukaemia cells. Brit. J. Haematol. 32, 13.
6. Salmon, S. E. and Seligmann, M. (1974) B cell neoplasia in Man. Lancet, *ii*, 1230.
7. Lukes, R. J. and Collins, R. D. (1975) New approaches to the classification of the lymphomata. Brit. J. Cancer, 31, Suppl. II, p. 1.
8. Edelson, R. L., Kirkpatrick, C. H., Sherach, E. M., Schein, P. S., Smith, R. N., Green, I. and Lutzner, M. (1974) Preferential cutaneous infiltration by neoplastic thymus derived lymphocytes. Ann. Int. Med., *80*, 685.
9. Flandrin, G., Brouet, J. C., Daniel, M. T. and Preud'homme, J. L. (1975) Acute leukaemia with Burkitt's tumour cells. A study of six cases with special reference to lymphocyte surface markers. Blood, *45*, 183.
10. Catovsky, D., Goldman, J. M., Okos, A., Frisch, B. and Galton, D. A. G. (1974) T lymphoblastic leukaemia: a distinct variant of acute leukaemia. Brit. Med. J., p. 643.
11. Borella, L. and Sen, L. (1973) T cell surface markers on lymphoblasts from acute lymphocytic leukaemia. J. Immunol., *111*, 1275.
12. Cuatrecasas, P. (1973) Gangliosides and membrane receptors for cholera toxin. Biochem., *12*, 3558.
13. Hakomori, S. (1975) Structures and organisation of cell surface glycolipids. Biochem. et Biophys. Acta., *417*, 55.

14. Mohanakumar, T., Metzgar, R. S. and Miller, D. S. (1974) Human leukaemia cell antigens: Serological characterisation with xeno-antisera. J. Nat. Cancer Inst., *52*, 1435.
15. Baker, M. A., Ramachandar, K. and Taub, R. N. (1974) Specificity of heteroantisera to human acute leukaemia associated antigens. J. Clin. Invest., *54*, 1273.
16. Greaves, M. F., Brown, G., Lister, T. A. and Rapson, N. T. (1975) Antisera to Acute Lymphoblastic Leukaemia cells. Clin. Immunol. Immunopath., *4*, 67.
17. Brown, G., Capellaro, D. and Greaves, M. F. (1975) Human leukaemia associated antigens. J. Nat. Cancer Inst. (in press).
18. Böyum, A. (1968) Separation of leukocytes from blood and bone marrow. Scand. J. Clin. Lab. Invest. *21*, Suppl. 97.
19. Bonner, W. A., Hulett, H. R., Sweet, R. G. and Herzenberg, L. A. (1972) Fluorescence activated cell sorting. Rev. Scientific Instr., *43*, 404.
20. Hulett, H. R., Bonner, W. A., Sweet, R. G. and Herzenberg, L. A. (1973) Development and applications of a rapid cell sorter. Clin. Chem., *19*, 813.
21. Revesz, T., Greaves, M. F., Capellaro, D. and Murray, R. K. Differential expression of cell surface binding sites for cholera toxin in acute and chronic leukaemias. Brit. J. Haematol. (in press).
22. Beard, M. E. J., Amess, J. L., Roberts, M., Kirk, B., Durrant, J. and Galton, D. A. G. (1976) Blast crisis of chronic myeloid leukaemia (CML) I. Presentation simulating acute lymphoblastic leukaemia (ALL) Brit. J. Haematol. (in press).
23. Janossy, G., Greaves, M. F., Revesz, T., Lister, T. A., Roberts, M., Durrant, J. and Beard, M. (1976) Blast crisis of chronic myeloid leukaemia (CML): II. Membrane marker characteristics. Brit. J. Haematol. (in press).
24. Critchley, D. R. and MacPherson, I. (1973) Cell density dependent glycolipids in NIL hamster cell derived transformed cell lines. Biochim. Biophys. Acta, *296*, 146.
25. Hollenberg, M. D., Fishman, P. H., Bennett, V. and Cuatrecasas, P. (1974) Cholera toxin and cell growth: role of membrane gangliosides. Proc. Natl. Acad. Sci., *71*, 4224.
26. Mathé, G., Tubiana, M., Calman, F., Schlumberger, J. R., Berumen, L., Choquet, C., Cattan, A. and Schneider, M. (1967) Les syndromes de leucemie aigue (SLA) appraisant au cours de l'evolution des haematosarcomes et des leucemies chroniques (analyse clinique). Nouv. Rev. Fr. Haematol., *7*, 543.
27. Boggs, D. R. (1974) Hematopoietic stem cell theory in relation to possible lymphoblastic conversion of chronic myeloid leukaemia. Blood, *44*, 449.
28. McCaffrey, R., Harrison, T. A., Parkman, R. and Baltimore, D. (1975) Terminal deoxynucleotidyl transferase activity in human leukaemic cells and in normal human thymocytes. New Engl. J. Med. p. 775.
29. Gallo, R. C. (1975) Terminal transferase and leukaemia. New Engl. J. Med., p. 804.
30. Brown, G., Hogg, N. and Greaves, M. F. (1975) A candidate leukaemia specific antigen in Man. Nature, 258, 454.
31. Teich, N. M., Weiss, R. A., Salahuddin, S. Z., Gallagher, R. E., Gillespie, D. H. and Gallo, R. C. (1975) Infective transmission and characterisation of a C-

type virus released by cultured human myeloid leukaemia cells. Nature, *256*, 552.

32. Wunderlich, J. R., Rosenberg, E. B. and Connolly, J. M. (1971) Human lymphocyte dependent cytotoxic antibody and mechanisms of target cell destruction in vitro. In 'Progr. in Immunology' p. 473 (Ed. B. Amos) Acad. Press, N.Y.

33. Davies, D. A. L and O'Neill, G. J. (1973) In vivo and in vitro effects of tumour specific antibodies with chlorambucil. Brit. J. Cancer, Suppl. 1, *28*, 285.

34. Greaves, M. F. and Brown, G. (1973) A human B lymphocyte antigen. Nature New Biol., *246*, 116.

35. Engelfriet, C. P., Diepenhorst, P., Giessen, M. V. D. and von Riesz, E. (1975) Removal of leucocytes from whole blood and erythrocyte suspensions by filtration through cotton wool. IV. Immunisation studies in rabbits. Vox Sang., *28*, 81.

Use of Immunological Reagents Prepared in Animals to Characterise the Surface of Leukaemic Cells

N. A. Mitchison

Department of Zoology University College London,
London, U. K.

Two central questions emerged concerning the immune response to leukaemia cell surface antigens. One concerns the relationship of such antigens to those on the surface of normal cells: are antigenic markers shared in common with normal cells of the T cell, B cell, or myeloid series, and if so, do the overlaps provide valid clues to the target cell of the malignant transformation? And if not, do we have truly tumour specific antigens which can be utilised for monitoring disease progress, for instance, in the prediction of relapse? The second concerns the role of viruses in leukaemia; can immunological procedures detect glycoproteins of viral origin on the surface of human leukaemic cells?

The contributions of Billings, Graeves, Kadin and Reyes bore mainly on the first of these questions. Two rather different approaches, both using specific antibodies raised in foreign species, are being employed. One (Greaves, Brouet) uses whole cells as immunogen, and relies either on coating the immunogen with antibody or on extensive absorptions to get round the problem of contamination of the desired reagent with irrelevant antibody. The most remarkable achievement of reagents produced in this way is to have divided ALL into two diseases, the less common characterised by the presence of T cell markers, and the more common by the presence of a unique ALL specific antigen. The second approach (Billings, Reyes) is to produce reagents by immunising with purified or partially purified molecules. Thus, specific anti-immunoglobulins can be used to detect immunoglobulin on the surface of CLL cells. Antibodies to less well-defined surface molecules can be used to detect partially leukaemia-specific antigens, but cross reactions with B cells are also detected with these reagents. Both types of reagent can usefully be conjugated to electron-dense molecules, such as ferritin, thus permitting the distribution of surface antigen to be examined in the electron microscope.

As regards the second question concerning viral antigens, the best data came from murine leukaemia virus tumours in rats and mice (Herberman). These indicate that the host repsonse is directed exclusively at viral antigens. The precice target of the response has not been fully established; ubiquitous immunity to endogenous viruses complicates the issue, and the role of the virus polypeptide P30 on the cell surface remains controversial. The unique antigen detected by Greaves on ALL has so far eluded attempts to identify it as a viral product.

Trends in the Treatment of Childhood Leukemia

By Joseph V. Simone, M. D.
Rhomes J. A. Aur, M. D.
H. Omar Hustu, M. D.
Manuel Verzosa, M. D.

Hematologie-Oncology and Radiotherapy Services, St. Jude Chrildren's Research Hospital, Memphis, Tennessee 38 101.

Introduction

The gratifying results now being obtained in the treatment of children with acute lymphocytic leukemia has had at least two major effects on the attitude of the medical community. First, these results have encouraged physicians to think of ALL as an eminentably treatable and, perhaps, curable disease, Second, physicians have become more aware of the obligation to avoid serious side effects that might compromise the otherwise good results. My purpose in speaking to you today is to review briefly some of the results obtained, mainly at our own institution, in the treatment of this disease and to point out some of the problems that have been encountered as result of treatment. Our data has been reported in some detail recently (19) so I will present only selected points rather than an exhausive review. Some of the results I will talk about today are preliminary and will require months or years before definitive conclusions can be made.

Materials and Methods

Definitions

Acute lymphocytic leukemia (ALL) is diagnosed on the basis of excessive numbers of lymphoblasts and/or "stem cells" in an aspirated bone marrow specimen. In practice, this diagnosis includes all children with leukemia that is not characterized by Auer rods or myelocytic or monocytic differentiation. Special cytochemical stains and histological specimens are sometimes helpful, but, ultimately, the diagnosis ist the concensus of at least three experienced investigators. Approximately 78 % of leukemia cases at this institution are diagnosed as ALL. Children with lymphoblastic or "stem cell" lymphosarcoma who had marrow involvement at diagnosis are considered to have ALL and are included in these studies.

Our definitions of remission, relapse and survival are described in detail elsewhere (15). Complete remission duration is the period free of all signs of ALL,

Supported by Cancer Research Center Grant CA-08480, Research Project Grants CA-07594 and CA-13050, and Training Grants CA-05176 and CA-08151 from the National Institutes of Health, by Project Grant CI-70 from the American Cancer Society and by ALSAC.

263

whether hematologic, visceral or in the CNS. CNS leukemia is diagnosed by the observation of leukemia cells in a Wright-stained centrifugate of cerebrospinal fluid (CSF). The appearance of leukemia cells in the bone marrow signifies hematologic relapse.

Methods

A brief outline of the treatment plan for the first seven studies is shown in Table 1. This shows some of the variations on the theme of therapy that has been used over the years. Basically however, treatment entails four phases: 1) remission induction, 2) preventive CNS therapy, 3) continuation (maintenance) chemotherapy, and 4) cessation of therapy.

Table I: Outline of Protocols

Remission Induction (4 to 6 weeks)
  Prednisone
  Vincristine
  + Daunomycin in Study VI (2)
  + Asparaginase in Study VIII
Preventive CNS Therapy (2 1/2 to 4 weeks)
  500–1200 rads Craniospinal in Studies I–III
  None in Study IV (16)
  2400 rads Cranial + I. T. Methotrexate in Studies V (4), VII (1), VIII
  2400 rads Craniospinal in Studies VI and VII
Continuation Chemotherapy (2 to 3 years)
  Mercaptopurine daily
  Methotrexate weekly
  Cyclophosphamide weekly
  + Vincristine weekly in Studies III, IV
  + Vincristine – Prednisone Pulses in Studies V, VI, VII
Cessation of Therapy after 2 to 3 years of Complete Remission (3)

Patients

These studies include a total of 549 children with ALL, of whom 363 entered studies I through VII, from 1962 through 1971. From 1972 to the present, 186 previously untreated children have entered study number VIII which is still under way. The initial features of a majority of these patients have been reported elsewhere (19).

Results

Remission Induction

Successful remission induction has been obtained in over 90 % of children with ALL. Vincristine and prednisone has been the treatment used in most of these studies and the addition of daunorubicin or asparaginase has not appreciably improved the remission induction rate. The reason for failure of patients to attain complete remission include: fatal infection in 2.5 %, usually due to gram-negative

264

sepsis in the first week of therapy; failure to respond to chemotherapy in 5 %; and leukemic pleocytosis in the cerebral spinal fluid on the day of first complete remission marrow in 1 %.

Preventive Central Nervous System Therapy

Attempts were made in earlier studies to prevent CNS leukemia from emerging by eradicating undetectable cells in the meninges early in remission. These early studies employed 500 or 1200 rads of craniospinal irradiation. However, these doses of irradiation did not reduce the frequency of CNS leukemia which terminated complete remission in 15 of 37 patients (18).

In 1967 it was decided that failure to prevent CNS leukemia in the earlier studies may have been due to inadequate dosage. Therefore, a study was designed in which 2400 rads of cranial radiation was given along with 5 doses of intrathecal methotrexate simultaneously (4). This form of treatment met with success since CNS leukemia terminated complete remission in only 3 of the 37 patients (19). Furthermore, over one-half of these patients remain in initial continuous complete remission for 6 years and have been off all therapy for three years.

The efficacy of preventive CNS irradiation was tested in a randomized control study before the results of the previous study were known (2). Patients were randomized to receive or not to receive 2400 rads craniospinal irradiation without intrathecal methotrexate. CNS leukemia terminated complete remission in only 2 of 45 patients who received preventive irradiation. However, CNS leukemia terminated complete remission in 33 of 49 patients who did not receive preventive irradiation. This study provided further evidence that CNS leukemia could indeed be prevented with adequate doses of irradiation. Another feature of this study was to determine whether CNS irradiation at the same dosage level would be as effective if given at the first sign of CNS relapse. Therefore, the 33 patients who developed CNS leukemia were given therapeutic craniospinal irradiation. Although the CSF was cleared of leukemic cells in all 33 patients, this second complete remission was terminated by recurrence of CNS leukemia in 13 patients and by simultaneous hematological and CNS relapse in 2. Only 9 of the 33 have had a lengthy second complete remission.

In a subsequent study, patients were randomized to receive either 2400 rads cranial irradiation with simultaneous intrathecal methotrexate or 2400 rads craniospinal irradiation (1). The results showed no significant difference between in the rate of CNS relapse with either form of therapy, which confirmed the historical controls of the two preceding studies.

Continuation (Maintenance) Chemotherapy.

In the above studies, patients received mercaptopurine daily and methotexate and cyclophosphamide weekly during the continuation phase of chemotherapy. A controlled study (16) has shown that these agents must be given in maximum tolerated dosage to achieve optimal results. Variations on this basic regimen have included the addition of vincristine once a week or periodic brief courses of rincristine plus prednisone.

With the overall improvement in results, it became important to try to learn the relative contribution of CNS therapy and continuation chemotherapy. The earlier studies, with apparently ineffective CNS therapy, had yielded a 17 % long-term leukemia-free survival rate. This had been improved to approximately 50 % in the studies using the higher dose of preventive CNS irradiation (19). In view of the major contribution of adequate CNS therapy, it was not known whether such aggressive chemotherapy during remission was necessary in view of its toxicity with a disturbing proportion of patients dying during initial continuous complete remission (21). An attempt to improve the therapeutic index of continuation chemotherapy by reducing toxicity was the major purpose behind the design of Total Therapy Study VIII. The preliminary results of this study are given here with the understanding that they are not definitive at this point, but do yield some important observations even at this early date.

The principal goal of Study VIII is to learn how the therapeutic index of chemotherapy during remission might be improved. Combination chemotherapy has been used to take advantage of different modes of action and lack of cross-resistance. The value of combination chemotherapy for inducing remission was established in 1951 with cortisone and methotrexate (6) and subsequently for other combinations (7, 8). Combinations of two or more drugs have also been given for continuing remission. For example, most of our studies employed a combination of mercaptopurine, methotrexate, and cyclophosphamide. There have been controlled studies of the cyclic (rotation of several drugs, one at a time) versus sequential (single drugs, each until relapse) chemotherapy (5, 12) and of the addition of one or another drug to a basic regimen (13). Controlled studies of different drug combinations began with the classical study by Acute Leukemia Group B (7a). The first controlled study of single versus combination chemotherapy, also performed by Group B, later showed that median durations of remission in childhood ALL were the same with mercatopurine, methotrexate, or both agents given simultaneously in the same dosages as in the single drug regimes (7). Since then, improved remission durations have been obtained in some studies using multiple-drug therapy (8, 20) leading to increasingly complex, multiple-drug regimens. For example, the L-2 protocol from Memorial Hospital employs eight drugs in cycles designed to take maximum advantage of estimated cellular kinetics (9).

However, individual drugs are not equally effective for prolonging remission of childhood ALL (8). Intermittent methotrexate is better than mercaptopurine and either is better than cyclophosphamide. Vincristine, cytosine arabinoside, daunomycin, asparaginase and other agents apparently are less effective. Most of these agents have overlapping toxicity, particularly myelosuppression and immunosuppression, often lowering the tolerable dosage limits of each drug in a multiple-drug regimen. In any given schedule, the effectiveness of single (8) or multiple (16) drugs is related to dosage. Thus, the critical question emerges: Does the advantage of multiple agent chemotherapy outweigh the disadvantage of dosage reduction of the more effective agents? An affirmative answer could lead one to employ all available agents (as many as six or ten) while a negative answer could lead to use of only the most effective agent (methotrexate) in maximum-tolerated dosage. Study VIII was designed to answer this question.

After successful remission induction and preventive CNS therapy, patients are randomized to receive one, two, three, or four drugs simultaneously during remission. The prescribed dosages are starting points only and in each regimen drug dosages are adjusted to the maximum tolerated by the patient. Upward or downward dosage adjustments are made proportionately for all prescribed drugs. To obtain valid conclusions it is essential that the dose-limiting toxicity be of comparable degrees in each group to avoid the "half-dosage effect" seen in Study IV (16). The principal guide for dosage for dosage adjustment ist maintenance of the leukocyte count between 2000 and 3500/mm³. Dosage reductions allowed for other predetermined degrees of toxicity, fever or infection are the same for all groups.

The preliminary results of Study VIII are given here mainly to illustrate the points of rationale and must not be viewed as conclusive at this early date. In the 33 months since beginning this study, 180 patients attained complete remission and received preventive CNS therapy. Thirty were given additional initial therapy due to the presence of features (CNS involved at diagnosis, mediastinal involvement, failure to attain remission after 4 weeks) associated with a poor prognosis and were not randomized. All received three drug maintenance. The remaining 150 were randomized to receive (1) methotrexate alone; (2) methotrexate + mercaptopurine; (3) methotrexate + mercaptopurine + cyclophosphamide; (4) methotrexate + mercaptopurine + cyclophosphamide + cytosine arabinoside. All agents except mercaptopurine were given by vein weekly.

At this time, the frequency of relapse has been approximately the same among patients receiving two drugs (6 of 44), three drugs (10 of 45) or four drugs (3 of 41 plus two deaths in remission). With methotrexate alone, 14 of 20 have relapsed and one patient died in initial remission. These early results show no systematic assocation of efficacy with the number of drugs but apparently indicate the superiority of multiple agents over methotrexate alone.

The smaller number of patients in the group receiving methotrexate alone is the result of discontinuing randomization to that arm of the study. This action was taken because the relapse rate was higher but, more importantly, a serious side effect was observed in this group. Eight of the twenty patients developed a neurological syndrome, not associated with CNS leukemia. It was characterized by disturbances of gait, speech and motor function. This syndrome was progressive and fatal in one child and left permanent residual damage in several others. The pathological lesion was found to be a severe leukoencepholopathy with myelin degeneration. This syndrome usually occurred in patients who had been receiving more than 50 mg per meter squared of methotrexate weekly for 6 months or more. A more detailed analysis of this problem is underway and will be reported in the near future. For the time being however, no patient who has received brain irradiation will be given more than 50 mg per meter squared per week of methotrexate by vein at this institution. This observation should serve to caution other investigators who are giving high doses of methotrexate to patients who had CNS irradiation.

Discussion

The efficacy and dangers of combined modality therapy of childhood ALL are reflected in these studies. The search by many investigative groups for more effective and less toxic modalities and combinations of therapy is illustrated by the scope of a few current studies. A recent Medical Research Council Study (28) has shown that CNS leukemia is effectively prevented by craniospinal irradiation with intrathecal methotrexate. A review of previous trials (25) and the anatomical nature of arachnoid leukemia (31) have led us to conclude that intrathecal methotrexate alone does not effectively prevent CNS leukemia. However, studies by Group B (10) and the Sothwest Oncology Group now in progress, as well as the L-2 Protocol at Memorial Hospital (9), should yield more information on the preventive value of intrathecal methotrexate. Since systemic chemotherapy in maximum-tolerated dosage delayed the onset of CNS leukemia in Study IV (11, 15, 16), the definitive results with even more aggressive systemic chemotherapy in the L-2 Protocol (9) will be of interest. Another approach under study by Children's Cancer Study Group A is a test of the value of extending irradiation of the CNS to include other organs such as liver, spleen, kidneys and gonads.

The question of when to stop therapy is an important one. It has been our practice to stop therapy after two to three years of complete remission. Our experience with this approach has been published recently (3).

Despite improvement in therapy, many old problems remain unsolved and new problems have emerged. Both patient and physician take little satisfaction in a longer survival unless it is of satisfactory quality, but, we must remind ourselves that the most important negative influence on quality of survival is the leukemia itself. By any standard of comparison, the cost of relapse and its complications in human and monetary resources far exceeds that of therapy. Nonetheless, the evolution of studies for childhood ALL demonstrates a keen awareness of the responsibility to minimize undesirable effects of therapy. This requires even more careful design of studies because with combined modality therapy, the side effects may not be due to a single agent but to the unfortunate synergism of several agents.

References

1. Aur, R. J. A., Hustu, H. O., Verzosa, M. S., Wood, A., and Simone, J. V.: Comparison of two methods of preventing central nervous system leukemia. Blood 42: 349–357, 1973.
2. Aur, R. J. A., Simone, J. V., Hustu, H. O., and Verzosa, M. S.: A comparative study of central nervous ystem irradiation and intensive chemotherapy early in remission of childhood acute lymphocytic leukemia. Cancer 29: 381–391, 1972.
3. Aur, R. J. A., Simone, J. V., Hustu, O., Verzosa, M. S., and Pinkel, D.: Cessation of therapy during complete remission of childhood acute lymphocytic leukemia. New Eng. J. Med. 291: 1230–1234, 1974.
4. Aur, R. J. A., Simone, J., Hustu, H. O., Walters, T., Borells, L., Pratt, C., and Pinkel, D.: Central nervous system therapy and combination chemotherapy of childhood lymphocytic leukemia. Blood 37:272–281, 1971.
5. Colebatch, J. H., Baikie, A. G., Clark, A. C. L., Jones, D. L., Lee, C. W. G., Lewis, I. C., and Newman, N. M.: Cyclic drug regimen for acute childhood leukemia. Lancet 1: 313–318, 1968.
6. Farber, S., Toch, R., Sears, E. M., and Pinkel, D.: Advances in chemotherapy of cancer in man. Advances Cancer Res. 4: 1–22, 1956.
7. Frei, E., III, Freireich, E. J., Gehan, E., Pinkel, D., Holland, J. F., et al.:

Studies of sequential and combination antimetabolite therapy in acute leukemia: 6-mercaptopurine and methotexate, from the Acute Leukemia Group B. Blood 18: 431–454, 1961.

7a. Frei, E., III, Holland, J. F., Schneiderman, M. A., Pinkel, D., Selkirk, G., Freireich, E. J., Silver, R. T., Gold, G. L., and Regelson, W.: A comparative study of two regimens of combination chemotherapy in acute leukemia. Blood 13: 1126, 1958.

8. Goldin, A., Sandberg, J. S., Henderson, E. S., Newman, J. W., Frei, E. III, and Holland, J. F.: The chemotherapy of human and animal acute leukemia. Cancer Chemother. Rep. 55: 309–507, 1971.

9. Hagbin, M., Tan, C. C., Clarkson, B. D., Mike, V., Burchenal, J. H., and Murphy, M. L.: Intensive chemotherapy in children with acute lymphoblastic leukemia (L-2 Protocol). Cancer 33: 1491–1498, 1974.

10. Holland, J. F., and Glidewell, O.: Chemotherapy of acute lymphocytic leukemia of childhood. Cancer 30:1480–; 1487, 1972.

11. Hustu, H. O., Aur, R. J. A., Verzosa, M. S., Simone, J. V., and Pinkel, D.: Prevention of central nervous system leukemia by irradiation. Cancer 32: 585–597, 1973.

12. Krivit, W., Brubaker, C., Thatcher, L. G., Pierce, M., Perrin, E., and Hartmann, J. R.: Maintenance therapy in acute leukemia of childhood: Comparison of cyclic vs. sequential methods. Cancer 21: 352–356, 1968.

13. Leikin, S., Brubaker, C., Hartmann, J., Murphy, M. L., and Wolff, J.: The use of combination therapy in leukemia remission. Cancer 24: 427–432, 1969.

14. Medical Research Council: Treatment of acute lymphoblastic leukaemia: Effect of "prophylactic" therapy against central nervous system leukaemia. Brit. Med. J. 2: 381–384, 1973.

15. Pinkel, D.: Five-year follow-up of "total therapy" of childhood lymphocytic leukemia. J.A.M.A. 216: 648–652, 1971.

16. Pinkel, D., Hernandez, K., Borella, L., Holton, C., Aur, R., Samoy, G., and Pratt, C.: Drug dosage and remission duration in childhood lymphocytic leukemia. Cancer 27: 247–256, 1971.

17. Price, R. A., and Johnson, W. W.: The central nervous system in childhood lymphocytic leukemia. I. The arachnoid. Cancer 31: 520–533, 1973.

18. Simone, J. V.: Treatment of children with acute lymphocytic leukemia. Advan. Pediat. 19: 13–45, 1972.

19. Simone, J.: Acute lymphocytic leukemia in childhood. Sem. Hemat. 11: 25–39, 1974.

20. Simone, J. V.: Aur, R. J. A., Hustu, H. O., and Pinkel, D.: "Total Therapy" studies of acute lymphocytic leukemia in children. Current results and prospects for cur. Cancer 30: 1488–1494, 1972.

21. Simone, J. V., Holland, E., and Johnson, W.: Fatalities during remission of childhood leukemia. Blood 39: 759–770, 1972.

The Therapy of Acute Leukemia in the Adult
A Progress Report

Peter H. Wiernik, M. D.

Section of Medical Oncology
National Cancer Institute,
Baltimore Cancer Research Center
at the
University of Maryland Hospital
Baltimore, Maryland, USA

Introduction

Complete remissions in adult patients with acute leukemia were unusual, if not rare, fifteen years ago. The discovery of highly effective antileukemic drugs such as cytosine arabinoside and daunorubicin and the development of more effective combinations of active chemotherapeutic agents largely through empiric clinical trial and error have dramatically changed that situation so that today 70 % or more of previously untreated patients achieve complete remission status. This improvement has been facilitated by major developments in supportive care. The use of allopurinol for the prevention of urate nephropathy has eliminated that serious complication of antileukemic therapy. Newer antibiotics active against *Pseudomonas aeruginosa* have allowed for the successful treatment of many life threatening infections which occur in the granulocytopenic leukemia patient. Laminar air flow rooms which provide essentially sterile air, and oral nonabsorbable antibiotics which sterilize the gastrointestinal tract, protect the leukemia patient in large measure from microbial hazards in his external and internal environments. Blood cell component therapy allows for replacement of platelets and granulocytes in cytopenic patients. It is the purpose of this paper to detail some of these achievements.

Reprint Requests to:
Peter H. Wiernik, M. D.
Baltimore Cancer Research Center
22 South Greene Street
Baltimore, Maryland 21201
USA ·

Induction Chemotherapy for Acute Nonlymphocytic Leukemia (ANLL)

The first drug combination that proved effective as therapy for acute non-lymphocytic leukemia was the POMP regimen, which consisted of high intravenous doses of prednisone, vincristine, methotrexate and mercaptopurine (1). This therapy was successful in producing complete remissions in approximately 25 % of adult patients and was the first clinical proof that combinations of effective drugs could be more active than single agents. Shortly after this demonstration, cytosine arabinoside (Ara C) became available for clinical trial and it soon proved to be a drug as active as the POMP combination (Table 1). The discovery of the clinical antileukemic activity of daunorubicin (DNM) shortly thereafter represents a turning point in the history of the therapy of acute nonlymphocytic leukemia. DNM alone will produce complete remissions in over 40 % of patients with ANLL (Table 1) and, more importantly, it (or a related anthracycline antibiotic, adriamycin) has become the cornerstone around which the most effective combination therapies to date have been built (Table 2). These new combinations have produced complete remissions in up to 70 % of previously untreated adults with ANLL.

Table I: Representative Results of Induction Therapy for ANLL using Cytosine Arabinoside or Daunorubicin alone in Previously Untreated Patients

Author	Ref	Regimen	CR rate
Wiernik	1	DNM 60mg/M^2 day 1–3	50 %
Wiernik	5	DNM 60mg/M^2 day 1–3	49 %
Wiernik (ALGB)	4	DNM 60mg/M^2 day 1–3	43 %
Ellison (ALGB)	12	Ara C 30mg/M^2 daily in 12 hr infusion to hypoplasia	24 %
Goodell	19	Ara C 40–70mg/M^2 in 4 hr infusion daily x 4	25 %
Armentrout	20	Ara C 4mg/kg in 8 hr infusion daily x 4–14 days	42 %
SWOG	14	Ara C 1.0gm/M^2 infused over 12 hrs	39 %

In an effort to achieve the greatest response rate with the least amount of induction therapy and, therefore, the least risk of serious (or even fatal) toxicity from induction therapy, a nonrandomized study has recently been initiated at the Baltimore Cancer Research Center in which patients are allocated to receive DNM 60 mg/M^2/dayx3, or Ara C 200 mg/M^2/dayx7 continuous IV infusion, or DNM 45 mg/M^2/day x 3, days 1–3 and Ara C 100 mg/M^2/day, days 1–7 continuous IV infusion, on the basis of certain biochemical tests performed on each patient's leukemic marrow cells. Patients whose cells have a high DNM reductase activity level (2)* but a low kinase:deaminase activity ratio (3)** receive DNM alone. Patients whose cells have a high kinase:deaminase activity ratio but a low DNM reductase activity level receive Ara C alone, and patients in whom both enzyme

Table II: Current Induction Therapy Results in Previously Untreated Patients with ANLL using Drug Combinations which include Cytosine Arabinoside and an Anthracycline Derivative

Author	Ref	Regimen	CR rate
Glucksberg	18	DNM 1.5mg/kg on day 1 VCR 1mg/M² on day 1 Pred. 1mg/kg day 1–5 Ara C 2mg/kg q 12 hr day 1–5 TG 2mg/kg q 12 hr day 1–5	59 %
Glucksberg	18	DNM 1.5mg/kg day 1–3 VCR 1mg/M² day 1 & 7 Pred. Ara C, TG as above	70 %
Brincker	17	DNM 80 mg q 5 days Ara C 150 mg daily Both given until hypoplasia	53 %
Masami	13	DNM 25mg/M² Ara C 80mg/M² 6-MPR 300mg/M² day 1–4 Pred. 60mg/M²	61 %
McCredie	15	ADM day 1 VCR day 1 Pred. days 5–9 Ara C days 1–9	70 %
Wiernik (ALGB)	4	DNM 100mg/M² day 1 TG 100mg/M² q 12 hr day 1–5 Ara C 100mg/M² 12 hr day 1–5	50 %
Wiernik	5	DNM 75mg/M² day 1 Ara C 75mg/M² q 12 hr day 1–5 TG 75mg/M² q12 hr day 1–5 Pyrimethamine 1mg/kg day 1–5	46 %
Yates	16	DNM 45mg/M² day 1–3 Ara C 100mg/M² day 1–7 (cont. IV infusion)	67 %
Rai (ALGB)	56	DNM 45mg/M² day 1–3 Ara C 100mg/M² day 1–7 (cont. IV infusion)	66 %*

* Some patients with M-1 marrows did not technically fulfill all requirements for CR because of drug induced peripheral cytopenia.

measurements are high, low or not performed for technical reasons receive both drugs. It is too early to evaluate this study since only 25 patients have completed therapy. It is evident already, however, that only about 25 % of patients will receive either Ara C or DNM alone when the above criteria for selection are applied. Thus far, with 35 patients who received both drugs evaluable, the complete remission rate is 70 % for that group of patients in the current BCRC study.

Maintenance Therapy for ANLL

Complete remission duration in adults with ANLL is disturbingly short and does not seem to vary greatly with induction or maintenance chemotherapy schemes. As an example, in a recent study of 3 induction regimens performed by Acute Leukemia Group B (protocol 7221) median complete remission duration was 5.5–6.6 months despite the use of monthly moderately intensive maintenance chemotherapy (4). It seems clear, however, that while such maintenance therapy commonly sustains complete remission for only approximately six months, the results are superior to those obtained when similar induction therapy is followed by no maintenance chemotherapy. In an early BCRC study (1) DNM 60 mg/M² daily x3 was used as an induction therapy and no maintenance treatment was given. The median duration of complete remission was 2.3 months. In a later BCRC study (5) and in the ALGB study referred to above (4) the same dose and schedule of DNM was used as an induction therapy option and moderately

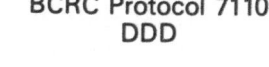

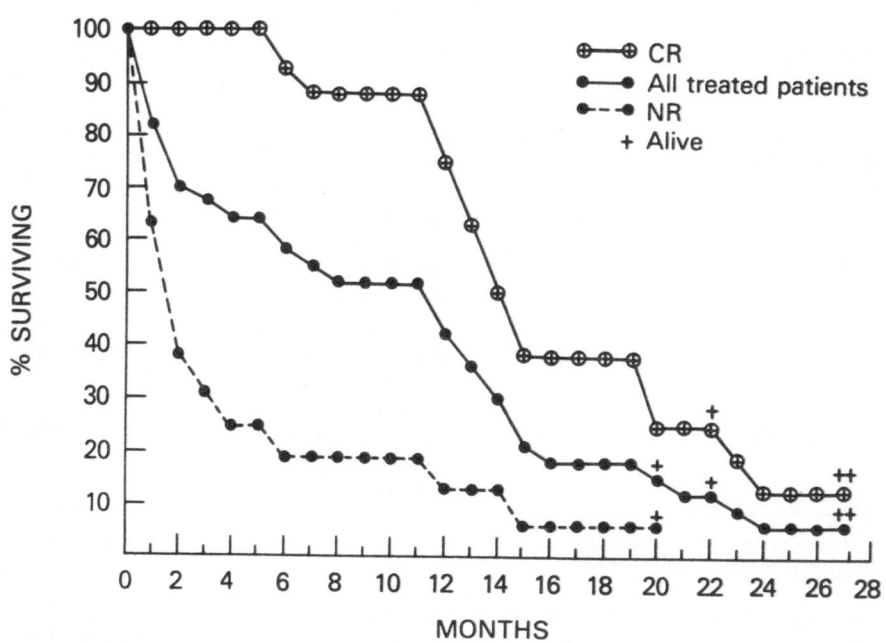

Fig. 1: Survival curves drawn by the life table method for patients with ANLL treated with daunorubicin alone for induction therapy in a recent BCRC study. The curves illustrate the significant survival advantage seen in all studies for patients who achieve complete remission.

intensive maintenance therapy was administered monthly. The median durations of remission in those studies were 6.8 and 6.2 months respectively.

Early data from Bodey, et al (6) suggest that when intensive re-induction courses of chemotherapy are given after a substantial complete remission has occurred, remission duration may be further prolonged. Such therapy is not without hazard, however, and results in significant morbidity and potential mortality.

The most significant contribution of immunology to clinical cancer therapy has been the development of immunotherapy maintenance regimes for ANLL. Studies in which BCG (7), the methanol extractable residue (MER) of BCG (8), or neuraminidase-treated allogenic leukemic cells (9) have been used for maintenance therapy of ANLL in conjunction with anti-leukemic drugs have all resulted in significant enhancement of remission duration of 2–3 fold over control patients maintained with chemotherapy alone. Such therapy is not innocuous and can result in severe local pain and disfigurement. However, although the mechanism of action of such agents is by no means clear, it *is* clear that they do favorably affect remission duration in ANLL. The clinical action of these substances derived from living unicellular material is reminiscent of "spontaneous" remission in acute leukemia observed rarely after bacterial infection (10).

Maintenance therapy with cyclophosphamide and 1, 3-bis (2-chloroethyl)-1-nitrosourea has recently been observed to produce a median duration of complete remission in ANLL comparable to that observed after immunotherapy (11). This observation has not yet been confirmed, however.

New Drugs for Induction Therapy of ANLL

Three new drugs currently under investigation for their antileukemic activity are of interest: 5-azacytidine, VP16-213, and neocarcinostatin.

5-azacytidine, a pyrimidine nucleotide analogue, produced a 28 % complete remission rate in one study (21) in which patients refractory to DNR, thioguanine, and Ara C were treated. The drug's mechanism of action is unclear and some data suggest (22) that it may act in a manner unlike any other antileukemic drug. Gastrointestinal, marrow, and mucous membrane toxicity are common with the drug. In addition a neuromuscular toxicity syndrome consisting of myalgia and weakness occasionally occurs. It has been suggested that this syndrome is due to hypophosphatemia secondary to hyperphosphaturia which results from a nephrotoxic action of 5-azacytidine (23).

VP16-213 (4-demethyl-epipodophyllotoxin-B-D-ethylidene glucoside) is a semi-synthetic derivative of podophyllotoxin. The drug prevents cells from accomplishing mitosis and has been shown to have antileukemic activity in certain animal systems. In one small study (24) a complete remission was obtained in one-third of patients with ANLL. A 50 % complete remission rate was obtained in a smaller group of patients who had a monocytic component to their leukemia. Marrow and gastrointestinal side effects are apparently less severe than with many other induction therapy drugs.

A remarkable 55 % complete remission rate with neocarcinostatin in patients with ANLL was reported from Japan (25). This drug, an acidic single chain polypeptide, is elaborated by *Streptomyces sp.* and has been shown to be active against a number of animal tumor systems. Further evaluation of this drug is clearly warranted.

Adult Acute Lymphocytic Leukemia (ALL)

Adult ALL is responsive to the same chemotherapeutic agents used successfully in childhood ALL but lower complete remission rates and shorter durations of remission have been the rule (26, 27). Thus, while almost 90 % of children with ALL achieve complete remission with vincristine and prednisone most therapeutic trials in adults have produced complete remission in less than 50 % of patients, and while the median duration of remission approaches 5 years in some childhood studies most adult studies have yielded median remission durations of 1 year or less.

Vincristine in combination with prednisone has been employed in virtually all programs for initial induction therapy in both childhood and adult ALL. Chemotherapeutic agents which have shown beneficial effects when combined with vincristine and prednisone for remission induction therapy include methotrexate and 6-mercaptopurine (POMP) (28), L-asparaginase (29), daunorubicin (27), and adriamycin (30).

ADULT ACUTE LYMPHOCYTIC LEUKEMIA
1965-72 VS. 1973-75

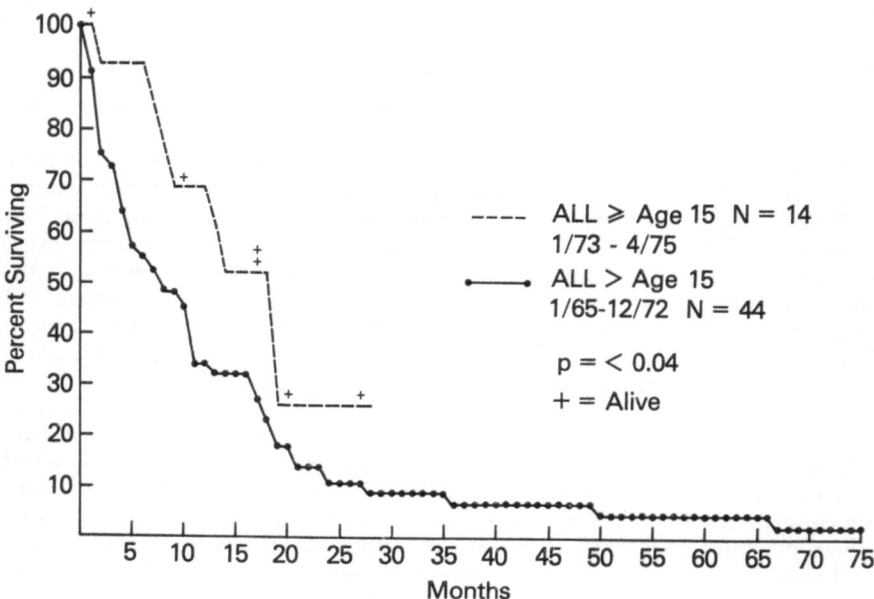

Fig. 2: Survival curves for all treated adults with ALL seen at the BCRC since 1965. The curves compare those patients treated most recently with those treated earlier and show a statistically significant advantage for the most recent patients (two-tailed analysis, method of Gehan (55)).

276

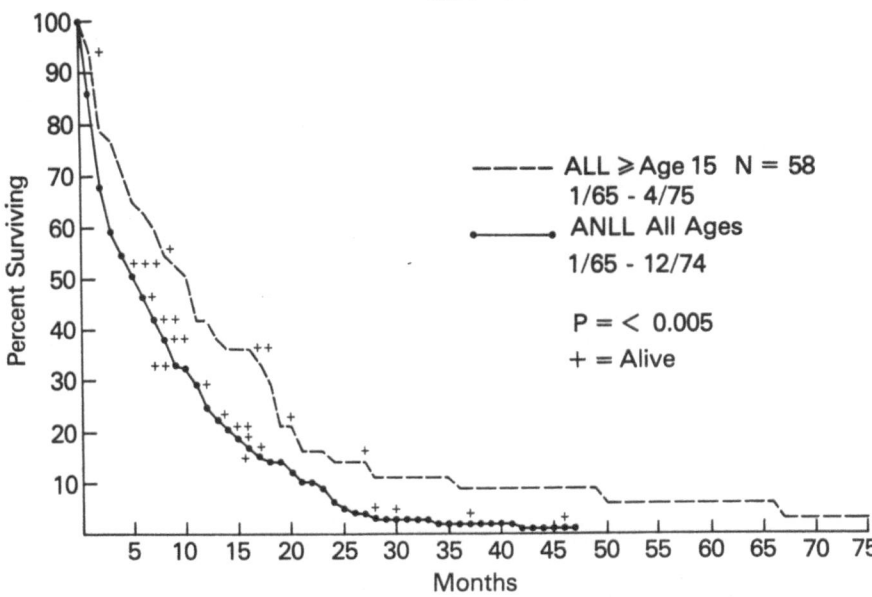

Fig. 3: Survival curves comparing all adult ALL patients with all ANLL patients (N = 276) treated at the BCRC since 1965. There is a highly significant advantage for the ALL patients (55).

In a recent study of induction therapy of adult ALL at the Baltimore Cancer Research Center 6-thioguanine, vincristine, dexamethasone and pyrimethamine were given in combination (31). Dexamethasone, a corticosteroid which increases the mobilization of granulocytes (32) was used for its potentially beneficial effect on infection in the induction period. Thioguanine, which has been shown to be as active as other purine antagonists in childhood ALL (33), was chosen instead of 6-mercaptopurine because its metabolism is not influenced by the concurrent administration of allopurinol. Pyrimethamine is a weak antifol that crosses the blood-brain barrier when given orally. The drug was reported to have activity against meningeal leukemia (34) and was studied in this regimen for its potential as a prophylactic meningeal leukemia agent. It has been clearly demonstrated in childhood ALL that prophylactic meningeal leukemia therapy significantly prolongs complete remission duration (26). In this study 53 % of adult patients achieved complete remission. However, severe infections occurred in more than half the patients and approximately one third developed meningeal leukemia. Thus, dexamethasone and pyrimethamine were not successful in this study. The median survival of all treated patients was more than 13 months, and complete responders had a median survival of 16+ months. These figures represent some improvement over earlier studies at this institution. Two recent investigations, one conducted

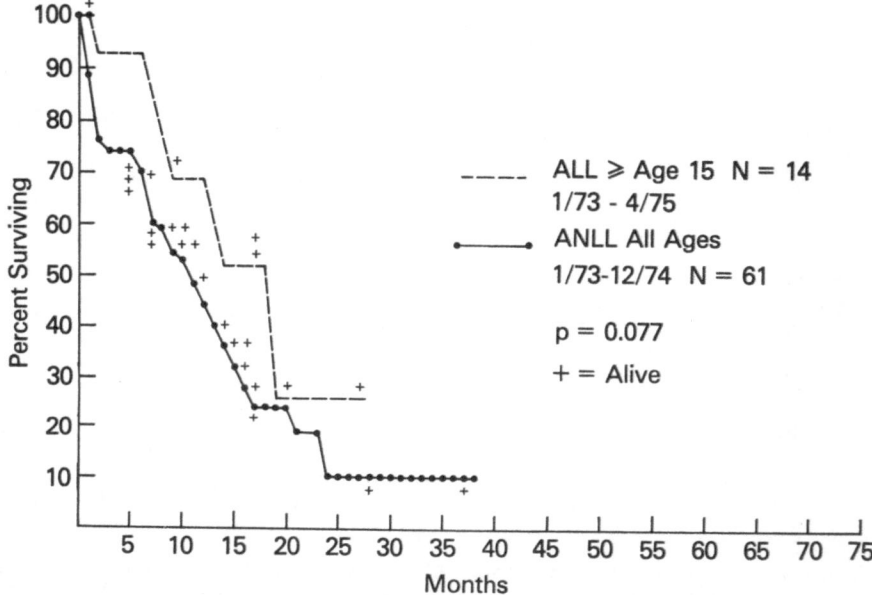

Fig. 4: Survival curves comparing the most recently completed study of therapy for ANLL with that for ALL at the BCRC. Significant improvement in the management of both diseases has lessened the heretofore significant survival difference between ALL and ANLL.

by Henderson for ALGB (29) and one reported by Capizzi, et al (35) are of special interest. In Henderson's study treatment with L-asparaginase for 10 days after several vincristine and prednisone courses has resulted in complete remission in 80 % of adults so treated. Based on kinetic data determined both in animal leukemia models and human lymphoblasts in vitro (36), Capizzi et al have studied asparaginase and methotrexate sequentially as induction therapy in previously treated adult ALL patients. Early results have indicated an 80 % complete response rate in such patients (35). It appears that asparaginase not only increases the sensitivity of leukemic cells to methotrexate by producing a rapid regrowth phase 9–10 days after asparaginase administration (36) but also that asparaginase diminishes methotrexate toxicity when given 24 hours after methotrexate. Marrow and mucous membrane toxicity were minimal in Capizzi's study but allergic reactions to asparaginase became a significant problem after several months of intermittent aspariginase treatment (35). Other data suggest that if an allergic reaction occurs with E-coli asparaginase patients can be safely treated subsequently with asparaginase prepared from Erwinia sp. (37). Capizzi, et al (35) have continued sequential methotrexate and asparaginase indefinitely during remission as maintenance therapy and have obtained a median duration of remission of approximately 1 year in previously treated patients. The Capizzi regimen obviously deserves a trial in previously untreated patients. A study recently initiated at the Baltimore Cancer Research Center for such patients incorporates the Capizzi regimen. In that study patients receive a 10 day induction course as follows: on day 1 methotrexate 100 mg/M² given rapidly IV., Vincristine 2 mg, is given on day 2 and asparaginase 500 IU/kg is given as a 30 minute infusion beginning 24 hours after the methotrexate injection. Dexamethasone 6 mg/M² p. o. is given daily for 10 days. Induction courses are repeated if necessary and methotrexate doses are augmented to tolerance in subsequent courses. Six courses of methotrexate followed by asparaginase in the above doses are given as consolidation therapy beginning with the onset of complete remission, with 10 days between courses. Following that therapy 12 monthly courses of vincristine, dexamethasone, high dose methotrexate (100 mg/kg) and citrovorum factor are planned. Therapeutic results are not yet available from this study. However, early experience with the induction regimen indicates that marrow and mucous membrane toxicity may occasionally be much more severe than that originally observed by Capizzi, et al.

The Blastic Phase of Chronic Myelocytic Leukemia (CML)

Most patients with CML die shortly after a blastic transformation of the disease occurs. After this transformation the disease takes on many of the characteristics of ANLL except for one important difference: while, as noted above, real progress has been made in the treatment of ANLL, the blast phase of CML is essentially refractory to all known antileukemic drugs. Recently, in a study of the Acute Leukemia Group B some benefit from the combination of vincristine, prednisone, hydroxyurea, and 6-mercaptopurine has been noted, with approximately one-third of patients showing a favorable response with few complete remissions (38). However, the median survival of all patients treated in that study (from the onset of treatment for the blastic phase) is still only approximately 4 months. This median survival is comparable to that of many other studies.

Several new drugs deserve critical evaluation in the blastic phase of CML because of their demonstrated antileukemic activity in that disease. Butocin, an ethyl ester derivative of buthiopurine synthesized by Semonsky in Prague (39) was reported by Cerny (40) to have a high degree of activity in the CML blast phase, with over 40 %of a small group of patients obtaining a complete or partial remission in a mean treatment time of approximately one month. The duration of maximal response varied from 10 to 37 weeks, and the total drug dose necessary to achieve maximal response varied from 219 to 2028 mg/kg. A large trial of this drug in the blastic phase of CML should have high priority in therapeutic research in CML.

Piperazinedione and VP16-213 are agents recently made available for clinical trial that have demonstrated some degree of activity in the blastic phase of CML, although the number of patients treated is small (41, 42). Further study of these drugs may be productive.

Supportive Care

Infectious Disease Considerations: Patients with acute leukemia are particularly predisposed to serious infection because of granulocytopenia caused by the disease and its therapy. Poor leukocyte function, and easy access of bacteria through oral or intestinal mucosal ulcerations often resulting from chemotherapy are contributing factors as are other iatrogenic provocations such as indwelling venous catheters. It seems clear from recent studies at the Baltimore Cancer Research Center that the major causes of serious infection in acute leukemia patients are hospital-acquired organisms (43). As an example of this problem, I cite the recent evidence associating aspergillus infections in leukemia patients with fire-proofing materials used in the construction of a new hospital (44). It is, therefore, critical to offer the patient maximal protection against the acquisition of potentially lethal pathogens while granulocytopenic. Ample evidence has now been gathered from a number of centers which strongly suggests that patients placed in a sterile air environment acquire fewer pathogens than control patients and have fewer significant infections. Such an environment is best provided by laminar air flow room reverse isolation units equipped with high-efficiency particulate air filters (45). The incidence of pneumonia in leukemia patients so treated has been reduced by 50 %. Since pneumonia is the most frequent infection observed in granulocytopenic leukemia patients who are hospitalized without the benefit of such specialized units, the importance of the unit is clear. The addition of orally administered non-absorbable antibiotics to this regimen may add a further measure of protection to the patient by sterilizing his gastrointestinal tract. Indeed high dose, frequently administered oral gentamicin, vancomycin, and nystatin has recently been shown to significantly reduce the frequency of gram-negative bacteremia even when used alone, without the laminar air flow isolation units (46).

Two significant disadvantages of laminar air flow rooms are their great expense and the permanent installation that they require. We have been evaluating simpler, less expensive, portable equipment that utilizes the same type of filter as the laminar air flow rooms (Med Assist Filters, Med-Assist Devices, Chestnut Hill, Mass.). Thus far 9 patients have been evaluated while undergoing treatment in regular hospital rooms equipped with the Med-Assist filter units. Surveillance cultures were regularly obtained from predetermined room and patient sites. Careful housekeeping routines and reverse isolation procedures were employed. The air filtration units were effective in markedly reducing the number of airborne organisms. The room never became contaminated by organisms brought into it initially by the patient, and only 2 of the 9 patients acquired any new organism while under treatment. Although this initial study was primarily designed to test environmental control by the Med-Assist filter units, it is also apparent that significant infections were reduced in this small group of patients and no pneumonias were observed (47). It therefore appears that the Med-Assist air filtration system can reduce airborne infection in granulocytopenic patients, and more studies are indicated to define the precise role of these units relative to standard laminar air flow rooms in the supportive care of granulocytopenic leukemia patients.

Although the measures discussed above have clearly served to reduce the incidence of serious infection in acute leukemia patients, infection is still the most frequent cause of death in patients with that disease. Many serious infections in granulocytopenic patients can be successfully resolved with early use of appropriate antibiotics. Since most infections in granulocytopenic patients are not accompanied by classic localizing signs such as abscess formation (48) it is imperative that the physician act quickly at the first observance of a fever of unexplained origin. To procrastinate often means death to the patient (49). The proper, proven reaction to such a fever is the institution of empiric, broad spectrum antibiotic therapy after blood, urine, sputum and rectal cultures have been obtained. The empiric therapy should include at least one antibiotic with significant activity against *Pseudomonas aeruginosa*, such as gentamicin or carbenicillin (50). In 24–48 hours, appropriate changes in antibiotic therapy can usually be made on the basis of culture results and clinical reassessment. Such practice is of proven life-saving value in the management of the febrile granulocytopenic leukemia patient.

Blood Component Therapy: There is no doubt that granulocyte transfusions have been on occasion life saving to the infected granulocytopenic leukemia patient (51), especially when large numbers of cells are transfused (52). Transfused granulocytes have been demonstrated to circulate and to localize in infected soft tissue, although they rarely result in a rise in the peripheral granulocyte count. Several devices have been developed for the procurement of granulocytes from normal donors and all utilize a differential centrifugation principle (53) or the ability of granulocytes to adhere to nylon fibers – a process that can be reversed by the lowering of the pH of the system (51). Granulocyte transfusion has gained widespread clinical acceptance in the last year or two.

It is generally accepted now that platelet concentrate transfusions administered prophylactically to markedly thrombocytopenic leukemia patients *prevent* bleeding, and that donor platelets HL-A matched to the recipient significantly delay the onset of platelet transfusion "resistance." This practice of prophylactic platelet transfusion has all but eliminated serious bleeding in leukemia patients so treated (54).

It should be clear from the foregoing summary that significant progress has been made in the management of adult patients with acute leukemia. It should also be clear that progress has been much less dramatic than that which has occurred in the management of children with ALL. However, new drug therapies currently under investigation, and new experimental modalities of therapy ("immuno" therapy) coupled with refinements in supportive care currently under evaluation may soon serve to more favorably alter prognosis for the adult patient with acute leukemia.

References

1. Wiernik, P. H., Serpick, A. A.: A randomized clinical trial of daunorubicin and a combination of prednisone, vincristine, 6-mercaptopurine, and methotrexate in adult acute non-lymphocytic leukemia. Cancer Res 32: 2033, 1972.
2. Greene, W., Huffman, D., Wiernik, P. H., et al: High dose daunorubicin therapy for acute nonlymphocytic leukemia: correlation of response and toxicity with pharmacokinetics and intracellular daunorubicin reductase activity. Cancer 30: 1419, 1973.

3. Steuart, C. D., Burke, P. J.: Cytidine deaminase and the development of resistance to arabinosyl cytosine. Nature New Biol 233: 109, 1971.
4. Wiernik, P. H., Glidewell, O. J., Holland, J. F.: Comparison of daunorubicin with cytosine arabinoside and thioguanine, and with a combination of all three drugs for induction therapy of previously untreated AML. Proc Amer Assn Cancer Res 16: 82, 1975.
5. Wiernik, P. H., Schimpff, S. C., Schiffer, C. A., et al: A randomized clinical comparison of daunorubicin alone with a combination of daunorubicin cytosine arabinoside, thioguanine and pyrimethamine for the treatment of acute nonlymphocytic leukemia. Cancer Treatment Rep 60: 41, 1976.
6. Bodey, G. P., Freireich, E. J., McCredie, K. B., et al: Late intensification chemotherapy for patients with acute leukemia in remission. Proc Amer Assn Cancer Res 14: 110, 1973.
7. Gutterman, J. V., Rodriguez, V., Mavligit, G., et al: Chemoimmunotherapy of adult acute leukemia. Prolongation of remission in myeloblastic leukemia with B.C.G. Lancet 2: 1405, 1974.
8. Cuttner, J., Holland, J. F., Bekesi, J. G., et al: Chemoimmunotherapy of acute myelocytic leukemia. Proc Amer Soc Clin Oncol 16: 264, 1975.
9. Bekesi, J. G., Holland, J. F., Yates, J. W., et al: Chemotherapy of acute myelocytic leukemia with neuraminidase treated allogenic leukemic cells. Proc Amer Assn Cancer Res 16: 121, 1975.
10. Wiernik, P. H.: "Spontaneous" regression of hematologic malignancy. Nat Cancer Inst Monogr, in press, 1976.
11. Manaster, J., Cowan, D. H., Curtis, J. E., et al: Remission maintenance of acute non-lymphoblastic leukemia with BCNU (NSC-409962) and cyclophosphamide (NSC-26271). Cancer Chemother Rep 59: 537, 1975.
12. Ellison, R. R., Holland, J. F., Weil, M., et al: Arabinosyl cytosine: a useful agent in the treatment of acute leukemia in adults. Blood 32: 507, 1968.
13. Masami, H., Akimitsu, M., Fujio, S., et al: Quadruple combination chemotherapy of acute leukemia using daunomycin, cytosine arabinoside, 6-mercaptopurine riboside and prednisone. Jap J Clin Hematol 13: 951, 1972.
14. Southwest Oncology Group: Cytarabine for acute leukemia in adults. Arch Int Med 133: 251, 1974.
15. McCredie, K. B., Bodey, G. P., Burgess, M. A., et al: The management of acute leuke. in adults. Proc 14th Ann Clin Conf, M. D. Anderson Hosp, in press, 1975.
16. Yates, J. W., Wallace, Jr. H. F., Ellison, R. R., et al: Cytosine arabinoside (NSC-63878) and daunorubicin (NSC-83142) therapy in acute nonlymphocytic leukemia. Cancer Chemother Rep 57: 485, 1973.
17. Brincker, H.: Treatment of acute myeloid leukemia with cytosine arabinoside and daunorubicin in combination. Scand J Haematol 9: 657, 1972.
18. Glucksberg, H., Buckner, C. D., Fefer, A., et al: Combination chemotherapy for acute non-lymphoblastic leukemia in adults. Cancer Chemother Rep 59: 1131, 1975.
19. Goodell, B., Leventhal, B., Henderson, E.: Cytosine arabinoside in acute granulocytic leukemia. Clin Pharmacol Ther 12: 599, 1971.
20. Armentrout, S. A., Burns, C. P.: Cytosine arabinoside as a single agent in the therapy of adult acute leukemia. Amer J Med Sci 268: 163, 1974.

21. Levi, J. A., Wiernik, P. H.: A comparative clinical trial of 5-azacytidine and guanazole in previously treated adults with acute nonlymphocytic leukemia. Cancer, in press, 1975.
22. Presant, C. A., Vietti, T., Valeriote, F.: Delayed dytotoxicity of 5-azacytidine (Aza C). Proc Amer Assn Cancer Res 16: 62, 1975.
23. Ho, M.: personal communication, 1975.
24. European Organization for Research on the Treatment of Cancer, Clinical Screening Group: Epipodophyllotoxin VP-16213 in treatment of acute leukemia, hematosarcomas, and solid tumors. Brit Med J 3: 199, 1973.
25. Kitajima, K., Kamimura, O., Hiraki, K.: Neocarcinostatin: A new chemotherapeutic approach to acute leukemia. Acta Haem Jap 37: 316, 1974.
26. Henderson, E. S.: Acute lymphoblastic leukemia, in Holland, J. F., Frei, E., eds: Cancer Medicine, Lea & Febiger, Phila 1973, pp. 1173–1199.
27. Jacquillat, C., Weil, M., Gemon, M., et al: Combination therapy in 130 patients with acute lymphoblastic leukemia (protocol 66 LA 66 – Paris) Cancer Res 33: 3278, 1973.
28. Henderson, E. S.: Combination chemotherapy of acute lymphocytic leukemia in childhood. Cancer Res 27:2570, 1967.
29. Henderson, E. S., Glidewell, O.: Combination therapy of adult patients with acute lymphocytic leukemia. Proc Amer Assn Cancer Res 15:407, 1974 and personal communication, 1975.
30. Shaw, M. T.: Successful induction therapy in adults with acute lymphocytic leukemia. Proc Amer Assn Cancer Res 16: 1031, 1975.
31. Smyth, A. C., Wiernik, P. H.: Combination chemotherapy of adult acute lymphocytic leukemia. Clin Pharmacol Ther 19: 240, 1976.
32. Peters, W., Holland, J. F., Senn, H. J., et al: Corticosteroid administration and localized leukocyte mobilization in man. N Engl J Med 286: 1972.
33. Ellison, R. R., Karnofsky, D., Burchenal, J. H.: Clinical evaluation of chloroquine and thioguanine. Proc Amer Assoc Cancer Res 2: 36, 1955.
34. Geils, G., Scott, C., Baugh, C., et al: Treatment of meningeal leukemia with pyrimethamine. Blood 38: 131, 1971.
35. Capizzi, R., Castro, O., et al: Treatment of acute lymphocytic leukemia (ALL) with intermittent high dose methotrexate and asparaginase. Proc Amer Assoc Cancer Res 15:793, 1974 and personal communication, 1975.
36. Capizzi, R.: Biochemical interaction between asparaginase and methotrexate in leukemia cells. Proc Amer Assoc Cancer Res 15: 308, 1974.
37. King, O. Y., Sutow, W. W.: Therapy with Erwinia L-asparaginase in children with acute leukemia after anaphylaxis to E. coli L-asparaginase. Cancer 33: 611, 1974.
38. Coleman, M.: personal communication, 1975.
39. Slavik, M.: personal communication, 1975.
40. Cerny, V.: Preliminary clinical trial with a purine analogue butocine. Neoplasma 18: 489, 1971.
41. Strauss, G. M., Slavik, M.: Piperazinedione (NSC-135758) Clinical Brochure. Investigational Drug Branch, Cancer Therapy Evaluation, Division of Cancer Treatment, National Cancer Institute (USA).
42. Wiernik, P. H.: unpublished observation.

43. Schimpff, S. C.: Diagnosis of infection in patients with cancer. Europ. J. Cancer 11: 529, 1975.
44. Aisner, J., Schimpff, S. C., Bennett, J. E. et al: Aspergillus infections in cancer patients: an association with fire-proofing materials in a new hospital. J Amer Med Assn 235: 411, 1976.
45. Schimpff, S. C., Greene, W. H., Young, V. M., et al: Infection prevention in acute nonlymphocytic leukemia. Laminar air flow room reverse isolation with oral, nonabsorbable antibiotic prophylaxis. Ann Int Med 82: 351, 1975.
46. Hahn, D., Schimpff, S. C., Fortner, C., et al: Changing spectrum of infection in acute leukemia patients receiving oral nonabsorbable antibiotic prophylaxis. Proc 15th Interscience Conf Antimicrob Agents and Chemother, Session 6, Wash., D.C., 1975.
47. Schimpff, S. C., Young, V. M.: Unpublished data.
48. Sickles, E. A., Greene, W. H., Wiernik, P. H.: Clinical presentation of infection in granulocytopenic patients. Arch Int Med 135: 715, 1975.
49. Wiernik, P. H.: Management of the acute leukemia patient. Conn Med 39: 681, 1975.
50. Greene, W. H., Schimpff, S. C., Young, V. M., et al: Empiric carbenecillin, gentamicin, and cephalothin therapy for presumed infection in patients with granulocytopenia and cancer. Ann Int Med 78: 825, 1973.
51. Schiffer, C. A., Buchholz, D. H., Aisner, J., et al: Clinical experience with transfusion of granulocytes obtained by continuous flow filtration leukopheresis. Amer J Med 58: 373, 1975.
52. Higby, D. J., Yates, J. W., Henderson, E. S., et al: Filtration leukopheresis for granulocyte transfusion therapy. New Engl J Med 292: 761, 1975.
53. Eyre, H. J., Goldstein, I. M., Perry, S., et al: Leukocyte transfusions: function of transfused granulocytes from donors with chronic myelogenous leukemia. Blood 36: 432, 1970.
54. Wiernik, P. H.: Advances in the management of acute nonlymphocytic leukemia. Arch Int Med, in press, 1976.
55. Gehan, E. A.: A generalized Wilcoxon test for comparing arbitrarily singly censored samples. Biometrika 52: 203, 1965.
56. Rai, K. R., Holland, J. F., Glidewell, O.: Improvement in remission induction therapy of acute myelocytic leukemia. Proc Amer Soc Clin Oncol 16: 265, 1975.

* Performed by Dr. Nicholas R. Bachur.
** Performed by Dr. Bruce Chabner.

Aids in the Management of Leukemia (Cellremoval by Continuous Flow Leukapheresis and Impulsecytophotometry)

P. Höcker, E. Pittermann, D. Lutz and A. Stacher

1st Med. Dept and the Ludwig-Boltzmann-Institute for Leukemia
Research and Hematologie
Hanusch-Krankenhaus, Vienna

During the last years the mechanical withdrawal of white blood cells (WBC) by a continuous flow cellseparator (CFC) was shown to be an effective method to treat chronic leukemias, especially in certain situations (1, 2, 3, 6, 7, 8). We want

Table I: Clinical datas of patients with CML and CLL submitted to leukapheresis

	NUMBER	FEMALE	MALE	AVERAGE AGE	LEUKOCYTES x 10³ /cmm	UNTREATED	PRETREATED
CML	20	9	11	51.05 (23-79)	228 (63-700)	17	3
CLL	12	8	4	67.3 (49-81)	267 (110-660)	6	6

Table II: Indication for leukapheresis in patients with CML and CLL

	CML	CLL
HIGH PERIPHERAL COUNT	11	2
INCIPIENT BLAST CRISIS	2	0
RESISTANCE AGAINST CYTOSTATICS	2	0
INCOMPATIBILITY OF CYTOSTATICS	2	4
INITIALTHERAPY	3	6
TOTAL	20	12

Table III: Results of leukapheresis therapy

	NUMBER OF LPH	MEAN DURATION OF A SINGLE PROCEDURE/HOURS	BLOOD VOLUME POSESSED PER PROCEDURE	LEUKOCYTE REDUCTION %	LEUKOCYTES REMOVED x 10^{11} PER PROCEDURE
CML	1o8	4,o3 1,5 -,5,2	7,95 2,7 - 11,8	56 21,6-88,4	3,o2 o,9 - 11,2
CLL	142	4,16 o,9 - 6,7	7,44 2,1 - 1o,2	77,o6 48,89-96,2	4,oo o,4 - 16,o7

to demonstrate our results obtained in 20 patients with CML and in 12 patients with CLL who underwent repeated leukapheresis using an AMINCO cellseparator.

The clinical datas were shown in tab. 1. The indication for leukapheresis was mainly high peripheral cell count with signs of hyperviscosity in some of the patients, resistance to cytostatic treatment or incompatibility of cytostatic drugs. Also untreated patients entered this study (tab. 2).

The results obtained by leukapheresis are shown in tab. 3. In all cases a quick decrease in the peripheral cell count could be obtained by a single serie of 3–4 subsequent procedures. The number of removed cells varied from $0,9 – 11,2 \times 10^{11}$ in cases of CML and from $0,4 – 16,7 \times 10^{11}$ in cases of CLL. A close relationship

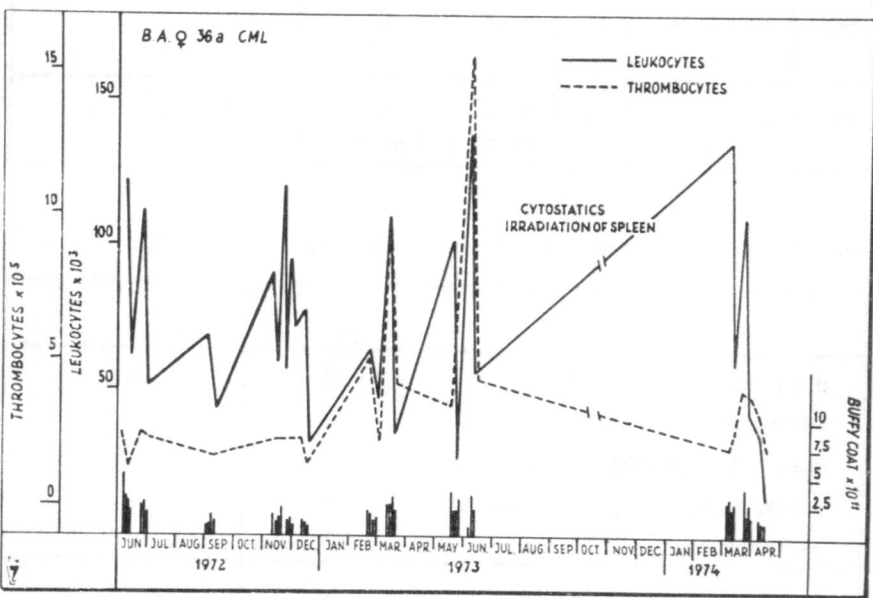

Fig. 1: Clinical course of a long time leukapheresis therapy in a patient with CML.

Table IV: Mean values of removed leukocytes in patients with CML and CLL with different pretreatment values

peripheral leukocyte count before Leucapheresis (10^3/mm^3)	CML			CLL		
	n	$\bar{x}$	s	n	$\bar{x}$	s
40 – 60	11	1,43	0,64	14	2.59	0.86
60 – 80	22	1.49	0.62	16	3.36	1.02
80 – 100	17	2.04	0.79	13	4.06	1.07
100 – 150	24	3.13	1.91	26	5.31	1.64
150 – 200	5	4.70	1.49	7	6.85	1.93

was seen between the initial cell count and the number of removed cells (tab. 4). The procedure itself was well tolerated and many of the patients were treated as out patients. One patient with CML was treated with 55 leukaphereses over a period of more than 2 years until her disease underwent malignant transforma-

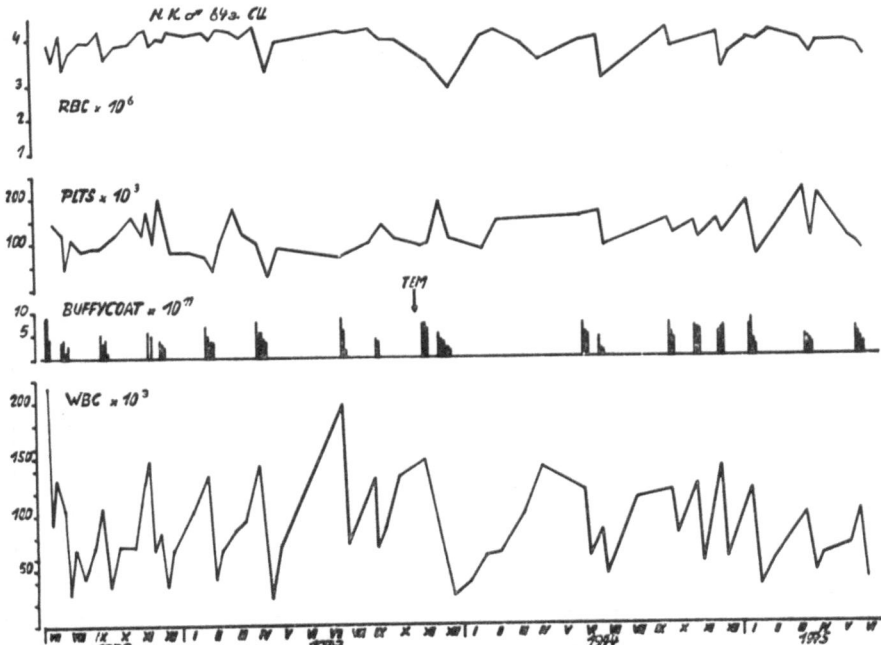

Fig. 2: Clinical course of a long time leukapheresis therapy in a patient with CLL.

287

Table V: Increase of the S and G_2+M fraction in the bone marrow and peripheral blood in a patient with CML after 4 subsequent leukaphereses

| K.R. ♂ CML | LI | DNA-histogram | | | Leuko | Enlarged | |
		G_1	S	G_2/M		Spleen	Liver
BLOOD	11.8%	60%	18%	22%	320000	+++	+
B.M.	4.5%	65%	17%	18%			
after 4 Leukaphereses (Cell separator)							
BLOOD	23.5%	51%	26%	23%	275000	++(+)	+
B.M.	13.6%	59%	21%	2o%			

tion (fig. 1). Another patient with CLL was also treated by 69 leukaphereses alone over a period of 3 years (fig. 2). This way a possibility is demonstrated to treat patients with chronic leukemia over a longer period of time without using any cytostatic drugs.

Kinetic studies were done by autoradiography and impulsecytophotometry in 6 cases of CML during a serie of 4 leukaphereses. Only in one case a slight increase of the S and G_2/M fraction was observed after the serie (tab. 5). This

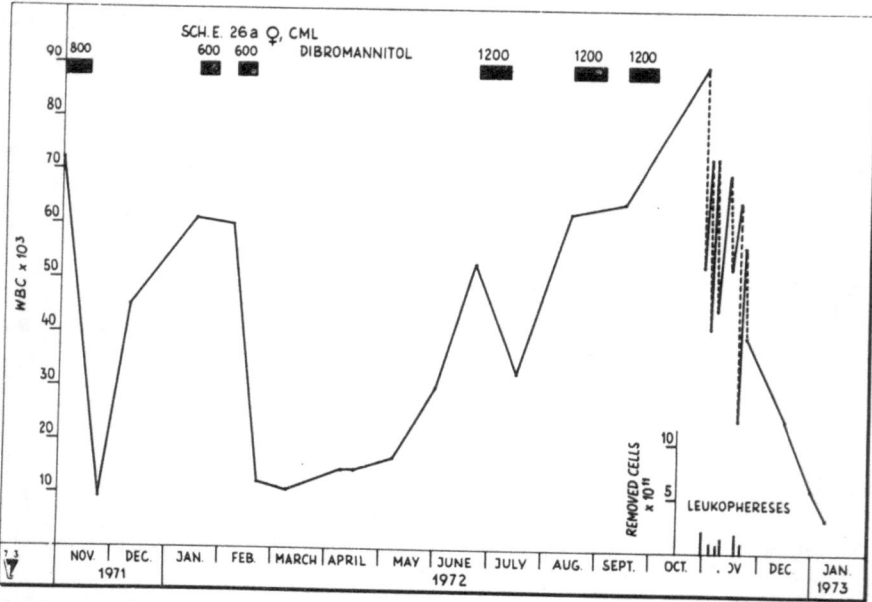

Fig. 3: Repeated leukapheresis in a patient with CML who developed resistance to dibromannitol.

Table VI: Loss of blood cells during leukapheresis

NUMBER OF LEUKAPHERESIS	LOSS OF PLATELETS %	LOSS OF ERYTHROCYTES %
67	28,57	4,98

Table VII: Side effects of leukapheresis

LOSS OF ERYTHROCYTES

LOSS OF THROMBOCYTES

HYPOVOLUMINIA

ANAPHYLACTOID REACTION CAUSED BY PLASMAEXPANDER

INCOMPATIBILITY AGAINST PROTAMIN

LOCAL THROMBOPHLEBITIS

proves that proliferation of leukemic cells is probably not enhanced by mechanical cellremoval. However, in one case of resistance to dibromannitol a good response to the same drug was seen after 6 leukaphereses had been performed (fig. 3).

In patients with CLL leukapheresis led to an increased blastic transformation rate and in some cases changes in the cytochemical findings were seen (4). Side effects were mainly the loss of platelets and the loss of erythrocytes which in some cases required a transfusion of packed red cells (tab. 6). Therefore patients with platelet counts below 20.000/cmm were not treated by leukapheresis. Sometimes anaphylactoid reactions to dextran and protamin were seen as well as local thombophlebitis (5) (tab. 7). According to our experience with leukaphereses by CFC in the treatment of chronic leukemias the following points might be taken into consideration (tab. 8). Leukapheresis is an expensive, time and personal consuming procedure which is accompanied by a loss of erythrocytes and platelets and which does not influence the basic disease. The benefits of the procedure are: it is well tolerated and side effects such as hyperuricemia and bone marrow aplasia

Table VIII:

DISADVANTAGES	ADVANTAGES OF LEUKAPHERESIS
EXPENSIVE PROCEDURE	WELL TOLERATED
LOSS OF ERYTHROCYTES	MINIMAL SIDE EFFECTS
BASIC DISEASE IS NOT INFLUENCED	NO BONE MARROW TOXICITY

Table IX: Indication for leukapheresis

A) HIGH PERIPHERAL CELL COUNTS WITH CLINICAL SYMPTOMS, WHICH REQUIRES BRISK CELL REDUKTION.

(INCREASED BLOOD VISCOSITY)

B) RESISTANCE AGAINST CYTOSTATICS

C) INCOMPATIBILITY OF CYTOSTATICS

D) PREGNANCY

are absent. It has also to be mentioned that large amounts of granulocytes can be obtained of patients with CML, wich permits granulocyte transfusions in leuko-penic patients. Leukapheresis should therefore be used in patients with a high peripheral cell count which requires a brisk cell reduction as well as in cases of resistance to cytostatic drugs and in cases of inability to use irradiation or cyto-static treatment, f. i. in pregnancy (tab. 9).

Since most cytostatic agents currently used in the treatment of acute leukemia are strongly cell cycle dependent, their cytotoxic effect correlates with the pro-liferation rate of a certain cell population. The proliferation kinetics of leukemic cells vary from one case to another, therefore the effect of the same kind of leukemia can be different. Also the proliferation pattern of a leukemic population is often changed after the application of cytostatic drugs. Therefore the knowledge of the proliferative parameters of a leukemic cell population might help to predict the response to a certain drug. The possibility presented by the flow system anal-ysis of impulsecytophotometry to obtain within a short time useful informations about the proliferative state of a given cell suspension is a considerable contri-bution to the cytostatic treatment of leukemic patients.

Blood and bone marrow samples are fixed with ethanol and stained with ethidium bromide. Ethidium bromide is a fluorescent dye which binds quantitatively the double stranded nucleic acids. The amount of ehtidium bromide bound per cell corresponds with the DNA content of each cell. Since the DNA content of a cell is a characteristic parameter in each phase of the cell cycle, it represents a good marker for determining the cellular proliferation kinetics. By this flow

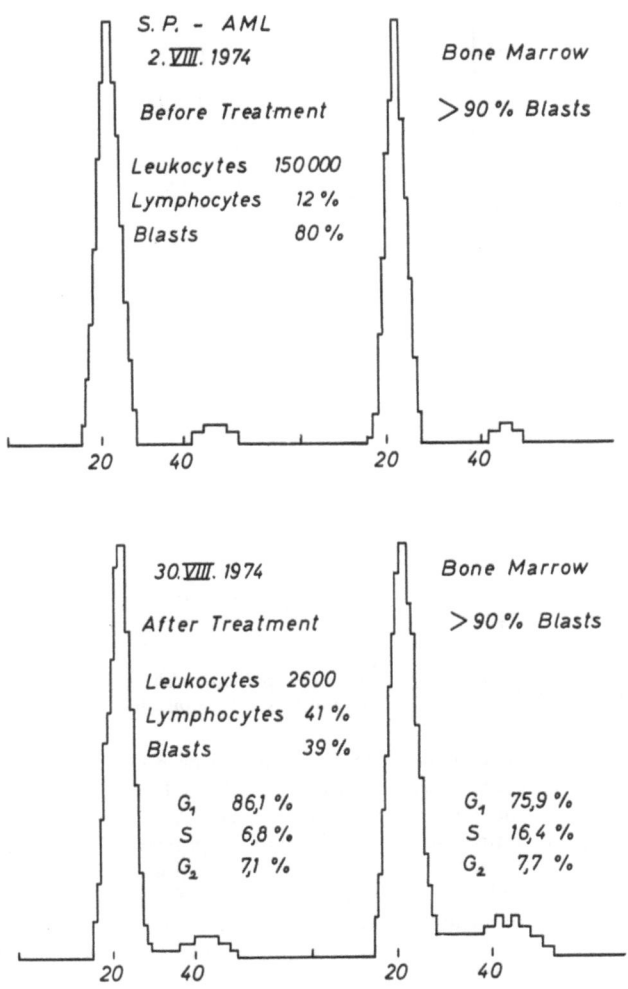

Fig. 4: Low proliferation activity of leukemic cells in a patient with AL, unchanged despite of the application of several cytotoxic drugs.

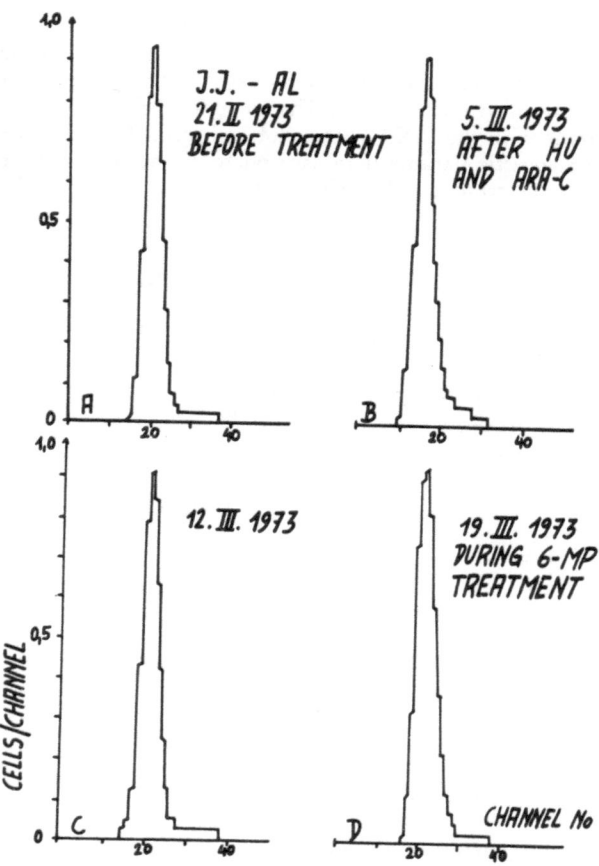

Fig. 5: Increase of proliferation activity in a patient with AL after 3 courses with Adriamycine and ARA-C, followed by a complete remission after two further courses.

system 50,000 to 100,000 cells in suspension are measured and each cell is recorded in a multichannel analyzer according to its ethidium bromide impulse intensity which corresponds to the DNA content of each cell. Such a measurement results in a DNA histogram representing the distribution pattern of measured cells according to their DNA content. The planimetric evaluation of the DNA histograms indicates the percentage of cells in the different phases of the cell cycle.

Using this method for measuring the proliferation pattern of peripheral blood and bone marrow cells in leukemic patients, the following observations were done:

1.) Patients suffering from acute leukemia with no changes in the blood and bone marrow histogram before and during therapy did not respond to various cytostatic drugs and had a bad outcome (fig. 4). This is in accordance with other informations in which the prognosis was better when the labelling index of the

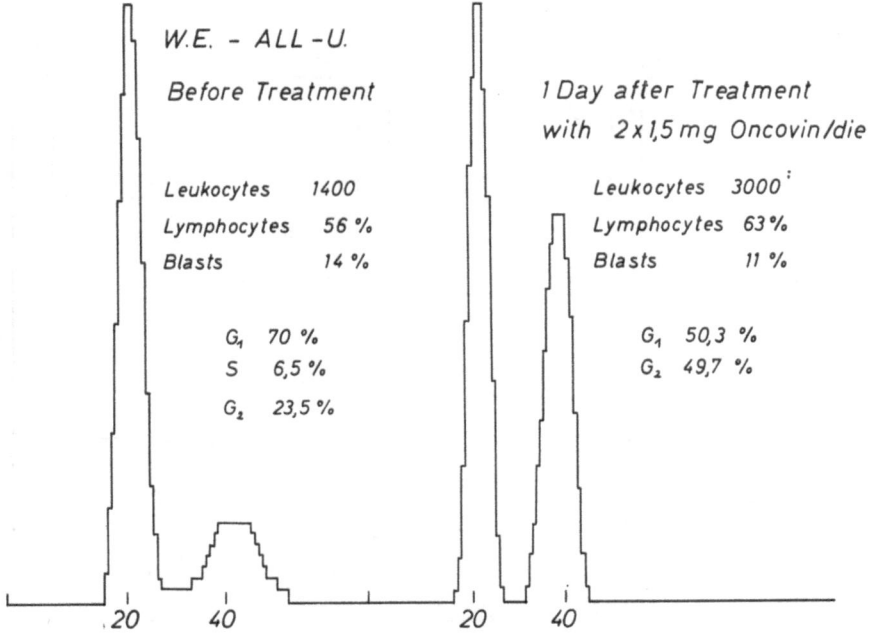

Fig. 6: Increase of the G₂ + M fraction after the application of vincristine.

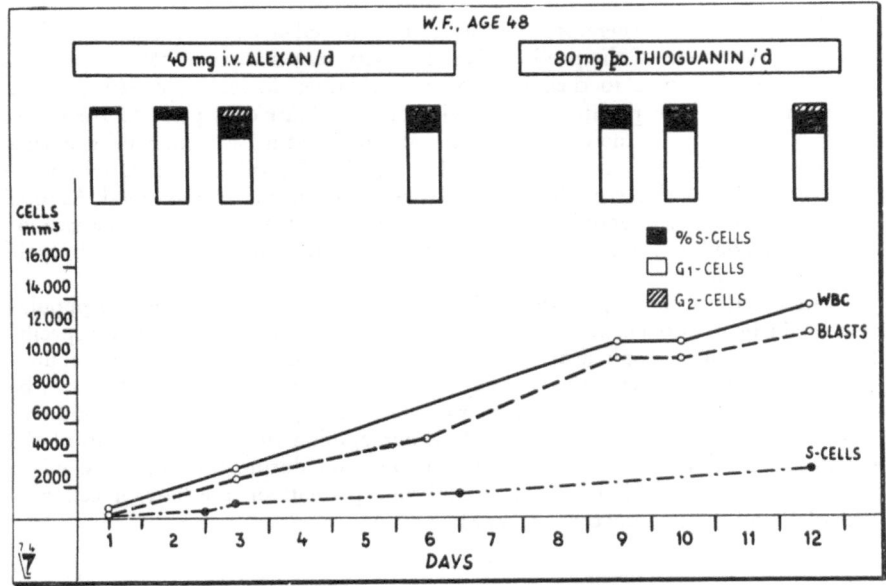

Fig. 7: Effect of a low dosage of thioguanine following to ARA-C Application leading to an increase of blastcells in the peripheral count and unchanged proliferation activity.

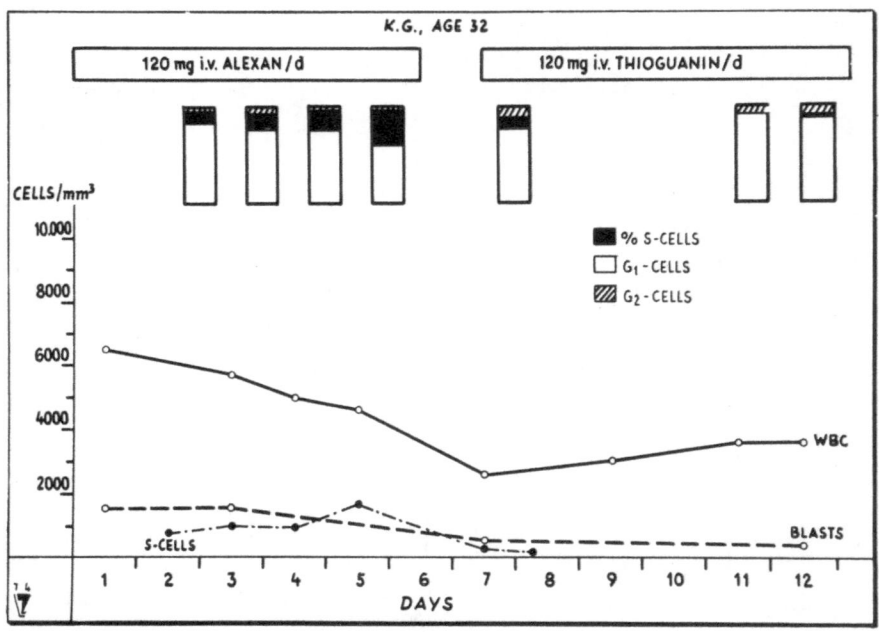

Fig. 8: Effect of high dosage of thioguanine following to ARA-C application leading to a decrease of blastcells in the peripheral count.

blood was increased. Therefore the success of any cell dependent drug should be related to the extent of the proliferative reactivity of a malignant cell population.

2.) A good response to chemotherapy was obtained in leukemic patients who either showed a high proliferative activity of their blast cells prior to treatment or who exhibited an increasing amount of proliferating leukemic cells during cytostatic therapy. In most cases such changes of the proliferation pattern were observed in the bone marrow histograms as well as in the peripheral blood. As soon as a high proliferative activity of leukemic blast cells was reached during chemotherapy, a good response was obtained by the cytotoxic treatment with cycle specific drugs (fig. 5).

Therefore the follow up of the proliferative activity of a leukemic cell population might be of prognostic importance. 4.) Cytokinetic changes which are specific for the action of an applied drug can be measured easily and rapidly by impulse-cytophotometry. This way the response of leukemic cells to a certain drug can be observed in each leukemic patient, so that individual changes of the chemotherapeutic treatment are possible (fig. 6). It is our opinion that the follow up of the proliferative activity of a leukemic cell population during chemotherapy might facilitate the individual treatment of leukemic patients on the base of cell proliferation and drug interaction (fig. 7, 8).

Acknowledgement: We are indepted to the late Federal President of Austria Dr. h. c. Franz Jonas for support of our work by means of his "Leukämieforschungsspende".
This research has been made by order of the Austrian Bundesministerium für Wissenschaft und Forschung.
Address of author: Dr. Paul Höcker, Ludwig Boltzmann-Institut für Leukämieforschung und Hämatologie, Hanusch Krankenhaus, Heinrich Collinstraße 30, 1140 Wien/Austria.

References:

1. Buckner, D., Graw, R. G., Robert, Jr., Eisel, J., Henderson, E. S. and Perry, S.: Leukapheresis by Continuous Flow Centrifugation (CFC) in Patients with Chronic Myelocytic Leukemia (CML). Blood *33*, 353 (1969).
2. Curtis, J. E., Hersh, E. M. and Freireich, E. J.: Leukapheresis Therapy of Chronic Lymphocytic Leukemia. Blood *39*, 163 (1972).
3. Hadlock, D. C., Mac Cullough, J. J., Deinard, A., Kennedy, B. J. and Fortuny, I. E.: Role of Continuous – Flow – Centrifugation (CFC) Leukapheresis in the Menagement of Chronic Myelogenous Leukemia (CML). Int. Congress about Cancer, Florenz 1974, p. 514 (Abstract).
4. Höcker, P., B. Haist, M. Goberts und A. Stacher: Die PHA-Stimulierung bei chronisch lymphatischen Leukämien vor und nach Leukapherese mit dem Zellseparator. 4. Arbeitstagung über Leukozytenkulturen "Lymphozytenfunktion in vitro", Innsbruck 1973 (Abstract).
5. P. Höcker, E. Pittermann, M. Goebets, A. Stacher: Treatment of patients with Chronic Myeloid Leukemia (CML) and Chronic Lymphocytic Leukemia (CLL) by Leukapheresis with a Continuous Flow Cell Separator. Int. Symp. on Leukocyte Separation and Transfusion, London, September 1974, in press.
6. Lowenthal, R. M. and Graubner, M.: Leukapheresis as Initial Therapy of chronic myeloid leukemia, In: 3. Int. Arbeitstagung "Proliferative Erkrankungen des myeloischen Systems" Wien, März 1975, in press.
7. Schwarzenberg, L., Mathe, G., Pouillant, P., Weiner, R., Locour, J., Genin, J., Schneider, M., de Vassal, F., Hayat, M., Amiel, J. L., Schlumberger J. R., Jasmin C. and Rosenfeld, C.: Hydroxyurea, Leukapheresis and Splenectomy in Chronic Myeloid Leukemia at the problastic phase. Brit. Med. J., *1*, 700 (1973).
8. Vallejos, C. S., Mac. Credie, K. B., Brittin, G. M. and Freireich, E. J.: Biological Effects of Repeated Leukapheresis of Patients with Chronic Myelogenous Leukemia. Blood, *42*, 925 (1973).

The Place of Immunological Methods of Treatment in the Management of Acute Leukaemia

R. L. Powles and J. A. Russell

Royal Marsden Hospital Blood Cell separator and
Immunotherapy
Unit Sutton, Surrey, U. K.

The development of the syngeneic animal system permitted tumour transplantation experiments to be conducted without interference from genetically determinaled antigens, and provided systems in which acquired 'neo-antigens' could be studied. Under carefully manipulated conditions several different immunological manouevres were shown to be capable of slowing the growth of tumours in experimental animals (see review, Alexander, 1974), and the two most promising methods that emerged which were applicable to man were non-specific stimulation of the immune system using agents such as B.C.G. (Halpern, et al 1959) and specific stimulation with tumour cells (Haddow and Alexander, 1964).

In all the animal experiments successful anti-tumour effects were only seen if the tumour load was very small. Leukaemia in man is therefore a particularly good model in which to test immunotherapy because patients in remission have undetectable numbers of cells remaining but if left untreated they ineviatably relapse. A prerequisite for active specific immunotherapy for leukaemia in man was the demonstration (see Powles review 1974a) using mixed cell cultures of surface components on human leukaemia cells which behaved like tumour specific transplantation antigens (T.S.T.A.'s). This provided a rationale for using killed leukaemia cells in addition to B.C.G. for immunotherapy in man. Thus, in the last ten years specific (killed tumour cells) and non-specific (B.C.G.) immunotherapy have been used in a number of controlled clinical trials in man.

The first comparative study was initiated by Mathé (Mathé, 1969), who selected a group of patients with A.L.L. who had been in remission for at least two years. For some all treatment stopped and the rest were given weekly Pasteur B.C.G., killed allogeneic A.L.L. cells, or both B.C.G. and cells. All 10 of the untreated patients relapsed within 130 days, whereas half of the 20 immunotherapy patients remained in remission for greater than 295 days, some of them for many years. The numbers were too small to decide which of the immunological regimes was best.

Several attempts have been made to confirm the value of B.C.G. alone in A.L.L. during remission. In Britain, the Medical Research Council arranged a trial (M.R.C. 1971) which compared the use of twice weekly Methotrexate with B.C.G. or no treatment. They found no benefit from the use of B.C.G. but it must be remembered that a different form of B.C.G. (i. e. Glaxo) was used. A similar study in the U.S.A. by Leukaemia Study Group A, (Heyn et al 1973) also failed to show benefit from B.C.G. More recently the Houston Group (Gutterman et al 1974) have used Pasteur B.C.G. for the maintenance of remission of all forms of adult leukaemia, and although they report benefit in A.M.L. (see below) there was no evidence that Pasteur B.C.G. prolonged remission in A.L.L. In the related disease Burkitt's Lymphoma, Ziegler (Ziegler and Magrath, 1974) used Pasteur B.C.G. given for a limited period by scarification and also found no therapeutic effect in maintaining remission in these children.

Table I: Bart's 2, 3, + 4 trial of maintenance chemotherapy versus maintenance chemotherapy plus immunotherapy.

Days	Proportion in remission		Proportion surviving*		Proportion Surviving after relapse	
	C**	C+I***	C	C+I	C	C+I
0	100	100	100	100	100	100
100	78	82	96	100	40	74
200	50	68	70	90	0	44
300	32	54	50	72	0	24
400	18	40	32	60	0	10
600	14	26	14	42	–	–
800	10	8	14	36	–	–
1000	10	4	10	14	–	–
No. pts.	22	28	22	28	20	27
No. Remaining	2	1	2	5	0	4
P. value**** difference C to C+I	N. S.		0.03		0.0005	

* From onset remission.
** C Chemo maintenance only.
*** C+I chemo plus immunotherapy maintenance.
**** Log rank non-parametric method (Peto and Peto, 1972).

At present, the place of immunotherapy for A.L.L. remains speculative since only Mathé has reported a therapeutic effect and no other study has done exactly as he did in giving Pasteur B.C.G. and cells. Whether it is at present necessary to use immunotherapy as a primary method of treatment for A.L.L. in the face of the outstanding results produced by intensive combination chemotherapy and prophylatic treatment of the central nervous system as developed by Pinkel and his colleagues (Simone, 1974) remains to be tested. Initially A L.L. was selected as the best disease to test immunotherapy because so few patients with Acute Myelognous Leukaemia A.M.L. obtained remission with chemotherapy and so it was impossible to conduct a trial. This situation, however, has changed.

A joint Barts Hospital/Marsden Hospital study (B. 2, 3, 4.) was started in

1970 to establish the effect of immunotherapy in the maintenance of patients with A.M.L. (Powles, et al 1973). This was a controlled trial in which all patients in remission were given 5 days maintenance chemotherapy every month for one year but a randomized group of these patients were also given weekly immunotherapy consisting of Glaxo B.C.G., administered percutaneously using a Heaf Gun, and allogeneic irradiated A.M.L. cells intradermally and subcutaneously in three other sites. Results, summarised in Table 1, show that remission length and overall survival was prolonged in those patients who received immunotherapy and there was also a very significant prolongation of survival of the immunotherapy patients after they relapsed. The mechanism of action is obscure because for technical reasons it has not been possible to measure the immune reaction of the host directed against the T.S.T.A. of A.M.L. although tests employing the mixed leucocyte reactions (Powles, et al, 1971) indicate that immunization with leukaemia cells increases the ability of A.M.L. patients to recognise their own leukaemia cells (which have been kept stored). Two possible mechanisms deserve consideration; the first is an increased immune reaction to T.S.T.A.'s produced by administration of cells which would account for the prolongation of first remission, but it is difficult to see how such a mechanism could be involved in the prolongation of survival after relapse. A second mechanism which could produce this latter effect is a non-specific stimulation of the bone marrow which permitted immunotherapy patients who had relapsed to tolerate the high doses of cytotoxic chemotherapy which were then required. Such an effect has been seen in animal systems (Wolmark et al 1974, Dimitrov et al 1975) and would be effective in man because patients who have relapsed usually die due to bone marrow failure.

An obvious question concerns the relative importance of the B.C.G. and cells and to answer this would require three arms to a trial, i. e. chemotherapy alone, chemotherapy plus B.C.G., and chemotherapy plus B.C.G. plus cells. This was not possible in the initial study because of the limited number of patients available.

Three other groups have documented the effects of giving various forms of immunotherapy to remission patients with A.M.L. and all described clinical benefit. The Manchester group (Freeman, et al, 1973) repeated exactly the sort of immunotherapy given in the Barts/Marsden study. Although their patients did well by contemporary standards they were not able to make this a controlled clinical trial due to the small number of patients available. This group did, however, comment on the ease of obtaining second remission in these patients and also remarked that survival after relapse appeared to be long.

The first report of B.C.G. alone as immunotherapy for maintaining patients with A.M.L. appeared last year from the U.S.A. (Vogler and Chan, 1974). They described the work of the South-East Co-operative Group for the study of leukaemia in which 41 patients in remission were treated with Methotrexate and 18 of these patients also received B.C.G. (Tice strain) twice weekly for 4 weeks. They noted in the initial follow-up period a significant prolongation of remission length in the immunotherapy group, but the use of Methotrexate alone to maintain remission only produced a remission length of 26 weeks which is inferior to recent chemotherapeutic programmes. It may be that this study, when it is completed, will show whether B.C.G. adds significantly to chemotherapy in prolonged remission. Another study involving the use of B.C.G. which was essentially similar to the Vogler report has been described by the Houston Group (Gutterman, et al 1974). In this they suggested that there was a distinct benefit to be obtained from the use of immunotherapy for maintaining A.M.L. patients in remission. However, criticism of the statistical analysis and data presented in this study (Peto and Galton, 1974) must lead to some reservations at present concerning the significance of its conclusions.

At the time the Barts/Marsden (B2, 3, and 4) study was commenced it was not ethical to have untreated remission patients with A.M.L. and so the only way to establish the controlled trial for immunotherapy was by giving them all maintenance chemotherapy. When the preliminary results of this trial suggested that immunotherapy might be of value, it was justified to test the effetcs of immunotherapy alone. Due to a need to obtain further information about methods of improving the drug regime to obtain remission in A.M.L., two new slightly different forms of induction chemotherapy were used (B.F.2, B.F.3) before starting the immunotherapy and so a direct comparison with the initial Barts/Marsden study (B234) was not possible. Table 2 shows the results obtained in such a group of

Table II: Remission duration and survival of patients receiving immunotherapy only for maintenance of remission. All patients receive weekly B.C.G., BF2 patients also receive weekly unirradiated cells, BF3* patients weekly irradiated cells.

Days	Proportion in remission		Proportion surviving	
	BF2	BF3	BF2	BF3
0	100	100	100	100
100	72	91	95	100
200	32	58	77	83
300	18	17	72	76
400	5	–	32	65
500	5	–	23	65
No. pts.	22	24	22	24
No. remaining	1	8	4	18

* BF3 was sequentially after BF2 so these patients have not had sufficient time to die.

patients with A.M.L. and it is important to point out that this was not a controlled trial. The immunotherapy was similar to that described in the B2, 3, and 4 study except that the cells had been both unirradiated (BF2). (Powles, 1974b) and irradiated (BF3) (Powles, 1973).

Although remission length in both groups of immunotherapy alone patients was shorter than those who had received immunotherapy plus chemotherapy, all three of these groups had similar overall survival and prolonged periods of survival after relapse. In this study there was no significant difference in results between the use of unirradiated and irradiated cells but more time must elapse before we can be definite about this because the two groups have been sequentially studied and B.F.3 has only been including patients for 1½ years.

Throughout the world there are now several other trials under way, the outcome of which should help identify the place of immunotherapy in A.M.L. As yet it is unclear whether intensive chemotherapy (Whitecar et al, 1972, Clarkson, 1972) is better for the patient than low dose intermittent chemotherapy and/or immunotherapy.

Some variations of the procedures just described are currently being studied clinically. There is experimental evidence to suggest that after sialic acid has been removed from tumour cell surfaces using neuraminidase they become more immunogenic (Currie and Bagshawe, 1968). A controlled trial is now under way for A.M.L. in which cells so treated are used for immunotherapy (Bekesi et al 1976).

Another approach is to use B.C.G. as a 'classical' adjuvant as has been tested with melanoma (Currie and Basham, 1974) and we are at present conducting a controlled trial using B.C.G. mixed with leukaemia cells for this purpose. In this study all patients receive weekly irradiated cells and B.C.G. as in the previous studies, but some of these patients also receive A.M.L. cells and B.C.G. mixed together intradermally during the first three months of remission. Preliminary results (Table 3) suggest there is no difference between these two groups for

Table III: Proportion of patients of two groups remaining in remission at various durations after starting weekly immunotherapy. In one group cells and B.C.G. are mixed together, in the other they are given at different sites

Days	Proportion in remission	
	Cells + B.C.G. (separate sites)	Cells + B.C.G. (mixed)
0	100	100
50	91	100
100	85	100
150	69	70
200	30	58
250	9	44
300	–	29
Total number	11	13
No. in remission (Sept. 75)	5	3

remission duration, but it is too early to examine the survival data. The possibility of treating patients whilst they still have detectable disease is also being explored and a preliminary study at Bart's (Hamilton-Fairley, 1975) indicates that this form of immunotherapy may help to obtain remission in patients who do not respond completely to induction chemotherapy.

There are three entirely new approaches which might soon deserve consideration in clinical studies. Specific xenogeneic antisera are now available for acute leukaemia cells (Mohanakumar et al 1974, Greaves et al, 1975) and although this has immediate application for monitoring the disease process, the possibility of using such materials for passive serotherapy should be considered as their specificity would overcome many of the problems previously encountered with such methods. Another recent development has been the isolation in human leukaemia cells of R.N.A. sequences (Gallo et al, 1974, Spiegelman et al, 1974), which appear to have a common identity with Simian R.N.A. virus particles. Once the relevance of these observations to pathogenesis has been established the possibility of an immunological (and chemotherapeutic) approach to their presence could be considered.

Finally, in a rat leukaemia model, Thymosin – a hormone extracted from the Thymus – has been found effective in bringing about total remission (Khaw and Rule, 1973) and when this material becomes available in larger quantities the possibility of clinical evaluation may not then be too distant.

Acknowledgements

We wish to thank the Leukaemia Research Fund of Great Britain for financing this research.

References

Alexander, P., (1974) Immunotherapy of Malignant Disease. In Handbuch der allgemeinen Pathologie. (Ed von H. W. Altmann) p 711. Springer-Verlag Berlin, Heidelberg, New York.

Bekesi, T. Roboz, T. P. and Holland, J. (1976) Therapeutic effectiveness of Neuromidase treated Tumour Cells as Immunogen in man and experimental animals with Leukaemia. Proc Nat, Acad. Sci. (In the press)

Clarkson, B. D., (1972) Acute Myelocytic Leukaemia in Adults. Cancer, N.Y. 6., 1572.

Currie, G. A., and Bagshawe, K. D., (1968) The role of Sialic Acid in Antigenic Expression: further studies of the Landschütz Ascites Tumour. British Journal of Cancer 22. 843.

Currie, G. A., and Basham, C. (1972) Serum Mediated Inhibition of the Immunological Reactions of the Patient to his own Tumour: A Possible Role for Circulating Antigens. British Journal of Cancer. 26. 427.

Dimitrov, N. V., Andre, S., Eliopoulos, G., and Halpern, B., (1975) Effect of Corynebacterium Parvum on Bone Marrow Cultures (38557). Proceedings of the Society for Experimental Biology and Medicine 148. 440.

Freeman, C. B., Harris, R., Geary, C. G., Leyland, M. J., Maciver, J. E., and Delamore, I. W., (1973) Active Immunotherapy used alone for Maintenance of Patients with Acute Myeloid Leukaemia. British Medical Journal. 4. 571.

Gallo, R. C., Gallagher, R. E., Sarngadharan, M. G., Sarin, P., Reitz, M., Miller, N., and Gillespie, D. H., (1974) The Evidence for Involvement of Type C, RNA Viruses in Human Adult Leukaemia. Cancer Vol. 34 No. 4 October Supplement p. 1398.

Greaves, M. S., Brown, G., Rapson, N. T., and Lister, T. A., (1975) Antisera to Acute Lymphoblastic Leukaemia Cells. Journal of Clinical Immunology and Immunopathology 4. 67.

Gutterman, J. U., Hersh, E. M., Rodriguez, V., McCredie, K. B., Mavligit, G.,

Reed, R., Burgess, M. A., Smith, T., Gehan, E., Bodey, G. P., and Freireich, E. J., (1974) Chemotherapy of Adult Acute Leukaemia. Prolongation of Remission in Myeloblastic Leukaemia with B.C.G. The Lancet 4. 1405.

Haddow, A., Alexander, P., (1964) An Immunological Method of Increasing the Sensivity of Primary Sarcomas to Local Irradiation with X-rays. Lancet, I, 452.

Halpern, B. N., Biozzi, G., Stiffel, G., and Mouton, D., (1959) Effet de la stimulation du systeme reticulo-endothelial par l'inoculation du bacille de Calmette-Guerin sur le developpement d'epithelioma atypique t-8 de Guerin chez le rat. Comptes Rendus des Semces de la Societe de Biologies et de Ses Filiales. 153. 919.

Hamilton-Fairley, G., (1975) Immunotherapy in the Management of Leukaemia. Proceedings of the International Society of Haematology; 3rd European and African Division. In the Press.

Heyn, R., Borges, W., Joo, P., Karon, M., Nesbit, M., Shore, N., Breslow, N., Weiner, J., and Hammond, D., (1973) B.C.G. in the Treatment of Acute Lymphocytic Leukaemia (A.L.L.). Proceedings of the American Association of Cancer Research, 14. 45.

Khaw, B. A., and Rule, A. H., (1973) Immunotherapy of the Dunning Leukaemia with Thymic Extract. British Journal of Cancer, 28. 288.

Mathe, G., (1969) Approaches to the Immunological Treatment of Cancer in Man. British Medical Journal. 4. 7.

Mohanakumar, T., Metzgar, R. S., and Miller, D. S., (1974) Human Leukaemia Cell Antigens, Serological Characterizations with Xenogeneic Antisera. Journal of the National Cancer Institute. 52. 1435.

M.R.C. Report on the Treatment of Acute Lymphoblastic Leukaemia (1971) British Medical Journal. 4. 189.

Peto, R., and Galton, D. A. G., (1975) Chemoimmunotherapy of Adult Leukaemia. Lancet 1. 454.

Peto, R., and Peto, J., (1972) Asympototically Efficient Rank Invariant Test Procedures. Journal of the Royal Statistical Society. Series A.2. In the Press.

Powles, R. L., Balchin, L. A., Hamilton Fairley, G., and Alexander, P., (1971) Recognition of Leukaemic Cells as Foreign Before and After Autoimmunization. British Medical Journal 1. 486.

Powles, R. L., (1973) Immunotherapy for Acute Myelogenous Leukaemia. Br. J. Cancer, 28. Suppl. I, 262.

Powles, R. L., Crowther, D., Bateman, C. J. T., Beard, M. E. J., McElwain, T. J., Russell, J., Lister, T. A., Whitehouse, J. M. A., Wrigley, P. F. M., Pike, M., Alexander, P., and Hamilton Fairley, G., (1973) Br. J. Cancer 28. 365.

Powles, R., (1974a) Tumour-Associated Antigens in Acute Leukaemia. In 'Advances in Acute Leukaemia' (Eds. F. J. Cleton, D. Crowther, and J. S. Malpas) p. 115 North-Holland American Elsevier.

Powles, R. L. (1974b) Immunotherapy for Acute Myelogenous Leukaemia. using irradiated and unirradiated leukaemia cells. Cancer. 34. 1558.

Simone, J., (1974) Acute Lymphocytic Leukaemia in Childhood. Seminar in Haematology XI. 25.

Spiegelman, S., Axel, R., Baxt, W., Kufe, D., and Schlom, J., (1974) Human Cancer and Animal Viral Oncology. Cancer. October Supplement. 34. 1406.

Vogler, W. R., and Chan, Y-K, (1974) Prolonging Remission in Myeloblastic Leukaemia by Tice-Strain Bacillus Calmette-Geierin. The Lancet. 2. 128.

Whitecar, J. P., Bodey, G. P., Freireich, E. J., McCredie, K. B., and Hart, J. S., (1972) Cyclophosphamide (NSC-26271) Vincristine (NSC-67574) Cytosine Arabinoside (NSC-63878) and Prednisone (NSC-10023) (COAP) Combination Chemotherapy for Acute Leukaemia in Adults. Cancer Chemotherapy. Reports. 56. 543.

Wolmark, N., Levine, M., and Fisher, B., (1974) The effect of a single and repeated administration of corynebacterium parvum on bone marrow macrophage colony production in normal mice. The Journal of the Reticuloendothelial Society. 16. 252.

Ziegler, J., and Magrath, I., (1973) B.C.G. immunotherapy in Burkitt's Lymphoma: Preliminary results of a randomised clinical trial. National Cancer Institute Monograph. No. 39. P. 199.

Perspectives and Prospectives in the Management of Acute Leukemia*

Edward S. Henderson, M. D.

Roswell Park Memorial Institute
666 Elm Street
Buffalo, New York 14263

The management of and outlook for patients with acute leukemia is strikingly different than it was 10 years ago. The introduction and refinement of empirically based combination chemotherapy in the early 1960's not only demonstrably improved the response and survival of acute leukemia victims, but equally stimulated basic scientists and clinicians alike to view this malady as an entity which could be cured within the foreseeable future. With this stimulus a remarkable amount of careful, and, often, inspired research has been conducted with the idea of better understanding and controlling this illness. In 1975, the task is not to stimulate interest in the pathogenesis and pathophysiology of leukemia, but to determine whether sufficient information is already available to consistently manage the disease, and, if so, how best to integrate current knowledge.

As with most illnesses, although progress has been made in parallel in the clinical and non-clinical spheres, and although clinical protocols have often been rationalized on the basis of pre-clinical studies, it is not clear that any therapeutic advance has directly and totally depended upon non-clinical observations. For example, the systematic determination of schedule dependency, independent mechanisms of action, and pharmacokinetics of individual drugs have provided models for and explanations of the increased effectiveness of drug combinations, but it is hard to imagine that without these studies individual drugs with anti-leukemic activity would not have been combined in much the same fashion as is the current practice without these ancillary investigations. Indeed historically many of the clinically most successful approaches were conceived and implemented before or concurrent with the non-clinical studies which provided their radionale. Furthermore, many unequivocal conclusions in animals cannot be (or at least as yet have not been) confirmed in man.

For example, studies in vitro of the scheduling of agents have suggested that a certain sequence of drug administration is optimal – and as a corollary, that the opposite sequence may be detrimental. Edelstein and his colleagues have shown that for greatest effect, cytosine arabinoside (ara-C) should preceed daunorubicin (DNR) (1), yet both Omura, et al (2) and Weil, et al. (3) have been unable to demonstrate such a difference in the clinical management of acute myelocytic

* Supported by USPHS grants CA-5834 and CA-2599 from the National Cancer Institute.

leukemia, while DNR for 3 days plus ara-C for 7 days (3 during, and 4 following) has been as good or better therapy as any evolved to date for this condition (4, 5).

Second, viral reinduction of leukemia has been documented in animals (6) and suggested in man (7), yet the few attempts at anti-virus therapy in patients with leukemia have either met with little or no success or clear evidence of failure (8, 9, 10).

This preamble is not intended as a criticism of basic pre-clinical research, but rather as an explanation of and introduction to the great dilemma of any conscientious clinician, namely when to abandon or modify effective modalities of management based on repeated laborious clinical observations, for new approaches of extreme intellectual attractiveness developed in a non-clinical setting. Such a consideration is most germane to a symposium such as this one, at which reports of significant recent advances in clinical chemotherapy, immunotherapy and combination modalities, empirically based and derivative are interspersed with reports of new insights and techniques of potentially revolutionary scope which have evolved peripheral to or in some cases exclusive of the clinicial arena. If, indeed, our clinical efforts had hitherto proved fruitless, it would be a simple matter to bear with those treatments we have, rather than flying to those we know not of. But clearly this is not our condition at present. Rather, therapy has made major strides in children during the last decade and in adults during the last 5 years. At every age, the most successful programs have been similar or identical (Table 1),

Table I: Remission Induction in acute leukemia*

Drugs	% Complete Remission	
	Adults	Children
Acute Lymphocytic Leukemia:		
Prednisone (P) + Vincristine (V)	50	88
P + Daunorubicin (D)		65
P + V + D	50–88	89–100
P + V + Asparaginase	74	87
P + V + Mercaptopurine + Methotrexate (POMP)	43–60	50–90
Acute Myelocytic Leukemia:		
Daunorubicin (D)	34	37
Cytosine Arabinoside (ara-C)	16–31	25
POMP	44	75
POMP/PVD	38	71
Ara-C + Thioguanine	35–36	43
Ara-C + D (5 days, 2 days)	43	56
Ara-C + D (7 days, 3 days)	77	–
Adriamycin + Ara-C + V + P	83	

* for references, and additional data, see reference 29.

although, in virtually all instances, age per se has proven to be the most critical determinant of response and survival. At the present time, perhaps 90 percent of children and 70 percent of adults with acute leukemia initially respond to optimal therapy, and up to 50 percent of children can be expected to survive, disease free, for 4 to 5 years or more following diagnosis. The long range effectiveness of treatment in adults is only now being assessed, but within the last 4 years the remission rates and median survival for both acute lymphocytic leukemia and acute myelocytic leukemia treated with the best available protocols has doubled, so that there is hope and optimism that the 2 % 5 year survival rates previously observed (Table 2) will be significantly increased.

Table II: Long term (≧ 5-Year) survival in acute leukemia in adults

Type	Number at Risk	Median Duration of Survival	Number Alive and Disease-Free for ≧ 5 Years
AML	97	5.5	3
ALL	40	8.5	0
TOTAL	137	6.5	3

What then are the clues from non-clinical research that may be so advantageously incorporated into future clinical management that we can abandon or significantly modify current practices? I can see only one at present, but several more are approaching the threshold of clinical experimentation. The available clinical modality is the use of non-cytocidal substances, chiefly bacteria or bacterial antigens, to stimulate natural immunity and/or hematopoiesis. This approach was spearheaded initially in acute lymphocytic leukemia (10), but has shown to more

Table III: Remission maintenance of acute myelocytic leukemia with chemotherapy ± immunotherapy (28)

Maintenance Treatment		No. of Patients	Median Months of Complete Remission
Chemotherapy	Immunotherapy		
OAP (V, P, Ara-C)	BCG	20	21
OAP (V, P, Ara-C)	None	33	11.5
Ara-C + D, Ara-C + TG	BCG + AML cells	23	11
Ara-C + D, Ara-C + TG	None	19	7
MT X ± (V + C)	BCG	22	11
MT X ± (V + C)	None	26	7.5
Ara-C + TG, Ara-C + D, Ara-C + C	Neuraminidase treated AML cells	7	16+
Ara-C + TG, Ara-C + D, Ara-C + C	None	10	5

consistent advantage as an adjuvant to chemotherapy in the remission maintenance phase of acute myelocytic leukemias (Table 3) (11, 12, 13, 14, 15). Dr. Raymond Powles, in this volume, has presented some of the difficulties in defining the mechanism(s) of action of this approach. What is clear is that first, use of the term "immunotherapy" for such approaches is at best premature and second, irrespective of the mode of action such explorations will and should continue both at the laboratory and clinical levels.

On the horizon shimmering with promise and backed by abundant data in animal models are the use of cell kinetics for drug selection, the exploitation of normal biological rhythms for drug scheduling, and the selection of drugs based on intracellular biochemical determinants of drug action. While clinical application of these approaches have been attempted in the past (16–19) with limited success, the obvious deficiencies in the methodology required for on-going studies may have abbrogated any striking clinical benefit. For example, most methods of determining intracellular DNA synthesis are either retrospective and limited to a few key determinations (e. g., radioautography) or are indirect and not specific for the most critical stem cell population (e. g., in vitro thymidine incorporation or spectrofluorometry). Recent progress in cell fractionation and real time analysis procedures, e. g., high-pressure liquid chromatography, should facilitate future studies in these areas.

The use of biological pharmacological stimuli to control cell replication and differentiation is perhaps the most intriguing new avenue for exploration. Without question both naturally produced and synthetic activities can induce strikingly quantitative and qualitative changes in both normal and malignant cell populations in vitro as amply reviewed in this symposium (20–24). How general is this phenomenon, and how effectively these activities can be isolated and successfully delivered to their cellular targets will determine the applicability of such an approach in vivo.

Evaluation of all modes of therapy present and future, would be greatly bolstered by the development of sensitive, specific assays of the extent of idsease involvement. Is initial therapy still appropriate? Must therapy be continued, and for how long? Do foci of leukemic cells (or leukemogenic agents) remain in the marrow, or in extramedullary sites such as the central nervous system or gonads? These are without question the most common questions asked by and of the leukemia therapist, and at present the answer is almost always "wait and see." The greatest frustration for the physician remains that only failure is established with certainty, while the greatest calamity of therapy is the injury or death of a patient through treatment which might not be necessary.

Unfortunatley no suitable asssay is currently available. Light microscopy is capable of assessing orders of magnitude of 10^9–10^{12} leukemic cells in a clinical setting although even within this range the specificity of morphological (and cytochemical) criteria are frequently suspect. Cytogenetic assays may occasionally extend this range, but are fraught with many technical and sampling variables not to mention the fact that approximately half of all leukemic cell lines go unrecognized with current karyotypic techniques. The production of muramidase, polyamines, uric acid, and lactic acid dehydrogenase are at present too non-specific and insensitive for clinical monitoring. For the above examples, and indeed for all other readily available tests, there is insufficient resolution to assess tumor extent or activity during the increasingly crucial period of complete remission.

There is reason to hope, however, that current research will shortly improve leukemic cell identification. Several of the most promising lines of investigation have been reviewed in this symposium. These include the development and utilization of antisera to leukemic cells, the identification of previously undescribed and possibly more specific metabolites of leukemia cells, and perhaps of greatest immediate value, the development of more rapid and precise techniques of cell separation, e. g., the fluorescence activated cell sorter. These separation techniques may well enhance the sensitivity of all leukemic cell identification procedures, both current, based on morphology, cytochemistry, and immunological characteristics and future, including the identification of oncorna virus footprints. The report in this volume by Greaves and co-workers (25) exemplifies the combination of a highly specific leukemia cell assay with sophisticated cell separation which should aid in clinical management and in the assessment of new treatments.

Finally, I would like to briefly summarize the observations made by my colleague at Roswell Park Memorial Institute, Dr. Alex Bloch, concerning the urinary excretion of cytidine 3', 5'-monophosphate (cyclic CMP). Dr. Bloch has recently identified not only this previously unrecognized cyclic nucleotide, but cytidyl cyclase as well, in murine leukemia L1210. In this model cyclic CMP stimulates rapid cell proliferation, shortening the lag phase of in vitro passaged L1210 from two hours to less than thirty minutes (26). Cyclic CMP is either in low concentration or absent in normal mouse tissues; however it becomes elevated in regenerating liver following partial hysterectomy. Based upon these observations, the urinary excretion of cyclic CMP was evaluated in 6 patients with active leukemia (2 ALL, 3 AML, and 1 CLL), whereas no cyclic CMP could be detected in individuals or pooled urines from normal urine samples, concentrations of 0.27 to 1.31 u moles were observed in the 24 hour urines collected from all leukemic patients (27). In the one patient studied serially, a fall in urine concentration of cyclic CMP paralleled the reduction of bone marrow and blood myeloblasts. Clearly this observation is most preliminary, and any further judgment must await the completion of the controlled assessments currently in progress. Nonetheless it is this type of non-invasive monitering which must be developed if therapeutic trials are to be safely and scientifically conducted.

In summary, the dilemma of the therapist is how far to pursue modifications of the empirical cytotoxic approach to leukemia therapy, and when and how to seek new avenues of leukemia control which have as yet no clinical substantiation. It is encouraging to note the continued interest and accomplishments of laboratory investigators in leukemia research, since despite remarkable progress during the last decade, leukemia remains incurable for the majority of those afflicted.

References

1. Edelstein, M., Vietti, T., and Valeriote, F.: Cancer Res. 34: 293, 1974.
2. Omura, G. A. Proc. AACR/ASCO 15: 266, 1975.
3. Weil, M., Jacquillat, C., and Bernard, J. Personal Communication.
4. Yates, J. W., Wallace, H. J., Ellison, R. R., and Holland, J. F. Cancer Chemother. Rep. 57: 485, 1973.

5. Rai, K. R., Holland, J. F., and Glidewell, O. Proc. AACR/ASCO 15: 265, 1975.
6. Skipper, H. E., Schabel, F. M., Jr., Trader, M. W. Cancer Chemother. Rep. 53: 345, 1969.
7. Fialkow, P. J., Thomas, E. D., Bryant, J. I., and Neiman, P. E. Lancet 1: 251, 1971.
8. Robinson, R. A., DeVita, V., Levy, H., Barron, S., Hubbard, S., and Levine, A. S., J. Natl. Cancer Inst., in press, 1976.
9. Mathe, G., Amiel, J. L., Schwarzenberg, L., Hayat, M., deVassal, F., Jasmin, C., Rosenfeld, C., Sakoohi, M., and Choay, J. Rev. Eur. Etud., Clin. Biol. 15: 671, 1970.
10. Mathe, G., Amiel, J. L., and Schwarzenberg, L. Rev. Eur. Etud. Clin. Biol. 16: 216, 1971.
11. Gutterman, J. V., Rodriguez, V., Maglavit, G., Burgess, M. A., Gehan, E., Hersh, E. M., McCredie, K. B., Reed, R., Smith, T., Bodey, G. P., Sr., and Freireich, E. J. Lancet 2: 1405, 1974.
12. Powles, R. L. These Proceedings.
13. Bekesi, J. G., Holland, J. F., Yates, J. W., Henderson, E., and Fleminger, R. Proc. AACR/ASCO 16: 121, 1975.
14. Vogler, W. R., and Chan, Y. K. Lancet 2: 128, 1974.
15. Weiss, D. W., Stupp, Y., Many, N., and Izak, G. Transplant. Proc. 7: 545, 1975.
16. Lampkin, B. C., McWilliams, N. B., and Mauer, A. M. Seminars in Hematol. 9: 211, 1972.
17. Klein, H. O., and Lennartz, K. J. Seminars in Hematology 11: 203, 1974.
18. Hall, T. C. NCI. Monograph 34: 145, 1971.
19. Halberg, F., Hans, E., Cardoso, S. S., Scheving, L. E., Kuhl, J. F. W., Shiotsuka, R., Rosene, G., Pauly, J. E., Runge, W., Spalding, J. F., Lee, J. K., and Good, R. A. Experientia 29: 909, 1973.
20. Till, J. E., Mak, T. W., Price, G. B., Senn J. S and McCulloch E A. These Proceedings.
21. Preisler, H. D. These Proceedings.
22. Iscove, N. N. and Sieber, F. (1975), Experimental Hematology, 3, 32.
23. Paul, G. These Proceedings.
24. Forget, B. G., Glass, J., and Housman, D. These Proceedings.
25. Greaves, M. F. These Proceedings.
26. Bloch, A. Biochem. Biol. Res. Com. 58: 652, 1974.
27. Bloch, A., Hromchak, R., and Henderson, E. S. Proc. AACR/ASCO 15: 91, 1975.
28. Henderson, E. S., in Hematology, 2nd edition, Williams, W. J., Beutler, E., Erslev, A. J., and Rundles, R. W., eds., McGraw-Hill, New York, 1976, in press.

Restricted Addition of Proviral DNA in Target Tissues of Chickens infected with Avian Myeloblastosis Virus

M. A. Baluda, M. Shoyab, M. Ali, P. D. Markham and
W. N. Drohan

University of California
Department of Microbiology & Immunology
Los Angeles, California USA 90024

Avian myeloblastosis virus (AMV) is an avian RNA tumor virus which can replicate in every cell from susceptible chickens but expresses its oncogenic effect only in specific target cells. In chickens, the BAI Strain A of AMV used in these studies gives rise to highly differentiated neoplasias, i. e., myeloblastic leukemia, chronic lymphoid leukemia, nephroblastoma and osteopetrosis. *In vitro*, AMV can transform cells from hematopoeitic tissues and from the Bursa of Fabricius (c. f. Baluda, 1962).

AMV, as all RNA tumor viruses do, replicates its RNA via a DNA template (v-DNA) (Temin, 1963, 1964; Bader, 1964, 1965; Baluda & Nayak, 1970; Baltimore, 1970; Temin & Mizutani, 1970). This was established by isolation of infectious DNA from virus transformed cells and by detection of viral specific DNA sequences in infected cells and of reverse transcriptase in virions (Baluda & Nayak, 1970; Baltimore, 1970; Temin & Mizutani, 1970; Hill & Hillova, 1971; Svoboda et al., 1972 Neiman, 1972; Shoyab et al., 1974). Furthermore, some strains of sarcoma viruses, avian and murine which do not contain active RNA directed DNA polymerases are noninfectious (Hanafusa & Hanafusa, 1971; May et al., 1972; Peebles et al., 1972). Due to the vertical transmission of endogenous proviral DNA, even apparently normal chicken cells contain DNA sequences which are complementary to the RNA of AMV (Baluda & Nayak, 1970; Baluda, 1972; Neiman, 1972; Shoyab et al., 1974 a, b, c; Shincariol et al., 1974; Varmus et al., 1972). After infection of chicken cells with an RNA tumor virus, the amount of viral specific sequences is increased due to the acquisition of qualitatively different virus specific sequences (Baluda, 1972 Shoyab et al., 1974 a, b). Addition of viral DNA after infection with avian oncornaviruses also takes place in mouse, rat or duck cells which do not contain DNA sequences homologous to the RNA of avian oncornaviruses (Baluda, 1972; Harel et al., 1972; Varmus et al., 1973; Shoyab et al., 1974; Shoyab et al., 1975).

Endogenous Viral DNA in Normal Chicken Cells. AMV RNA hybridizes with normal chicken DNA 50–65 % as much as with DNA from leukemic cells transformed by AMV (Baluda, 1972; Shoyab et al., 1974 a, b, c). We had postulated that hybridization between AMV RNA and normal chicken DNA might be due to homology between AMV RNA and the RAV-0 like endogenous virus genome.

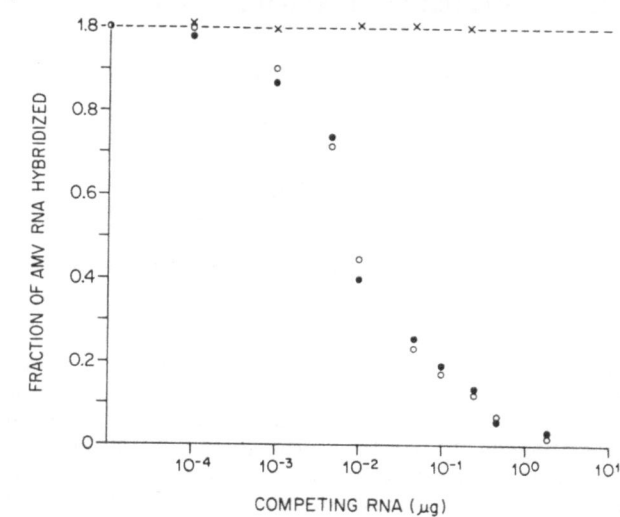

Fig. 1: Inhibition of hybridization between ³H-35S AMV RNA and normal chicken DNA by 35S RAV-0 RNA: The hybridization mixture contained 1.6 mg of sonicated DNA, 6 x 10⁻⁴ µg of ³H-labeled 35S viral RNA (specific activity: 1.9 x 10⁶ cpm per µg), 0–2 µg of unlabeled 35S viral RNA and 0.1 % SDS in 0.4 ml of 0.4M phosphate buffer pH 6.8. The hybridization mixture was placed in tightly silicone-stoppered tubes, boiled for 3 minutes in a water ethylene-glycol bath, quickly transferred to a water bath at 65 C and incubated for 64 h to reach a Cot of approximately 15,000 (concentration of nucleotides in moles per liter x time in seconds). The mixture was then diluted with cold water and processed to determine the fraction of ³H-labeled RNA which became RNase resistant. Viral RNA which hybridized with embryonic mouse DNA under similar conditions (6 %) was subtracted from the experimental values. The values obtained in the presence of yeast RNA but in the absence of unlabeled viral RNA were normalized to 100 percent and competition presented as percent of maximum hybridization.

    ○——○ Competition by 35S AMV RNA
    ●——● Competition by 35S RAV-0 RNA

That is the case as shown in Figure 1; 35S RNA from RAV-0 inhibited by 98 % hybrid formation between normal chicken DNA and 35S AMV RNA.

Similar conclusions are obtained with another competition hybridization technique (Table I). If normal chicken DNA is first hybridized with an excess of unlabeled 70S RAV-0 RNA, there is no subsequent hybridization with ³H-35S AMV RNA. If yeast RNA replaced RAV-0 RNA in the first hybridization, 288 cpm of AMV RNA hybridized with normal chicken DNA. Also, 70S RAV-0 RNA inhibits by 84 % hybridization between ³H-labeled 35S AMV RNA and DNA from leukemic chicken myeloblasts. This findings is in agreement with other work which shows that there is approximately 70 % homology between the genomes of RAV-0 and AMV. This was determined by RNA excess competition of DNA driven RNA-DNA hybridization. Hybridization between ³H-labeled 35S AMV RNA and

Table I: Filter hybridization of ^{3}H-35S AMV RNA with normal or leukemic chicken DNA with or without prehybridization with unlabeled 70S RAV-0 RNA

DNA	CPM Hybridized/100 µg DNA Prehybridized With:		
	Unlabeled 70S RAV-0 RNA (A)	Yeast RNA (B)	$\frac{A}{B}$
Normal Chicken Embryos	0	288 ± 5	0
Leukemic Chickens	97 ± 7	616 ± 8	0.16

Two hybridization vials were used. In the first vial, the hybridization mixture contained 10 µg/ml of 70S unlabeled RAV-0 RNA and .05 % SDS in 4 X SSC. In the second vial, yeast RNA replaced RAV-0 RNA. At the end of the first cycle of hybridization at 70 °C for 20 h, the filters were directly transferred to different vials containing 1.05 X 10^6 cpm of 35S ^{3}H-AMV RNA, 7.5 mg of yeast RNA in 1.5 ml of 4 X SSC plus 0.05 % SDS. After the second hybridization performed for 12 h at 70 °C, the filters were washed, treated with ribonucleases A and T$_1$ and processed as described earlier (Baluda & Nayak, 1970). Cpm bound to each mouse DNA filter (12 cpm when RAV-0 RNA was used as competitor or 21 cpm when cold yeast RNA was used in the first cycle of hybridization) were deducted from cpm hybridized to experimental filters.

DNA from leukemic chicken myeloblasts was inhibited 92 % by 2 µg per 0.4 ml of unlabeled 35S AMV, and 68 % by 2 µg of unlabeled 35S RAV-0 RNA. Conversely, hybridization between ^{3}H-labeled 35 S RAV-O RNA and leukemic chicken DNA was inhibited 96 % by unlabeled 35S RAV-0 RNA and 67 % by unlabeled 35S AMV RNA.

Appearance of Viral DNA After Infection of Chick Embryo Fibroblasts with Prague Strain of Rous Sarcoma Virus (PR-RSV) or Avian Myeloblastosis Virus (AMV). Proviral DNA is synthesized early after infection. This has been shown by hybridization of ^{3}H-labeled 70S AMV RNA with DNA from chick embryo fibroblasts (CEF) infected with either AMV or PR-RSV (Ali & Baluda, 1974). It was possible to separate v-DNA newly synthesized after infection from the endogenous viral DNA integrated into high molecular weight cellular DNA by the Hirt fractionation procedure. The fractionation of v-DNA into Hirt's supernate (low molecular weight DNA) and pellet (high molecular weight DNA) from cells infected with AMV at a high input multiplicity of infection showed an enrichment of viral DNA in the Hirt supernate as early as 1 h after infection. The synthesis of small molecular weight viral DNA continued for approximately 72 hours (Figure 2). Alkaline sucrose velocity sedimentation analysis of v-DNA in the Hirt supernate suggests that v-DNA is synthesized as molecules equivalent to copies of the 3 X 10^6 daltons viral RNA subunit. Lagging a few hours behind the increase in free v-DNA, there was an increase in the pellet (integrated) v-DNA until it reached a maximum approximately 72 hours after infection (Figure 2).

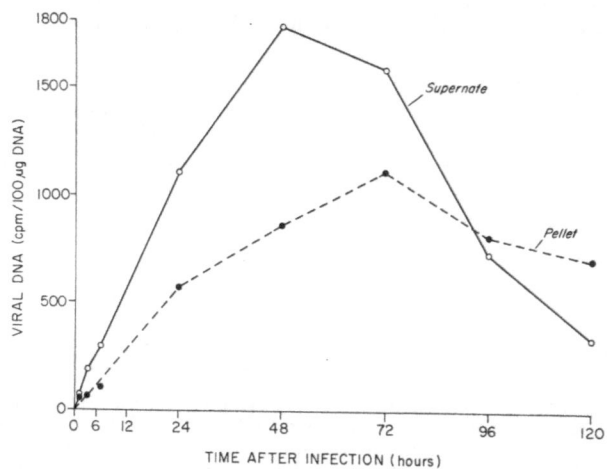

Fig. 2: Proviral DNA synthesis in cells infected with AMV or PR-RSV: CEF cultures were infected with AMV or PR-RSV at input multiplicities of 4 or more and were subjected to Hirt fractionation at various time intervals after infection. Hirt fractionation separates DNA of large molecular weight from DNA of small molecular weight. The cells were lysed in 0.6 % SDS, 0.01M Tris-HCl (pH 7.4) and 0.01M EDTA. The lysate was made 1M with NaCl, allowed to precipitate at 0 °C for 16 hours and centrifuged at 35,000 xg for 1 hour. DNA from supernate or pellet was then extracted, purified, denatured, immobilized on nitrocellulose filters and hybridized at 70 °C for 10 hours with ³H-labeled 70S AMV-RNA (10⁶ cpm per ml) in 4 x SSC containing 3 mg of mouse RNA per ml and 0.05 % SDS. After hybridization, the amount of DNA attached to each filter was determined by the Burton diphenylamine reaction.

Three to five filters were made with DNA from each fraction. ³H-AMV-RNA bound by mouse DNA filter was deducted from each experimental filter and the amount of ³H-AMV RNA hybridized per 100 µg of DNA was determined. The ³H AMV RNA hybridized to endogenous viral DNA in noninfected cells was deducted from the cpm hybridized at various time intervals for each fraction. Cpm in the Hirt supernate were also divided by the enrichment factor, i.e., ratio of DNA recovered in the pellet to that recovered in supernate calculated from the respective absorbancy at 260 mµ.

The newly synthesized viral DNA from the Hirt supernatant fraction was subjected to neutral cesium chloride-ethidium bromide density equilibrium sedimentation and 10–20 % of v-DNA sedimented at a density of 1.58–1.60 g/cc, demonstrating the existence of circular molecules. The presence of supercoiled circular molecules was also detected by velocity sedimentation in alkaline sucrose gradients. The free linear and circular viral DNA which is detected early after infection in oncornavirus infected avian cells appears to be synthesized for a short time only after infection, approximately 72 hours.

The sedimentation profiles of minimally sheared cellular DNA in alkaline sucrose velocity gradients suggest that v-DNA is synthesized as small molecules which subsequently are covalently linked to high molecular weight cellular DNA. Table II shows that 60 hours after infection of CEF with PR-RSV, 50 % of the newly synthesized v-DNA still appears as free molecules. By contrast, in leukemic

Table II: Alkaline sucrose velocity sedimentation of virus specific DNA isolated from CEF 60 hours after infection with PR-RSV

Fraction (range of sedimentation values)	DNA[a] per fraction (µg)	Cpm viral RNA hybrizided per 100 µg DNA[b]	Newly synthesized v-DNA %
(0– 18)S	24.8	3,273 ± 35	9.0
(18– 28)S	16.8	7,324 ± 621	27.6
(28– 40)S	14.4	5,331 ± 608	14.6
(40– 80)S	33.1	2,780 ± 380	6.8
(80–122)S	167.8	2,925 ± 232	42.1
Total DNA (uninfected)		2,133 ± 353	0
Total DNA (infected)		4,221 ± 373	

[3]H-labelled DNA from various fractions of the gradients was purified, denatured, immobilized on filters and hybridized with ^{32}P-labeled 70S AMV RNA in large excess.
a Determined from ^{3}H radioactivity before hybridization.
b Mean of 2–5 filters ± standard deviation. An average background of 131 cpm per filter of ^{32}P RNA hybridized to mouse DNA filters has been subtracted.

cells several weeks after infection, or in normal cells, 100 % of the v-DNA seems to be integrated (Markham & Baluda, 1973).

Integration of Oncornavirus DNA in Normal Chicken Cells and in Leukemic Cells Transformed by AMV. The integration of proviral DNA into host DNA had been postulated to explain the persistence of the viral genome in cells transformed by oncornaviruses (Bentvelzen et al., 1970; Temin, 1962, 1971). Also, genetic analysis suggested a close association between the cell genome and genetic information responsible for expression of virus specific products (c. f. Markham & Baluda, 1973).

The integration of v-DNA into normal chicken cell DNA and in leukemic myeloblasts transformed by AMV several weeks earlier was demonstrated by the formation of alkali stable bonds between v-DNA and nuclear cellular DNA of large molecular weight (Sambrook et al., 1968; Markham & Baluda, 1973). The sedimentation profile in alkaline sucrose gradients of minimally sheared DNA from leukemic myeloblasts transformed several weeks earlier showed that viral DNA sedimented with high molecular weight cellular DNA (Figure 3). There is no detectable free viral DNA. The presence of viral DNA in pools I and II is due to partial degradation of cellular DNA into fragments containing v-DNA, since the concentration of v-DNA per 100 µg of cellular DNA was similar in pools I, II, III and IV. If some v-DNA had existed in a free state of lower molecular weight, it would have become more concentrated in pools I and II since there was a 3-to-4-fold enrichment of smaller sized DNA in these pools as compared to pools III and IV.

The existence of v-DNA as supercoiled circular molecules of relatively small size with a high sedimentation coefficient, i. e., greater than 93S, can also be ruled

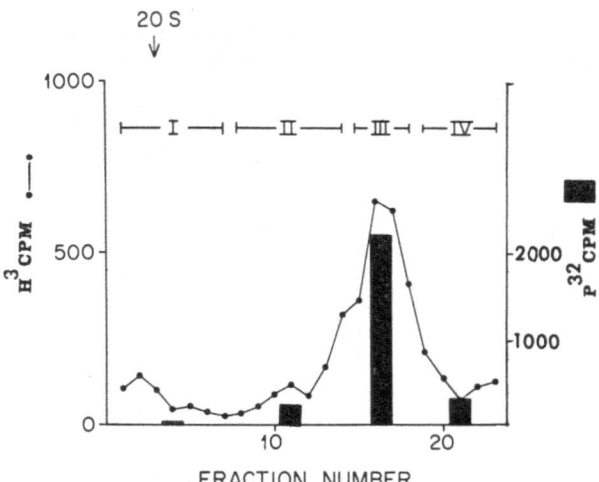

Fig. 3: Hybridization of ^{32}P-labeled 70S AMV RNA with ^{3}H-labeled DNA from cells fractionated by alkaline sucrose velocity sedimentation: Cultured leukemic cells were labeled for 8 h with ^{3}H-thymidine (2 µCi/ml), washed, and incubated in normal medium for an additional 16 h. Cells (2–3 x 10^6) were layered on the top of each alkaline sucrose gradient. The cells were lysed at 4 C for at least 12 h, then the gradients were centrifuged for 7 h at 22,000 rpm at 4 C in a Beckman SW-27 rotor. Fractions were collected from the top of each gradient by pumping 70 % sucrose into the bottom of the centrifuge tube. Samples from each fraction were precipitated with 5 % trichloroacetic acid, filtered, washed, dried, and counted in toluene scintillation fluid. Direction of sedimentation is from left to right. For each cell type, 72 gradients were run, and the DNA was pooled from 60 to 72 gradients according to specified sedimentation values and neutralized with 2 N HCl in 0.4M Tris, pH 7.4. Soluble yeast RNA was added as carrier (5 µg/ml), and the DNA was concentrated by ethanol precipitation, phenol extracted, treated with alkali (0.3 N KOH, 18 h at 37 C), dialyzed, denatured, and trapped on nitrocellulose membrane filters. DNA filters were hybridized with 1.2 x 10^6 counts per min per ml of ^{32}P 70S RNA (specific activity, 5.4 x 10^5 counts per min per µg). The histograms represent cpm of ^{32}P-70S AMV RNA hybridized to each pool of DNA with specified sedimentation values.

out. After neutral cesium chloride-ethidium bromide density equilibrium sedimentation, all the viral DNA was present as linear, double-stranded DNA not separable from linear chicken DNA. In addition, after extraction by Hirt's procedure, the viral DNA precipitated with high molecular weight cellular DNA. Similar results were obtained for endogenous v-DNA in normal chicken cells showing that all the endogenous v-DNA is integrated in nuclear cellular DNA of large molecular weight (Markham & Baluda, 1973).

Integration may be a great advantage for RNA tumor viruses since the DNA provirus becomes part of the cellular genome and stability of infection is insured (Temin, 1971). Also, since the viral information has an RNA phase, activation of viral replication can occur without excision of the integrated viral DNA. Oncornaviruses, therefore, avoid the need for many complicated regulatory mechanisms to control DNA replication, transcription and excision such as those required by temperate phages (Borek & Ryan, 1973; Echols, 1971).

Table III: Filter hybridization of 35S [³H] AMV RNA with DNA from various tissues of normal and leukemic chickens[a]

	CPM Hybridized per 100 µg DNA[b] from								
	Brain	Thigh Muscle	Heart	Liver	Lung	Spleen	Kidney	RBC	Leukemic Myeloblasts
Normal Chickens	1415±78	1249±99	1049±25	1221±105	1209±67	1123±68	1232±57	1201±93	2810±134
Leukemic Chickens	1286±60	1335±108	2038±110	1831±112	1903±70	1662±84	3374±394	2820±240	

a. Various tissues from 12 normal and from 12 leukemic 3–5 week old chickens were removed and pooled. DNA was isolated, purified, trapped on nitrocellulose filters and hybridized for 10 h at 70 °C. Five filters were hybridized in each vial which contained 5 x 10⁵ cpm of ³H-35S AMV RNA (specific activity: 1.9 x 10⁶ cpm per µg) and 1.5 mg of mouse RNA in 0.5 ml of 4 x SSC plus 0.05 % SDS. After hybridization and processing, each filter contained between 30–40 µg of DNA. ³H-RNA bound to mouse DNA (15–20 cpm per filter) was subtracted as background from each experimental filter.

b. Counts per minute ± standard deviation.

Table IV: Hybridization of 70S AMV ^{3}H-RNA to DNA from different tissues of chickens with kidney tumors[a]

Chicken Number	Cpm hybridized per 100 µg DNA from [b]								
	Breast Muscle	Heart	Liver	Lung	Spleen	RBC	Normal Kidney	Kidney Tumor No. 1	Kidney Tumor No. 2
16307	533±36	530±51	550±50	728±27	Atrophied[c]	976±27	595±53	1083±36	1385±36
16322	710±36	657±36	621±44	666±44	604±36	923±36	1376±27	1085±36	1331±63
16343	675±44	n.d.	515±53	n.d.	746±44	911±41		1811±71	

[a] One-day old chicks were injected intraperitoneally with AMV, and three that developed kidney tumors (embryonal nephromas) detected by abdominal palpation were sacrificed on day 102. Chicken 16307 had a nephroma confined to the upper lobe of the right kidney (kidney tumor no. 1); the other lobes of the right kidney and the entire left kidney (normal kidney) were not affected. Chickens 16322 and 16343 had bilateral kidney tumors. Chicken 16322 had a large cystic tumor involving the entire left kidney (kidney tumor no. 1) and a smaller cystic tumor of the top lobe of the right kidney (kidney tumor no. 2); the other two lobes of the right kidney appeared normal (normal kidney). Chicken 16343 had a teratoma involving the entire left kidney (kidney tumor no. 1) and a cystic tumor involving the entire right kidney (kidney tumor no. 2); there was no detectable normal kidney tissue.

DNA was isolated from each organ, purified, treated with .3N KOH, denatured, trapped on nitrocellulose filters, and hybridized at 70 °C for 10 hr with 70S AMV ^{3}H-RNA. Each vial contained five experimental filters from one organ in 1 ml of 4 x saline citrate with 0.05 % sodium dodecyl sulfate, 3.0 mg of mouse embryo RNA, and 1 x 10^6 counts per min of AMV ^{3}H-RNA (specific activity of 8.1 x 10^5 counts per min per µg). The counts per minute shown represent ^{3}H radioactivity hybridized per 100 µg of DNA.

[b] Mean of five filters ± standard deviation.

[c] At postmortem it was noted that the spleen of this chicken (16307) was devoid of pulp.

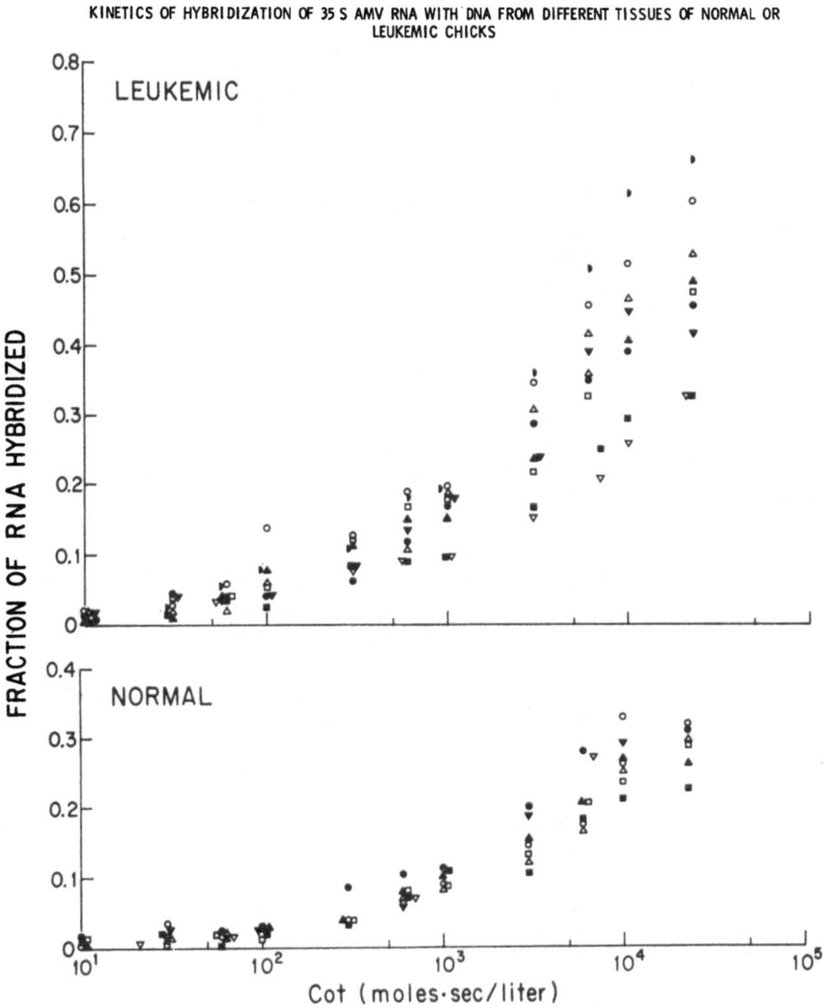

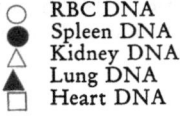

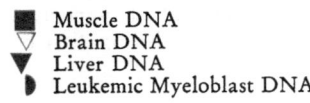

Fig. 4: Hybridization kinetics of ^{3}H-labeled 35S AMV RNA with excess DNA from various tissues of normal and leukemic chickens: Tissues from six normal or from six leukemic chickens were pooled and DNA isolated. The hybridization mixture contained per ml 4 mg of cellular DNA sheared to a fragment size of 6–7S, 2,500 cpm of sonically treated ^{3}H-labeled 35S AMV RNA (size 8 to 10S, specific activity 1.9 x 10^6 cpm per μg) in 0.4M phosphate buffer, pH 6.8 plus 0.1 % SDS. The hybridization was carried out at 65 C in tightly silicone-stoppered tubes. After boiling for 3 min in a waterethylene glycol bath, the mixture was quickly transferred to a water bath at 65 C. Samples of 0.25 ml were taken at different time intervals and diluted with cold water in an ice-water bath. One-half of each sample was then treated with pancreatic A and T_1 ribonucleases to determine the fraction of viral RNA rendered ribonuclease resistant. A background of 2 % obtained a Cot 0 was deducted from all experimental values.

○ RBC DNA
● Spleen DNA
△ Kidney DNA
▲ Lung DNA
□ Heart DNA
■ Muscle DNA
▽ Brain DNA
▼ Liver DNA
◗ Leukemic Myeloblast DNA

Acquisition of Viral DNA in Target Tissues of AMV Infected Chickens. DNA-RNA hybridization studies were carried out to investigate: i) the distribution of vertically transmitted endogenous viral DNA in various tissues of normal chickens, and ii) the distribution of AMV provirus in various tissues of chickens which developed neoplasias after infection with AMV. Two types of nucleic acid hybridization were used: i) denatured cellular DNA immobilized on filters was hybridized to an excess of viral RNA to quantitate the cellular concentration of viral DNA sequences in different tissues, and ii) 35S viral RNA was hybridized to an excess of cellular DNA to determine the proportion of the AMV genome that is present in different tissues.

Filter Hybridization in RNA Excess. Our findings demonstrate that in normal chickens the endogenous viral DNA is present at the same cellular concentration in every tissue that was tested (Table III). This demonstrates the constancy of vertically transmitted endogenous viral DNA in every organ and probably in every cell of normal chickens. By contrast, after injection of AMV into one-day old chicks, AMV specific DNA appears to be acquired only by tumor cells and by target cells in leukemic chickens (Table III). The tissues from leukemic chickens can be divided into three groups: 1) muscle and brain in which the cellular concentration of viral DNA remains the same as before infection with AMV, 2) heart, lung, liver and spleen in which the concentration of v-DNA is increased approximately 50 %, 3) leukemic myeloblasts, RBC and kidneys in which there is a 2–2.5-fold increase in v-DNA. The latter group of tissue contains about the same amount of viral DNA. These tissues are known to contain target cells which can be converted to neoplastic cells by AMV (Baluda & Jamieson, 1961; Baluda et al., 1963; Walter et al., 1962).

AMV-induced kidney tumors provide well defined, localized carcinoma tissue and apparently normal tissues can be obtained from the same chicken due to the absence of metastases. Consequently, 1-day-old chicks were injected intraperitoneally with AMV, and 3 months later three female survivors that had enlarged abdomens with a palpable tumor mass were sacrificed. Examination of their peripheral blood revealed that all three chickens had slightly immature (blue-gray) erythrocytes. In addition to the RBC, six apparently normal tissues (breast muscle, heart, liver, lung, spleen, and kidney) were removed, and their DNA was tested for viral DNA content (Table IV). Tissues known to contain target cells for tumor induction by AMV showed an increase in the average cellular concentration of viral DNA, whereas non-target tissues did not. The lungs, which may be considered a partial target tissue because they contain a large number of leukocytes and erythrocytes, showed a small, but significant (at the 0.01 level using the t test) increase in viral DNA content.

Liquid Hybridization in DNA Excess. To determine what proportion of the AMV genome was present in the various tissues of normal and leukemic chickens, 35S AMV RNA was hybridized in liquid to an excess of cellular DNA (Shoyab et al., 1974). Cellular DNA from every organ of normal chickens tested contained viral DNA sequences which represented approximately the same fraction of the AMV RNA genome (Figure 4). The amount of input viral RNA made RNase resistant by DNA from various tissues of normal chicken varied between 23 to 32 %. This represents hybridization of AMV-RNA with RAV-0 like endogenous viral

320

DNA. The kinetics of hybridization are almost the same for every normal tissue and are identical to the kinetics of hybridization between AMV RNA and DNA from individual whole normal chicken embryos (Shoyab et al., 1974). These results indicate that the endogenous oncornavirus DNA sequences, estimated at two to three copies per diploid cell genome, are quantitatively and qualitatively similar in every organ of normal chickens.

Unlike the findings obtained with tissues from normal chickens, the kinetics of hybridization of AMV RNA with DNA from tissues of leukemic chickens varied with different tissues (Figure 4). Maximum hybridization was obtained with DNA from leukemic myeloblasts or RBC (64 to 67 %). Hybridization obtained with kidney DNA was about 10 % lower than with DNA from leukemic myeloblasts or RBC. DNA from muscle or brain hybridized 33 % of input viral RNA, the same fraction hybridized by DNA from uninfected chickens. DNA from heart, liver, lung, or spleen hybridizes a fraction (42 to 50 %) of viral RNA intermediate between the first two groups of tissues. These data indicate that there are 4 to 6 DNA copies of the viral genome per leukemic myeloblast.

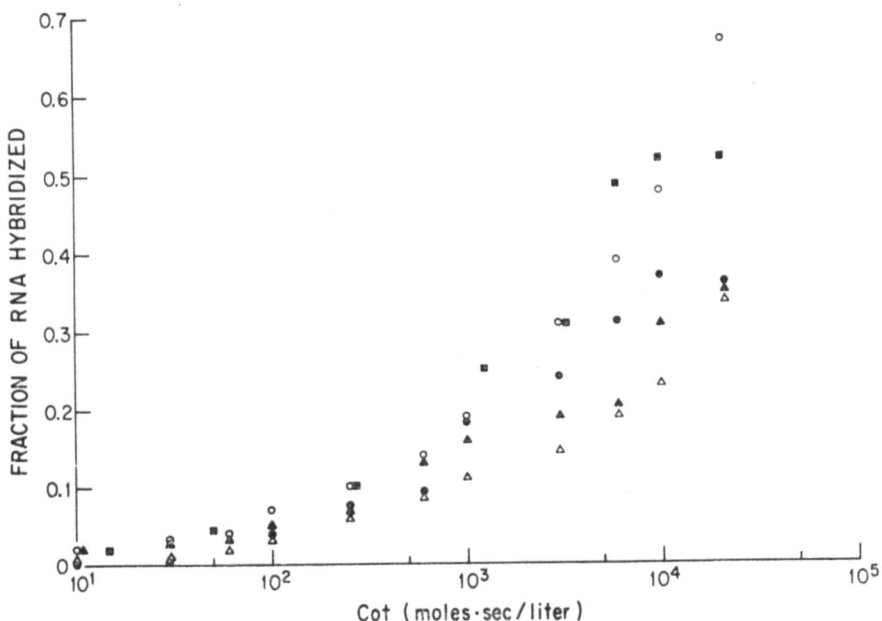

HYBRIDIZATION OF 35 S AMV RNA WITH DNA FROM DIFFERENT TISSUES OF CHICKENS WITH KIDNEY TUMORS

Fig. 5: Hybridization kinetics of ³H-labeled 35S AMV RNA with excess DNA from various tissues of chickens with kidney tumors: The conditions of hybridization were identical to those in Figure 1.

○ Kidney Tumor DNA   ● Spleen DNA
△ Liver DNA   ▲ Lung DNA
■ Apparently normal kidney DNA

321

The intermediate increase of viral DNA sequences in some tissues, e. g., heart, liver, lung, and spleen, may reflect either a mixture of noninfected and infected cells, infiltration of the organ by leukemic myeloblasts and RBC, or addition of fewer or incomplete DNA copies of the AMV genome in certain types of cells.

The data in Table IV show that the cellular concentration of AMV DNA increases as much in kidney tumor cells as it did in leukemic myeloblasts or in RBC of leukemic chicks but that there is no increase in non-target organs such as muscle or liver. To determine whether the increase in AMV DNA content represented the acquisition of new complete DNA copies of the AMV genome or amplification of preexisting endogenous sequences, ^{3}H-AMV RNA was hybridized in an excess of cellular DNA from various tissues of kidney tumor-bearing chickens. The results (Figure 5) show that DNA from kidney tumors hybridizes approximately twice as much viral RNA (67 %) as does DNA from spleen, lung or liver. DNA from the latter tissues hybridizes with AMV RNA to the same extent (33–36 %) as DNA from the tissues of uninfected chickens. The kinetics of hybridization indicate that entire DNA copies of AMV RNA have been acquired by kidney tumor cells and that there are 4–6 copies of viral DNA per diploid cell genome.

To demonstrate more directly the presence of viral DNA sequences in neo-

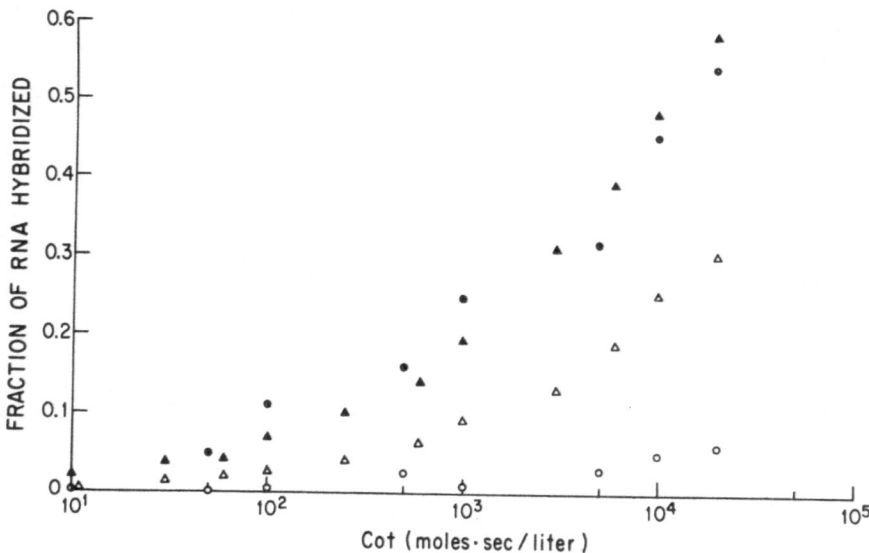

KINETICS OF HYBRIDIZATION OF 35 S AMV RNA WHICH DID NOT HYBRIDIZE WITH NORMAL DNA

Fig. 6: Kinetics of hybridization in excess of DNA of ^{3}H-labeled 35S AMV RNA and 35S AMV RNA which failed to hybridize with normal chicken embryonic DNA. The conditions of hybridization were the same as those described in Figure 1.
    △ Hybridization of 35S AMV RNA with normal chicken embryo DNA
    ▲ Hybridization of 35S AMV RNA with chicken kidney tumor DNA
    ○ Hybridization of residual AMV RNA with normal chicken embryo DNA
    ● Hybridization of residual AMV RNA with chicken kidney tumor DNA

plastic tissues, e. g., leukemic myeloblasts and kidney tumor cells that are not present in normal tissue, sonicated 35S AMV RNA was hybridized exhaustively with an excess of DNA from normal chicken cells to remove all viral RNA sequences homologous to endogenous viral DNA in normal cells. The unhybridized AMV RNA was then isolated and rehybridized with excess DNA from normal or neoplastic kidney tissues. The kinetics of the second hybridization are shown in Figure 6, which also includes for comparison hybridization of untreated 35S AMV RNA with DNA from the same tissues. At Cot 20,000 kidney tumor DNA hybridized 59 % of untreated 35S AMV RNA whereas normal embryonic chicken DNA hybridized only 30 % of the viral RNA. The residual AMV RNA fraction that failed to hybridize with DNA from normal chickens hybridized only 6 % with DNA from normal cells. In contrast, the kinetics of hybridization of the residual AMV RNA with the kidney tumor DNA was similar to the kinetics of untreated 35S RNA and 54 % of the residual RNA became RNase resistant. These results provide direct evidence that kidney tumor DNA contains new AMV DNA sequences acquired after infection with AMV. Similar results were obtained with DNA from leukemic myeloblasts.

Conclusions

Proviral DNA is synthesized within an hour after infection of chicken cells with an avian oncornavirus and is integrated into nuclear cellular DNA within a short time. The viral DNA appears to be synthesized as double-stranded molecules of approximately 6×10^6 daltons some of which are converted into supercoiled circles perhaps as a requisite for integration.

The endogenous v-DNA in normal chicken cells and both the endogenous and AMV v-DNA in leukemic chicken myeloblasts are covalently linked with chromosomal DNA. There is no detectable free DNA either circular or linear present in leukemic cells several weeks after infection. The endogenous v-DNA which is transmitted vertically from parents to offspring is uniformly and stably distributed in all chicken organs. There are about 1–2 copies of endogenous provirus per haploid genome of all normal cells. This DNA is very closely related to RAV-0 RNA. After infection with AMV it seems that target cells such as leukemic myeloblasts, RBC and nephroblasts acquire complete copies of AMV DNA. Interestingly, only these target cells can be converted to neoplastic cells in the chicken as well as *in vitro*. The target cells acquire 1–2 copies of AMV specific DNA per haploid genome in addition to the endogenous v-DNA.

All the available evidence shows that leukemic and kidney tumor cells have acquired AMV v-DNA. It remains to be elucidated whether the newly added viral DNA is alone responsible for neoplastic changes or does so in conjunction with endogenous viral information.

Acknowledgements

The work described here was supported by USPHS Grant CA-10197 from the National Cancer Institute and by contract CP-33283 within the Virus Cancer Program of the National Cancer Institute.

References

Ali, M. and M. A. Baluda (1974) Synthesis of avian oncornavirus DNA in infected chicken cells. J. Virol. *13*: 1005–1013.

Bader, J. P. (1964) The role of deoxyribonucleic acid in the synthesis of Rous sarcoma virus. Virology 22: 462–468.

Bader, J. P. (1965) The requirement for DNA synthesis in the growth of Rous sarcoma and Rous-associated viruses. Virology 26: 253–261.

Baltimore, D. (1970) Viral RNA-dependent DNA polymerase. Nature *226*: 1209–1211.

Baluda, M. A., I. E. Goetz and S. Ohno (1963) Induction of differentiation in certain target cells by avian myeloblastosis virus: an *in vitro* study. In 17th Annual Symposium on Fundamental Cancer Research, M. D. Anderson Hospital. Viruses, Nucleic Acids and Cancer. Baltimore, William & Wilkins Co., pp. 387–400.

Baluda, M. A. and P. P. Jamieson. (1961) *In vivo* infectivity studies with avian myeloblastosis virus. Virology *14*: 33–45.

Baluda, M. A. and D. P. Nayak (1970) DNA complementary to viral RNA in leukemic cells induced by avian myeloblastosis virus. Proc. Nat. Acad. Sci. USA *66*: 329–336.

Bentvelzen, P., J. H. Daams, P. Hageman and J. Calafat (1970) Genetic transmission of viruses that incite mammary tumors in mice. Proc. Nat. Acad. Sci. USA *67*: 377–384.

Borek, E. and A. Ryan (1973) Lysogenic induction. Prog. Nuc. Acid. Res. & Mol. Biol. *13*: 249–300.

Echols, H. (1971) Lysogeny: viral repression and site-specific recombination. Ann. Rev. Biochem. *40*: 827–857.

Hanafusa, H. and T. Hanafusa (1971) Noninfectious RSV deficient in DNA polymerase. Virology *43*: 313–316.

Harel, L., J. Harel and G. Frezouls (1972) DNA copies of RNA in rat cells transformed by Rous sarcoma virus. Biochem. Biophys. Res. Comm. *48*: 796–801.

Hill, M. and J. Hillova (1972a) Virus recovery in chicken cells tested with Rous sarcoma cell DNA. Nature New Biology *237*: 35–39.

Hill, M. and J. Hillova (1972) Recovery of the temperature-sensitive mutant of Rous sarcoma virus from chicken cells exposed to DNA extracted from hamster cells transformed by the mutant. Virology *49*: 309–313.

Hirt, B. (1967) Selective extraction of polyoma DNA from infected mouse cell culture. J. Mol. Biol. *26*: 365–369.

Markham, P. D. and M. A. Baluda (1973) Integrated state of oncornavirus DNA in normal chicken cells and in cells transformed by avian myeloblastosis virus. J. Virol. *12*: 721–732.

May, J. T., K. D. Somers and S. Kit (1972) Defective mouse sarcoma virus deficient in DNA polymerase activity. J. Gen. Virol. *16*: 223–226.

Neiman, P. E. (1972) Rous sarcoma virus nucleotide sequences in cellular DNA: measurement by RNA-DNA hybridization. Science *178*: 750–753.

Peebles, P. T., D. K. Haapala and A. F. Gazdar (1972) Deficiency of viral ribonucleic acid-dependent deoxyribonucleic acid polymerase in noninfectious virus-like particles released from murine sarcoma virus-transformed hamster cells. J. Virol. 9: 488–493.

Sambrook, J., H. Westphal, P. R. Srinivasan and R. Dulbecco (1968) The integrated state of viral DNA in SV-40 transformed cells. Proc. Nat. Acad. Sci. USA 60: 1288–1295.

Schincariol, A. L. and W. K. Joklik (1973) Early synthesis of virus specific RNA and DNA in cells rapidly transformed with Rous sarcoma virus. Virology 56: 532–548.

Shoyab, M., M. A. Baluda and R. M. Evans (1974) Acquisition of new DNA sequences after infection of chicken cells with avian myeloblastosis virus. J. Virol. 13: 331–339.

Shoyab, M., P. D. Markham and M. A. Baluda (1974) Reliability of the RNA-DNA filter hybridization for the detection of oncornavirus-specific DNA sequences. J. Virol. 14: 225–230.

Shoyab, M., R. M. Evans and M. A. Baluda (1974) Presence in leukemic cells of avian myeloblastosis virus-specific DNA sequences absent in normal chicken cells. J. Virol. 14: 47–49.

Shoyab, M., P. D. Markham and M. A. Baluda (1975) Host induced alteration of avian sarcoma virus B-77 genome. Proc. Nat. Acad. Sci. USA 72: 1031–1035.

Svoboda, J., I. Hlozanek and O. Mach (1972) Detection of chicken sarcoma virus after transfection of chicken fibroblasts with DNA isolated from mammalian cells transformed with Rous virus. Folia Biologia 18: 149–153.

Temin, H. M. (1962) Separation of morphological conversion and virus production in Rous sarcoma virus infection. Cold Spring Harbor Sym. Quant. Biol. XXVII, 407–414.

Temin, H. M. (1963) The effect of actinomycin D on growth of Rous sarcoma virus in vitro. Virology 20: 577–582.

Temin, H. M. (1964) Nature of the provirus of Rous sarcoma. Nat. Cancer Inst. Monogr. 17: 557–570.

Temin, H. M. and S. Mizutani (1970) RNA-dependent DNA polymerase in virions of Rous sarcoma virus. Nature 226: 1211–1213.

Temin, H. M. (1971) Mechanism of cell transformation by RNA tumor viruses. Ann. Rev. Microbiol. 25: 609–648.

Varmus, H. E., P. K. Vogt and J. M. Bishop (1973) Integration of deoxyribonucleic acid specific for Rous sarcoma virus after infection of permissive and nonpermissive hosts. Proc. Nat. Acad. Sci. USA 69: 576–580.

Varmus, H. E., H. Suzanne and J. M. Bishop (1974) Use of DNA-DNA annealing to detect new virus specific DNA sequences in chicken embryo fi-roblast after infection by avian sarcoma virus. J. Virol. 14: 895–903.

Walter, W. G., B. R. Burmester and C. H. Cunningham (1962) Studies on the transmission and pathology of a viral-induced avian nephroblastoma (embryonal nephroma). Avian Diseases 6: 455–477.

Sequences and Functions of Rous Sarcoma Virus RNA

Peter H. Duesberg, Lu-Hai Wang, Karen Beemon,
Sadaaki Kawai* and Hidesaburo Hanafusa*

Virus Laboratory and Department
of Molecular Biology, University of California,
Berkeley, California 94720
and
* Rockefeller University, New York, N. Y. 10021

Abstract

A procedure has been developed to map the genetic elements of avian tumor virus RNA, which has a molecular weight of about 3×10^6 daltons and a poly(A) sequence at the 3' end. For this purpose, about 30 RNase T_1-resistant oli gonucleotides were ordered relative to the 3'-poly(A) terminus of the RNA, to construct an oligonucleotide map of viral RNAs. A cluster of seven envelope gene (env)-specific oligonucleotides, identified by their absence from the other- wise very similar oligonucleotide map of an envelope-defective deletion mutant (which lacks the major viral glycoprotein), mapped at a distance of 0.9 to 1.6×10^6 daltons from the poly(A) end of sarcoma virus RNA. A cluster of three sarcoma gene (src)-specific oligonucleotides, identified by their absence from the other- wise nearly identical oligonucleotide map of a transformation-defective deletion mutant mapped at a distance of 0.2 to 0.6×10^6 daltons from the poly(A) end of sarcoma virus RNA. The oligonucleotide maps of sarcoma viruses and of related deletion mutants were the same from the poly(A) end up to 0.2×10^6 daltons and included one terminal oligonucleotide, termed C, which is found in all avian tumor viruses tested so far. Preliminary mapping experiments ordering the src-specific and env-specific oligonucleotides of recombinants, selected for sarcoma and en- velope genes of different parents, agree with those obtained by comparing maps of wild type viruses and deletion mutants. A partial genetic map consistent with these results suggests that the src gene maps between the env gene and the 3'-poly(A) end of viral RNA. This map reads: poly(A)-src-env-(pol, gag).

a) *Introduction*

The genome of avian tumor viruses is probably a 60–70S RNA complex (1, 2). It consists of predominantly two 30–40S RNA subunits (3) with an approximate molecular weight of 3×10^6 daltons each (3, 4, 5, 6). Genetic (7) and biochemical (5, 6) studies suggest that these 30–40S subunits are very similar, perhaps identical. This implies that the viral genome is diploid.

The 30–40S RNA of nondefective (nd) avian sarcoma viruses carries at least four different genetic elements (8): (i) a gene for cell transformation, termed *src* (17), [the previous term *onc* is replaced here by *src* since so far a transformation gene has only been found in sarcoma viruses (4, 7, 9, 10, 12, 13). By contrast oncogenicity is a more general term and applies to transformation by both sarcoma and leukemia viruses]. (ii) a gene for the viral envelope glycoprotein, termed *env*, (iii) a gene for the viral DNA polymerase, termed *pol* and (iv) a gene for the viral group-specific antigen, termed *gag*.

It is the purpose of our experiments to identify chemically RNA sequences of these genes on 30–40S tumor virus RNAs and to map these sequences on the viral RNA relative to its 3'-poly(A) terminus (9, 10).

b) *Chemical identification of src-specific and env-specific sequences of avian tumor virus RNA*

RNA sequences of the *src* and *env* genes of nondefective (nd) sarcoma viruses can be chemically identified, because they are missing from certain related deletion mutants. For example, transformation-defective (td) deletion mutants, which lack the *src* gene, were also shown to lack 15 % of the RNA present in corresponding nd sarcoma virus RNA (4, 10, 13). Chemical identification of these and other sequences of tumor virus RNA was based on the large RNase T_1-resistant oligonucleotides which they contain. These are prepared by exhaustive digestion of viral [^{32}P]RNA with RNase T_1, which cleaves only after G residues. These large RNase T_1-resistant oligonucleotides consist of 15–40 nucleotides, including C, A, and U, and have one G at the 3' hydroxyl end. They represent altogether about 5 % of the RNA (5). The large oligonucleotides form a unique pattern, which is termed a fingerprint, after two-dimensional resolution by electrophoresis and chromatography (11). Twenty to thirty such large oligonucleotides are found in avian tumor virus RNA. Since these oligonucleotides are rather evenly distributed over the RNA, an average 5 % segment of the RNA carries one such oligonucleotide and can be so identified. An RNA segment can be identified unambiguously by two or more such oligonucleotides.

Autoradiographs of fingerprint analyses of the 60–70S RNAs of three nd sarcoma viruses, Rous sarcoma virus (RSV) Prague B (PR-B), Prague C (PR-C) and B77, and of their td counterparts are shown in Fig. 1. It can be seen that, in agreement with earlier studies (13), fingerprint patterns of each nd sarcoma virus and its corresponding td deletion mutant are very similar. Identical numbers were used to designate presumably homologous (same composition and size) spots in corresponding patterns of nd and td viruses. Because two fingerprint analyses of the same digest never run completely identically (11), visual identification of presumably homologous oligonucleotides, by triangulation with neighboring spots, is relatively subjective. Therefore definitive identification of oligonucleotides in different fingerprint patterns was based on partial sequence analyses of oligonucleotides. These were obtained by eluting oligonucleotides from the DEAE-cellulose thin layer and digesting them with RNase A. The resulting fragments of most oligonucleotides were then resolved by electrophoresis on DEAE paper (11) and have been described elsewhere (10).

Each nd virus tested in Fig. 1 contained two oligonucleotide spots (numbered 9 and 12 in PR-B, 8 and 10 in PR-C, and 8 and 10 in B77) which were not present

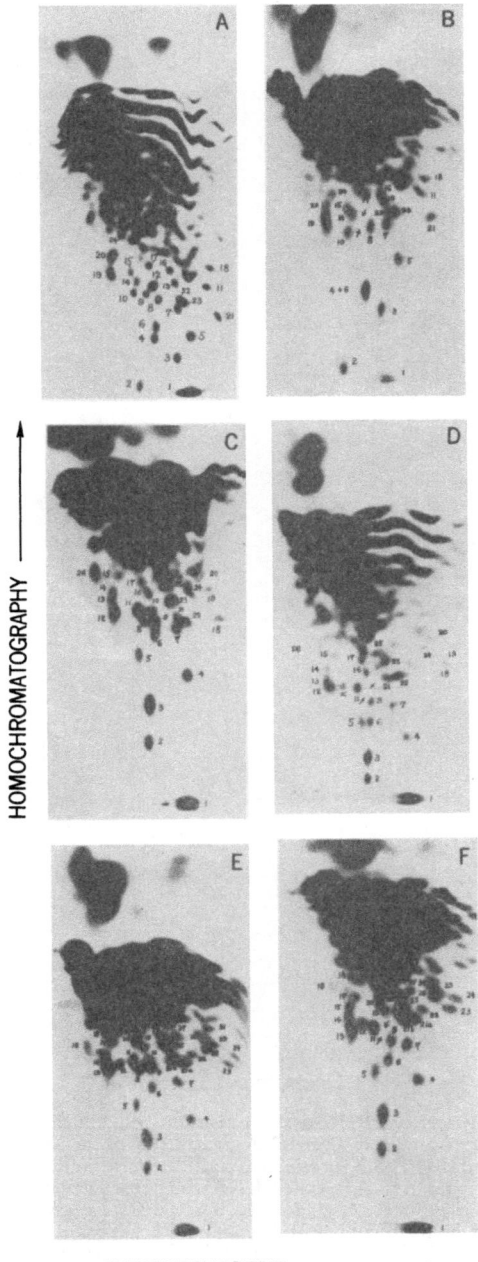

HOMOCHROMATOGRAPHY

ELECTROPHORESIS

Fig. 1: Autoradiographs of two-dimensional fingerprint analyses of RNase T₁-digested 60–70S [³²P]RNAs from different nd and td viruses (10): PR-B (A), td PR-B (B), PR-C (C), td PR-C (D), B77 (E), td B77 (F). Conditions for the preparation of viral [³²P]RNAs, digestion with RNase T₁ and fingerprinting by electrophoresis and homochromatography were described (10). The arrows in B, D, F denote the locations where sarcoma spots would appear.

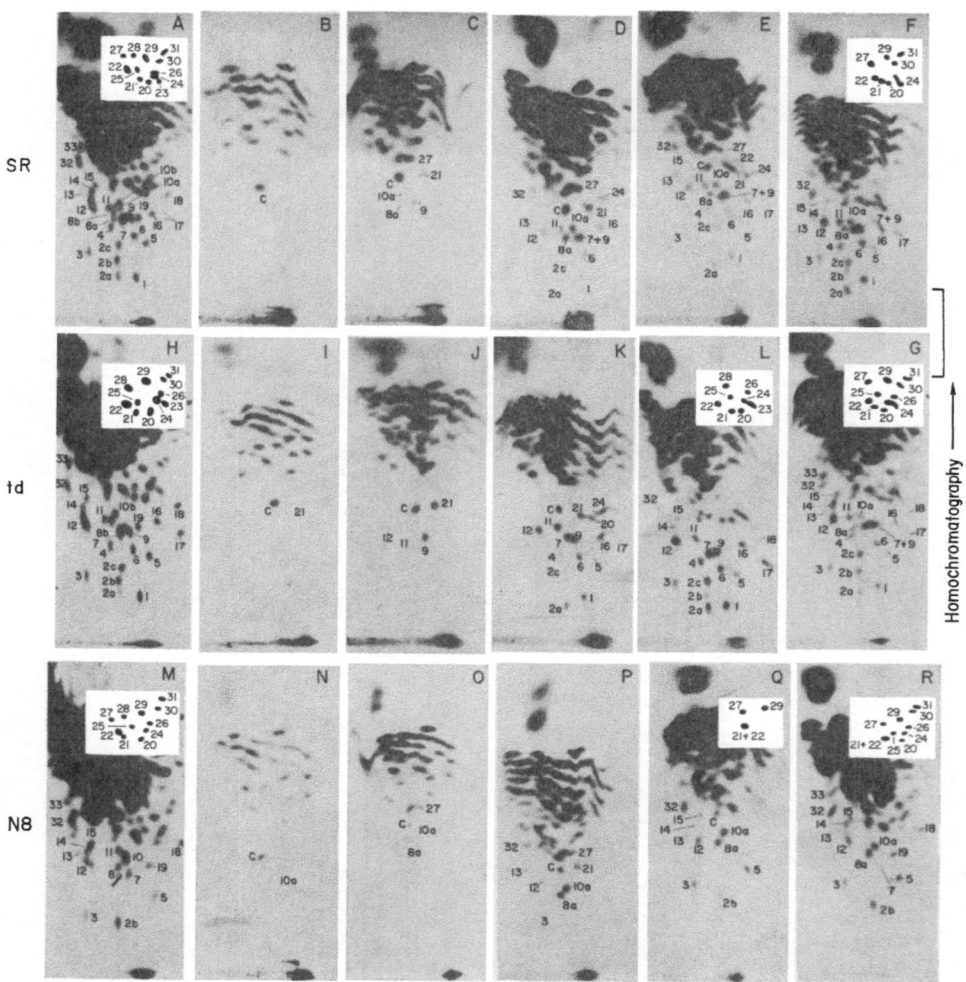

Homochromatography ⟶

Electrophoresis ⟶

Fig. 2: Fingerprint patterns of RNase T₁-resistant oligonucleotides of 60–70S viral [^{32}P]RNAs and poly(A)-tagged [^{32}P]RNA fragments of nd SR, td SR and SR N8 (17). Preparation of viral [^{32}P]RNA, selection and sucrose gradient fractionation of poly-(A)-tagged fragments from alkali-degraded RNA and subsequent fingerprint analysis have been described previously (9, 10, 17). Homologous spots were given identical numbers in all fingerprint patterns. Some oligonucleotide spots which were still detectable and numbered in the original autoradiographs are no longer visible in the reproductions shown here. The inserts in some panels show tracings and numbers of spots appearing in the center right region of the respective fingerprint pattern. SR: Fingerprints of 60–70S nd SR RNA (A) and poly(A)-tagged RNA fragments of 4–10S (B), 10–14S (C), 14–18S (D), 18–22S (E), 22–26S (F) and 26–30S (G). Approximately 35 x 10⁶ cpm of [^{32}P]RNA was degraded at

330

in the fingerprint pattern of the corresponding td virus. These oligonucleotide spots are sarcoma-specific and are thought to come from sarcoma-specific sequences of nd virus RNA. They had homologous positions in each of the three sarcoma viruses compared here. Biochemical analyses indicated that they also contained the same RNase A-resistant fragments and that the faster chromatographing sarcoma-specific oligonucleotide spot of each nd sarcoma virus (no. 12 PR-B, no. 10 PR-C, no. 10 B77) consisted of two chromatographically overlapping oligonucleotides (10). We conclude that three out of about twenty-five large RNase T$_1$-resistant oligonucleotides of the nd sarcoma viruses are from sarcoma-specific sequences. Sarcoma-specific sequences of nd sarcoma viruses had been estimated previously to represent about 450,000 daltons or about 15 % of the mass of the 30–40S RNA (4, 10, 13).

Identification of envelope-specific sequences of viral RNA was accomplished in an analogous fashion by comparing the RNA of an envelope-defective deletion mutant of Schmidt-Ruppin RSV, termed SR N8, to that of the wild type, nd SR. Since SR N8 expresses *gag*, *pol* and *src* genes (it transforms fibroblasts like the wild type) but lacks an envelope glycoprotein (14), it is likely that its defect is a partial or complete deletion of the *env* gene. Due to this defect it can enter cells only in the coat of a helper virus or by fusion with UV-inactivated Sendai virus (14). Thus, envelope-specific sequences of nd SR RSV RNA are defined as those which are missing in SR N8 RNA.

We have shown that the RNA of SR N8 is 21 % smaller than that of the wild type (16) and that all of its obligonucleotides had homologous counterparts (same numbers Fig. 2A, M) in nd SR RNA (16, 17). However 8 out of about 33 oligonucleotides present in nd SR (nos: 1, 2a, 2c, 4, 6, 9, 16 and 17) where absent from SR N8 (Fig. 2A and M). These are thought to be from the 21 % of the nd SR RNA that was deleted to generate SR N8. Fig. 2H shows a fingerprint pattern of td SR RNA. Two oligonucleotide spots, 8a and 10a, present in nd SR are absent from td SR and are thought to be from sarcoma-specific sequences of nd SR.

c) *Mapping of src-specific, env-specific and other sequences on avian*
   tumor virus RNA

Src-specific and *env*-specific sequences were mapped on RSV RNA by determining the location of *src*-specific and *env*-specific oligonucleotides on an oligonucleotide map. For this purpose viral RNA was randomly degraded by alkali.

pH 11 at 50° for 3 min. Sixteen percent of the starting RNA was recovered as poly(A)-tagged fragments after two cycles of binding and elution from oligo(dT)-cellulose (9, 10). These fragments had a broad distribution with a peak at about 21S after sucrose gradient fractionation (10) done to obtain the size cuts (B-G). td: Fingerprints of 60–70S td SR RNA (H) and of poly(A)-tagged RNA fragments of 4–10S (I), 10–15S (J), 15–20S (K) and 20–28S (L). About 7 x 10⁶ cpm of 60–70S [³²P]RNA was fragmented for 6 min as described above, and approximately 11 % was recovered as poly(A)-tagged RNA fragments with an average sedimentation coefficient of 16S. SR N8: Fingerprints of 60–70S SR N8 RNA (M) and of poly(A)-tagged RNA fragments of 4–9S (N), 9–15S (O), 15–20S (P), 20–25S (Q) and 25–30S (R). About 5 x 10⁶ cpm of 60–70S [³²P]RNA was degraded for 3 min as above, and 18 % was recovered as poly(A)-containing RNA fragments with an average sedimentation coefficient of 22S.

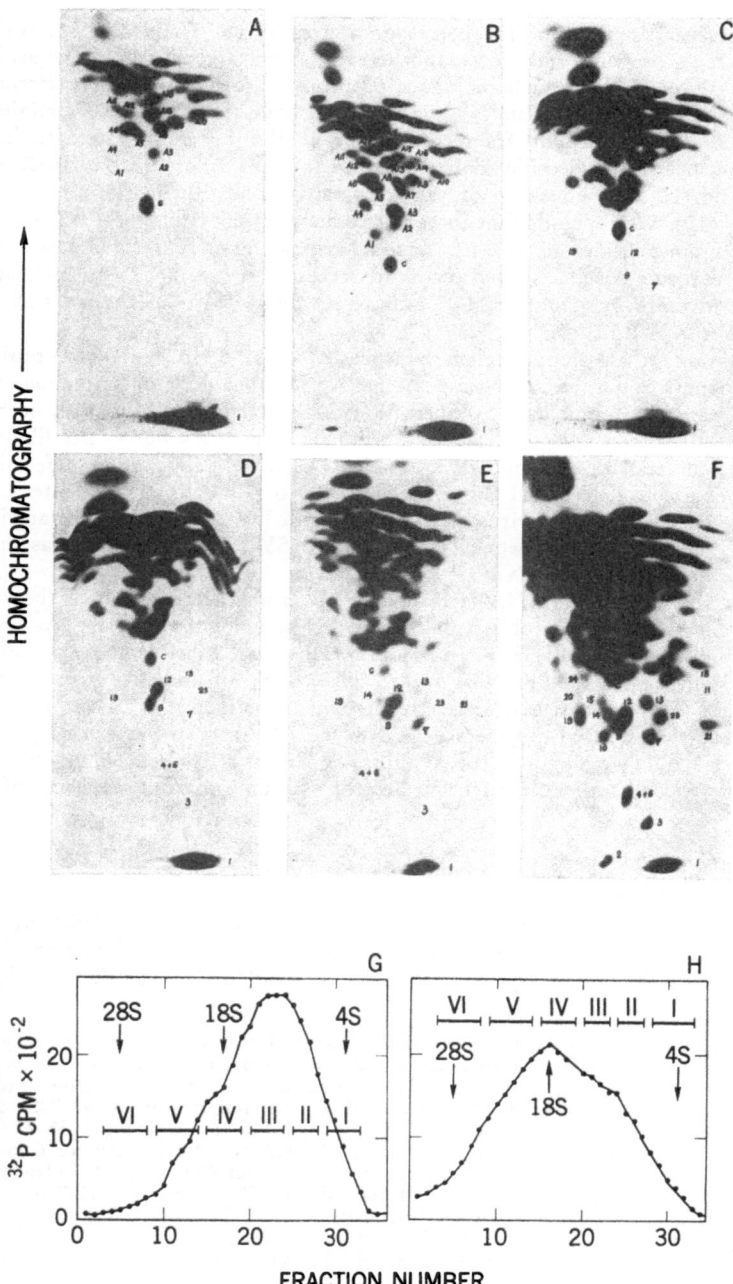

Fig. 3: Autoradiographic fingerprint analyses of poly(A)-tagged PR-B RNA fragments of

Poly(A)-tagged RNA fragments were selected by binding to oligo (dT)-cellulose, fractionated according to size and fingerprinted to detect their oligonucleotides (compare Figs. 2, 3, 5, 7). The map position of a given oligonucleotide relative to the poly(A) end of viral RNA was then deduced from the size of the smallest poly(A)-tagged RNA fragment from which it could be isolated. In this fashion, 20 to 30 large RNase T_1-resistant oligonucleotides were ordered on the basis of their distance grom the 3'-poly(A) end of the RNA to construct oligonucleotide maps (Figs. 2–6). The method has been described in detail (9, 10, 17). Examples of the fractionation of poly(A)-tagged fragments of PR-B RNA and their finger-prints are shown in Fig. 3, and the fingerprints of poly(A)-tagged fragments of nd SR RNA, td SR RNA and SR N8 RNA are shown in Fig. 2. These finger-prints demonstrated clearly that in all cases examined an approximately linear relationship existed between the size of poly(A)-containing fragments and the number of RNase T_1-resistant oligonucleotides they contained. We could deduce the approximate location of each oligonucleotide relative to the 3'-poly(A) end of the RNA from the size of the smallest poly(A)-tagged RNA fragment from which it could be isolated (9, 10). In this way the oligonucleotide maps of nd PR-B, td PR-B, nd PR-C, nd B77 and td B77, shown in Fig. 4, were derived.

It can be seen in Fig. 4 that the *src*-specific oligonucleotides of PR-B (no. 9 and 12), PR-C (no. 8 and 10) and B77 (no. 8 and 10), respectively, cluster together and map very near the poly(A) end of each viral RNA. The same appears to be true for spots 8a and 10a which are thought to be *src*-specific spots of nd SR (Fig. 6). It is concluded that the *src*-gene-specific sequences map near the poly(A) end of viral RNA. It can also be seen in Fig. 4 that the oligonucleotide maps of PR-B and td PR-B, as well as those of B77 and td B77, are the same as far as determinded with the exception of the *src*-specific oligonucleotides which are absent from the td viruses. This implies that the gene order of the nd and corresponding td viruses is the same. A few oligonucleotides of PR-B, PR-C and B77 were found to have homologous chromatographic locations and chemical compositions [compare fingerprints of Fig. 1 and biochemical analyses of Wang *et al.* (10)]. The

various sizes after exhaustive digestion with RNase T_1 as described (10). Approximately 25×10^6 to 30×10^6 cpm of 60 to 70S [^{32}P]PR-B RNA were partially degraded with Na_2 CO_3 at pH 11. and 50 C for 8 min to yield RNA fragments with a peak at 12S (G) and for 4 min to yield RNA fragments with a peak at 18S (H). Poly(A)-tagged fragments were selected by two consecutive cycles of binding to and elution from membrane filters (Millipore Corp.) (10). About 7.3 % of the radioactive RNA was recovered as poly(A)-tagged fragments if degradation was for 4 min (H), and 5.2 % of the radioactive RNA was recovered if degradation was for 8 min (G). Poly(A)-tagged RNA fragments selected from the 8 min (G) and 4 min (H) degradation mixture were fractionated according to size by sedimentation in sucrose gradients as described (10). The radioactivity was determined from an appropriate aliquot of each gradient fraction (G, H). The poly(A)-tagged viral RNA fragments were divided into several discrete pools (I→VI) indicated by horizontal bars in (G) and (H). Sedimentation coefficients of these pools were estimated from the positions of 28S, 18S and 4S chicken cell RNA standards analyzed in a parallel gradient and indicated in (G) and (H) by arrows. Pools of RNA fragments from the two gradients with the same range of sedimentation coefficients were combined, and the RNA of each pool was fingerprinted. The fingerprints of pools I→VI are shown in A→F, respectively. Some oligonucleotide spots which were still detectable and were numbered in the original autoradiographs are no longer visible in the reproductions shown here and in Fig. 2 and Fig. 5.

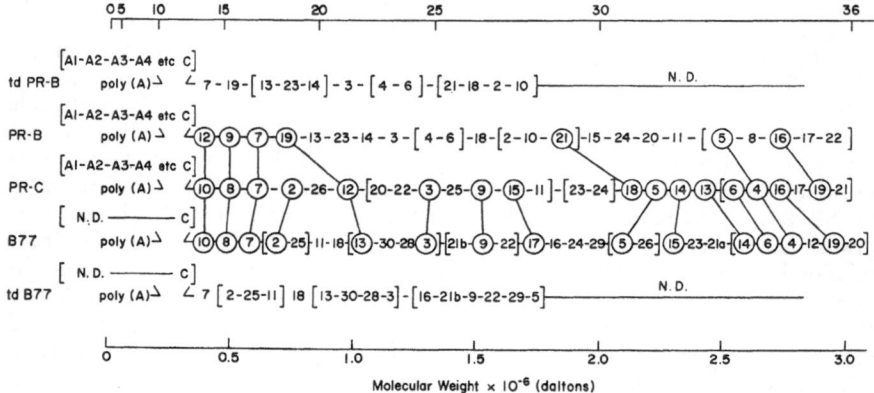

Maps of RNase T1-Resistant Oligonucleotides of 30-40S Viral RNAs

Fig. 4: Maps of RNase T₁-resistant oligonucleotides of 30 to 40S viral RNAs (10). RNase T₁-resistant oligonucleotides of td PR-B, PR-B, PR-C, B77, and td B77, numbered as in the fingerprints shown in Fig. 1, 3, 5 were arranged linearly relative to the poly(A) end. The map position of a given oligonucleotide was determined from the smallest poly(A)-tagged RNA fragment from which it could be obtained. The relative positions of several oligonucleotides, which first appeared together within a given 5 to 10S cut of poly(A)-tagged fragments (Fig. 3), were estimated by quantitating their molarities. The higher the molarity of a given oligonucleotide, the closer it was placed toward the poly(A) end of a given size cut (see text). Oligonucleotides whose relative map positions within a certain sedimentation range could not be estimated are in parentheses. ND: Not determined. The top scale represents the size of the viral RNA or RNA fragments in S values and the bottom scale represents a molecular weight scale derived from the respective S values by Spirin's formula: molecular weight = $1,550 \cdot S^{2.1}$ (15). Those oligonucleotides of the three nd sarcoma viruses that have very similar or identical compositions and sequences (Fig. 1, ref. 10) are circled and connected by vertical lines. The portions of these maps which include the poly(A) segments and the terminal heteropolymeric sequences of about 140,000 daltons, containing the oligonucleotides A1→A4 and C (in parenthesis), are not strictly proportional to the scale of the remaining RNA segments.

oligonucleotides shared by these viruses are circled in the maps of Fig. 4 and connected by lines. Again it can be seen that homologous oligonucleotides also have homologous map locations in the three viral RNAs compared in Fig. 4. This implies that the gene orders of these three different strains of viruses are also closely related.

Given the location of *src*-specific sequences near the poly(A) end of viral RNA, a simple mechanism could be suggested to explain the occurrence of td-deletion mutants from nd sarcoma viruses. This mechanism postulates that the deletion could result from late initiation during transcription from viral RNA to proviral DNA (2) or premature termination during transcription from proviral DNA to viral RNA. If this were correct, one would predict that the terminal heteropolymeric sequences at the 3'-poly(A) end of nd and corresponding td viruses should be different. A small poly(A)-tagged fragment, with the approximate size of the *src*-specific sequences (∼ 450,000 daltons, see above and Fig. 4),

334

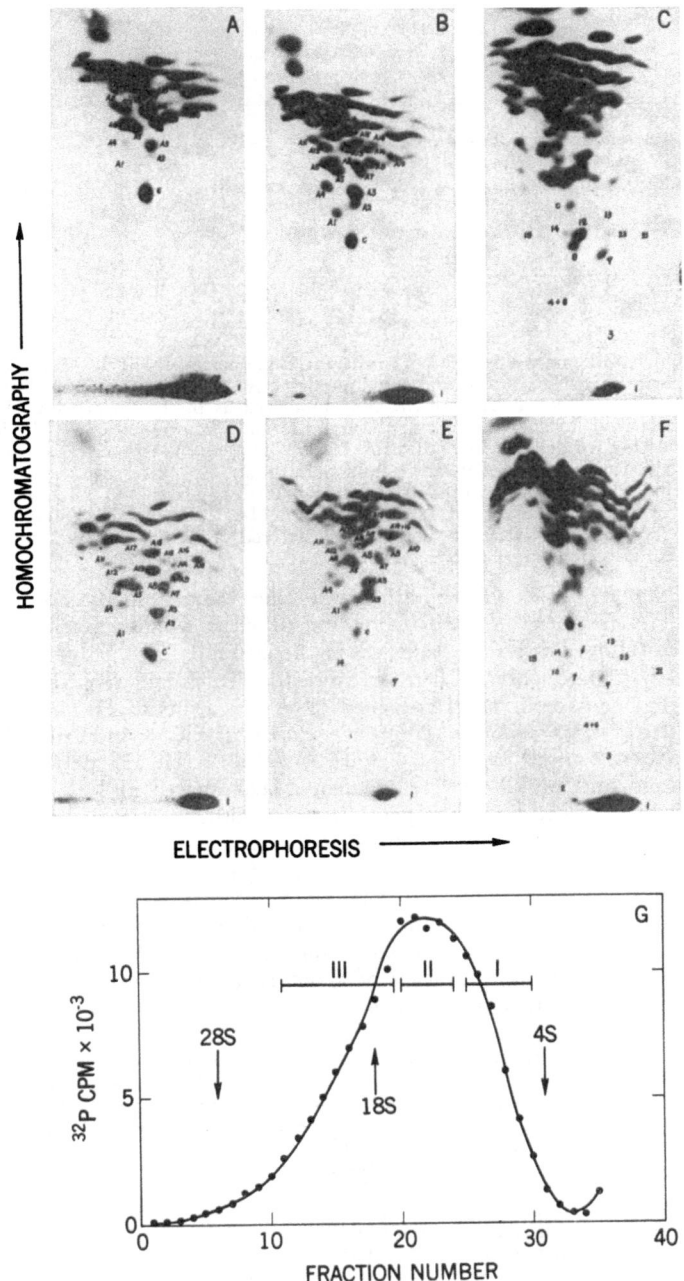

Fig. 5: Fingerprint patterns of RNase T₁-resistant oligonucleotides of small poly(A)-tagged fragments of PR-B and td PR-B RNAs (10). 60–70S [³²P]PR-B RNA was degraded for

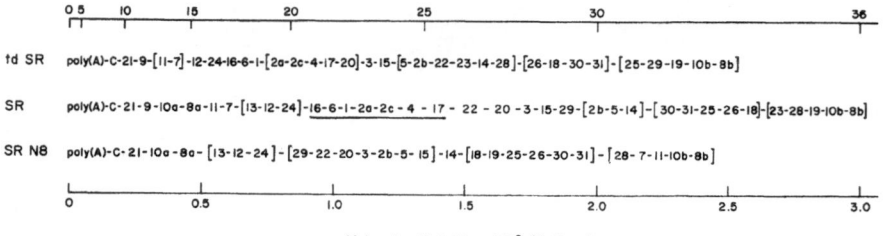

Maps of RNase TI-Resistant Oligonucleotides of 30-40S Viral RNAs

Sedimentation Coefficient (S)

Fig. 6: Oligonucleotide maps of R Nase T_1-resistant oligonucleotides of 30–40 RNAs of nd SR, transformation-defective(td) SR and envelope-defective SR N8 (17). RNase T_1-resistant oligonucleotides of nd SR, td SR and SR N8, numbered as in the fingerprints shown in Fig. 2, were arranged linearly relative to the poly(A) end. Determination of the location of a given spot has been described (see also ref. 16, 17). Those spots whose relative locations could not be determined accurately are put in parentheses. A cluster of seven, probably envelope-specific, oligonucleotides present in nd SR but absent from SR N8 is underlined. The top scale represents the size of viral RNA or RNA fragments in S units and the bottom scale represents a molecular weight scale derived from the S values by Spirin's formula (molecular weight = $1{,}550 \cdot S^{2.1}$ (15).

of nd sarcoma RNA would contain *src*-specific sequences. By contrast, an analogous RNA fragment of a corresponding td virus would contain those sequences which follow *src*-specific sequences in the nd viral RNA but which would be directly adjacent to poly(A) here (because td viruses lack *src*). To test this hypothesis, analogous small poly(A)-tagged RNA fragments of nd and td PR-B were compared by fingerprinting. The result, shown in Fig. 5, indicated that the fingerprint patterns of up to 10S ($\sim$ 200,000 daltons, ref. 15) poly(A)-tagged fragments of nd and td PR-B were the same. They shared at least five intermediatesized oligonucleotides at the poly(A) end, which were termed C, A1, A2, A3 and A4 (10). This implies that the deletion of sarcoma-specific sequences (which generated td PR-B) was not from the very end of the nd viral RNA but was internal and that some 3'-terminal heteropolymeric sequences of the nd virus had been conserved in the deletion mutant. It would follow that the RNA of the nd sarcoma viruses studied here is arranged in this order: poly(A) of about 60,000 daltons (9), a heteropolymeric sequence of about 150,000 daltons which is shared by nd and corresponding td viruses (Fig. 4, 6), about 450,000 daltons of *src*-specific

8 min with Na_2CO_3 and analyzed as described for Fig. 3. Poly(A)-tagged fragments sedimenting between 4 to 7S (A), 7 to 10S (B), and 15 to 20S (C) were fingerprinted after digestion with RNase T_1. About 9×10^6 cpm of 60 to 70S td PR-B [^{32}P]RNA was partially degraded with Na_2CO_3 at 50° for 8 min. About 6.6 % of the starting radioactivity was recovered after two cycles of binding and elution from membrane filters (10). Sedimentation of the poly(A)-tagged fragments is shown in (G). Three pools of poly(A)-tagged fragments were prepared: I (4 to 7S), II (8 to 13S), and III (13 to 23S). Fingerprint analyses of RNase T_1-digested pools I→III are shown in D→F. The arrows in F denote the locations where the sarcoma-specific spots would appear. The homomixture b used here was preincubated at 60° for 24 hr (10).

336

Possible structures of recombinants between nondefective (nd) sarcoma
and transformation-defective (td) leukosis viruses.*

Parents	Recombinants

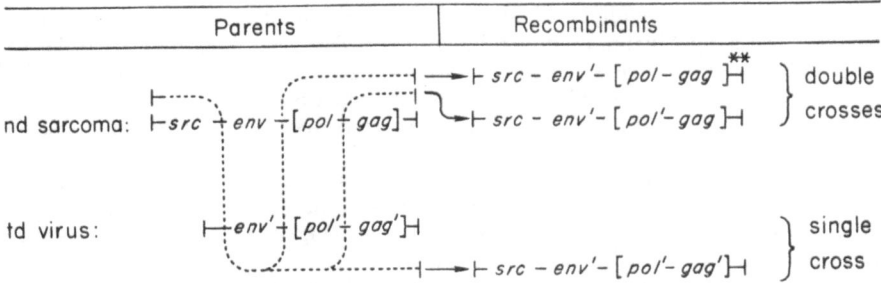

Fig. 7: *Recombinants were selected for the *src* gene of nd sarcoma viruses and the *env* gene of td viruses. Intragenic crossovers and multiple crossovers are not depicted. **Relative map location of *pol* and *gag* genes is unknown.

sequences (Fig. 4), and the remaining 2.4 x 10⁶ daltons which should contain *env*, *pol*, and *gag* sequences.

We have used SR N8, the envelope-defective deletion mutant of nd SR, to map *env*-specific sequences in nd SR RNA. The method was the same as that described to map the *src*-specific sequences. Fingerprint patterns of poly(A)-tagged RNA fragments of nd SR, SR N8 and also of td SR of various sizes are shown in Fig. 2, and the resulting oligonucleotide maps are shown in Fig. 6. It can be seen in Fig. 6 that seven out of eight presumably *env*-specific oligonucleotides map together (nos. 16, 6, 1, 2a, 2c, 4 and 17) in a cluster that is about 0.9–1.6 x 10⁶ daltons away from the poly(A) end. It may be concluded that *env*-specific sequences of nd SR map in this region of the RNA. In addition *src*-specific oligonucleotides of nd SR (nos. 8a, 10a in Fig. 2, 6), like those of other nd sarcoma viruses (Figs. 3, 4, ref. 10), appear to map near the poly(A) end of viral RNA. It would follow that *src*-specific sequences map between the poly(A) end and *env*-specific sequences of nd SR. Since we do not know whether SR N8 is a complete or perhaps only a partial deletion of the *env* gene, we can only define a minimal map segment for the *env* gene with this virus. Further deletion mutants or recombinants (see below) would be required to determine the exact map segment of the *env* gene. The remaining oligonucleotide (no. 9) which is present in nd SR but absent from SR N8 may be the result of a point mutation that set apart the two viruses after the original deletion had occurred (16, 17).

In summary, we may deduce the partial map, poly(A)-*src-env*-, for nd sarcoma virus RNAs by comparing their oligonucleotide maps to those of related deletion mutants.

Fingerprint analyses of short poly(A)-tagged RNA fragments of nd SR, SR N8 and td SR were found to look very similar, and all contained oligonucleotide spot C (compare Figs. 2B, I, N and C, J, O). This is analogous to the finding described above that nd sarcoma viruses and corresponding td viruses also have the same terminal heteropolymeric sequences (Fig. 4) (compare also refs 10 and 17).

337

d) *Distribution of env-specific and src-specific sequences from different parents in the RNAs of avian tumor virus recombinants*

Recently we have started to map genes of avian tumor virus recombinants (5) by comparing the oligonucleotide maps of recombinants to those of their parents. The recombinants used had inherited an *env* gene from a td or leukosis virus parent and a *src* gene from a nd sarcoma virus parent. *Src* and *env*-specific oligonucleotides of the recombinants can be identified by correlating parental and recombinant *src* or *env* markers with the respective segments of their oligonucleotide maps.

All of these recombinants must have at least one crossover point between the *src* gene (which is near the end of the nd virus) and the *env* gene which appears to be close to *src*, but is perhaps not exactly adjacent (Fig. 5, ref. 17). The crossover point between the *src* and the *env* genes should approximately define the 5' end of the *src* gene and the 3' end of the *env* gene. If double crosses occurred, the 5' end of the *env* gene could be approximately defined by analysis of the second crossover point as outlined in the scheme on Fig. 7.

Preliminary mapping experiments of several recombinants between Prague RSV-A and leukosis virus RAV-2, and Prague RSV-B and leukosis virus RAV-3 (5), suggest that all recombinants selected for the *src* gene of the nd virus and the *env* gene of the leukosis virus parent contain a cluster of three to four *src*-specific oligonucleotides mapping in about the first 0.6×10^9 daltons away from the 3' end of their RNAs. The remainder of the oligonucleotide map of some recombinants was completely colinear with that of the leukosis virus parent which had donated the *env* gene. Another recombinant RNA contained leukosis virus-specific oligonucleotides only between 0.6 and 1.5×10^6 daltons from the poly(A) end, its remaining oligonucleotides mapping between 1.5×10^6 daltons and the 5' end of the RNA were again derived from the sarcoma parent. It would appear that this recombinant was generated by a double cross between parents and that the leukosis virus-specific oligonucleotides between 0.6 and 1.5 daltons from the poly(A) end include the leukosis virus-specific *env* gene. Based on the analyses of these recombinants their *env* and *src* genes can be tentatively ordered to yield the partial map: poly(A)-*src*-*env*-. This map is in good agreement with that derived above from comparative analyses of nd viruses and their deletion mutants.

Discussion

A genetic map of avian tumor viruses: A tentative map emerges from the experiments described here for nd avian sarcoma viruses, beginning at the poly(A) coordinate in molecular weight units ($\times 10^{-5}$): 0–0.6, poly(A); 0.6–2, heteropolymeric sequences shared with corresponding td and envelope-defective viruses; 2–6.5, *src*-specific sequences; 6.5–9, a segment of RNA which may have a distinct function or may be part of the envelope gene (Nd SR and SR N8 share oligonucleotides (nos. 12 and 24, Fig. 6) in this map position, but SR N8 may not represent a complete deletion of the *env* gene.); 9–16, *env*-specific sequences; 16–30, *pol*-specific and *gag*-specific sequences which have not been mapped so far. Further experiments analyzing different deletion mutants and viral recombinants will be used to map the functions described more precisely and to map the two remaining genes, *pol* and *gag*, of tumor virus RNA.

Generation of deletion mutants: It was observed that the oligonucleotide maps of all td-deletion mutants and of the *env*-defective mutant SR N8 show deletions from within the RNA, rather than from the ends as would be expected for deletions arising from transcriptional errors. This suggests that the deletion mutants we have analyzed may be the products of recombinational events occurring at the level of proviral DNA. A proviral DNA intermediate could, by formation and subsequent elimination of loops, delete any sequences from the genome with equal probability.

Acknowledgements

The recent research upon which this article is based was supported by Public Health Service research grants CA 11426 and CA 14935, and Postdoctoral Fellowship CA 05085, from the National Cancer Institute, and by the Cancer Program-National Cancer Institute under Contracts Nos. NO1 CP 43212 and NO1 CP 43242.

Note added in proof: More complete data on mapping *src* and *env*-genes in vival-recombinants have since been published by us (18, 19). In addition we have mapped the *pol*-gene of a temperature-sensitive polymerase mutant and of recombinants derived from it and have proposed poly(A)-*src-env-pol-gag* as the complete genetic map of nd RSV (19).

References

1. Duesberg, P. H. (1970 *"Current Topic Microbiol. and Immunology"* 51, 79–104.
2. Tooze, J. (1973) in *The Molecular Biology of Tumour Vuruses.* Cold Spring Harbor Laboratory, Cold Spring Harbor, New York, N.Y.
3. Mangel, W. F., Delius, H., and Duesberg, P. H. (1974) *Proc. Nat. Acad. Sci. USA 71,* 4541–4545.
4. Duesberg, P. H., and Vogt, P. K. (1973) *J. Virol 12,* 594–599.
5. Beemon, K., Duesberg, P. H., and Vogt, P. K. (1974) *Proc. Nat. Acad. Sci. USA 71,* 4254–4258.
6. Billeter, M. A., Parsons, J. T., and Coffin, J. M. (1974) *Proc. Nat. Acad. Sci. USA 71,* 3560–3564.
7. Duesberg, P. H., and Vogt, P. K. (1973) *Virology 54,* 207–218.
8. Baltimore, D. (1974) *Cold Spring Harbor Symposium 39,* 1187–1200.
9. Wang, L. H., and Duesberg, P. H. (1974) *J. Virol. 14,* 1515–1529.
10. Wang, L. H., Duesberg, P. H., Beemon, K., and Vogt, P. K. (1975) *J. Virol. 16,* 1051–1070.
11. Barrell, G. G. (1971) in *Procedures in Nucleic Acid Research* (eds. S. L. Cantoni and D. R. Davis) Vol. 2, Harper and Row, New York, N.Y.
12. Duesberg, P. H., and Vogt, P. K. (1970) *Proc. Nat. Acad. Sci. USA 67,* 1673–1680.
13. Lai, M. M-C., Duesberg, P. H., Horst, J., and Vogt, P. K. (1973) *Proc. Nat. Acad. Sci. USA 70,* 2266–2270.
14. Kawai, S., and Hanafusa, H. (1973) Proc. Nat. Acad. Sci. USA 70, 3493–3497.
15. Spirin, A. S. (1963) *Prog. Nucleic Acid. Res. 1,* 301–345.

16. Duesberg, P. H., Kawai, S., Wang, L. H., Vogt, P. K., Murphy, H. M., and Hanafusa, H. (1975) *Proc. Nat. Acad. Sci, USA 72*, 1569–1573.
17. Wang, L. H., Duesberg, P. H., Kawai, S., and Hanafusa, H. (1976) PNAS *73*, 447-451.
18. Wang, L. H., Duesberg, P. H., Mellon, P. and Vogt, P. K. (1976) Proc. Nat. Acad. Sci., USA *73*, 1073-1077.
19. Duesberg, P. H., Wang L. H., Mellon, P., Mason W. S. and Vogt, P. K. (1976) in: Proceedings of the ICN-UCLA Symposium (1976) on Animal Virology, eds. Baltimore, D., Huang, A. and Fox, F. (Academic Press, New York), in press.

Infection of Developing Mouse Embryos with Murine Leukemia Virus: Tissue Specificity and Genetic Transmission of the Virus

Rudolf Jaenisch, Jessica Dausman, Virginia Cox and Hung Fan

The Salk Institute
San Diego, California 92112
and
Byron Croker
Scripps Clinic & Research Foundation
La Jolla, California 92037

Abstract

The tissue specificity of Moloney leukemia virus (M-MuLV) was studied by infecting mice at two different stages of development. Either newborn mice which can be considered as essentially fully differentiated animals were infected with M-MuLV or preimplantation mouse embryos were infected *in vitro* at the 4–8 cell stage, a stage of development before any differentiation has taken place. After surgical transfer to the uteri of pseudopregnant surrogate mothers, the latter developed to term and adult mice. In both cases, animals were obtained that had developed an M-MuLV induced leukemia.

Molecular hybridization tests for the presence of M-MuLV-specific sequences were conducted on DNA extracted from different tissues of leukemic animals to determine which tissues were successfully infected by the virus. Mice which were infected as newborns carried M-MuLV-specific DNA sequences in "target tissues" only, i. e., thymus, spleen, lymph nodes or in organs infiltrated by tumor cells, whereas "non-target tissues" did not carry virus-specific sequences. In contrast, when leukemic animals derived from M-MuLV-infected preimplantation embryos were analyzed, virus-specific sequences were detected in target tissues as well as in non-target tissues, such as liver, kidney, brain, testes and the germ line.

To study the expression of the viral DNA integrated in target and non-target organs, RNA was extracted from different tissues of an animal infected at the preimplantation stage. Fifty to 100 times more M-MuLV-specific RNA was detected in tumor tissues than was found in non-target organs. Since all organs contained the same amount of virus-specific DNA, these results indicate that the integrated virus genome can be differentially expressed in different tissues. The organ-tropism of RNA tumor viruses is discussed in view of these findings.

Mice that were infected at the preimplantation stage were found to have M-MuLV integrated into their germ line. Virus transmission from the father to the offspring occurred according to simple Mendelian expectations. Molecular hybridization tests revealed that in the animals studied, the virus was integrated into the germ line at only one out of two or three possible integration sites. During the development of leukemia amplification of this virus copy was observed in the target tissues only, but not in the non-target tissues.

Introduction

In principle, two different classes of RNA tumor viruses can induce murine leukemia: endogenous and exogenously or horizontally infecting C-type viruses. The genetic information of endogenous viruses is present in all somatic and germ cells of all animals in a given mouse strain and the endogenous virus is transmitted genetically according to Mendelian expectations (1). One of the best characterized examples of an endogenous oncogenic leukemia virus is found in the AKR strain of mice with a high incidence of leukemia (2). Virus production in AKR mice is controlled by two dominant loci, one of which has been mapped on linkage group I (3). This locus has been shown to represent the structural gene of the AKR virus by molecular hybridization techniques (4).

In contrast, the genetic information of horizontally infecting or exogenous viruses is not transmitted genetically from the father to the offspring (5, 6, 7). This is readily understood since infection of newborn animals with leukemia virus leads to integration of viral DNA into a few "target tissues" only whereas most other tissues, notably the germ line, do not become infected (8, 9). One of the goals of this work was to study the basis of this "organ-tropism" of murine leukemia viruses.

The second aim of the experiments described in this paper was to obtain mice that carry an exogenously infecting virus in their germ line. This would allow us to study genetic transmission of an exogenous virus, to map its integration site and to compare this site with the known loci of endogenous viruses.

One way to obtain an animal carrying exogenous virus genes in every cell including the germ line would be to infect the animals at a very early stage of embryonic development before any differentiation has taken place, for example at the preimplantation stage. At this stage of development, cellular infection might not be restricted by the organ-tropism of a given virus and therefore all cells of the embryo might become successfully infected. An animal derived from such an infected embryo should contain virus information in each cell and the expression of the virus information and of virus-induced oncogenesis should depend on regulatory events in individual cells which, in turn, might be influenced by the differentiated state of a given cell. Indeed, it has been shown recently that adult mice derived from blastocysts infected with SV40 DNA carried SV40-specific sequences in some of their organs (10, 11).

We report here the successful infection and development of Moloney virus (M-MuLV) infected embryos into mature adult mice and the experimental recovery of M-MuLV-specific DNA sequences from the tissues of some of these animals. Our experiments indicate chromosomal integration and genetic transmission of M-MuLV. Some of the experiments described below have been published recently (9).

Materials and Methods

1. *Virus*-M-MuLV clone No. 1 was grown and purified as described (12, 13). Virus stocks were titered by endpoint dilution using the XC plaque test (14).

2. *cDNA*-Virus-specific DNA probes were prepared from purified M-MuLV stock in the presence of 25 or 100 µg/ml actinomycin D (12). ^{32}P-labeled dCTP and/or TTP at a specific activity of 100 Ci/mm (NEN) was used as radioactive precursor. The DNA synthesized had a specific radioactivity of 60–120 x 10^6 cpm/µg and sedimented between 5.5 and 6S in alkaline sucrose gradients. It annealed up to 90 % to M-MuLV 60–70S RNA.

3. *Isolation and infection of mouse embryos* – Four-eight cell stage embryos were isolated from BALB/c females mated with 129J males and the zona pellucida was removed with pronase (15). The embryos were infected with 10^8 PFU/ml of M-MuLV in medium containing 2 µg/ml polybrene for 5 hr and subsequently cultured in medium for 24 hr. At this time, they were surgically transplanted to the uterine horns of pseudopregnant ICR foster mothers (15).

4. *Extraction of nucleic acids* – Mouse tissues were removed and extracted as described (9, 10). In some experiments, the nucleic acids were extracted by the Kirby method (16), the DNA was banded in ethidium bromide CsCl gradients, sonicated and boiled in 0.2 M NaOH for 10 min. The DNA used for hybridization sedimented with approximately 6S in alkaline sucrose gradients. RNA was purified as described previously (12).

5. *Molecular hybridization* – DNA-DNA and DNA-RNA hybridizations were carried out as described previously (9, 12). The cell DNA was in a 2–10 x 10^6 fold excess over the ^{32}P-labeled M-MuLV cDNA. Input radioactivity was 400–800 cpm per experimental point.

6. *Histology* – Sections of the major organs were fixed, sectioned and stained by standard histological techniques (14). Each organ was then evaluated for the extent of lymphomatous infiltration.

7. *Serum analysis* – Mice were bled from the retro-orbital plexus and the serum was analyzed for p30 (14).

Results

1. *Infection of preimplantation mouse embryos with M-MuLV.*

Preimplantation mouse embryos at the 4–8 cell stage were infected with M-MuLV as described in Materials and Methods, washed extensively and incubated in medium at 37°. After 24 hr the virus-infected embryos, as well as the uninfected control embryos, had developed to the blastocyst stage (32–64 cell stage). At this time, they were washed again in medium and transplanted to foster mothers to insure further development *in utero* (see next section).

In order to determine whether infectious virus could be detected on blastocysts, two types of experiments were performed. First, the blastocysts were co-cultivated with BALB/c or NIH Swiss 3T3 cells for six days, the cultures were passed two or three times and all the tissue culture supernatants were tested for M-MuLV by the XC cell assay. Five separate attempts to recover infectious virus were negative. Second, infected blastocysts were fixed, sectioned and prepared for electron microscopy. No C-type particles were observed in five embryos examined.

These observations suggest that the input M-MuLV used for the primary infection of the 4–8 cell embryos did not survive in infectious form during the *in vitro* cultivation period and that the infected embryos did not produce detectable virus at the preimplantation stage.

a) *Induction of leukemia after M-MuLV infection:* Of 29 embryos that were infected at the 4–8 cell stage with M-MuLV and transferred to foster mothers, 15 developed to term and into apparently healthy young mice. The survival rate to birth was therefore 50 % and is comparable to the survival rate of uninfected embryos (50–70 % in this laboratory).

At two months of age, the animals were bled and the serum tested for the presence of murine p30 protein by radioimmune assay. Whereas 14 animals were negative in this test (less than 0.03 µg/ml serum), one mouse showed a high level of 1.9 µg p30 per ml serum. Two weeks later this animal was sacrificed. Autopsy revealed a typical lymphatic leukemia with enlarged spleen and lymph nodes.

The foster mothers used in this experiment were bled four and twelve weeks after delivery and tested for murine p30. The serum contained less than 0.03 µg/ml p30, suggesting that no virus infection of the mother via the embryos was detectable.

b) *Histology and isolation of virus:* Histological examinations of sections of different organs revealed massive infiltration of lymph nodes, spleen and kidneys with lymphoma cells, intermediate infiltration of the thymus and relatively little infiltration of the liver. The lung, brain and testes did not show any tumor cell

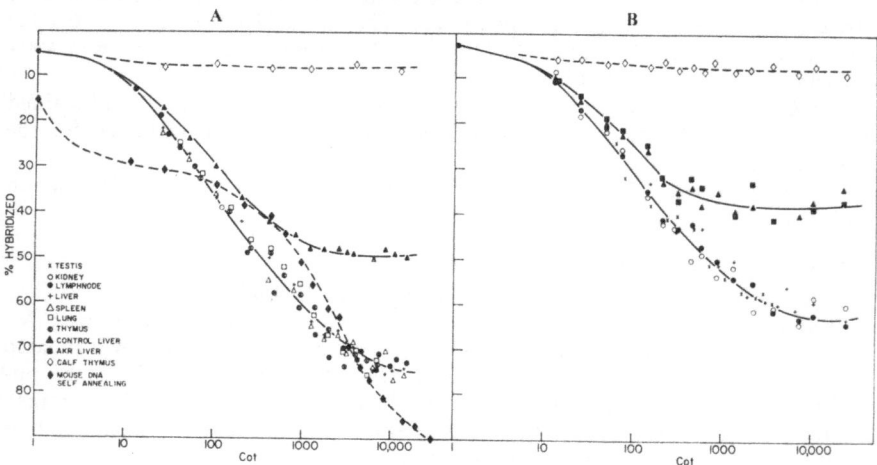

Fig. 1: Association kinetics of ^{32}P-labeled M-MuLV cDNA with mouse cellular DNA derived from various organs of the mouse infected at the 4–8 cell stage with M-MuLV, from control mice (BALB/c 129 and AKR) or from calf thymus. The reaction mixture containing 0.5 ng/ml of ^{32}P-labeled M-MuLV cDNA (1.2×10^8 cpm/µg), 4 mg/ml mouse or calf thymus DNA in 0.01 M Tris-HCl, pH 7.0, 1 mM EDTA, 1M NaCl, was heat denatured and incubated at 68°. Per cent hybridization is plotted as a function of Cot, corrected to standard annealing conditions (25). The cDNA probes used annealed to 80 % (A) or 70 % (B) to M-MuLV 60–70S RNA.

344

infiltration (Table 1). The lymphoid tumors and infiltrates were composed of sheets of uniform large lymphoblasts.

The serum was tested for infectious virus on B and N type cells. Virus was found and titered equally well on both test cells and the TCID 50/ml serum was 2 x 10⁴ on B cells and 3 x 10⁴ on N cells. Virus recovered from infected BALB/c cells also titered equally well on NIH Swiss and B type cells, indicating that the virus isolated was N-B tropic similar to the infecting M-MuLV.

c) *M-MuLV specific sequences in mouse DNA:* The presence of M-MuLV specific sequences in cellular DNA was determined by annealing the M-MuLV cDNA probe with DNA extracted from various tissues of the M-MuLV-infected mouse, control BALB/129 and AKR mice. The reassociation kinetics are shown in Figs. 1a and b. In Fig. 1a, up to 75 % of the cDNA probe (up to 63 % in Fig. 1b) hybridized to the DNA extracted from the different tissues of the M-MuLV-infected mouse; with BALB/c 129 control or AKR DNA, the maximum hybridization observed was 50 % (37 % in Fig. 1b) and essentially no hybridization was detected to calf thymus DNA. The different maxima of hybridization observed for the same cellular DNA preparations in Figs. 1a and b are attributable to different cDNA probes used with different levels of maximal hybridization to virion 60–70S RNA. In Fig. 1a the reassociation kinetics of total mouse cell DNA is also plotted.

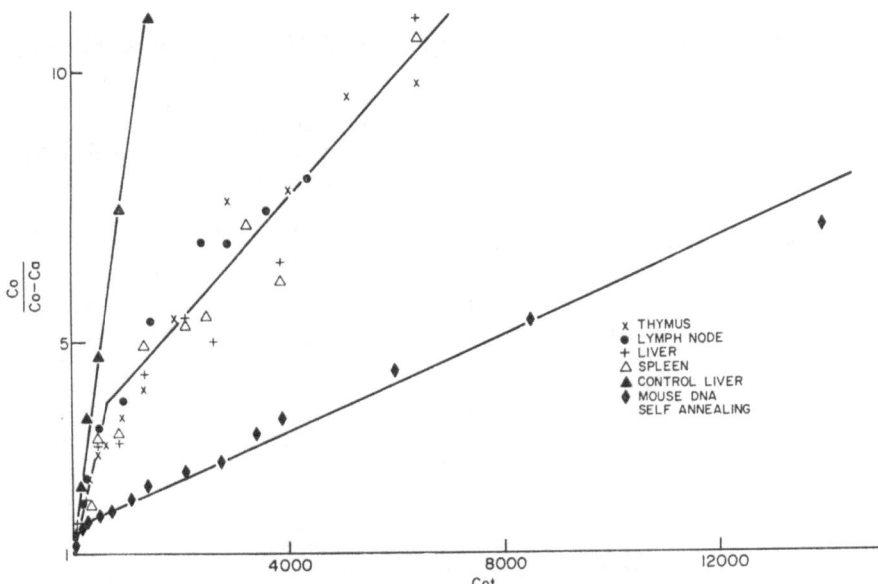

Fig. 2: Analysis of the association kinetics of ³²P-labeled M-MuLV cDNA with mouse DNA by the method of Wetmur and Davidson (17). The results are plotted as the reciprocal of the fraction of DNA remaining single-stranded as a function of C_0t. The maximum observed hybridization was normalized to 100 %. (Co = fraction of single-stranded DNA at time 0, Ca = fraction of single-stranded DNA at different times.) The data are taken from Fig. 1A.

The results indicate that uninfected control mice (BALB/129 and AKR) carry some sequences (up to 50 %) homologous to M-MuLV cDNA. In addition, the Moloney virus-infected mouse acquired M-MuLV-specific sequences which are not present in uninfected animals. All tissues tested contained the same amount of M-MuLV-specific DNA.

In order to examine more closely the kinetics of reassociation and to determine the number of virus copies present, the data in Fig. 1a was plotted as the reciprocal of the fraction of unhybridized probe versus the C_0t normalized to 100 % hybridization (4, 17). If all virus-specific sequences are present in the cellular DNA in equal numbers, the results would be a single straight line with a slope proportional to the number of copies of that set of sequences. On the other hand, if several sets of virus-specific sequences were present, each in different proportions, the curves would describe several slopes. It can be seen that the viral probe anneals with the DNA extracted from the M-MuLV-infected mouse as though there were two distinct sets of virus-specific sequences in the cell DNA (Fig. 2). The $C_0t_{1/2}$ for each component was calculated, giving a value of 1,100 mole·sec/liter for the slow annealing component of M-MuLV-specific sequences and a value of 80–100 mole·sec/liter for the fast annealing sequences in comparison to a $C_0t_{1/2}$ of 2,200 for unique cell DNA. The slopes of this slow annealing set of sequences in Fig. 2 is about 2.5 times steeper and the slope of the fast annealing set about 15

Table I: Detection of M-MuLV-specific DNA and RNA in tissues of the Moloney virus-infected mouse.

Organ	Histology: extent of infiltration with lymphoma cells	No. of M-MuLV specific sequences		M-MuLV specific RNA %
		Fast annealing set	Slow annealing set	
lymph node	High	15–30	2–3	0.43
kidney	High	15–30	2–3	0.41
spleen	High	15–30	2–3	0.31
thymus	Medium	15–30	2–3	0.088
liver	Low	15–30	2–3	0.005
lung	None	15–30	2–3	0.19
testis	None	15–30	2–3	0.017
brain	None	(+)*	(+)*	0.005
control liver, spleen, kidney	n. t.	15–30	0	0
AKR liver	n. t.	15–30	0	n. t.

Table1: Detection of M-MuLV specific DNA and RNA in various tissues of the Moloney virus-infected mouse.
The number of M-MuLV-specific DNA copies in haploid mouse genomes was calculated from the $C_0t_{1/2}$ values of each class of virus-specific sequences relative to the $C_0t_{1/2}$ of unique DNA (Figs. 1 and 2). The concentration of M-MuLV-specific RNA was calculated from the $C_rt_{1/2}$ values in Fig. 3.
* The brain DNA was positive for M-MuLV-specific DNA but no quantitation was possible due to the small amount of brain DNA isolated.

times steeper as compared to the self-annealing of cellular DNA. These values and the $C_0t_{1/2}$ values suggest about 2–3 copies per haploid genome for the slow annealing component and about 15–30 copies for the fast annealing component of sequences complementary to M-MuLV. Thus, the Moloney virus-infected animals acquired 2–3 copies of Moloney virus-specific sequences not present in control animals (Table I).

d) *Differential transcription of M-MuLV specific sequences in different organs:* M-MuLV cDNA was annealed with RNA extracted from eight organs of the M-MuLV-infected mouse and also with RNA from some organs of control mice (Fig. 3). RNA extracted from the various organs of the experimental animal

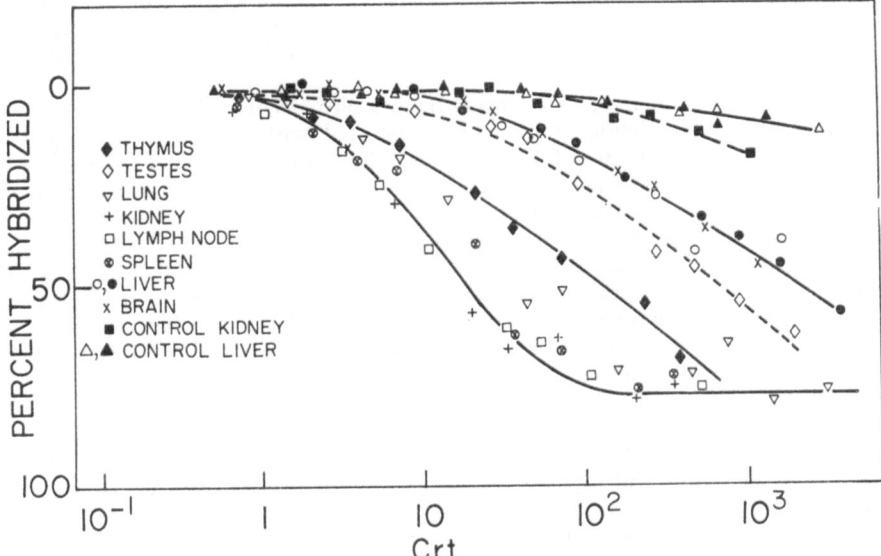

Fig. 3: Annealing of labeled M-MuLV cDNA with cellular RNA from different organs of the M-MuLV infected and control mice. Annealing in conditions of RNA excess was performed as described (12). Per cent hybrid formation is displayed as a function of C_rt, corrected to standard annealing conditions (25).

efficiently hybridized with the M-MuLV cDNA, while control RNA annealed only small amounts at extremely high C_rt values. Maximal hybridization for the M-MuLV cDNA was 75 % as determined by annealing to purified M-MuLV 60–70S RNA.

The amount of M-MuLV specific RNA present in the various organs was determined from the half-saturation values of hybridization $(C_rt_{1/2})$ (12), and was found to vary over a wide range (Table 1). Between 0.3 and 0.43 % of the total RNA extracted from spleen, lymph nodes and kidney was virus-specific, whereas liver, testes and brain contained approximately 50–100-fold less M-MuLV-specific RNA. The thymus and the lung showed intermediate levels of virus-specific RNA. With the exception of the lung, the levels of M-MuLV-specific RNA appeared to correlate roughly with the degree of infiltration of a given organ with lymphoma cells (see Table 1). These results indicate that although all tissues contained the same number of M-MuLV DNA copies, these virus genes were expressed at different levels in different organs.

II. *Genetic transmission of M-MuLV.*

The previous experiments established that infection of preimplantation mouse embryos can lead to animals carrying M-MuLV-specific DNA sequences in many, if not all, the tissues of the adult. We were interested in studying whether integration of the virus into the germ line could take place since this would allow us to map the integration site of an exogenously infecting virus and to compare this site with the known integration sites of endogenous viruses. Therefore, we investigated whether genetic transmission of M-MuLV from a viremic father to its offspring can occur.

The male used for these experiments (mouse No. 339 in Table 2) was derived from a 4–8 cell preimplantation embryo infected with M-MuLV. The animal showed moderately elevated levels of serum p30 (0.8–1.0 µg/ml) at six weeks of age and was bred with unexposed females. Of 80 progeny tested so far, seven had infectious M-MuLV in the serum at 4–5 weeks of age. This observation suggests either that approximately 10 % of the sperm of the father carried virus-specific information in its genome and transmitted it genetically to his offspring or that about 10 % of the offspring were congenitally infected from the viremic father via the mother (as opposed to genetic transmission, 18). Earlier observations seem to rule out the latter explanation since leukemic males infected *in utero* or after birth with M-MuLV do not transmit the disease to their offspring (5–7). If, on the other hand, germ line transmission had occurred, two testable predictions should be fulfilled.

1) The number of M-MuLV-specific DNA copies in the viremic N-1 animals should be constant in all organs of individual animals (in contrast to animals infected after birth, see below).

2) Viremic N-1 males mated to uninfected females should transmit the virus according to simple Mendelian expectations to the next generations.

a) *M-MuLV-specific DNA sequences in N-1 animals:* The first 25 progeny of the viremic male infected at the preimplantation stage with M-MuLV were tested for both infectious virus in their serum as well as for M-MuLV-specific DNA sequences in some of their organs. Four of these 25 animals showed infectious virus with titers between 10^2–10^3 XC PFU/ml. Only in DNA extracted from these four XC positive animals were M-MuLV-specific DNA sequences found, whereas in the other 21 animals, no M-MuLV-specific DNA could be detected. Figure 4 shows the annealing kinetics of ^{32}P labeled M-MuLV cDNA with DNA extracted from five different organs of one of these animals. The slopes of the annealing kinetics for non-target organs, i. e., brain, liver, kidney and muscle, are identical, whereas the spleen, a target organ of M-MuLV infection, anneals with M-MuLV cDNA four times faster. The number of virus-specific DNA copies was calculated to be one-half copy per haploid mouse genome equivalent for the non-target organs and two copies for the spleen. Hybridization experiments with the other three viremic N-1 animals gave identical results.

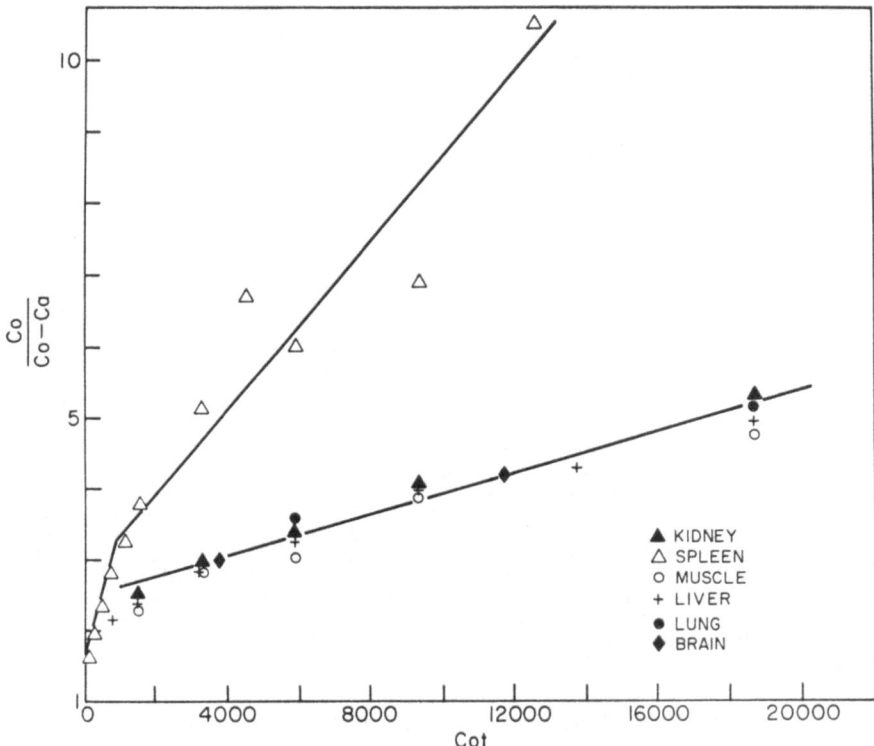

Fig. 4: Analysis of the annealing kinetics of ^{32}P-labeled M-MuLV cDNA with mouse DNA extracted from an N-1 animal derived from mating mouse No. 339 (Table 2) with an uninfected female. The reaction mixture containing 0.2 ng/ml of ^{32}P-labeled M-MuLV cDNA (1.5×10^8 cpm/µg) and 5 mg/ml of mouse DNA extracted from different organs was annealed as described in Fig. 1 and the data plotted as described in Fig. 2. The cDNA probe used annealed up to 92 % to M-MuLV 60–70S RNA.

These observations indicate that whenever M-MuLV DNA sequences were transmitted from the father to its offspring (in four out of 25 N-1 animals tested) the virus information was expressed as infectious virus in the serum. Secondly, the number of M-MuLV-specific DNA copies found in all non-target organs of these animals was identical and increased four-fold in the target tissues during the development of leukemia.

b) *Transmission of M-MuLV to the N-2 generation: The* hybridization results described above indicate that the viremic N-1 animals carried one-half copy of M-MuLV per haploid mouse genome equivalent in each cell, suggesting that these animals may have been heterozygotes for one integration site of M-MuLV. This would predict a 50 % transmission of M-MuLV to the N-2 generation.

One viremic N-1 male and two viremic N-2 males were used to test this hypothe-

Table II: Genetic Transmission of M-MuLV

Mouse No.		Mode of Infection with M-MuLV	Transmission of M-MuLV to Offspring when Mated with Uninfected Females	
			No. of Viremic Offspring	%
339	♂	4–8 cell preimplantation stage	7/80	9 %
921	♂	N-1 of No. 339	19/30	63 %
901–3	♂		4/ 8	50 %
901–10	♂	N-2 of No. 339	6/20	30 %
			Total 29/58	50 %
1	♂		0/35	0 %
2	♂	Infected as new-	0/29	0 %
4	♂	borns with	0/32	0 %
9	♂	M-MuLV	0/25	0 %
			Total 0/121	0 %

Table 2: Genetic transmission of M-MuLV.
Four–eight cell embryos were infected with M-MuLV and transplanted to foster mothers as described in the text. One viremic mouse derived from these embryos (male No. 339) was bred with uninfected BALB/c females and the resulting N-1 generation was analyzed for infectious virus in the serum. Viremic N-1 males were bred with normal BALB/c females to yield N-2 and N-3 animals. Furthermore, newborn mice were infected with M-MuLV and bred with BALB/c females after development of viremia. All the progeny were tested for infectious M-MuLV in the serum by the XC assay.
Figure Legends

sis. The N-1 male (No. 921, Table 2) was derived by mating mouse No. 339 with an uninfected BALB/c female. The N-2 males (No. 901–3 and 901–10 in Table 2) were derived from a viremic daughter of mouse No. 339 mated with an uninfected BALB/c male. Annealing kinetics of DNA extracted from various organs of this female with M-MuLV cDNA have been described in Fig. 4. These three viremic males were mated to uninfected females and the resulting N-2 and N-3 generations were tested for infectious virus in the serum. The results in Table 2 indicate that of a total of 58 N-2 and N-3 animals tested, 29 were positive for infectious M-MuLV. These data strongly favor the hypothesis that M-MuLV was integrated into the germ line of these mice and was transmitted genetically to the offspring according to simple Mendelian expectations.

Table 2 also contains breeding data of viremic males infected with M-MuLV at birth. None of these animals transmitted the virus to the offspring, confirming earlier observations (5–7).

III. *Infection of newborn mice with M-MuLV.*
The experiments described above have shown that after infection of an animal at the preimplantation stage with M-MuLV, virtually all tissues of the resulting adult can carry the same amount of virus-specific sequences per cell, regardless of whether the tissue represents a "target" tissue for the virus or not. The situation

might be very different when infection takes place at a later developmental stage, i. e., after birth, when all cells of the animal are fully differentiated. To investigate this possibility, newborn mice were infected with M-MuLV and following development of viremia and leukemia, the DNA from different organs was analyzed for the presence of virus-specific sequences. The results obtained with one of these animals are described below.

When sacrificed at four months of age, this animal appeared terminally ill with extensive tumor cell infiltration in many organs. Radioimmunoassay revealed 2 µg/ml serum of murine p30. Histological examination demonstrated almost 100 % lymphoma cell infiltration in the highly enlarged thymus and spleen, approximately 30–50 % infiltration in the liver and less than 10 % infiltration in the kidneys. Brain and muscle had little if any signs of lymphoma cell infiltration.

The DNA was extracted from all these tissues and annealed with ³²P-labeled M-MuLV cDNA (Fig. 5). The slopes of the DNA annealing kinetics revealed two sets of virus-complementary sequences comparable to the results described in Fig. 2. But, in contrast to the results obtained with the animal infected at the preimplantation stage (Figs. 1, 2) or in animals with genetically transmitted virus (Fig. 4), the curves indicate that different amounts of the slow annealing set of

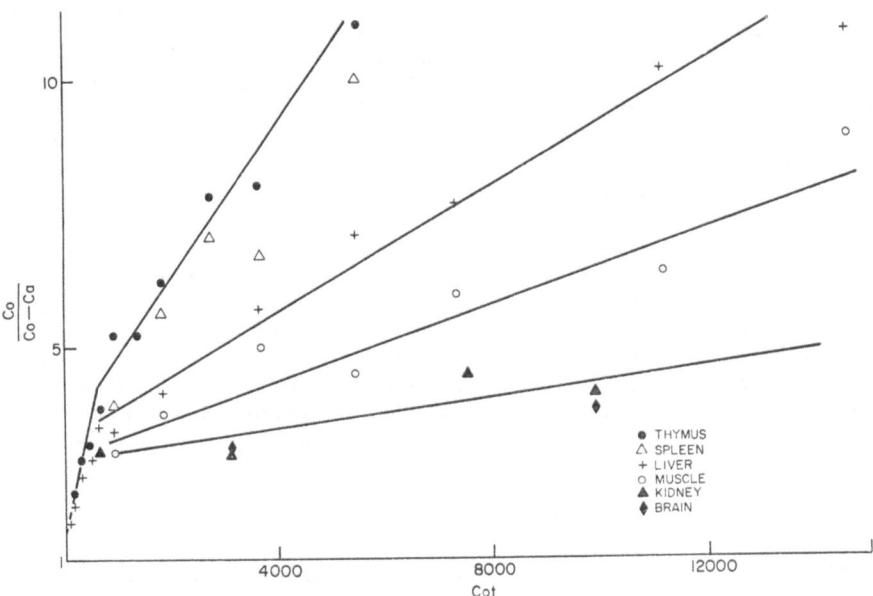

Fig. 5: Analysis of the association kinetics of ³²P-labeled M-MuLV DNA with mouse DNA extracted from an animal infected after birth with M-MuLV. The reaction mixture containing 0.2 ng/ml of ³²P-labeled M-MuLV cDNA (8 x 10⁷ cpm/µg) and 6 mg/ml of mouse DNA extracted from different organs was annealed as described in Fig. 1, and the data are plotted as described in Fig. 2. The cDNA probe used annealed up to 90 % to M-MuLV 60–70S RNA.

M-MuLV-specific sequences were present in the different organs. Spleen and thymus showed the highest concentration of virus-specific DNA, comparable to the concentration found in each of the organs of the animal described in Figs. 1 and 2. On the other hand, the slow annealing M-MuLV cDNA sequences annealed more slowly with the DNA extracted from the other organs. From the slopes of these curves, it can be calculated that in comparison to the thymus and spleen, the concentration of M-MuLV-specific DNA present in the liver was only about 0.4 times as much, in the muscle about 0.25 and in brain and kidneys approximately 0.05–0.1 times as much. With the exception of the muscle, these values roughly correlate with the extent of histological detected lymphoma cell infiltration. This suggests that the virus-specific DNA sequences detected in the DNA of the different organs was derived primarily from the infiltrating tumor cells and not from the parenchymal cells. This correlation does not hold for the muscle and may be due either to extensive tumor cell infiltration of the skeletal muscles undetected in the limited number of histological sections examined, or to muscle cells being susceptible to virus infection (in contrast to other parenchymal cells).

Discussion

Murine leukemia induced by exogenously infecting M-MuLV or by the endogenous Gross virus develops as a typically thymus-derived disease. Other RNA tumor viruses, such as Friend virus or murine mammary tumor virus, are characterized by a different organ-tropism, i. e., they transform spleen erythroblasts or mammary gland cells, respectively, but not the thymus derived lymphoblasts. One of the aims of this investigation was to study the possible basis of the organ-tropism of a given tumor virus.

We, therefore, compared the type of tissues that can be infected by M-MuLV at different stages of development. We have chosen two extreme stages of development for infection, the preimplantation 4–8 cell embryo and the newborn mouse. At the 4–8 cell stage of development, no differentiation or commitment of the single blastomers can be recognized (19), whereas the newborn mouse can be considered as an essentially fully differentiated organism. By testing for the presence of M-MuLV-specific DNA sequences in different tissues of the adult leukemic mouse, we were able to demonstrate that the developmental stage of an animal at which the infection takes place indeed determines which tissues can be infected and which tissues are not susceptible to infection. Furthermore, we studied the expression of M-MuLV genetic information present in target and non-target organs.

I. *Tissue distribution of M-MuLV specific sequences.*

The leukemic animal described in this paper infected at the 4–8 cell stage with M-MuLV (Figs. 1 and 2, Table 1) was derived from a BALB/c 129 cross, both of which are low leukemia incidence strains. The animal had developed the leukemia at two months of age and the pathology of this disease was typical for a Moloney virus-induced lymphatic leukemia and distinctly different from the pathology of a spontaneous leukemia in these mouse strains. This, together with the isolation of N-B tropic virus from the serum, tends to exclude the possibility that the animal developed a spontaneous leukemia but rather indicates that this leukemia was induced by the infecting M-MuLV. This conclusion is further supported by the hybridization studies.

The DNA-DNA hybridization experiments revealed one class of M-MuLV complementary sequences in uninfected animals and two classes of sequences in the Moloney virus-infected animal (Figs. 1 and 2). The more abundant class of M-MuLV complementary sequences was present at approximately 15–30 copies per haploid genome in infected and uninfected animals. A second less frequent set of Moloney virus-specific sequences was found only in the experimental animal at a frequency of 2–3 copies per haploid mouse genome.

Multiple copies of the endogenous C-type viruses have been detected in a variety of species (1, 4, 20, 21) and the number of copies of endogenous viruses varies considerably, depending on the system studied and the viral probe used. The class of M-MuLV complementary sequences we have detected in uninfected animals may represent sequences of endogenous viruses that are homologous to part of the M-MuLV cDNA.

Eight different tissues derived from all three germ layers of the Moloney virus-infected animal carried the same number of M-MuLV specific DNA copies, regardless of whether the respective organ was infiltrated with lymphoma cells or not. This observation suggests that the virus DNA was integrated into the host genome, possibly at specific sites, rather than existing as an independently replicating plasmid. That chromosomal integration of RNA tumor viruses occurs following exogenous infection has been demonstrated recently (22, 23).

The tissue distribution of viral DNA sequences following infection at the pre-implantation stage is in sharp contrast to the situation found after infection of newborn animals with leukemia virus. In chicks infected with avian myeloblastoma virus at one day of age, virus-specific DNA sequences occurred only in cells from tumors or tumor cell infiltrated organs, whereas tumor cell free "non-target" tissues did not contain viral specific sequences (8). The experiments described in Fig. 5 showed similar results. When newborn mice were infected with Moloney virus, virus-specific sequences were found primarily in leukemia target tissues such as thymus and spleen. The amount of virus-specific sequences found in other organs was correlated to the extent of infiltration with lymphoma cells of the respective organ, suggesting that the parenchymal cells did not become infected with virus, although muscle tissue was a possible exception. These observations suggest that susceptibility of the different cells of an animal to virus infection may be determined by the developmental stage of the animal at the time of infection. Once the animal has developed to birth, i. e., to a fully differentiated stage, only certain target tissues are susceptible or accessible to leukemia virus infection. In contrast, when the animal is infected at the 4–8 cell stage, i. e., prior to any detectable cell differentiation, the organ-tropism of the virus does not determine which cells become infected and consequently virus infection can result in animals carrying the virus information in possibly all the differentiated cells of the adult.

II. *Genetic transmission of M-MuLV.*

The experiments discussed above suggest that infection of newborn animals should not lead to germ line integration of the virus. Indeed, in experiments done previously germ line transmission of leukemia virus introduced into mice by transplacental infection or by infection after birth was never observed (5–7, Table 2). The experiments described in Fig. 4 and Table 2 indicate that infection of preimplantation embryos, on the other hand, can lead to virus integration into the germ line and to genetic transmission of the exogenously infecting virus. The data in Fig. 4 suggest that only one copy of M-MuLV DNA was transmitted vertically, thus resulting in an N-1 animal carrying only one-half copy of M-MuLV-specific DNA per haploid mouse genome. It is likely that the male used for these studies (mouse No. 339 in Table 2) carried the virus integrated at only one site in approximately 10 % of his sperm, suggesting that this animal is characterized by germ line mosaicism analogous to allophenic mice (24). The 50 % transmission of M-MuLV from the N-1 to the N-2 and N-3 generations indicates that the integrated virus behaved essentially like a Mendelian dominant gene. Experiments are presently being conducted to map the integration site.

The observation that non-target organs of viremic N-1 animals carried one-half copy of M-MuLV DNA per haploid mouse genome but target organs like the spleen and the thymus carried two copies per haploid mouse genome (Fig. 4) indicates that during the development of leukemia an amplification of the germ line transmitted virus DNA had taken place. It is not known if this amplification is due to reintegration of the virus into the mouse genome or if the observed amplification is the result of selective chromosomal duplication in the transformed cells. In any event, these observations and the results described in Figs. 1 and 2 and Table 1 suggest that the maximum number of virus copies that can integrate is 2–3 copies per haploid mouse genome. The viremic animals derived from mouse No. 339 (Table 2) might therefore carry M-MuLV integrated into their germ line at only one out of two or three possible integration sites.

III. *Expression of M-MuLV.*

The animal described in Figs. 1 and 2 carried equal amounts of M-MuLV-specific DNA in all tissues tested. This enabled us to compare the expression of the virus information in target and non-target organs of M-MuLV infection.

The virus information present in the cells was expressed to very different extents in the various tissues. For most tissues, the amount of virus-specific RNA found roughly correlated with the degree of infiltration with lymphoma cells in the respective organs. RNA from brain, liver and testes, which histologically showed little or no infiltration contained 50–100 times fewer viral sequences than RNA from the highly infiltrated spleen, lymph nodes and kidneys (Table 1). The lung was the only clear exception in this correlation with no tumor cell infiltration observed in the histological specimen but nevertheless with a relatively high concentration of viral-specific RNA expressed. The contribution in these measurements of viral-specific RNA from virus particles present in the serum has not yet been determined.

Several interrelated aspects of known gene expression and ontogeny may explain these results. One possibility is that viral DNA was transcribed into RNA in lymphoma cells only. The amount of virus-specific RNA found in different tissues would then reflect the extent of infiltration. In any case, it is evident that M-MuLV transcription is one manifestation of differential gene expression in different tissues. All tissues contained the same amount of M-MuLV DNA, so it is likely that the M-MuLV virus gene came under control of host regulatory elements such as those involved in normal tissue differentiation.

These experiments suggest a second control mechanism involved in the organ-tropism of RNA tumor viruses. If, as in these experiments, an M-MuLV gene is introduced into the DNA of all cells in an animal, its expression still appears to be repressed in all cells except the target cells. Therefore, in addition to organ-tropism at the level of adsorption, penetration or integration of the virus (as shown by the data on M-MuLV infected newborn animals), a second level of organ-tropism appears to be operating at the level of the expression of the inte-grated virus genome.

Acknowledgements

We thank Mrs. Carolyn Goller for her assistance in preparing the manuscript. This work was supported by National Institutes of Health Grants Nos. CA-15561-02 and CA-15747-02 and by National Science Foundation Grant No. GB 38656. B. C. received a postdoctoral fellowship, J-241, from the American Cancer Society.

References

1. Todaro, G., Benveniste, R., Callahan, R., Lieber, M., and Sherr, C. (1974) Cold Spring Harbor Symp. Quant. Biol. *39*: 1159.
2. Gross, L. (1974) Proc. Nat. Acad. Sci. USA *71*: 2013.
3. Rowe, W. (1972) J. Exp. Med. *136*: 1272.
4. Chattopadhyay, S., Lowy, D., Teich, N., Levine, A., and Rowe, W. (1974) Cold Spring Harbor Symp. Quant. Biol. *39*: 1085.
5. Rubin, H., Fanshier, L., Cornelius, A., and Hughes, W. (1962) Virology *17*: 143.
6. Buffet, R., Grace, J., DiBerardino, L., and Mirand, E. (1969) Cancer Res. *29*: 588.
7. Law, L., and Moloney, B. (1961) Proc. Soc. Exp. Biol. Med. *108*: 715.
8. Baluda, M., and Drohan, W. (1972) J. Virol. *10*: 1002.
9. Jaenisch, R., Fan, H., and Croker, B. (1975) Proc. Nat. Acad. Sci. USA 72, 4008.
10. Jaenisch, R., and Mintz, B. (1974) Proc. Nat. Acad. Sci. USA *71*: 1250.
11. Jaenisch, R. (1974) Cold Spring Harbor Symp. Quant. Biol. *39*: 375.
12. Fan, H., and Baltimore, D. (1973) J. Mol. Biol. *80*: 93.
13. Fan, H., and Paskind, M. (1974) J. Virol. *14*: 421.
14. Croker, B., DelVillano, B., Jensen, F., and Dixon, F. (1974) J. Exp. Med. *140*: 1028.
15. Mintz, B. (1971) *in* Methods in Mammalian Embryology (Daniel, J., ed) (Freeman, San Francisco), pp. 189–214.
16. Kirby, K. (1966) *in* Methods in Enzymology 22: 87.
17. Wetmur, J., and Davidson, N. (1968) J. Mol. Biol. *31*: 349.
18. Tooze, J. (1973) *in* The Molecular Biology of Tumor Viruses (Cold Spring Harbor Laboratory, Cold Spring Harbor, New York) p 617.

19. Herbert, M., and Graham, C. (1974) *in* Current Topics in Develop. Biol. *8*: 151.
20. Weiss, R. (1975) Perspect. Virol. *9*: 165.
21. Benveniste, R., and Todaro, G. (1974) Nature *252*: 170.
22. Varmus, H., Guntaka, R., Fan, W., Heasley, S., and Bishop, M. (1974) Proc. Nat. Acad. Sci. USA *71*: 3874.
23. Gianni, A., Smotking, D., and Weinberg, R. (1975) Proc. Nat. Acad. Sci. USA *72*: 447.
24. Mintz, B. (1968) J. Animals Science *27*, Supplement 1, 51.
25. Britten, R., Dale, G., and Neufeld, R. (1974) *in* Methods in Enzymology *29*: 363.

Type C Virogenes: Modes of Transmission and Evolutionary Aspects

George J. Todaro, M. D.

Viral Leukemia and Lymphoma Branch
National Cancer Institute
National Institutes of Health
Bethesda, Maryland 20014

Introduction

Extensive evidence has demonstrated that type C RNA viruses are active agents in the causation of naturally occuring cancers. Type C RNA viruses are a distinct class of vertebrate viruses which share a common morphology, protein composition, and viral life cycle. They are spherical particles containing a large single-stranded RNA as their viral genome complexed with a RNA-directed DNA polymerase (reverse transcriptase) in a central, symmetric, electron dense core surrounded by a unit membrane. During viral replication the nucleoid condenses beneath the surface of the cytoplasmic cell membrane with subsequent "budding" of the virus from the cell surface.

Type C RNA viruses have been isolated from many vertebrate species. They have been shown to cause a variety of naturally occurring vertebrate neoplastic diseases, including leukemias and sarcomas of chickens, lymphomas and related hematopoietic neoplasms and sarcomas of mice, lymphosarcomas and fibrosarcomas of domestic cats, and leukemias and sarcomas of some primates. Type C viruses have also been isolated from other mammalian species such as rats, guinea pigs, hamsters, cattle, domestic pigs, woolly monkeys, gibbon apes, and baboons (Table 1). Recently there have been reports of isolates from human tissues (see below). As yet, in some of these species, the relationship between these viruses and neoplastic diseases of their host species has not been clarified. There have also been reports of electron microscopic observations of typical type C viral particles in tissues from some other mammalian species, including dogs, horses, rhesus monkeys, and in certain human tissues, but such viruses have not yet been isolated in vitro and biochemically characterized. Type C RNA viruses exhibit varying biological activity. Some have no known pathological effect and others are extremely efficient in producing neoplasias. Also, transformation may occur either with complete or incomplete virus expression. Type C viruses have also been detected in normal tissues; embryonic and placental tissues show more type C viral expression than other differentiated tissues. The viruses produced by both normal and tumorigenic

357

Table I: Mammalian type C RNA virus isolates

Species	Description
Mouse (*Mus musculus*)	Many well-studied laboratory strain leukemia and sarcoma viruses (MuLV, MSV). Large variety of endogenous viruses.
Mouse (*Mus caroli*)	Antigenically related to gibbon and woolly monkey viruses (see text).
Rat (*Rattus norvegicus*)	Endogenous viruses released from numerous rat cell lines in culture. Poorly infectious.
Chinese hamster (*Cricetulus griseus*) and Syrian (or Golden) hamster (*Mesocricetus auratus*)	Poorly infectious viruses released from cells in culture.
Guinea pig (*Cavies spp.*)	Type C virus induced from cultured cells and associated with spontaneous and transmissable leukemia. Some consider it more like a type B virus.
Domestic cat (*Felis catus*)	Two distinct classes: (a) Feline leukemia and sarcoma viruses (FeLV, FeSV); (b) RD-114/CCC family of endogenous feline viruses.
Pig (*Sus scrofa*)	Endogenous viruses released from both normal and leukemic cell lines in culture. Poorly infectious.
Cattle (*Bos taurus*)	Infectious type C viruses isolated from lymphosarcoma tissue.
Woolly monkey (*Lagothrix ssp.*)	Simian sarcoma virus (SSV-1).
Baboon (*Papio cynocephalus* and other *Papio* species)	Endogenous viruses which replicate well in cells of heterologous species.
Gibbon ape (*Hylobates lar.*)	Gibbon lymphosarcoma virus (GLV).

tissues are very similar to one another in their morphology, biochemical and immunological properties (1, 2).

Transmission of virogenes

The spontaneous appearance of complete, infectious type C RNA viruses in animals of certain mammalian species and in cultured cells derived from these animals led to the hypothesis that the information for the production of such viruses might be transmitted genetically from parent to progeny along with other cellular genes (virogene-oncogene hypothesis) (3, 4). Activation of this normally repressed, genetically transmitted, type C endogenous virogene information, rather than infection from outside the animal was proposed as the most common mechanism by which type C RNA tumor viruses produce naturally occurring cancers.

Table II: Species where a COMPLETE virogene is known to be present in normal cells

Chicken	Mouse *(Mus musculus)*	Cat
Chinese Hamster	Mouse *(Mus caroli)*	Pig
Syrian Hamster	Rat	Baboon

Vertical transmission from generation to generation rather than infection from animal to animal was postulated to be the primary means by which the viral genes have been maintained in animal populations. Much subsequent experimental work supports this, the most important being that "virus-free" cell cultures (Table 2) derived from chicken, mouse, hamster, rat, pig, cat, and baboon tissues (reviewed in 5) can begin to secrete either spontaneously or after treatment with chemical inducing agents, typical complete type C viruses (6, 7). Cocultivation of the virus producing cell cultures with appropriate permissive cell lines from heterologous species has been needed to detect and increase virus production in several of these systems (8–10). The properties characterizing such endogenous mammalian type C RNA viruses which are products of the genetically transmitted virogenes are summarized in Table 3.

Table III: Properties of endogenous type C virogenes

1. DNA of all somatic and germ cells of all the animals in a species contain viral gene sequences.
2. Multiple related but not identical copies present in the cellular DNA, more than DNA from a heterologous cell that is actively producing virus.
3. Virus expression (RNA, gs antigen, polymerase, complete particles) under cellular control. Expressed in certain tissues at certain times during development.
4. Clonal lines either spontaneously or after induction are capable of releasing complete virion.
5. Cells generally resistant to exogenous infection by the homologous endogenous virus.

The endogenous type C virogenes are those sets of gene sequences that are an integral part of the host species' chromosomal DNA and code for the production of type C viruses. These gene sequences contained in normal cellular DNA should be distinguished from type C viral DNA sequences which can be added to the animal's genome from the outside by "exogenous" viral infection and subsequent integration (provirus formation) (11). Endogenous type C virogenes should also be distinguished (Table 4) from those gene sequences not originally present in the genome, that are postulated to arise by gene duplication and/or recombination mediated by the reverse transcriptase mechanism (12, 13) (protovirus formation (14)).

The endogenous virogenes and the oncogenes (those cellular genes responsible for transforming a normal cell into a tumor cell which may or may not be present

Table IV: Major differences between virogene and protovirus models

Virogene	Protovirus
1. Viral copies present in germ cells and somatic cells.	1. Germ cells lack virus information. Generated in rare somatic cells by chance.
2. Genes maintained in population by normal cellular replication. Reverse transcriptase *not required*.	2. Reverse transcriptase plays essential role in generating new viruses.
3. Transformation results from activation of normally latent cellular genes associated with and/or part of the viral gene sequences.	3. Transformation results from the generation of new gene sequences that do not preexist in normal cellular DNA.

as a part of the genome of type C viruses (4)) are normally repressed, but can be activated by a variety of intrinsic (genetic, hormonal) as well as extrinsic (radiation, chemical carcinogens, other infecting viruses) factors (Table 5). Regulatory genes and environmental factors determine the extent of virogene transcription.

Table V: Implications of the virogene-oncogene hypothesis

Virogenes
1. All somatic cells of a species have DNA homologous to type C virus RNA of that species (virogenes).
2. Type C viruses derived from closely related species should have closely related specific antigens, e. g., gs antigens, polymerase and their nucleic acid sequences should be more related to one another than are those viruses released by distantly related species (virogene evolution).

Oncogenes
3. The transformation specific sequences of RNA tumor viruses should be present in normal cellular DNA (oncogenes).
4. Spontaneous, chemically induced and viral induced transformed cells and tumor cells should have RNA as well as DNA sequences homologous to the transforming specific sequences found in tumor viruses (oncogene expression).

Type C virogene sequences offer several distinct advantages for the study of evolutionary relationships. As cellular genes, type C virogenes are subject to the pressures of mutation and selection; thus, closely related animal species would be expected to have closely related, but not identical, endogenous type C virogenes. Type C virogenes are unique from all other known cellular genes in their ability to give rise to the production of infectious type C virus particles. The complete expression of virogenes, at least in some species, with concomitant production of type C viruses containing specific viral proteins, a reverse transcriptase, and a high molecular weight RNA, offers a unique possibility for the isolation of a discrete set of cellular genes and their products. Single-stranded ^{3}H-DNA transcripts that represent the viral RNA sequences, synthesized in vitro by the viral reverse transcriptase, can be used to detect information in the cellular DNA of related species. Mammalian type C viruses are present in cellular DNA in multiple complete copies (five to fifteen per haploid genome) as a family of related, but not identical, gene sequences (15). These sets of type C virogenes appear to evolve more rapidly than the unique sequence cellular genes, possibly because of their presence in multiple copies in each genome (16). This apparent faster rate of evolutionary divergence of the primate type C viral genes allows a fine degree of discrimination among the various primate species. It is thus possible to establish taxonomic relationships among closely related species that are not revealed by methods involving the annealing of *entire* unique sequence DNA. The use of such viral probes clearly indicates that virogene evolution has followed the pattern of overall species evolution (16). In contrast, infectious, horizontally transmitted primate viruses spread from animal to animal and are completely unrelated by molecular and antigenic criteria to endogenous, genetically transmitted primate viruses. The properties of infectious viruses traveling from animal to animal can become rapidly altered, thereby obscuring their origin. Genetically transmitted viruses have remained stable enough to make it possible to detect events which occurred millions of years ago, and precisely determine the species from which they originated. The inability to detect viral-related sequences in more distantly related species reflects extensive changes in base sequences that have accumulated in the virogene since divergence (17).

Endogenous primate type C viruses

It has only been within the last year or two that endogenous type C viruses have been successfully propagated from primates, man's closest relatives. Several isolates from different tissues and from different species of baboons have been obtained in this laboratory. They are morphologically and biochemically typical of mammalian type C viruses, are closely related by host range, viral neutralization and interference and by immunologic and nucleic acid hybridization criteria, but are distinctly different from all other previously studied type C viruses (10, 18). ^{3}H-DNA transcripts prepared from three of the baboon type C virus isolates hybridize completely to DNA extracted from various tissues of several different healthy baboons (18). These type C virus isolates satisfy all the criteria for endogenous, genetically transmitted viruses of primates. The finding of DNA sequences in normal tissues is one of the strongest pieces of evidence that the viral information is maintained in the population as cellular genes.

If the baboon type C viruses were truly endogenous primate viruses (10) and had evolved as the species evolved, then it appeared reasonable to suspect that other Old World monkeys that are close relatives to the baboon would have related virogene sequences in their DNA. Primate species more distantly related taxonomically to baboons would be expected to have more extensive mismatching of their virogene DNA sequences as measured by the thermal stability of nucleic acid hybrids formed or by the final extent of hybridization (19, 17).

The study of the evolutionary relationships of type C viral gene sequences is especially favorable in primates since much is known about the evolutionary relationships between primates: the fossil record has been intensively studied as *Homo sapiens* have been particularly interested in their own origins. The Old World monkeys (which include the baboon species) have been separated from the great apes and man for 30 to 40 million years. The New World monkey branch diverged from the common stem leading to both the apes and the Old World monkeys, approximately 50 million years ago while the prosimians evolved from primitive mammalian stock roughly 60 to 80 million years ago.

Hybridization studies employing a DNA copy of the baboon virus RNA were used to detect type C viral nucleic acid sequences in primate cellular DNA. Multiple copies of viral gene sequences related to the RNA genomes of the baboon type C viruses are found in all other Old World monkey species, higher apes, and are also found in man. However, no homology can be detected in various New World monkey DNAs (17). The degree of relatedness of the virogene sequences closely correlates with the txonomic relatedness of the monkey species based upon anatomic criteria and the fossil record. The results establish that, within the primates, type C viral genes have evolved as the species have evolved, with virogenes from more closely related genera and families showing more sequence homology than those from distantly related taxons. That such species as the baboon and rhesus monkey, which have diverged genetically and have been geographically separated for several million years, still retain related virogene sequences, and the low, but consistently observed, hybridization to ape (chimpanzee) DNA with the baboon viral probe, demonstrates that this virogene information has been conserved in the primate stock during the course of evolution as stable cellular elements for at least 30 to 40 million years (17). The ubiquitous presence of endogenous type C virogenes among anthropoid primates and their evolutionary preservation suggest that such genes provide functions with a selective advantage to the species possessing them.

Virogene information is not only present in other Old World primates, but is also normally expressed. Probes from the baboon virus isolates have detected viral-specific RNA in rhesus monkey, stumptail and green monkey liver tissue; and p30 antigen has been found in normal stumptail spleen tissue and in a rhesus ovarian carcinoma (20). Two human tumors, an ovarian carcinoma and a lymphocytic lymphoma, have also been found to contain primate type C viral p30 antigen (21). These genes, therefore, are not inactive, but are normally expressed; the level, however, varies from animal to animal and from tissue to tissue in a given animal.

Interspecies transfer of type C virogenes

Type C viruses have also, under natural conditions, been transferred between species that are only remotely related phylogenetically. In some instances, type C virogenes have escaped host control as virus particles infectious to other species. These viruses can be transmitted from one species to another with integration of their information into the DNA and subsequent perpetuation through the germ line of the recipient species. Because of the stability of the viral gene sequences when they are incorporated into cellular DNA, events that have occurred millions of years ago still can be recognized by examining the genetic information of the virus and that of the host cell. One can assess the relatedness of a given virus to the host it is associated with by comparing (using molecular hybridization) the match between the viral RNA genome and the DNA of cells from an animal of the species with which the virus is associated. Endogenous viruses from one species horizontally transmitted to another species are related to, but distinct from, one another by many different criteria: nucleic acid sequence homology, antibody inhibition of polymerase activity, antigenicity of the p30 protein, viral interference and viral neutralization. Three known examples of trans-species infections by endogenous type C genes are discussed below.

One example involves the transfer of an endogenous primate type C virus into the germ line of the ancestor of the domestic cat (22, 23). Results have shown that domestic cat DNA contains sequences partially related to endogenous baboon type C viral sequences, even though unique sequence baboon and cat *cellular* DNA show no homology. Since other mammals do not contain those related sequences, the finding of baboon type C viral sequences in the distantly related domestic cat *(Felis catus)* cannot be explained strictly on evolutionary grounds (17).

Domestic cat DNA contains type C virogenes which can lead to the production of endogenous RD-114/CCC viruses (24, 25). In comparing the endogenous primate viruses to this feline group of viruses we found that they are related to each other, but can be distinguished by biologic and immunologic criteria and by partial nucleic acid sequence homology. Endogenous viruses from one group of mammals (primates) are concluded to have infected and become a part of the germ line of an evolutionary distant group of animals, progenitors of the domestic cat (22, 23) and thus have had a common ancestor even though they now behave as endogenous viruses of two taxonomically distant mammalian species.

Genes related to the nucleic acid of an endogenous domestic cat type C virus (RD-114/CCC) are found in the cellular DNA of anthropoid primates while at the same time many members of the cat family Felidae lack these sequences (Table 6).

Table VI: Relationship between cat and baboon endogenous type C virus

1. The cat (RD-114/CCC) and baboon virus groups are *related but distinct* from one another by:
   a. Viral DNA-RNA hybridization,
   b. Inhibition of polymerase activity by antibody,
   c. Antigenicity of the p30 protein,
   d. Viral interference,
   e. Viral neutralization.
2. Cat and baboon unique sequence DNA markedly different, species diverged from one another over 80 million years ago.
3. Cat (RD-114/CCC) virus DNA transcripts hybridize to the DNAs of *all* Old World Monkeys and apes, and to the DNAs of domestic cats and certain other *Felis* species.
4. Baboon (M7/M28) virus DNA transcripts hybridize to the DNAs of all Old World Monkeys, higher apes, and man, and to DNAs of those *Felis* species which contain RD-114 related sequences.

From the relatives of the domestic cat that have RD-114/CCC viral genes and from those that did not acquire them, we have concluded that the infection occurred 3 to 10 million years ago, in Africa or in the Mediterranean Basin region before the Old World monkeys had significantly diverged. This absence of RD-114/CCC related information in other cats is consistent with acquisition of this virus relatively recently in feline evolution.

Experiments have shown that, besides the RD-114/CCC cat viruses which were transmitted from primates to cats (as described above), another distinct class of type C RNA virus was acquired by cats and is now present in their germ line. These feline leukemia viruses (FeLV) were transmitted from an ancestor of the rat to ancestors of the domestic cat and their close relatives (26). The relationships observed between FeLV and the endogenous viruses of rodents are similar to those between endogenous feline viruses of the RD-114/CCC group and endogenous primate type C viruses. FeLV-related gene sequences are found not only in the cellular DNA of domestic cats but also in the DNA of three other closely related Felidae *(Felis sylvestris, F. margarita, F. chaus)*. More distantly related *Felis* species lack FeLV-related virogenes, while the cellular DNA of rodents, in particular rats, contains related virogene sequences. This suggests that FeLV-related genes were introduced into the *Felis* lineage following trans-species infection(s) by type C viruses of rodent origin. The absence of FeLV-related DNA sequences in most of the Felidae indicates that these genes were acquired subsequent to the initial Felidae divergence in evolutionary history but prior to the radiation of the above four *Felis* species. It is interesting that cats which contain sequences related to RD-114/CCC genes also contain FeLV-related genes, while other members of the *Felis* species lack both sets of sequences. Both groups of viral genes appear to have been introduced to the cat germ cells from distinctly different groups of animals (rodents and primates) (26).

The third example of trans-species infection is that of an endogenous virus acquired by an ancestor of the domestic pig from an ancestor of the mouse (27). Pig cell cultures produce type C viruses (28–31) that are genetically transmitted and present in all pig tissues in multiple copies in the cellular DNA (31, 15). Partially homologous viral gene sequences are also found in rodent, in particular Muridae, cellular DNA (27). Close relatives, such as the European wild boar and the African bush pig, have closely related viral genes in their DNA. The nucleic acid homology between the endogenous pig type C viral RNA and murine cellular DNA suggests that the endogenous viruses had a common ancestor. It can be shown that this virus was acquired by an ancestor of the pig from a small rodent related to the mouse (27). From the extent of hybridization of the pig type C viral DNA probes to rodent cellular DNA, the type C virogenes were introduced into the Suidae lineage by trans-species infection from members of the family Muridae after the mouse had separated from the rat, but before the different species of mice had diverged from each other. Rodent viral genes thus gave rise to infectious particles that became incorporated into the porcine germ line. The rate of evolution of the virogene sequences in the pig appears to be much slower than that of genes that have remained in the rodent lineage; this may be a consequence of transfer from a shorter-lived animal (the rodent) to a longer-lived one (the pig) (27). The time of gene transmission is estimated as occurring 5 to 10 million years ago and it is concluded

Table VII: Examples of transmission of type C virus genes between species

Donor	Recipient	Genetically Transmitted in Recipient
Primate (Old World monkey)	*Felis* (Ancestor of the domestic cat)	Yes
Rodent (Mouse ancestor)	Pig ancestor	Yes
Rodent (Rat ancestor)	*Felis* (Ancestor of domestic cat)	Yes (but also horizontally transmitted in *Felis catus*)
Rodent (*M. caroli* or close relatives)	Primates	No

that the present-day porcine type C virogenes most closely approximate the viral genes as they were 4 to 6 million years ago in the rodent lineage (27).

The data as summarized in Table 7 demonstrate that *viral genes from one group of animals can give rise to infectious particles that not only can integrate into the DNA of animals of another species, but can also be incorporated into the germ line (germ line inheritance of acquired virus genes).* Clearly, if viral gene sequences can be acquired in this way, it is possible that type C viruses have served to introduce other genes from one species to another, and may provide an important mechanism by which species stably acquire new genetic information.

The infectious primate type C RNA virus group

Infectious primate type C viruses have recently been recovered from several colonies of gibbon apes with various hematopoietic neoplasms, especially myelogenous and lymphoid leukemias (32), and from one woolly monkey with a spontaneous fibrosarcoma (a New World primate) (33, 34). GALV (gibbon ape leukemia virus) and SSV-SSAV (simian sarcoma virus-simian sarcoma associated virus) spread from animal to animal under natural conditions and induce tumors when inoculated into other primates (34–36). These viruses are related to one another by several immunologic criteria and contain related RNA genomes (37). Gene sequences homologous to those of the RNAs of GALV and SSAV have not been detected in the cellular DNA of normal primates studied thus far (38, 19). Thus, unlike the baboon type C virus, these two viruses are *not* endogenous viruses of primates.

The type C viruses of the GALV-SSAV group are poorly controlled by the primate host and appear readily capable of producing neoplastic disease. Infection by such viruses can cause local epidemics of lymphoproliferative tumors in infected gibbon colonies (39). The ability to isolate viruses from gibbons, however, is not restricted to animals with tumors. Recently, three isolates have been obtained from the brains of normal gibbons (animals without tumors) from a single colony in the United States (37). Based on immunologic assays and interference tests, the group of infectious type C viruses of primates contains many members, all partially related to one another. At present, the infectious primate type C viruses can be classified into four distinct subgroups (see Table 8) based on hybridization studies

Table VIII: Infectious primate type C viruses; isolation and partial characterization

Proposed Subgroup	Isolates	Reference
A Woolly monkey	SSV/SSAV	(34)
B Gibbon type 1	GALV-1	(32)
C Gibbon type 2	GALV-SEATO	(39)
D Gibbon type 3	GBr-1, GBr-2, GBr-3	(37)

which show extensive mismatching of the gene sequences when the different gibbon isolates were compared to one another and to SSAV (37). It is probable that additional subgroups will be defined as new isolates are obtained.

In studying the relationships between the various mammalian type C viruses using nucleic acid hybridization it was noted that the infectious primate viruses, GALV and SSAV, share a significant degree of nucleic acid sequence homology with endogenous type C viruses from the laboratory mouse, *Mus musculus* (40). Several homologous proteins of these two major groups of viruses also share unique interspecies determinants (41). These unexpected findings suggested the possibility that the infectious primate viruses of the GALV-SSAV group were derived from endogenous mouse viruses or from a type C virus of a rodent closely related to the mouse. Primates can, therefore, possess both endogenous and exogenous type C viruses. The ease with which type C viruses can be isolated from an Asian primate, the gibbon, and their relationship to *Mus musculus* cellular DNA suggested that an Asian species of *Mus* might have a more closely related endogenous virus. For these reasons, we chose to study type C viruses from several feral Asian subspecies of *Mus musculus*. Ten of thirteen single cell clones of the distantly related Thai mouse species *Mus caroli* are inducible for a xenotropic type C virus. This virus, unlike the isolates from other *Mus musculus* subspecies, was found to be closely related antigenically to a group of infectious primate type C viruses (gibbon and woolly monkey type C viruses) and only weakly related to and distinctly different from previously studied type C viruses of *Mus musculus*. The polymerase of the *Mus caroli* virus is antigenically more similar to the primate viral enzymes than to the enzymes of all *musculus* type C viruses tested (Table 9). It shares cross-reactive p30 antigens, and cross-interferes with the infectious primate type C viruses (42). The p30 protein of the *Mus caroli* virus is more closely related antigenically to viruses of the GALV-SSAV group than to *Mus musculus* type C viruses. By immunologic and interference criteria, then, the virus isolated from *Mus caroli* cells is unique among the murine viruses characterized thus far in its close relationship to infectious viruses isolated from primates. These results lead to the conclusion that

Table IX: Inhibition of viral reverse transcriptase Activity by antisera to viral polymerases

Virus From:	μg Needed For 30 % Inhibition	
	Anti-MuLV	Anti-SSAV
Mouse		
Rauscher	[0.8]	>30
Moloney	0.8	>30
AKR	1.2	>30
BALB/c	1.0	>30
Mus musculus (wild mouse)	0.9	>30
Mus caroli	>60	3.6
Primate		
SSAV	>60	[0.7]
GALV-1	>60	1.2
GALV-SEATO	>60	1.2
GBr-1	>60	1.0
GBr-2	>60	0.9
GBr-3	>60	1.3

a group of infectious, type C viruses horizontally transmitted among primates originated by trans-species infection(s) of certain primates (gibbon, woolly monkey, and perhaps other apes and monkeys) by an endogenous type C virus from *Mus caroli* or another closely related species. This trans-species infection appears to be a relatively recent, perhaps contemporary, event with the viruses not yet being incorporated into the genomes of the recipient primate species.

Type C RNA viruses and human neoplasia

The studies of type C virogenes in primate populations as described above are unusually significant: first, they are the first isolates of type C viruses from primates; second, some of these viruses have been proven to be oncogenic; third, they provide the closest model of animal neoplasia for man; and fourth, it is possible that one, the other, or both of these two primate virus groups (GALV and SSAV) may be involved in human neoplasia.

Since the horizontally transmitted primate viruses described above are infectious for and can cause tumors in primates, the possibility exists that this group of viruses may be involved in the etiology of human cancer. This is supported by data obtained using different experimental procedures in a number of laboratories. An enzyme with biochemical properties related to those of type C viruses and with antigenic properties similar to polymerases of the woolly monkey type C virus (SSAV) and the gibbon ape leukemia virus (GALV) has been detected in human acute leukemia cells (43, 44). The DNA products of endogenous reactions from the "virus-like" particulate fraction of acute leukemia cells hybridize preferentially to viral RNA from SSAV and GALV (45, 46). Using radioimmunoassays, antigens related to the major structural proteins (p30) of type C viruses have been detected in peripheral white blood cells from five patients with acute leukemia (47). These results suggest that viruses of this group, known to be infectious for and tumorigenic in other primates, may also be associated with acute leukemia in man.

Recently, several laboratories have reported the isolation of complete infectious type C viruses from human materials (48–51). Most information is available on the isolate designated HL-23, obtained from a cell culture derived from a woman with acute myelogenous leukemia. It appears to be closely related to the woolly monkey virus, SSAV (50), and thus may belong to one of the four previously described subgroups of infectious primate viruses. A virus closely related to baboon type C viruses was also isolated from patient HL-23 (52). Since two different type C viruses also related to the same primate viruses as HL-23 have recently been found in the human embryo cells described by Panem et al. (49), isolation of *one* infectious virus from human material now appears to be an unusual rather than common occurrence. Additional isolates of HL-23 virus have recently been reported from separate clinical specimens obtained at different intervals from the same patient (53). The significance of these isolations, however, requires further evaluation. The careful characterization of additional isolates made by other laboratories from human tissues and cell cultures, then, is awaited with keen interest.

Primates, including man, are known to contain endogenous type C viral sequences in their genome which are related to those found in endogenous baboon viruses (16). Endogenous virogenes may be partially expressed in humans and other primates as evidenced by the detection of RNA sequences (20), and antigens related to the p30 proteins (20, 21) of endogenous baboon viruses. The expression of endogenous viral-related antigens is found in carcinomas and lymphomas (21) as well as in leukemias (47); viral p30 antigen expression has also been reported in certain normal human tissues (54).

If infectious type C RNA viruses are important agents in cancer causation in man, it is critical to know how the viral information is transmitted, normally controlled, and maintained in the population. Are they contained in an animal reservoir or do they spread solely from primate to primate? Finding this reservoir(s), if it exists, provides a chance of disrupting the process. If human leukemia involves the spread of an infectious agent from individual to individual as is clearly shown to be the case for cat leukemia (55) and bovine leukemia (56), then identification of the agent and its mode of spread would provide one set of approaches to prevention of the disease. If, on the other hand, activation of genetically transmitted virus by extrinsic (chemical and physical agents) as well as by various intrinsic factors leads to tumor development and there is no contagious virus involved, the approaches to the prevention of the disease would be quite different. The endogenous primate type C virogenes, present in human cells, would appear to be the more logical candidate virus for involvement in the generality of human cancer.

Possible normal functions of type C viruses

The presence of genetically transmitted viral genes in so many vertebrate species and the evidence that they have been conserved through evolution in several distinct vertebrate lineages suggests that they may provide normal function(s)

Table X: Possible functions of genetically transmitted virogenes in normal cells

1. Activation of oncogenic information, while inappropriate in adult tissue, plays a normal role during differentiation and development.
2. The integrated virus serves to protect the species against related, more virulent infectious type C viruses.
3. Virus activation, being linked to transformation, protects the animal by altering the cell membrane. The released virus could alert the immune system making the transformed cells more susceptible to immunologic control.
4. They may have had an evolutionary role as conveyors of genetic information not only within a species but also between species. Only this group of viruses has been shown to transmit genes between germ cells of different species under natural conditions.

advantageous to the species carrying them (Table 10). The first suggested role, derived from studies on the expression of viral antigens during the course of development, was that such viral expression during the early stages of differentiation was a normal part of the developmental process (3). If this were the case, the expression of cancer genes later in life would be an inappropriate manifestation of a normal developmental function. If viral genes provide a function critical for normal development, they clearly would be conserved during evolution.

The acquisition of viral genes by cats from both primates and rodents, and by pigs from rodents, along with the fact that they have been maintained for millions of years suggests the possibility that the newly acquired viral genes, once integrated, might have been beneficial to the recipient species if they were able to provide resistance to related, but more virulent viruses. Animals that successfully integrated the genomes would have been at a selective advantage relative to those that did not, if the integrated genome protected against infection, and if infection led to cancer or other type C viral-mediated diseases. Genes that provide protection against disease, especially against epidemic diseases, would be at a strong selective advantage in natural populations. This may well explain the success of the transmission between species as described above. For example, in our laboratory we have shown that those species of the genus *Felis*, including the domestic cat, that have acquired primate type C viral genes are resistant to infection by the endogenous baboon viruses, while those *Felis* species that have not acquired the viral information are still susceptible to baboon viral information.

A third possible role for endogenous viruses arises if viral activation was closely linked to the transformed state in the cell. Expression of the endogenous virus under natural circumstances, may be protective on an immunological basis against cancer, rather than the virus acting as the etiological agent. The activated virus could alter the cell membrane and thus alert the host immune system, conveying information as to the number and location of transformed cells in the body. This possibility is supported by the observation that transformed cells in culture, whether transformed spontaneously, by chemical carcinogens, or by other viruses, release their endogenous type C viruses more readily than do their normal, untransformed counterparts (57–59). Transformed cells that are releasing high titers of type C virus have been reported to be much less able to produce tumors when inoculated into immunocompetent animals of the same species (60). Partial viral expression where viral antigens are introduced into the cell surface may be sufficient to alter its antigenicity and facilitate rejection of these cells.

One final possibility that should be considered is that type C viruses have played an important evolutionary role as transmitters of genetic information, not only between cells of an animal, and animals of a species, but also between species. That viruses can transmit themselves between the germ cell DNAs of very different species has been established as a result of experiments in the past year. That they can recombine with cellular gene sequences and transmit these genes to new cells of a different species also has been clearly demonstrated (61, 62). That this transmission of cellular gene information between species has been a major force in evolution, however, remains a speculation.

This suggestion that viruses may have had a major role in evolution is not a new one (63). Viruses are unique in that they can serve to carry information between genetically isolated species. Classical Darwinian evolution deals with changes which occur within the genetic information of a species; which can be changed and rearranged by mutation and selection, duplication and rearrangements, but not added to from the outside. Viruses, however, offer the possibility of additions of new gene sequences to a species. The type C viruses as a group, are uniquely suited for this role since they must incorporate into the cellular DNA in order to replicate (14) but they do not kill the cells that they infect. Each time they move from cell to cell they may carry with them host cell genes providing a means of communication between cells of different species and different phyla. They serve to keep a species in contact or in communication with its neighbors-ecologic neighbors as well as genetic neighbors.

Of course they can transmit information that may disrupt normal cellular control, and by so doing, lead to the development of cancer in the individual. Instances of genetic significance, however, occur when new genes are incorporated into the germ line. From this perspective, the fact that these viruses cause cancer would then be viewed as a pathological manifestation of normal processes. While the viral genes may well be etiologic agents in cancer causation, either as exogenous or endogenous viruses, and this may be of profound significance to the affected individuals, these relatively rare and sporadic cases may not be of great evolutionary significance.

References

1. Kalter, S. S., Helmke, R. J., Panigel, M., Heberling, R. L., Felsburg, P. J. and Axelrod, L. R.: Observations of apparent C-type particles in baboon *(Papio cynocephalus)* placentas. Science 179: 1332–1333, 1973.
2. Schidlovsky, G. and Ahmed, M.: C-type virus particles in placentas and fetal tissues of rhesus monkeys. *J. Natl. Cancer Inst.* 51: 225–233, 1973.
3. Huebner, R. J. and Todaro, G. J.: Oncogenes of RNA tumor viruses as determinants of cancer. *Proc. Natl. Acad. Sci. USA* 64: 1087–1094, 1969.
4. Todaro, G. J. and Huebner, R. J.: The viral oncogene hypothesis: New evidence. *Proc. Natl. Acad. Sci. USA* 69: 1009–1015, 1972.
5. Lieber, M. M. and Todaro, G. J.: Mammalian type C RNA viruses. In: *Can-*

cer: A Comprehensive Treatise, Vol. II. Becker, F. F. (Ed.), Plenum Press, New York, 1975, pp. 91–130.

6. Lowy, D. R., Rowe, W. P., Teich, N. and Hartley, J. W.: Murine leukemia virus: High-frequency activation in vitro by 5-iododeoxyuridine and 5-bromodeoxyuridine. *Science* 174: 155–156, 1971.

7. Weiss, R. A., Friis, R. R., Katz, E. and Vogt, P. K.: Induction of avian tumor viruses in normal cells by physical and chemical carcinogenesis. *Virology* 46: 920–938, 1971.

8. Livingston, D. M. and Todaro, G. J.: Endogenous type C virus from a cat cell clone with properties distinct from previously described feline type C viruses. *Virology* 53: 142–151, 1973.

9. Benveniste, R. E., Lieber, M. M. and Todaro, G. J.: A distinct class of inducible murine type C viruses which replicate in the rabbit SIRC cell line. *Proc. Natl. Acad. Sci. USA* 71: 602–606, 1974.

10. Benveniste, R. E., Lieber, M. M., Livingston, D. M., Sherr, C. J., Todaro, G. J. and Kalter, S. S.: Infectious type C virus isolated from a baboon placenta. *Nature* 248: 17–20, 1974.

11. Temin, H. M.: Mechanism of cell transformation by RNA tumor viruses. *Annual Review of Microbiology* 25: 609–648, 1971.

12. Baltimore, D.: RNA-dependent DNA polymerase in virions of RNA tumour viruses. *Nature* 226: 1209–1211, 1970.

13. Temin, H. M. and Mizutani, S.: RNA-dependent DNA polymerase in virions of Rous sarcoma virus. *Nature* 226: 1211–1213, 1970.

14. Temin, H. M.: The RNA tumor viruses – background and foreground. *Proc. Natl. Acad. Sci. USA* 69: 1016–1020, 1972.

15. Benveniste, R. E. and Todaro, G. J.: Multiple divergent copies of endogenous type C virogenes in mammalian cells. *Nature* 252: 170–173, 1974.

16. Benveniste, R. E. and Todaro, G. J.: Evolution of type C viral genes: I. Nucleic acid from baboon type C virus as a measure of divergence among primate species. *Proc. Natl. Acad. Sci. USA* 71: 4513–4518, 1974.

17. Benveniste, R. E., Sherr, C. J., Lieber, M. M., Callahan, R. and Todaro, G. J.: Evolution of primate type-C viral genes. In: *Fundamental Aspects of Neoplasia.* Gottlieb, A. A., Plescia, O. J. and Bishop, D. H. L. (Eds.). Springer-Verlag, New York, 1975, pp. 29–53.

18. Todaro, G. J., Sherr, C. J., Benveniste, R. E., Lieber, M. M. and Melnick, J. L.: Type C viruses of baboons: Isolation from normal cell cultures. *Cell* 2: 55–61, 1974.

19. Benveniste, R. E., Heinemann, R., Wilson, G. L., Callahan, R. and Todaro, G. J.: Detection of baboon type C viral sequences in various primate tissues by molecular hybridization. *J. Virol.* 14: 56–67, 1974.

20. Sherr, C. J., Benveniste, R. E. and Todaro, G. J.: Type C viral expression in primate tissues. *Proc. Natl. Acad. Sci. USA* 71: 3721–3725, 1974.

21. Sherr, C. J. and Todaro, G. J.: Type C viral antigens in man. I. Antigens related to endogenous primate virus in human tumors. *Proc. Natl. Acad. Sci. USA* 71: 4703–4707, 1974.

22. Benveniste, R. E. and Todaro, G. J.: Evolution of C-type viral genes: Inheritance of exogenously acquired viral genes. *Nature* 252: 456–459, 1974.

23. Todaro, G. J., Benveniste, R. E., Callahan, R., Lieber, M. M. and Sherr, C. J.: Endogenous primate and feline type C viruses. *Cold Spring Harbor Symp. Quant. Biol.* 39: 1159–1168, 1974.

24. Baluda, M. A. and Roy-Burman, P.: Partial characterization of RD114 virus by DNA-RNA hybridization studies. *Nature New Biol.* 244: 59–62, 1973.

25. Neiman, P. E.: Measurement of RD114 virus nucleotide sequences in feline cellular DNA. *Nature New Biol.* 244: 62–64, 1973.

26. Benveniste, R. E., Sherr, C. J. and Todaro, G. J.: Evolution of type C viral genes: Origin of feline leukemia virus. *Science* 190: 886–888, 1975.

27. Benveniste, R. E. and Todaro, G. J.: Evolution of type C viral genes. III. Preservation of ancestral murine type C viral sequences in pig cellular DNA. *Proc. Natl. Acad. Sci. USA* 72: 4090–4094, 1975.

28. Breese, S. S.: Virus-like particles occurring in cultures of stable pig kidney cell lines. *Archiv Gesamte Virusforsch* 30: 401–404, 1970.

29. Strandström, H., Veijalainen, P., Moennig, V., Hunsmann, G., Schwarz, H. and Schäfer, W.: C-type particles produced by a permanent cell line from a leukemic pig. I. Origin and properties of the host cells and some evidence for the occurrence of C-type-like particles. *Virology* 57: 175–178, 1974.

30. Todaro, G. J., Benveniste, R. E., Lieber, M. M. and Sherr, C. J.: Characterization of a type C virus released from the porcine cell line PK(15). *Virology* 58: 65–74, 1974.

31. Lieber, M. M., Sherr, C. J., Benveniste, R. E. and Todaro, G. J.: Biologic and immunologic properties of porcine type C viruses. *Virology* 66: 616–619, 1975.

32. Kawakami, T. G., Huff, S. D., Buckley, P. M., Dungworth, D. L., Snyder, S. P. and Gilden, R. V.: C-type virus associated with gibbon lymphosarcoma. *Nature New Biol.* 235: 170–171, 1972.

33. Theilen, G. H., Gould, D., Fowler, M. and Dungworth, D. L.: C-type virus in tumor tissue of a woolly monkey *(Lagothrix ssp.)* with fibrosarcoma. *J. Natl. Cancer Inst.* 47: 881–889, 1971.

34. Wolfe, L. G., Deinhardt, F., Theilen, G. H., Rabin, H., Kawakami, T. G. and Bustad, L. K.: Induction of tumors in marmoset monkeys by simian sarcoma virus, type I *(Lagothrix)*: A preliminary report. *J. Natl. Cancer Inst.* 47: 1115–1120, 1971.

35. Parks, W. P., Scolnick, E. M., Noon, M. C., Watson, C. J. and Kawakami, T. G.: Radioimmunoassay of mammalian type C polypeptides. IV. Characterization of woolly monkey and gibbon viral antigens. *Int. J. Cancer* 12: 129–137, 1973.

36. Kawakami, T. G., Buckley, P. M., McDowell, T. S. and DePaoli, A.: Antibodies to simian C-type virus antigen in sera of gibbons *(Hylobates sp.)* *Nature New Biol.* 246: 105–107, 1973.

37. Todaro, G. J., Lieber, M. M., Benveniste, R. E., Sherr, C. J., Gibbs, C. J. Jr., and Gajdusek, D. C.: Infectious primate type C viruses: Three isolates belonging to a new subgroup from the brains of normal gibbons. *Virology* 67: 335–343, 1975.

38. Scolnick, E. M., Parks, W., Kawakami, T., Kohne, D., Okabe, H., Gilden, R. and Hatanaka, M.: Primate and murine type C viral nucleic acid association

kinetics: Analysis of model systems and natural tissues. *J. Virol.* 13: 363–369, 1974.

39. Kawakami, T. G. and Buckley, P. M.: Antigenic studies in gibbon type-C viruses. *Transplantation Proc.* 6: 193–196, 1974.

40. Benveniste, R. E. and Todaro, G. J.: Homology between type-C viruses of various species as determined by molecular hybridization. *Proc. Natl. Acad. Sci. USA* 70: 3316–3320, 1973.

41. Sherr, C. J., Fedele, L. A., Benveniste, R. E. and Todaro, G. J.: Interspecies antigenic determinants of the reverse transcriptases and p30 proteins of mammalian type C viruses. *J. Virol.* 15: 1440–1448, 1975.

42. Lieber, M. M., Sherr, C. J., Todaro, G. J., Benveniste, R. E., Callahan, R. and Coon, H. G.: Isolation from the Asian mouse *Mus caroli* of an endogenous type C virus related to infectious primate type C viruses. *Proc. Natl. Acad. Sci. USA* 72: 2315–2319, 1975.

43. Todaro, G. J. and Gallo, R. C.: Immunological relationship of DNA polymerase from human acute leukaemia cells and primate and mouse leukaemia virus reverse transcriptase. *Nature* 244: 206–209, 1973.

44. Gallagher, R. E., Todaro, G. J., Smith, R. G., Livingston, D. M. and Gallo, R. C.: Relationship between RNA-directed DNA polymerase (reverse transcriptase) from human acute leukemic blood cells and primate type-C viruses. *Proc. Natl. Acad. Sci. USA* 71: 1309–1313, 1974.

45. Miller, N. R., Saxinger, W. C., Reitz, M. S., Gallagher, R. E., Wu, A. M., Gallo, R. C. and Gillespie, D.: Systematics of RNA tumor viruses and virus-like particles of human origin. *Proc. Natl. Acad. Sci. USA* 71: 3177–3181, 1974.

46. Mak, T. W., Kurtz, S., Manaster, J. and Housman, D.: Viral-related information in oncornavirus-like particles isolated from cultures of marrow cells from leukemic patients in relapse and remission. *Proc. Natl. Acad. Sci. USA* 72: 623–627, 1975.

47. Sherr, C. J. and Todaro, G. J.: Primate type C virus p30 antigen in cells from humans with acute leukemia. *Science* 187: 855–857, 1975.

48. Gallagher, R. E. and Gallo, R. C.: Type C RNA tumor virus isolated from cultured human acute myelogenous leukemia cells. *Science* 187: 350–353, 1975.

49. Panem, S., Prochownik, E. V., Reale, F. R. and Kirsten, W. H.: Isolation of type C virions from a normal human fibroblast strain. *Science* 189: 297–299, 1975.

50. Nooter, K., Aarssen, A. M., Bentvelzen, P., de Groot, F. G. and van Pelt, F. G.: Isolation of infectious C-type oncornavirus from human leukaemic bone marrow cells. *Nature* 256: 595–597, 1975.

51. Gabelman, N., Waxman, S., Smith, W. and Douglas, S. D.: Appearance of C-type virus-like particles after co-cultivation of a human tumor-cell line with rat (XC) cells. *Int. J. Cancer* 16: 355–369, 1975.

52. Teich, N., Weiss, R. A., Salahuddin, S. Z., Gallagher, R. E., Gillespie, D. H., Gallo, R. C.: Infective transmission and characterization of a C-type virus released by cultured human myeloid leukaemia cells. *Nature* 256: 551–555, 1975.

53. Gallagher, R. E., Salahuddin, S. Z., Hall, W. T., McCredie, K. B. and Gallo,

R. C.: Growth and differentiation in culture of leukemic leukocytes from a patient with acute myelogenous leukemia and reidentification of a type-C virus. *Proc. Natl. Acad. Sci. USA* 72: 4137–4141, 1975.

54. Strand, M. and August, J. T.: Type-C RNA virus gene expression in human tissue. *J. Virol.* 14: 1584–1596, 1974.

55. Hardy, W. D. Jr., Old, L. J., Hess, P. W., Essex, M. and Cotter, S.: Horizontal transmission of feline leukaemia virus. *Nature* 244: 266–269, 1973.

56. Olson, C., Miller, L. D., Miller, J. M. and Hoss, H. E.: Transmission of lymphosarcoma from cattle to sheep. *J. Natl. Cancer Inst.* 49: 1463–1468, 1972.

57. Todaro, G. J.: "Spontaneous" release of type C viruses from clonal lines of "spontaneously" transformed Balb/3T3 cells. *Nature New Biol.* 240: 157–160, 1972.

58. Lieber, M. M. and Todaro, G. J.: Spontaneous and induced production of endogenous type-C RNA virus from a clonal line of spontaneously transformed Balb/3T3. *Int. J. Cancer* 11: 616–627, 1973.

59. Rapp, U. R., Nowinski, R. C., Reznikoff, C. A. and Heidelberger, C.: Endogenous oncornaviruses in chemically induced transformation. I. Transformation independent of virus production. *Virology* 65: 392–409, 1975.

60. Barbieri, D., Belehradek, J. Jr., and Barski, G.: Decrease in tumor-producing capacity of mouse cell lines following infection with mouse leukemia viruses. *Int. J. Cancer* 7: 364–371, 1971.

61. Scolnick, E. M., Rands, E., Williams, D. and Parks, W. P.: Studies on the nucleic acid sequences of Kirsten sarcoma virus: A model for formation of a mammalian RNA-containing sarcoma virus. *J. Virol.* 12: 458–463, 1973.

62. Weiss, R. A., Mason, W. S. and Vogt, P. K.: Genetic recombinants and heterozygotes derived from endogenous and exogenous avian RNA tumor viruses. *Virology* 52: 535–552, 1973.

63. Anderson, N. G.: Evolutionary significance of virus infection. *Nature* 227: 1346, 1970.

Bovine Leukemia Virus: An Exogenous RNA Oncogenic Virus?

R. Kettmann*†, D. Portetelle*†, M. Mammerickx††, Y. Cleuter*,
D. Dekegel**, M. Galoux*†, J. Ghysdael*, A. Burny*† and
H. Chantrenne*.

* Département de Biologie Moléculaire, Université Libre de
  Bruxelles, Belgique.
† Faculté Agronomique; Gembloux, Belgique.
†† Institut National de Recherches Vétérinaires, Uccle, Bruxelles,
  Belgique.
** Vrije Universiteit Brussel and Institut Pasteur du Brabant,
  Bruxelles, Belgique.

Abstract

Short term cultures of bovine leukemic lymphocytes release virus particles with biochemical properties of RNA oncogenic viruses. These particles, tentatively called Bovine Leukemia Virus (BLV) have a high molecular weight-reverse transcriptase complex and a density averaging 1.155 g/ml in sucrose solutions. Molecular hybridizations between BLV-^{3}H cDNA and several viral RNAs show that BLV is not related to Mason-Pfizer Monkey Virus (MPMV) Simian Sarcoma Associated Virus (SSV-1) Feline Leukemia Virus (FeLV) or Avian Myeloblastosis Virus (AMV). Rauscher Leukemia Virus (RLV) exhibits a slight but reproducible relatednesse to BLV. The high preference of BLV reverse transcriptase for Mg^{++} as the divalent cation suggests that BLV might be an atypical mammalian leukemogenic type C virus. Hybridization studies using BLV ^{3}H cDNA as a probe suggest that the DNA of bovine leukemic cells contains viral sequences that cannot be detected in normal bovine DNA.

Abbreviations: Eagle MEM: Eagle minimum essential medium – SDS: sodium dodecyl sulfate – MMTV: mouse mammary tumor virus.

Introduction

Bovine leukemia is a lymphoproliferative disease appearing in cattle herds under several forms (1). The following observations lead to the conclusion that viruses are the most probable etiological agents of the onzootic form of the disease:

(a) Bovine leukemia often appears in geographically localized foci. It spreads by horizontal as well as by vertical transmission (Mostly from mother to offspring) (2, 3, 4).

(b) Infected animals develop antibodies directed against an antigen present in the virus fraction of leukemic lymphocyte cultures. This antigen can be detected by immunofluorescence, immunodiffusion or complement fixation (5-9).

(c) Virus particles are occasionally seen in milk and tissues of leukemic animals (10, 11).

(d) Cultures of bovine leukemic material produce virus particles generally considered as type C (11-15) although they are morphologically somewhat different from typical type C viruses (16-17).

(e) Whole blood from leukemic animals transfers the disease with high frequency when fed to newborn calves (18, 3) or sheep (18, 19, 20). Successful infections are also obtained with the viral concentrate from short term cultures (21, 22).

Considering all these observations, it seems to us of basic interest to identify biochemically Bovine Leukemia Virus, to determine by molecular hybridization to what extent it could be related to other known type C viruses and finally and mostly to characterize it as an exogenous or an endogenous bovine virus.

Materials and Methods

Animals.

Our experimental herd was established from animals diagnosed as leukemic by hematological test (key of Göttingen). A sample of leukocytes from each animal was submitted to short term culture (see below) and examined by electron microscopy for the presence of "C type" virus. Every culture derived from a leukemic animal produced virus particles while cultures made of normal leukocytes remained negative (4).

Cell cultures.

Blood was collected from the jugular vein; clotting was prevented by the use of 3 ml of 1 % heparine for each 150 ml of blood anticipated to be taken. Leukocytes were separated by the distilled water 1.7 % saline method, as applied by Stock and Ferrer (21). After the red blood cells were lysed by hypotonic shock, the cells were adjusted to 3.0×10^6/ml of Eagle MEM supplemented with 20 % inactivated (30 min at 56 °C) fetal calf serum and maintained as stationary cultures. Penicillin (100 units/ml) and streptomycin (100 µg/ml) were added to the media. These short term cultures were incubated for 72-96 hours at 37 °C.

Virus concentration.

A. – *From short term culture supernatants.*

The medium was clarified by centrifugation at 1500 x g for 45 min at 3 °C and the virus was purified according to Bishop et al. (24) except that TNE (0.01 M Tris-HCl, pH 8.3; 0.15 M NaCl; 0.001 M EDTA) was used instead of MEM or Tris-HCl pH 7.5.

B. – *From cells.*

3 g of cultured lymphocytes were homogenized with an ultra-turrax homogenizer (Janke and Kunkel, type ZF) at full speed for 3 x 20 seconds in 4 volumes of TNE at 4 °C. The homogenate was then processed as the virus suspension.

Assay of 60–70S RNA directed DNA polymerase : simultaneous detection test.

Pellets obtained after equilibrium density gradient centrifugation of BLV were resuspended in 0.01 M Tris-HCl, pH 8.3 at a protein concentration of 3 mg/ml. Triton X-100 was adjusted to a final concentration of 0.03 % and a simultaneous detection test was performed (25).

Preparation of BLV ^{3}H cDNA.

The 60–70S RNA-^{3}H DNA complex of a BLV simultaneous detection test was recovered by alcohol precipitation, treated with alkali to destroy RNA and chromatographed on hydroxyapatite to purify single stranded ^{3}H cDNA molecules (26, 27).

Preparation of ^{3}H cDNA probes of AMV, SSV-1, RL Vand FeLV.

The reaction conditions were those previously described (28) except for RLV and feLV where Mg^{++} was replaced by Mn^{++} at a final concentration of 0.001 M.

Preparation of viral RNAs.

Viral proteins were solubilized and digested by a mixture of SDS and proteinase K (Merck, Darmstadt) at final concentrations of 0.5 % and 0.2 mg/ml respectively. The digested mixture was extracted twice at room temperature with phenol-cresol-chloroform (6:1:7). 60–70S RNA was recovered from the aqueous phase by ethanol precipitation and purified by sedimentation in sucrose gradient.

Preparation of DNAs.

DNA from leukemic and normal cells was isolated according to Sweet et al. (29). All DNAs were reduced to a sedimentation constant of 6–8S by ultrasonic vibration. DNAs extrated by this method had an A$_{260}$/A$_{280}$ nm ratio of 1.85–1.95.

Hybridization reactions.

^{3}H cDNA (2000 cpm) was added to indicated amounts of RNA (or DNA) in a final volume of 56µl of 0.4 M NaCl, 0.001 M EDTA, 0.1 % SDS and 0.01 M Tris-HCl, pH = 7.7. The mixture was incubated at 68 °C for various periods of time. The extent of hybrid formation was estimated either by Cs$_2$SO$_4$ equilibrium density gradient centrifugation (28) (for DNA-RNA hybrids) or S$_1$ nuclease digestion (30) (for DNA-DNA hybrids).

Results

Characterization of a 60–70S RNA and reverse transcriptase.

BLV particles released in the culture supernatant were concentrated as described in Methods and used as a source of template-primer and reverse transcriptase in an RNA dependent DNA synthesis reaction. The reaction proceeded linearly for at least 30 minutes. In some cases, linear incorporation lasted for as long as 2 hours. As a rule, reactions were stopped after 30 min. and analyzed by the simultaneous detection technique (25). We systematically searched for optimum conditions for cDNA recovery. Incubation of the reaction mixture with proteinase K (Merck, Darmstadt) before phenol-chloroform extraction improved the cDNA yield by at least 70 %.

Fig. 1 shows the outcome of a simultaneous detection test. Fractions 5 to 15 represent the region where 60–70S viral RNA-³H cDNA complexes sediment. The presence of these complexes per se is a strong indication that BLV contains a high molecular weight RNA and reverse transcriptase, molecules characteristic of

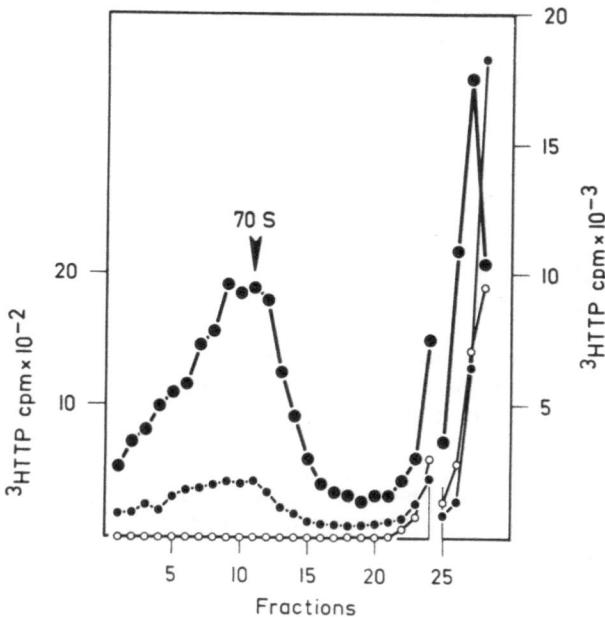

Fig. 1: Detection of the 60–70S RNA-³H cDNA complex of BLV from culture supernatants. Twelve hundred ml bovine lymphocyte culture supernatant were processed as described under "virus concentrations" and "simultaneous detection" (see Methods). The virus concentrate was divided into three equal parts. A standard RNA-directed DNA polymerase reaction was performed on one part. The RNA-³H cDNA product was sized on sucrose gradient (●——●). A second part of the virus concentrate was used in a reaction mixture lacking dATP (·——●). The third part of the virus concentrate was incubated in the complete reaction mixture supplemented with 100 µg/ml of RNase A (○——○).

378

RNA oncogenic viruses. The synthesis of 60–70S RNA-³H cDNAhybrids is dependent on the presence of the four deoxytriphosphates in the incubation medium. Leaving out dATP reduced the ³H TMP incorporation to about 20 % of the control value.

In the presence of RNAse A, ³H TMP incorporation is reduced to a background level.

The same experimental technology was applied to virus detection in cultured leukemic lymphocytes. The same positive outcome of the simultaneous detection test was obtained. Similar results were also obtained when leukemic lymphocytes from sheep infected by bovine leukemic blood were examined (data not shown). This indicates that the observed endogenous DNA polymerase activity is both RNA dependent and not due to an end addition enzyme activity.

Requirements of the BLV-reverse transcriptase reaction:
1/ Non ionic detergent.

In contrast to avian RNA tumor viruses (28, 31, 32) mammalian oncornaviruses (25, 26) require no detergent (33) or very limited concentrations of detergents for optimal rate of DNA synthesis. BLV endogenous synthesis of DNA was performed in the presence of various concentrations of NP40 or Triton X-100. At

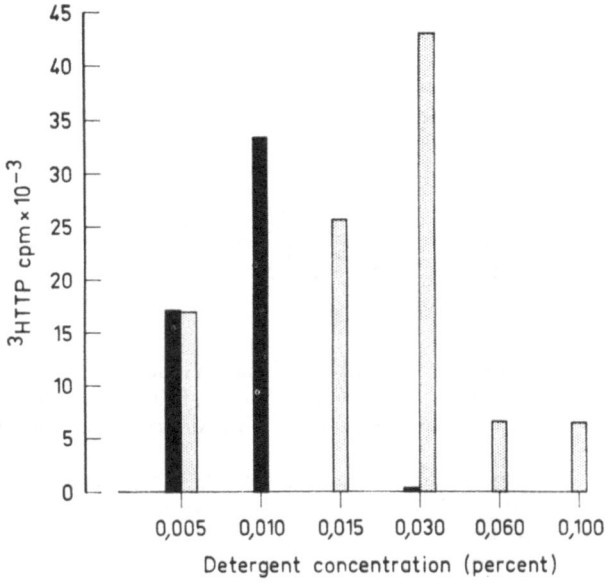

Fig. 2: *Panel A.*
BLV-DNA polymerase activity as a function of detergent concentration. ³H cDNA syntheses were run in the presence of the indicated concentrations of Triton X-100 (□) or NP-40 (■) and analyzed by sucrose gradient sedimentation. Results are expressed as TCA precipitable counts in the 60–70S region of the gradient versus indicated detergent concentration.

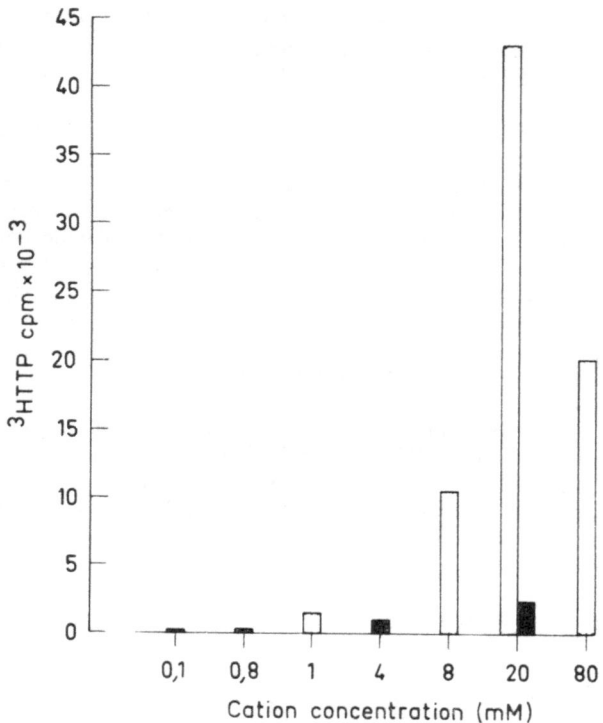

Panel B. BLV-DNA polymerase activity as a function of Mg^{++} ($\square$) or Mn^{++} ($\blacksquare$) con-centration in the reaction mixture. ^3H cDNA syntheses were run in the presence of the indicated concentrations of Mg^{++} or Mn^{++} and analyzed by sedimentation in sucrose gradients. Results are expressed as TCA precipitable counts in the 60–70S region of the gradient versus indicated cation concentration.

the protein concentration used (3 mg/ml) maximum synthesis of 60–70S ^3H cDNA occurred at 0.01 % of NP40 or 0.03 % of Triton X-100 in the reaction mixture. Higher detergent concentrations practically abolish the reaction (Fig. 2a).

2/ *Divalent cation.*

The preference of viral polymerase for Mg^{++} or Mn^{++} depends on the template-primer that is being used (34, 35). It has been shown also (36) that more similarity exists between the DNA polymerases from viruses of the same type than between the polymerases from viruses of different types but from closely related species. Divalent cation requirement may therefore be informative for the biochemical characterization of new oncornaviruses.

Endogenous ^3H cDNA synthesis was run in the conditions described in Methods except for divalent cation concentration. ^3H cDNA counts associated with high molecular weight RNA after sucrose gradient sedimentation were recorded in Fig. 2b as functions of divalent cation concentration used. As can be seen, no

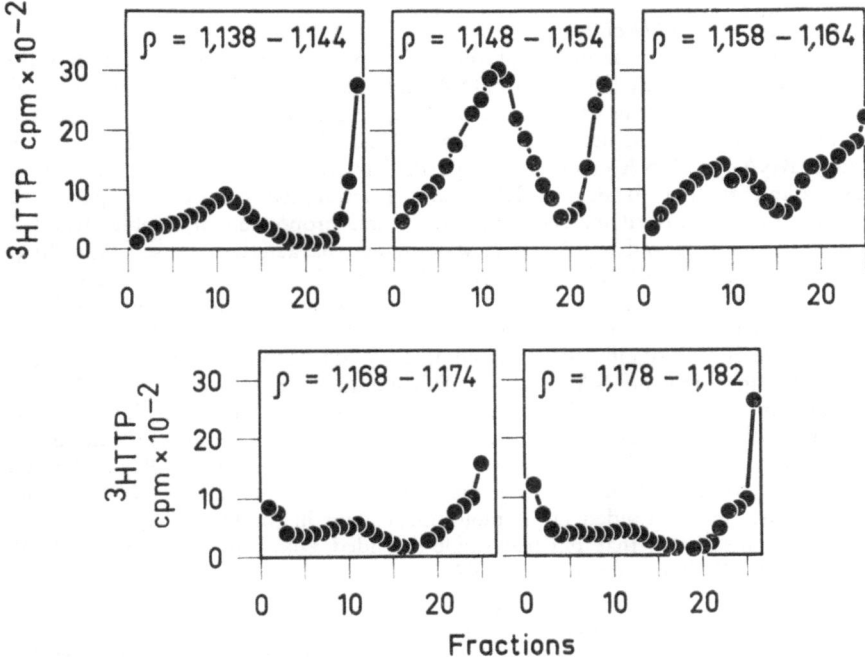

Fig. 3: Determination of BLV equilibrium density in sucrose solutions.
A BLV concentrate, prepared from short term culture supernatant (1200 ml) as described in Methods, was suspended in TNE buffer, layered on a linear gradient 20–50 sucrose in TNE buffer and centrifuged overnight at 25000 rpm in a Spinco SW 27 rotor at 4 °C. Fractions within regions of the indicated densities were pooled and assayed by the simultaneous detection test as described in Methods.

notable incorporation of ^{3}H TMP into DNA occurred at any of the Mn^{++} cation concentrations tested. Mg^{++}, on the other hand, clearly stimulated BLV reverse transcriptase. The optimum concentration for the reverse transcriptase activity in this assay was 20 mM Mg^{++}.

Buoyant density in sucrose gradients.
The buoyant density values of oncornaviruses in sucrose solutions vary according to the virus type (37). The B-type MMTV equilibrates at a density of 1.18 g/ml in sucrose while C type viruses have a density of 1.16 g/ml in sucrose.
In order to determine the density values of BLV, the virus released in the supernatant of 1200 ml of culture was processed as described in the legend to Fig. 3. The simultaneous detection profiles obtained reveal that BLV equilibrates in these conditions between 1.148 and 1.164 g/ml, the density region of C type viruses.

Preparation of BLV ³H cDNA.

Once the optimum conditions of the BLV reverse transcriptase reaction were determined, we prepared BLV ³H cDNA and tested it for its representativity of the BLV genome. A virus concentrate was prepared from five liters of lymphocyte culture supernatant and used to generate an ³H-DNA probe. The high molecular weight RNA-³H cDNA complex was purified by sucrose gradient centrifugation (25), alkali treated to destroy RNA and fractionated on hydroxyapatite to separate single stranded material from the small proportion of double stranded molecules. Single stranded ³H cDNA was further characterized by self annealing, annealing to globin mRNA and to BLV 60–70S RNA. Fig. 4a shows a Cs_2SO_4 equilibrium density profile of the self annealed single stranded material. All the ³H counts band as a sharp peak in the density region where DNA is expected. This profile is not significantly altered if BLV ³H cDNA has been previously hybridized to globin mRNA (Fig. 4b). This eliminates the possibility of BLV ³H cDNA contamination by poly thymidylic acid stretches. After annealing to BLV high molecular weight RNA (Fig. 4c), all the ³H cDNA counts equilibrate in the Cs_2SO_4 gradient in a broad density region from 1.66 g/ml (he RNA density region) up to 1.48 g/ml covering the whole region of RNA-DNA hybrids. Virtually no single stranded DNA molecule remains in the DNA region. This set of experiments shows that purified single stranded DNA molecules of the BLV probe specifically hybridize to BLV RNA sequences.

Relatedness of BLV to other RNA oncogenic viruses.

A constant amount (2000 cpm; SA = 2 x 10⁷ cpm/μg) of single stranded molecules was annealed to increasing amounts of BLV RNA. Percentages of hybrid-

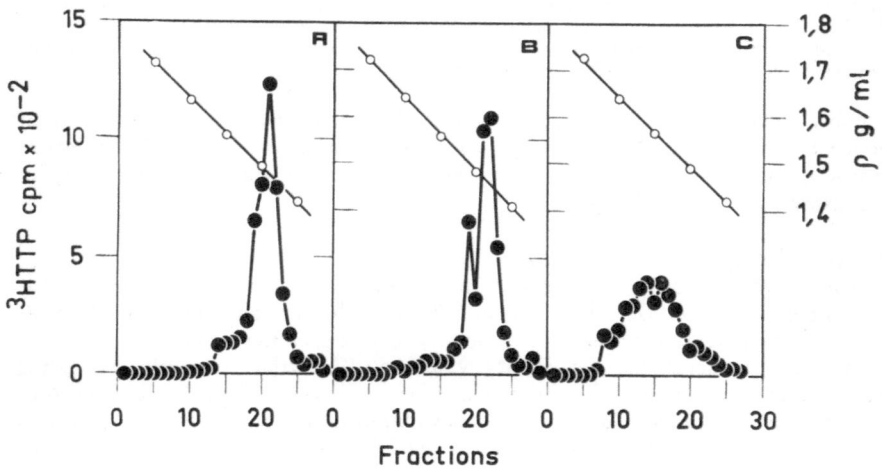

Fig. 4: Characterization of BLV cDNA probe.
Cs_2SO_4 equilibrium density gradient centrifugation of the purified BLV-cDNA alone (a) and after annealing at 68 °C for 3 days to 4.5 μg of globin 9S mRNA (b) and 0.16 μg of BLV 70S RNA (c) ● = cpm; ○ = density.

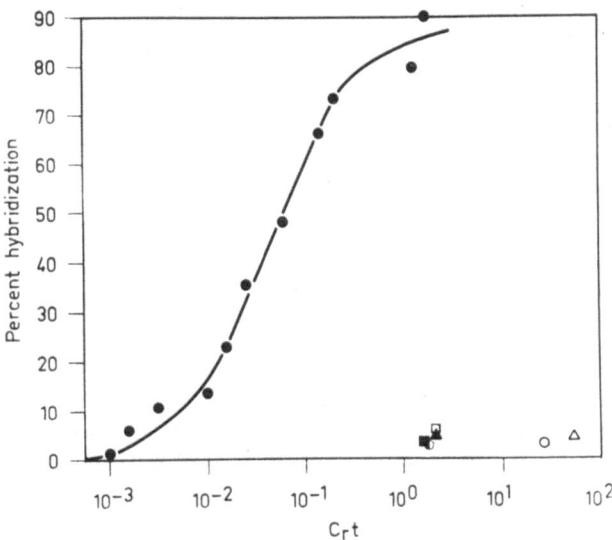

Fig. 5: Kinetics of annealing of BLV-cDNA to 60–70S BLV RNA. Crt is the product of nucleic acid concentration (in OD_{260}) and hybridization time (in hours/2). No corrections were made for salt concentrations. The hybridization mixtures contained from 0.078 ng to 160 ng of BLV 70S and were all incubated at 68 °C for 3 days. The extent of hybridization was determined by S_1 nuclease treatment (●——●).

Hybridizations with hemoglobin messenger RNA as a control (△); RLV 70S RNA (□) MPMV 70S RNA (■) AMV 70S RNA (○) SSV-1 70S RNA (▲) FeLV 70S RNA (◐) were run up to indicated Crt values.

ization were calculated from the ratios of S_1 resistant counts over total ³H cDNA counts in the controls. The values obtained were recorded (Fig. 5) as functions of Crt (concentration of viral RNA in moles/liter times time in seconds (38). Crt $1/2$ equals 7×10^{-2} moles x sec/liter. In similar experiments with AMV and RLV, values such as 3×10^{-2} (39) and 1.5×10^{-2} (40) were reported. The somewhat higher value obtained here in the BLV system is probably due to some contamination of BLV 60–70S RNA. As BLV is produced by degenerating cells, contamination of the 60–70S region of sucrose gradients by cellular nucleic acid cannot be ruled out. Such a Crt curve also shows that 90 % of the cDNA engaged in the reaction was hybridized at Crt values of 1 and above. Annealing experiments tending to detect an hypothetical relatedness between BLV and other known RNA oncogenic viruses must be carried out up to, at least, Crt values of 1. Such experiments were performed with globin mRNA as control and MPMV, RLV, FeLV, AMV, SSV-1, RNAs. Within the limits of our experiments, we can conclude that 4 of the 5 viruses tested do not share common RNA sequences with BLV. RLV, however, showed a slight but reproducible relatedness to BLV. BLV ³H cDNA systematically showed some 2 to 3 % of hybridization to RLV RNA. A control experiment was then performed where BLV 60–70S RNA was annealed to ³H DNA synthesized in the above five viruses tested (Table 1). Again, MPMV,

Table I: % Hybridization of ³H cDNA probes synthesized in various RNA viruses with globin mRNA (as control) and various viral 60–70S RNAs*.

³H cDNA probes	globin mRNA	AMV	SSV-1	RNAs MPMV	FeLV	RLV	BLV
BLV	4.3	3.1	4.9	3.6	–	6.1	85.1
SSV-1	0.0	–	90.0	–	–	–	0.3
AMV	0.0	90.2	–	–	–	–	2.6
RLV	0.0	–	–	–	–	80.1	8.8
FeLV	0.0	–	–	–	43.1	–	0.8

* Hybridizations were run at Crt values $\geq$ 2.

AMV, SSV-1, FeLV appeared to be unrelated to BLV but RLV ³H cDNA repeatedly hybridized to some extent (3 % to 8 %) to BLV-RNA.

BLV genome sequences in DNA from normal bovine cells and bovine lymphosarcoma cells.

A constant amount (2000 cpm; SA = 2 x 10⁷ cpm/μg) of single stranded BLV ³H cDNA was annealed to increasing amounts of normal and leukemic bovine

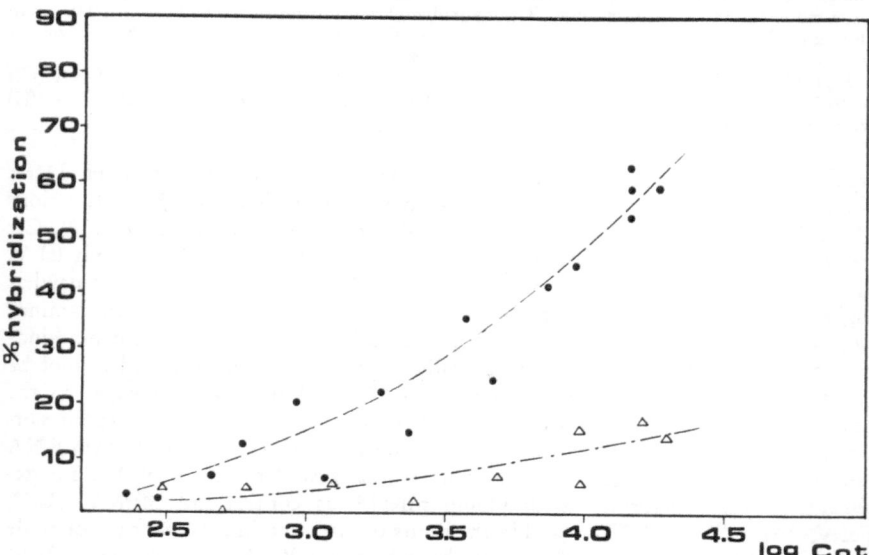

Fig. 6: Hybridization kinetics of BLV ³H cDNA with normal ($\triangle$——$\triangle$) and leukemic bovine DNA ($\bullet$——$\bullet$). Hybridization reactions were carried out with 2000 input counts/min of BLV ³H cDNA at a specific activity of 2 x 10⁷ cpm/μg, at 68 °C in Tris-HCl, 0.01 M, pH = 7.7; NaCl : 0.4 M; EDTA : 0.001 M; SDS : 0.1 %. The dashed lines are not mathematically derived, but simply fit to the data for illustrative purposes.

DNA. After about 20 days, the percentages of hybridization were determined and recorded as functions of Cot. Fig. 6 shows the kinetics of hybridization of BLV x ^{3}H cDNA with normal ($\triangle-\triangle$) and leukemic bovine DNA ($\bullet-\bullet$). About 60 % of the radioactive probe enters S_1 nuclease-resistant hybrids after annealing with bovine leukemic DNA. The same probe formed hybrids with normal bovine DNA at a much slower rate, reaching only 15 % at log Cot values of about 4.5.

These observations are consistent with the proposition that BLV contributes genome sequences to the leukemic cell which are not detectable by this technique, in normal bovine DNA. Definite proof that this proposition is indeed correct must await further experimental evidence. Recycling experiments (29, 41, 42) and thermal stability analysis of the hybrids are presently under way.

Discussion

Bovine leukemia is by far the best known natural model system from epidemiological studies. As outlined in the introduction of this report, the disease spreads by horizontal and vertical transmission. In the latter case, however, experiments strongly suggest that transmission of the disease is most probably due to perinatal infection (3). It was therefore of obvious interest to try to identify the putative agent, and characterize it, biologically and biochemically. A major step towards this goal was accomplished when virus production was achieved in short term cultures of leukemic lymphocytes. We report here on our attempt to study biochemical features of the virus. The positive outcome of simultaneous detection tests, the sensitivity of the reaction to ribonuclease treatment, and the strict requirement for the four deoxyribonucleoside triphosphates (Fig. 1) practically identifies BLV as an RNA tumor virus. The definite proof, however, that BLV possesses a high molecular weight RNA-reverse transcriptase complex could only be obtained through back hybridization of the DNA synthesized in vitro with the viral 60–70S RNA. Fig. 4 and 5 show that this is, indeed, the case.

Parameters of the endogenous reverse transcriptase reaction were then determined. As a rule, reverse transcriptases from mammalian leukemogenic viruses are extremely sensitive to non-ionic detergent concentrations (32). According to our titration experiments, BLV reverse transcriptase exhibits maximum activity when Triton X-100 reaches a concentration of 0.03 % in the solution where protein concentration averages 1.5 mg/ml. In the same conditions of protein concentration, the optimal NP-40 concentration is 0.01% (Fig. 2).

It could also be informative to investigate the metal requirements of BLV endogenous DNA synthesis. The optimum Mg^{++} concentration averages 20 mM while Mn^{++} is ineffective at any of the concentrations tested (Fig. 3). As pointed out by Waters and Yang (35), divalent metal requirements of a given reverse transcriptase reaction depends primarily on the template-primers used. If, however, the endogenous synthesis of DNA on an RNA template is considered, the following rules seem to obtain:

– Mammalian type C viruses: DNA synthesis proceeds equally well in the presence of Mg^{++} or Mn^{++} provided optimal concentrations are used. The reaction may even be stimulated if both cations are present at a given concentration (36).

– Type B viruses: Mg^{++} is a mandatory requirement for DNA synthesis (43).

385

– MPMV (36, 43), GPV (43), BLV: they are morphologically different from type B viruses but share their divalent cations requirements.

Further characterization of BLV included an equilibrium density gradient centrifugation in sucrose gradients. The simultaneous detection tests performed on material banding at the indicated densities (Fig. 4) show that BLV equilibrates between 1.148 and 1.164 g/ml, a density region characteristic of type C virus particles.

The potential relatedness of BLV to other known RNA oncogenic viruses was screened by hybridization of the various viral RNAs to BLV [3]H cDNA (Fig. 5) and, *mutatis mutandis,* of bovine viral RNA to the various viral [3]H cDNAs. The results of this double check are quite clearcut: AMV, MPMV, FeLV and SSV-1 are unrelated to BLV. Surprisingly enough, RLV showed in both tests a slight but reproducible relatedness to BLV (some 3 to 8 %) (Table 1). A comparable situation obtains when RLV ^{3}H DNA probes are used to search viral sequences in human leukemias, lymphomas and Hodgkin diseases (44, 45, 46). One would obviously want to understand the exact significance of this observation.

Epidemiological and experimental evidence strongly suggests bovine leukemia to be an infectious disease. It was therefore of crucial interest to try to classify BLV as an exogenous or an endogenous virus. The biochemical strategy of such experiments has been designed (41) and includes a recycling step. The recycling step is a mandatory prerequisite before classification of a virus, if the normal cell DNA of the species studies contains, at least, one copy equivalent of the viral genome. In this case indeed one could interpret leukemogenesis as an amplification of existing DNA sequences.

That viral transformation implies *de novo* insertion of viral DNA sequences into the genome of the infected host, is easy to demonstrate in cells transformed by a non-indigenous virus (47–49). That the same phenomenon holds true for cells infected by an indigenous virus, was clearly demonstrated by Baxt and Spiegelman (41) in the case of human leukemias. From studies on the leukemic member of identical twins (42), it was further concluded that leukemia specific information must have been inserted subsequent to fertilization. These facts observed in human systems have been extended to avian lymphoma (50) and leukemia (51). The data we present here (Fig. 6) about bovine leukemia, a "field" leukemia, suggest that leukemia specific sequences are present in the DNA of the leukemic cell. Further evidence in support of this proposition are presently being sought, i. e. recycling of BLV [3]H cDNA on normal bovine DNA, thermal stability analysis of the hybrids . . .

What is the information carried by the extra-sequences? From studies with a transformation defective mutant of Prague RSV-C, it has been suggested (52) that the sarcoma virus adds transformation specific sequences to the DNA of normal cells. The clearcut identification of the viral sequences responsible for each viral function should help answering the question.

In conclusion, we tend to believe, without having at the present time the definite proof, that bovine leukemia is an infectious disease both on epidemiological as well as on biochemical grounds. It seems also highly probable that it will be the first natural system in which Koch's postulate will be fulfilled.

Acknowledgements

The authors wish to thank Dr. M. Janowski for providing the purified S_1 nuclease and P. Ridremont, G. Vandendaele, J. Severs and L. Vanheule for skillfull assistance.

They warmly thank Dr. J. Gruber from the NCI, Office of Program Resources and Logistics for a generous gift of SSV-I and RLV and Dr. J. Schlom for a generous gift of FeLV and MPMV.

This work was made possible through the generous financial support of the Belgian Ministry of Agriculture, the "Caisse Générale d'Epargne et de Retraite" and the State Contract "Actions concertées".

R. K. is "Aspirant FNRS", D. P. is "Assistant C. G. E. R.". J. G. holds a fellowship from IRSIA.

References

1. Bendixen, H. J. (1963) Leukosis enzootica bovis: diagnostik, epidemiologi; bekaempelse. Thesis Copenhagen, 164 pp.
2. Croshaw, J. E., Abt, D. A., Marshak, R. R., Hare, W. C. D., Switzer, J., Ipsen, I. and Dutcher, R. M. (1963). Ann. N.Y. Acad. Sci., 108, 1193–1202.
3. Mammerickx, M. (1972) An. Med. Vet., 116, 647–659.
4. Mammerickx, M. and Dekegel, D. (1975) Zbl. Vet. Med. B., 22, 411–419.
5. Miller, J. M. and Olson, C. (1972) J. Nat. Canc. Inst., 49, 1459–1462.
6. Ferrer, J. F., Avila, L. and Stock, N. D. (1972) Cancer Res., 32, 1864–1970.
7. Paulsen, J., Rudolph, R. and Miller, J. M. (1974) Med. Microbiol. Immunol., 159, 105–114.
8. Miller, J. M. and van der Maaten, M. J. (1974) (A complement-fixation test for the bovine leukemia (C type) virus). J. Nat. Canc. Inst., 53, 1699–1702.
9. Mammerickx, M., Portetelle, D., Kettmann, R., Ghysdael, J., Burny, A. and Dekegel, D. (1976) Europ. J. of Canc. in press.
10. Dutcher, R. M., Larkin, E. P. and Marshak, R. R. (1964) J. Nat. Canc. Inst., 33, 1056–1064.
11. Wittmann, W. and Urbaneck, D. (1969) (Leukose des Rindes: Handbuch des Virus. Infektionen bei Tieren. Band V) Gustav Fischer, Jena, 41–174.
12. Miller, J. M., Miller, L. D., Olson, C. and Gillette, K. G. (1969) J. Nat. Canc. Inst., 43, 1297–1305.
13. Dutta, S. K., Larson, V. L., Sorensen, D. K., Perman, V., Weber, A. F., Hammer, R. F. and Shope, R. E. (1969) In "Comparative Leukemia Research". Bibliotheca Haematologica, 36, 548–554.
14. Kawakami, T. E., Moore, A. L., Theilen, G. H. and Munn, R. J. (1969) In "Comparative Leukemia Research". Bibliotheca Haematologica, 36, 471–475.
15. Olson, C., Hoss, H. E., Miller, J. M. and Baumgartener, L. E. (1973) J. Amer. Vet. Med. Assn., 163, 355–360.
16. van der Maaten, M. J., Miller, J. M. and Boothe, A. D (1974) J. Nat. Canc. Inst., 52, 491–497.
17. Calafat, J., Hageman, P. C. and Ressang, A. A. (1974) J. Nat. Canc. Inst., 52, 1251–1257.

18. Wittmann, W. and Urbaneck, D. (1969) Arch. Exp. Vet. Med., *23*, 709–713.
19. Mammerickx, M. (1967 to 1973) Rapports d'activité. Institut National de Recherches Vétérinaires. Uccle (Bruxelles).
20. Mammerickx, M. (1970) Experimentation animale, *4*, 285–293.
21. Miller, L. D., Miller, J. M. and Olson, C. (1972) J. Nat. Canc. Inst., *48*, 423–426.
22. Olson, C., Miller, L. D., Miller, J. M. and Hoss, H. E. (1972) J. Nat. Canc. Inst., *49*, 1463–1467.
23. Stock, N. D. and Ferrer, J. F. (1972) J. Nat. Canc. Inst., *48*, 985–996.
24. Bishop, D. H. L., Ruprecht, R., Simpson, R. W. and Spiegelman, S. (1971) J. Virol., *8*, 730–741.
25. Schlom, J. and Spiegelman, S. (1971) Science, *174*, 840–843.
26. Manly, K. F., Smoler, D. F., Bromfield, E. and Baltimore, D. (1971) J. Virol., *7*, 106–111.
27. Varmus, H. E., Levinson, W. E. and Bishop, J. M. (1971) Nature New Biol., *223*, 19–21.
28. Spiegelman, S., Burny, A., Das, M. R., Keydar, I., Schlom, J., Travnicek, M. and Watson, K. (1970) Nature, *227*, 563–567.
29. Sweet, R. W., Goodman, N. C., Cho, J. R., Ruprecht, R. M., Redfield, R. R. and Spiegelman, S. (1974) Proc. Natl. Acad. Sci. U. S., *71*, 1705–1709.
30. Vogt, V. M. (1973) Eur. J. Biochem., *33*, 192–200.
31. Temin, H. M. and Mizutani, S. (1970) Nature, *226*, 1211–1213.
32. Green, M. and Gerard, G. F. (1974) Progr. Nucl. Ac. Res. Mol. Biol., *14*, 188–322.
33. Baltimore, D. (1970) Nature, *226*, 1209–1211.
34. Scolnick, E., Rands, E., Aaronson, S. A. and Todaro, G. J. (1970) Proc. Natl. Acad. Sci. U.S., *67*, 1789–1796.
35. Waters, L. C. and Yang, W. K. (1974) Cancer Res., *34*, 2585–2593.
36. Abrell, J. N. and Gallo, R. C. (1973) J. Virol., *12*, 431–439.
37. Sarkar, N. H. and Moore, D. H. (1974) J. Virol., *13*, 1143–1147.
38. Britten, R. J. and Kohne, D. E. (1968) Science, *161*, 529–540.
39. Ghysdael, J. – in preparation.
40. Fan, H. and Baltimore, D. (1973) J. Mol. Biol., *80*, 93–117.
41. Baxt, W. G. and Spiegelman, S. (1972) Proc. Nat. Acad. Sci. U.S., *69*, 3437–3741.
42. Baxt, W. G., Yates, J. W., Wallace, H. J. Jr., Holland, J. F. and Spiegelman, S. (1973) Proc. Natl. Acad. Sci. U.S., *70*, 2629–2632.
43. Michalides, R., Schlom, J., Dahlberg, J. and Perk, K. (1975) – J. Virol. 16, 1039–1050.
44. Hehlmann, R., Kufe, D. and Spiegelman, S. (1972) Proc. Natl. Acad. Sci. U.S., U.S., *69*, 1727–1731.
45. Hehlmann, R., Kufe, D. and Spiegelman, S. (1972) Proc. Natl. Acad. Sci. U.S., *69*, 1727–1731.
46. Kufe, D., Peters, W. P. and Spiegelman, S. (1973) Proc. Natl. Acad. Sci. U. S., *70*, 3810–3814.
47. Baluda, M. A. (1972) Proc. Natl. Acad. Sci. U. S., *69*, 576–580.
48. Varmus, H. E., Vogt, P. K. and Bishop, J. M. (1973) J. Mol. Biol., *74*, 613–626.

49. Goodman, N. C., Ruprecht, R. M., Sweet, R. W., Massey, R., Deinhardt, F. and Spiegelman, S. (1973) Int. J. Cancer, *12*, 752–760.
50. Neiman, P. E., Purchase, G. H. and Okazaki, W. (1975) Cell, *4*, 311–319.
51. Shoyab, M., Evans, R. M. and Baluda, M. A. (1974) J. Virol., *14*, 47–49.
52. Neiman, P. E., Wright, S. E., McMillin, C. and MacDonnell, D. (1974) J. Virol., *13*, 837–846.

Molecular Evidence for the Association of RNA Tumor Viruses with Human Mesenchymal Malignancies

S. Spiegelman

Institute of Cancer Research, College of Physicians & Surgeons, Columbia University, 99 Fort Washington Avenue, New York, N.Y. 10032

I. The Strategy of the Search for RNA Tumor Viruses in Human Malignancies

Our overall purpose has been and remains to explore the possible involvement of RNA tumor viruses as etiologic or cofactor agents in human neoplasias and to exploit any leads that emerge that could be of any conceivable use in the prevention, diagnosis, or therapy of human cancer.

The task of identifying the existence and the causative role of the animal RNA tumor viruses was inadvertently made easier by breeding high cancer incidence animal strains. In the process, a homogeneous genetic background was created that was permissive for viral replication. As a consequence, virus particles reached levels that made their detection inevitable. Those who are concerned with human neoplasias are for the most part faced with the same difficulties encountered by the early animal oncologists prior to the availability of inbred strains. It follows that a search for putative human viral agents requires more sensitive devices than those which sufficed to establish their presence in the genetically homogeneous animal systems. In the quest for such tools, we quite naturally turned to molecular hybridization and the other methodologies developed by molecular biologists in the past several decades.

Our investigations evolved through a number of stages that are conveniently identified by the questions we posed for experimental resolution:

1) Do human neoplasias contain RNA molecules possessing detectable homology to the RNA of tumor viruses known to cause similar cancers in other mammals?

2) If a positive outcome is obtained, do the RNA molecules identified in tumors possess the size and physical association with reverse transcriptase that characterize the RNA of the animal oncornaviruses?

3) If such RNA exists in human tumors, is it encapsulated in a particle possessing the density and size of the RNA tumor viruses?

4) Is the RNA of human tumor particles homologous to the RNA of the viruses causing the corresponding disease in animals?

5) The "virogene-oncogene" concept proposes that all animals prone to cancer carry in their germ line a complete copy of the information required to convert a cell from normal to malignant for the production of tumor virus particles. Is this concept valid for randomly bred populations and, in particular, for the human disease?

II. The Animal Models as a Point of Departure

When we began our investigations, there were relatively few animal oncorna-viruses available in amounts adequate for the sort of biochemical experiments re-quired. Table I lists these and records certain relevant features that served as a

Table I: Comparsion of Some Representative Oncornaviruses

Virus	Indigenous Host	Homology*					Disease
		AMV	RSV	MuLV	MSV	MMTV	
AMV	Chicken	+	+	−	−	−	Leukemia
RSV (RAV)	Chicken	+	+	−	−	−	Sarcoma
MuLV	Mouse	−	−	+	+	−	Leukemia, lymphoma
MSV (MuLV)	Mouse	−	−	+	+	−	Sarcoma
MMTV	Mouse	−	−	−	−	+	Breast cancer

* The results of molecular hybridizations between [^{3}H]DNA complementary to the various RNAs and the indicated RNAs. The plus sign indicates the hybridizations were positive and the negative sign indicates none could be detected.

guide in these expermients. There are two avian viruses, myeloblastosis virus (AMV) and the Rous sarcoma virus (RSV), that cause mesenchymal malignancies in chickens. In addition, we have the murine leukemia virus (MuLV) and the murine sarcoma virus (MuSV) that induce similar diseases in mice. Finally, we have the murine mammary tumor virus (MMTV), which is the unique etiologic agent for mammary tumors.

When these viruses are examined for sequence homologies amongst their nucleic acids, a rather informative pattern emerges. It will be noted that the two chicken agents have sequences in common, but do not show detectable homology with any of the murine agents. Turning to the murine viruses, we find that the nucleic acids of the leukemia, lymphoma, and sarcoma agents are homologous to one another, but not to either of the two avian agents or to the mammary tumor virus. Finally, the mouse mammary tumor virus has a singular sequence homologous only to it-self.

It is important to understand that a plus sign does not indicate identity, but simply sufficient similarity to be detectable by the relaxed hybridization conditions used in these initial studies. Similarly, a negative sign does not imply the complete absence of sequence homology, but rather that none was observable by the proce-dures used.

If analogous, or similar, virus particles are associated with the corresponding human diseases, certain predictions may be hazarded on the basis of the specificity patterns exhibited in Table I, and they may be listed as follows:

(a) In view of the lack of homology between the avian and murine agents, it is unlikely, from simple evolutionary considerations, that human agents, should they exist, would show more homology to the avian group than to the murine oncorna-viruses.

(b) It follows that the murine tumor viruses would represent the more hopeful source of the molecular probes required to search for similar information in the analogous human cancers.

(c) If particles are found to be associated with human mesenchymal tumors (in leukemias, sarcomas, and lymphomas), their RNAs might show homology to one another and possibly to that of the murine leukemia virus.

(d) If RNA particles are identified in human breast cancer, they should not exhibit homology to the RNA of virus-like particles associated with the human mesenchymal neoplasias or to MuLV RNA, but might exhibit some homology to the RNA of the murine mammary tumor virus.

On the basis of both availability and the specificity considerations outlined above, it is clear why the murine agents were initially chosen for producing the necessary molecular probes to look for corresponding information in the human disease. Furthermore, the desire to monitor the biological consistency of our findings dictated that we examine in parallel the human neoplasias listed. Such a parallel examination would permit us to determine whether our findings in humans mir-rored biologically what was known from the animal experimental models. For this purpose, we focused our efforts on the mesenchymal neoplasias and on breast cancer.

III. Molecular Hybridization with Radioactive DNA Probes

The DNA-RNA hybridization procedure we used to answer the question whether human tumors contain viral-related RNAs was one that we had designed (1) some fifteen years ago to answer questions of almost precisely this nature in the case of virus-infected bacteria. The method depends on the ability of any piece of single-stranded DNA to find its complementary RNA and form, under the proper conditions, a double-stranded hybrid structure. The reaction is highly spe-cific and has proved to be of considerable value in molecular biology over the past decade.

The required radioactive DNA was synthesized by supplying detergent-disrupted virus preparations with magnesium and the deoxyriboside triphosphates, with one of them being labeled with tritium. When the synthesis is completed, the protein and the RNA present are eliminated, and the residual radioactive DNA is purified to completion. Each [^{3}H]DNA preparation is then rigorously examined for specific hybridizability to its appropriate template and for its inability to complex with irrelevant RNAs. After satisfying the specificity criteria, the purified viral-specific tritiated DNA is mixed with cytoplasmic RNA prepared from a variety of tumors and annealed under the conditions described in Figure 1. The hybridizations are always carried out with a vast excess of tumor RNA. Since the viral-specific tritiated DNA is small compared with the RNA, any complexes formed between them will behave physically more like RNA than DNA. Such complexes are readily detected by isopynic separation in equilibrium density gradients of cesium sulfate. At the end of the centrifugation, the distribution of the tritiated DNA is examined across the gradient. Any uncomplexed DNA will remain at a density correspond-

MOLECULAR HYBRIDIZATION OF TUMOR p-RNA
AND VIRAL SPECIFIC ^{3}H-DNA

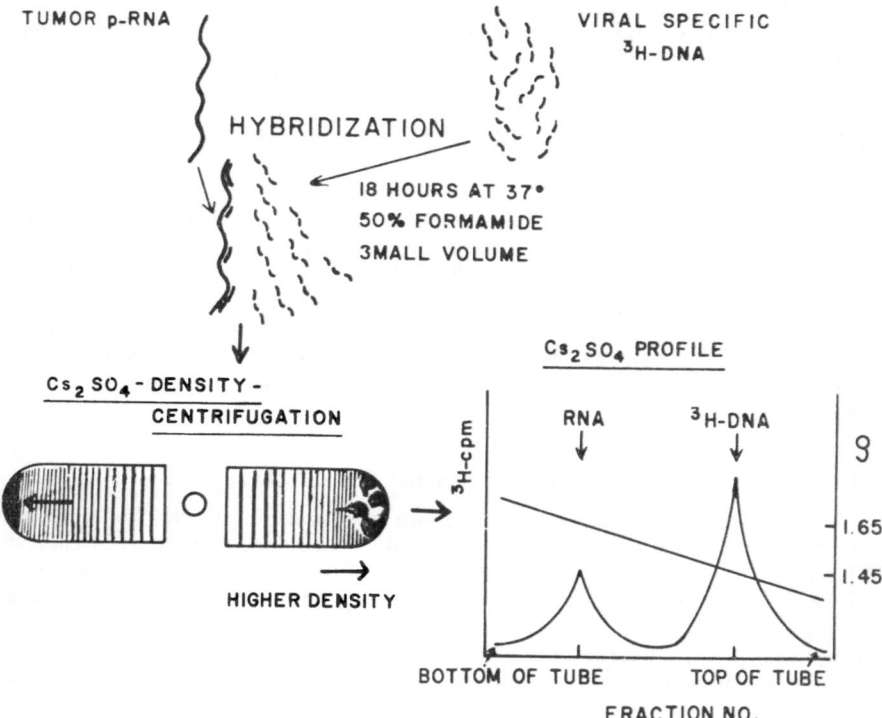

Fig. 1: Molecular hybridization and detection with viral-specific [^{3}H]DNA and tumor RNA (see text for further details).

ing to about 1.45. The DNA molecules that have annealed either partially or completely to RNA will band at or near the density of RNA ($\varrho = 1.65$). The movement of the tritiated DNA from the DNA density region to the RNA density region is then the signal that the probe used has found complementary sequences in the tumor RNA with which it is being challenged.

The human neoplasias examined included adenocarcinoma of the breast (2–4), the leukemias (5), the sarcomas (6), and the lymphomas (7). The leukemias encompassed both acute and chronic varieties of the lymphatic and myelogenous types. The human sarcomas studied included fibro, osteogenic, and liposarcomas. The lymphoma series contained Hodgkin's disease, Burkitt's tumors, lymphosarcomas, and reticulum cell sarcomas. Control adult and fetal tissues were always examined in parallel, and these were invariably negative. In the case of breast tissue, the two benign diseases, fibroadenoma and fibrocystic disease, were also included and were found to be negative.

Table II summarizes in diagramatic form the outcome of the survey of human neoplasias with the animal virus probes. The pluses signify that the corresponding

Table II: Homologies among Human Neoplastic RNAs and Animal Tumor Viral RNAs

	Human neoplastic RNAs			
Viral RNAs	Breast Cancer	Leukemia	Sarcoma	Lymphoma
MMTV	+	–	–	–
RLV	–	+	+	+
AMV	–	–	–	–

The results of molecular hybridization between [³H]DNA complementary to the various viral RNAs and pRNA preparations from the indicated neoplastic tissues. The plus sign indicates that hybridizations were positive and the negative sign, that none could be detected (5).

tritiated DNA complexed with the indicated tumor RNAs and the minuses, that no such complexes were detected. The positives in these earlier studies ranged from 67 % for breast cancer to 92 % for the leukemias. What is most noteworthy of the pattern exhibited in Table II is its concordance with predictions deducible from the murine system. Thus, human breast cancer contains RNA homologous only to that of the murine mammary tumor virus. The human leukemias, sarcomas, and lymphomas all contain RNA sharing sufficient homology to that of the Rauscher murine leukemia virus (RLV) to make a stable duplex. These mesenchymal neoplasias contain no RNA homologous to the MMTV RNA. Finally none of the human tumors contains RNA detectably related to that of the avian myeloblastosis virus. The homology of leukemic RNA to that of RLV and the homology of RNA from human breast cancer to that of MMTV have been confirmed (8, 9).

In summary, the specificity pattern of the unique RNA found in the human neoplasias is in complete agreement with what has been described for the corresponding virus-induced malignancies in the mouse.

IV. The Simultaneous Detection Test

The existence of RNA in human tumors having sequence homology to virus particles causing homologous diseases in mice does not of course establish a viral etiology for these diseases in man. The next step requires the performance of experiments designed to answer the second and third questions raised in the introductory paragraphs, i. e., those relating to the size of the RNA being detected and whether it is associated with the reverse transcriptase in a particle possessing other features of complete or incomplete oncornaviruses.

What we sought was a method of detecting the presence of particles similar to the RNA tumor viruses that would be simple, sensitive, and sufficiently discriminating so that a positive outcome could be taken as an acceptable signal of the presence of a viral-like agent. To achieve this goal, we devised a test that depended on the simultaneous detection of two diagnostic features of the animal RNA tumor viruses.

The oncornaviruses exhibit two identifying characteristics. They contain a large (1×10^7 daltons in molecular weight and composed of subunits each of which is 3×10^6 daltons) single-stranded RNA molecule having a sedimentation coefficient of 70S, or 35S if the 70S molecule has broken down into its subunits. They also have reverse transcriptase (10, 11), an enzyme that can use the viral RNA as a template to make a complementary DNA copy.

The possibility of a concomitant test for both the enzyme and its template was suggested by our prior experience with RNA transcriptase in which we found (12) that the growing RNA chain could be detected as a complex with its DNA template on removal of the protein from the reaction mixture. Similar observations were made in examinations of the early reaction intermediate (13, 14) of the reverse transcriptase reaction.

It was on this basis that Schlom and Spiegelman (15) developed the simultaneous detection test that was used to demonstrate (16) the presence in human milk of particles containing 70S RNA and the reverse transcriptase. The test was modified (17) to be applicable to tumor tissue using the mouse mammary tumor as the experimental model.

Figure 2 diagrams the procedure used. Tumor cells are first broken by the use of the Dounce homogenizer and nuclei, mitochondria, and large cell membrane fragments removed by low speed centrifugation. The supernatant is subjected to trypsin digestion to inactivate any nucleolytic enzymes and the trypsin is neutralized by trypsin inhibitor. The supernatant is then centrifuged at 150,000 X g to yield a cytoplasmic pellet containing virus particles, if present. The resulting pellet is then banded isopycnicly in a sucrose density gradient and the fraction between 1.16 and 1.19 g/ml is collected by centrifugation. The recovered pellet is then treated with a nonionic detergent (NP40) to disrupt possible viral particles, and the disrupted preparation is used in a brief endogenous reverse transcriptase reaction. The product of the reaction, with its RNA template, is freed of protein and analyzed in a glycerol velocity gradient to determine the sedimentation coefficient of the tritiated DNA. In addition, the product is subjected to equilibrium centrifugation in a Cs_2SO_4 gradient to determine its density.

The presence of particles encapsulating 70S RNA and a reverse transcriptase will be indicated by the appearance of a peak of newly synthesized DNA traveling at a speed corresponding to either a 70S RNA or a 35S RNA molecule. That the apparently large size of the [³H]DNA is due to its being complexed to an RNA molecule can be readily verified by subjecting the purified nucleic acid to ribonuclease prior to velocity examination. The disappearance of the 70S and 35S [³H]DNA peaks following RNase treatment proves that the [³H]DNA was complexed to large RNA molecules. Similarly, if the reaction is positive, newly synthesized DNA should appear in the RNA and/or hybrid regions of the Cs_2SO_4 gradient, and these peaks should again be eliminated by prior treatment with ribonuclease.

The simultaneous detection test was first applied to human breast cancer (18) in

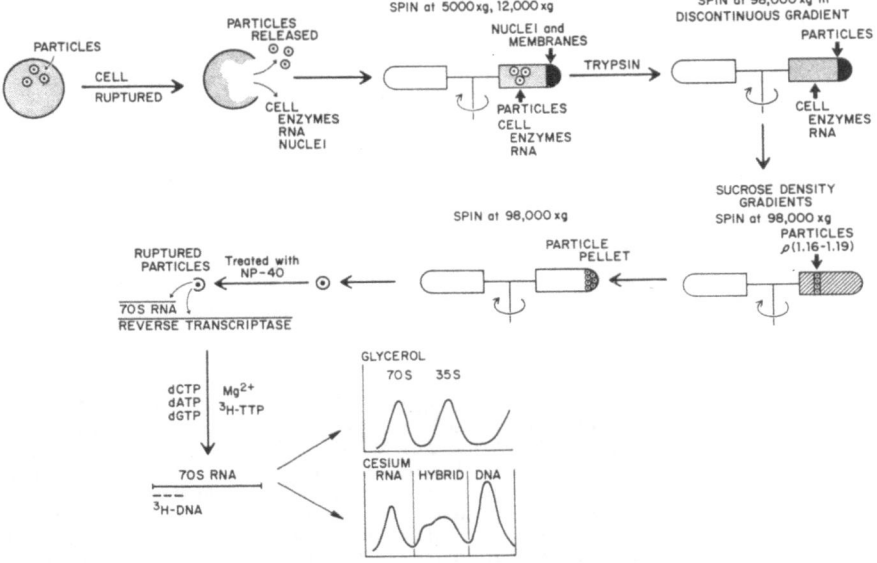

Fig. 2: Simultaneous detection test for 70S RNA and reverse transcriptase in neoplastic tissue (see text for further details).

a series including 38 adenocarcinomas and ten non-malignant controls. It was found that 79 % of the malignant samples were positive for the simultaneous detection reaction and all of the control samples from normal and benign tissue were negative. It was further shown that the particles possessing the reverse transcriptase activity and its 70S RNA template localize at a density between 1.16 and 1.19 g/ml, the density characteristic of the oncogenic viruses.

The data obtained therefore indicate that one can, with a high probability, find in human breast cancers particulate elements of the right density that encapsulate RNA-instructed DNA polymerase and a 70S RNA.

V. Application of the Simultaneous Detection Test to Mesenchymal Tumors

In our initial study of the leukemias (19), peripheral leukocytes were prepared from the buffy coats of both leukemic and nonleukemic control patients. Cells were disrupted and fractionated as described in Figure 2. Representative experiments examining the effects of ribonuclease treatment of the product and omission of one of the deoxytriphosphates during the reaction are shown in Figure 3. We see the telltale 70S peaks of DNA synthesized by the pellet fractions from the leukocytes of patients with acute lymphoblastic and acute myelogenous leukemias. The elimination of the complex by prior treatment with ribonuclease (Figure 3A) shows

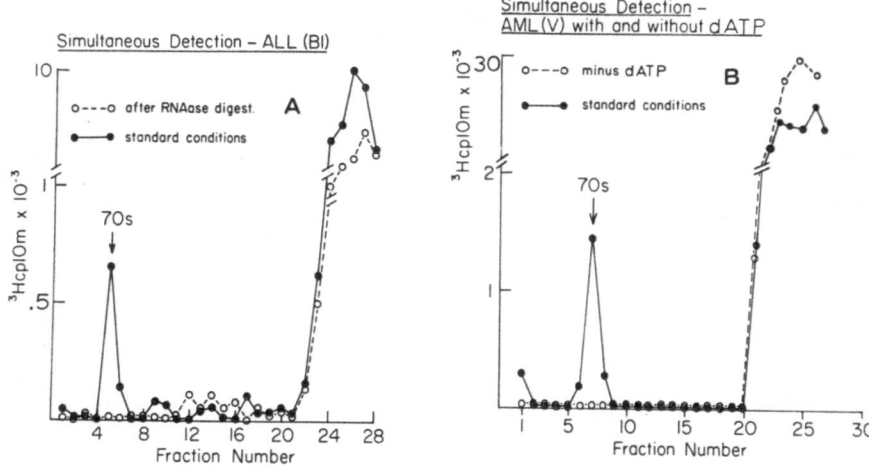

Fig. 3: Detection of 70S RNA [³H]DNA complex in human leukemic cells. 1 gm of leukemic WBC was washed in 5 ml of 0.01 M NaCl, 0.01 M Tris-HCl, pH 7.4, resuspended in 4 ml of 5 per cent sucrose, 0.005 M EDTA, 0.01 M Tris-HCl, pH 8.3, and ruptured with three strokes of a Dounce homogenizer. The nuclei were removed by low speed centrifugation (2,000 g, 5 min, 2°). The supernatant was brought to a final concentration of 1 mg/ml trypsin (Worthington) and incubated at 37° for 30 min. A tenfold excess of lima bean trypsin inhibitor (Worthington) was added (final concentration 3 mg/ml) and the solution again centrifuged at 2,000 g for 5 min at 2°. The supernatant was then centrifuged at 45,000 rpm for 60 min at 2°. The resulting cytoplasmic pellet was resuspended in 0.5 ml of 0.01 M Tris-HCl, pH 8.3, brought to 0.1 per cent Nonidet P-40 (Shell Chemical Co.) and incubated at 0° für 15 min. DNA was synthesized in a typical reverse transcriptase reaction mixture (final vol 1 ml) containing: 50 µmol of Tris-HCl, pH 8.3, 20 µmol NaCl, 6 µmol MgCl₂, 100 µmol each of dATP, dGTP, dCTP, and 50 µmol-[³H]dTTP (Schwarz Biochemical, 800 cpm per pmol). 50 µg/ml actinomycin D were added to inhibit DNA-instructed DNA synthesis. After incubation at 37° for 15 min, the reaction was adjusted to 0.2 M NaCl and 1 per cent SDS, and deproteinized by phenol-cresol extraction. The aqueous phase was layered on a 10 to 30 per cent gradient of glycerol in TNE buffer (0.01 M Tris-HCl, pH 8.3, 0.1 M NaCl, 0.003 M EDTA) and centrifuged in a SW-41 rotor Spinco at 40,000 rpm for 180 min at 2°. Fractions were collected from below and assayed for TCA-precipitable radioactivity. In this, as in all sedimentation analysis, 70S RNA of the avian myeloblastosis virus was used as a marker.

(A) One aliquot of product was run on the gradient as a control and the other was pretreated with 20 µg of RNase 1 (Worthington) for 15 min at 37° prior to sedimentation analysis. (B) Reactions with and without dATP (19).

that the tritiated DNA is indeed complexed to a 70S RNA molecule. Further, the omission of dATP (Figure 3B) leads to a failure to form the 70S complex, a result expected if the reaction is in fact leading to the synthesis of a proper heteropolymer. In similar experiments, it was shown that omission of either dCTP or dGTP also resulted in the absence of the 70S RNA-[³H]DNA complex, all of which argues against nontemplated end addition reactions.

In some cases leukemic cells were obtained in amounts adequate to permit a more complete characterization of the product. Hybridization of the human product to the appropriate viral RNAs provides the most revealing information since it tests sequence relatedness to known oncogenic agents. We summarize in Table III the results of examining the peripheral leukocytes of 23 patients, all in the active phases of their disease, including both acute and chronic leukemias. Of the 23 leukemic patients examined, 22 showed clear evidence that their peripheral leukocytes contained particles mediating a reaction leading to the appearance of endogenously synthesized $\overline{D}NA$ in the 70S region of a glycerol gradient. Nine of these were tested for ribonuclease sensitivity and in all cases the complexes were destroyed. In nine others, the DNA was recovered from the complex and annealed to RLV RNA and

Table III: Simultaneous Detection of 70S RNA and Reverse Transcriptase in Leukemic Cells (19)

Leukemias	Simultaneous detection cpm	RNase sensitivity	Hybridization to RLV-RNA	Hybridization to AMV-RNA or MMTV-RNA
Acute Lymphatic				
1	400	+	NT	NT
2	95	+	NT	NT
Acute Lymphatic/ Lymphosarcoma				
3	805	+	+	−
4	200	NT	+	−
5	185	+	NT	NT
6	105	+	NT	NT
Acute Myelogenous				
7	170	+	NT	NT
8	985	+	+	−
9	305	+	NT	NT
10	1295	+	+	−
11	1010	NT	+	−
12	115	NT	+	−
13	415	NT	+	−
14	400	NT	+	−
15	605	+	NT	NT
16	215	+	+	−
17	285	+	NT	NT
18	0	NT	NT	NT
19	1400	NT	+	−
Chronic Lymphatic				
20	200	+	NT	NT
Chronic Myelogenous				
21	405	NT	+	−
22	390	NT	+	−
23	600	NT	+	−

NT = Not Tested

to either MMTV RNA or AMV RNA. In all nine, hybridizations occurred with RLV RNA and not to either of the unrelated MMTV RNA or AMV RNA. In four patients, enough DNA complex was formed to permit a complete characterization of the product. In all four, the DNA complexes were destroyed by ribonuclease and the purified DNA hybridized uniquely to RLV RNA.

In addition to this initial group, we subsequently examined 85 leukemic patients and 38 patients with lymphomas (20, 21), including Hodgkin's disease, African Burkitt's lymphoma, lymphosarcoma, and reticulum cell sarcoma. The results of the simultaneous detection tests on these and corresponding control tissues are summarized in Table IV. It is noteworthy that positive outcomes were observed

Table IV: Simultaneous Detection on Mesenchymal Tissues

The simultaneous detection test was carried out as described in Figure 2. Peripheral white blood cells (WBC) were used in the leukemias, acute myelogenous (AML), chronic myelogenous (CML), acute lymphocytic (ALL) and chronic lymphocytic (CLL).

Tissue	Positives No. (Avg. cpm)	Negatives No. (Avg. cpm)	% Positives
Malignant			
AML	58 (985)	1 (10)	98
CML	18 (520)	0	100
ALL	25 (790)	0	100
CLL	4 (350)	0	100
Hodgkin's Disease (spleens)	22 (379)	6 (14)	79
Burkitt's Lymphoma	9 (369)	2 (14)	82
Other Lymphomas	7 (347)	1 (24)	88
Normal or Benign			
WBC	0	48 (12)	0
Spleens	0	34 (15)	0

in more than 99 % of the leukemic patients, whether they were acute or chronic, lymphocytic, or myelogenous. Thus despite their disparate clinical pictures and differing cellular pathologies, these various types of leukemias are associated with virus-like particles containing RNA with similar, though probably not identical, viral-related information. In the leukemias, we always dealt with peripheral white blood cells from patients with active disease, and this may account for almost total lack of negative responses. In the lymphomas, we were confined to examining spleens and lymphomatous tumor material where control over the content of malignant cells is more difficult to exercise. However, even here the proportion of positives is high, ranging from 79 % to 88 %. In contrast with these results are those obtained with the control series of 48 white blood cell samples and 34 spleens. The non-neoplastic samples included some with elevated white blood cell counts (in the range of 25,000/mm^3) due to a variety of disorders. None of the 82 samples from cancer-free patients exhibited any evidence of positive reactions. The difference in average cpm of positives and negatives is such that a diagnostic decision is unambiguous.

VI. Implications of Simultaneous Detection Tests on Human Breast Cancer and the Mesenchymal Tumors

The experiments we have just summarized on human breast cancer and the leukemias were designed to probe further the etiological significance of our exploratory investigations (2, 5), which identified in these neoplasias RNA homologous to those of the corresponding murine oncornaviruses. The data obtained with the simultaneous detection test established that at least a portion of the tumor-specific virus-related RNA we were detecting was a 70S RNA template physically associaed with a reverse transcriptase in a particle possessing a density between 1.16 and 1.19 g/ml, three of the diagnostic features of the animal RNA tumor viruses. Further, the DNA synthesized in the particles from both classes of neoplasias hybridized uniquely to the RNA of the corresponding oncornavirus. Note that this last result is complementary to and completes the logic of our experimental approach. We started out by using animal tumor viruses to generate [³H]DNA probes that were used to find related RNA in human neoplastic tissue. We concluded by using analogous human particles to generate [³H]DNA probes, which were then used to determine sequence relatedness to the RNA of the relevant oncornaviruses. None of the human probes hybridized to the avian viral RNA. The probe generated by the particles from human breast cancer was homologous only to the RNA of mouse mammary tumor virus, whereas the human leukemic probe was related in sequence only to RLV RNA, the murine leukemic agent. The biologically logical consistency of these results adds further weight to their probable relevance to the human disease.

VII. On the Problem of Germ-line Transmission of Viral Information

We now come to grips with the fifth question raised in the introductory paragraphs, the virogene-oncogene concept (22), which derives from animal experiments and argues that all animals prone to cancer contain in their germ line at least one complete copy of the information necessary and sufficient to convert a cell from normal to malignant and produce the corresponding tumor virus. This hypothesis presumes that the malignant segment normally remains silent and that its activation by intrinsic or extrinsic factors leads to the appearance of virus and the onset of cancer.

There are various ways of testing the validity of the virogene-oncogene hypothesis, but the pathways differ in the technical complexities entailed. One approach commonly used attempts to answer the question: Does every normal cell contain at least one complete copy of the required viral-related malignant information? The methodologies used included the techniques of genetics, chemical viral induction, and molecular hybridizations. However, for a variety of reasons, none of these gave, or could give, globally conclusive answers. Genetic experiments do not readily distinguish between susceptibility genes and actual viral information. Further, even if genetic data succeeded in identifying some structural viral genes, it would still be necessary to establish that *all* the viral genes are represented in the genome. Attempts to settle the question by demonstrating that *every* cell of an animal can be chemically induced to produce viruses have thus far, for obvious reasons, not been tried. The best that has been achieved along these lines is to show that *cloned* cells do respond positively. However, the proportion of clonable cells is small and *clonability may well be a signal for prior infection with a tumor virus*.

Finally, the quantitative limitations of molecular hybridization make it almost impossible to provide definitive proof that each cell contains one complete viral copy in its DNA. Although it is not very difficult to show that 90 % of the information is present, it is the last 10 % that constitutes the insurmountable barrier and 10 % of 3×10^6 daltons amounts to a far from trivial 3×10^5 daltons, the equivalent of about one gene.

A useful way to obviate these technical difficulties is to invert the problem. Instead of asking whether one complete copy exists in normal cells, the question can be phrased in the following terms: Does the DNA of a malignant cell contain viral-related sequences that are *not* found in the DNA of its normal counterpart? Phrasing the issue in this manner leads to the design of experiments that avoid the uncertainties generated by the demonstrated fact that many indigenous RNA tumor viruses share, completely or partially, *some* sequences with the normal DNA of their natural hosts (23). The crucial point is of course whether *all* of the viral sequences are to be found in normal DNA. The approach we adopted requires removal of those viral sequences that are contained in non-neoplastic DNA by exhaustive hybridization of the viral probe to normal DNA in vast excess. Any unhybridized residue can then be used to determine whether malignant DNA contains viral-related sequences not detectable in normal tissue.

We first investigated this question in the case of the human leukemias (24) and the strategy, as diagrammed in Fig. 4 (a and b), may be outlined in the following steps:

a) Isolate from leukemic cells the fraction enriched for the particles encapsulating the 70S RNA and RNA-directed DNA polymerase;

b) Use this fraction to generate [³H]DNA endogenously synthesized in the presence of high concentrations of actinomycin D to inhibit host and viral DNA-directed DNA synthesis;

c) Purify the [³H]DNA by hydroxyapatite and Sephadex chromatography with care being exercised to remove by self-annealing and column chromatography all self-complementary material in the tritiated probe;

d) Use the resultant [³H]DNA to detect complementary sequences in normal and leukemic leukocyte DNA;

e) If viral-related sequences are detected in *both*, remove those found in normal leukocytes by exhaustive hybridization to normal DNA; and

f) Test the residue for specific hybridizability to leukemic DNA.

In carrying out the recycling and test hybridizations, it is imperative that conditions be chosen to account for the possibility that the leukemia-specific sequences are present in only one copy per genome, a possibility which is in fact realized (24). To this purpose, the concentration in moles per liter (C_0) of DNA and the time (t in seconds) of annealing is adjusted to C_0t values of 10,000, which are adequate to locate unique sequences.

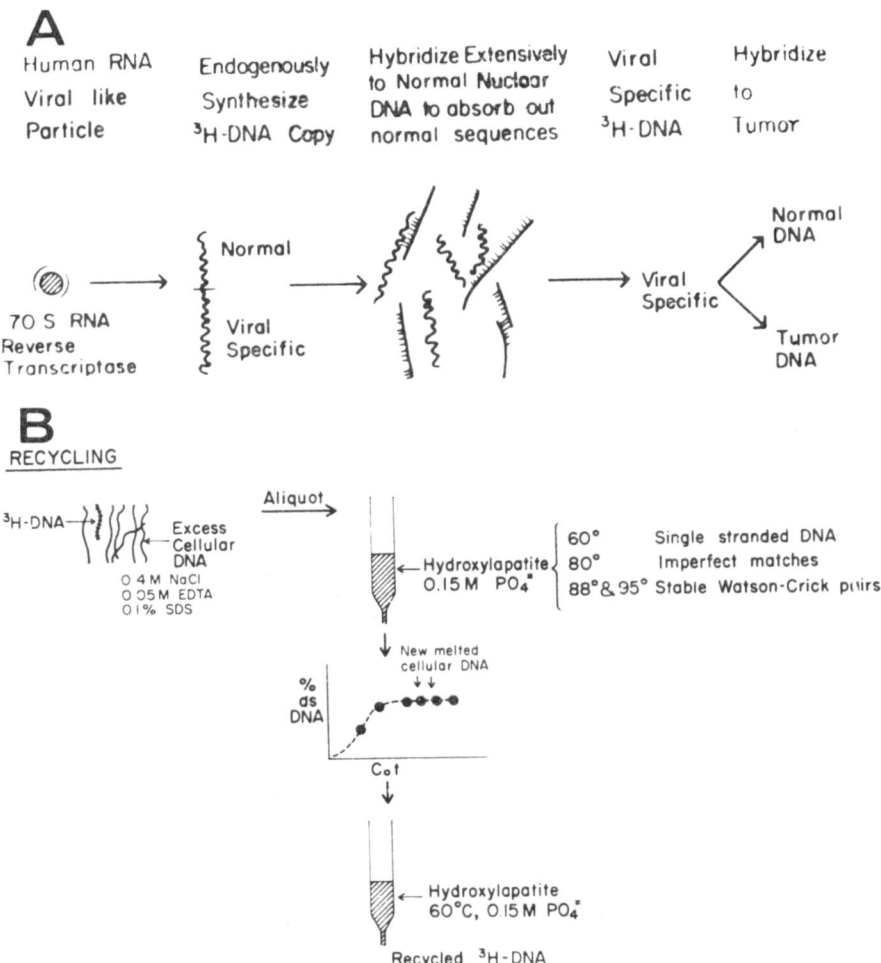

Fig. 4: (A) Generation of [³H]DNA by human leukemic particles and hybridization of sequences shared with normal DNA. (B) Separation of leukemia-specific sequences by hydroxyapatite chromatography. See text for further details.

A typical outcome of hybridizing such recycled tritiated DNA to normal and leukemic DNA is shown in Fig. 5. It is evident that no complexes stable at temperatures above 88° are formed with normal DNA. On the other hand, 57 % of the recycled [³H]DNA probe forms well-paired duplexes with leukemic DNA. A series of such experiments was performed with particle-generated [³H]DNA and nuclear DNA obtained from 8 untreated patients with either acute or chronic myelogenous leukemia. In every case (Table V), the [³H]DNA, after being sub-

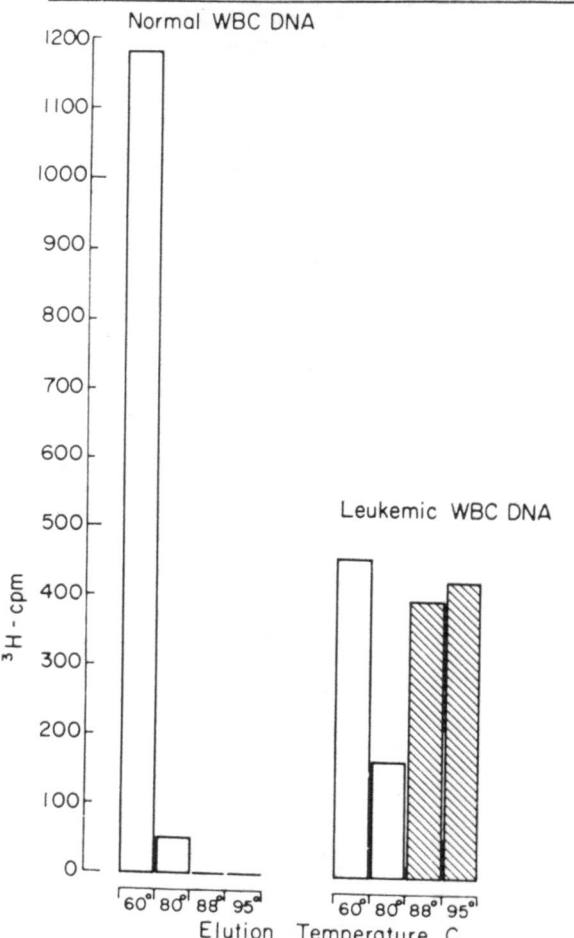

HYBRIDIZATION WITH RECYCLED ³H-DNA
LEUKEMIC PROBE

Fig. 5: Hydroxyapatite elution profile of a hybridization reaction of recycled leukemic [³H]DNA to nuclear DNA from normal leukocytes and from leukemic leukocytes of the patient from which the [³H]DNA was derived.

jected to exhaustive annealing to normal DNA, yielded a residue that forms stable duplexes only with leukemic DNA, in agreement with the experiment of Fig. 5.

In estimating the implication of these results, it must be recalled that the leukemia-specific sequences found (24) in leukemic cells are present as nonreiterated copies per genome. This was established by the C_0t values (concentration of nucleotides X time) required to detect them. The sensitivity used to examine

**Table V: Exhaustive Hybridization of [³H]DNA Probe Synthesized by Leu-
kemic Particles with Normal-leukocyte Nuclear DNA, Followed by
Hybridization of the Nonhybridizing Recycled Leukemic [³H]DNA
Probe to Normal DNA and to Leukocyte Nuclear DNA from the same
Leukemic Patient (24).**

| | | Leukemic [³H]DNA hybridized to normal-leukocyte DNA | | Recycled leukemic [³H]DNA hybridized to leukocyte DNA | | | |
| | | | | Leukemic | | Normal | |
		cpm	% Hy-bridization	cpm	% Hy-bridization	cpm	% Hy-bridization
1	(AML)	3020	61	523	56	0	0
2	(CML)	1350	40	1020	51	0	0
3	(CML)	2580	51	431	35	3	0
4	(CML)	510	45	101	36	0	0
5	(AML)	1100	43	303	48	4	0
6	(AML)	4520	49	1130	46	1	0
7	(AML)	390	42	45	69	0	0
8	(AML)	1450	49	510	52	0	0

Background was 30 cpm and all counts recorded represent cpm above background. CML
= Chronic myelogenous leukemia. AML = Acute myelogenous leukemia.

normal cells for the leukemia-specific sequences was such that 1/50th of an equivalent of that found in leukemic cells would have been readily detected. Consequently, one may conclude that the vast majority of normal cells do not contain
this particular stretch of malignant-associated information and it cannot therefore
be represented in the germ line of nonleukemic individuals.

VIII. Unique Sequences in Hodgkin's and Burkitt's Lymphomas and their Relatedness

We have already noted that, like the leukemias, Hodgkin's and Burkitt's
lymphomas have particles containing reverse transcriptase and a 70S RNA template related in sequence to that of RLV. It was of obvious interest to determine
whether the lymphomas also parallel the leukemias in possessing a unique sequence
not detectable in normal tissue. If they do, one can in addition ascertain whether
the sequences found in Hodgkin's and Burkitt's lymphomas are related to each
other. The outcome has evident significance for the possible relevance of the sequence to malignancy.

[³H]DNA probes were synthesized with particles isolated from four Burkitt's
tumors and three Hodgkin's disease specimens. Sequences shared with normal DNA
(between 35 % and 40 %) were then removed as described for the leukemias (24)
to yield the recycled [³H]DNA probes (25).

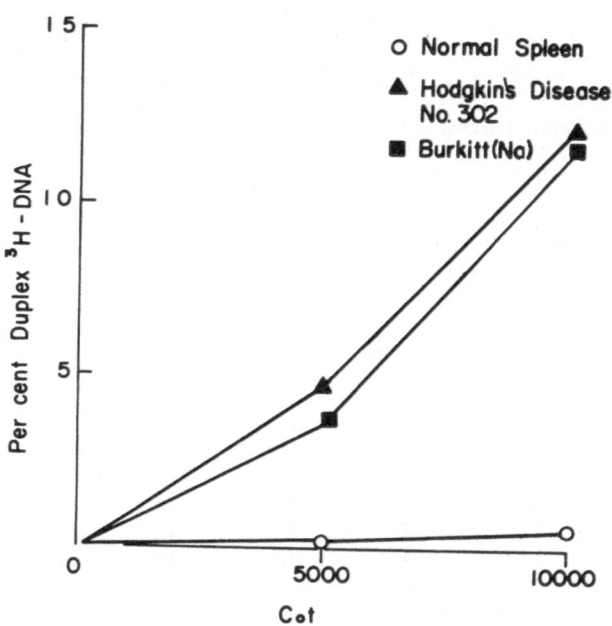

Fig. 6: Hybridization of recycled Hodgkin's disease #302 [³H]DNA to nuclear DNA isolated from normal spleen (0–0), Hodgkin's disease #302 (▲ – ▲), and Burkitt's lymphoma (NA) (■ – ■). Equal aliquots were removed from the hybridization vessel at each Cot value and hybrid formation was analyzed by hydroxyapatite chromatography. The input counts for each point were 1,500–2,000 cpm and only those duplexes eluting at 88° and above are counted as stably hybridized.

Figure 6 shows the outcome of challenging recycled Hodgkin's disease [³H]DNA with nuclear DNAs from normal spleen, Hodgkin's disease spleen, and from Burkitt's lymphoma. Few, if any, stable duplexes are formed with normal DNA. Note, however, that although the probe was made with Hodgkin's disease particles, the [³H]DNA hybridized to Burkitt's lymphoma nuclear DNA virtually as well as it complexed to DNA from Hodgkin's spleen. The converse is also true, as may be seen from Table VI, which summarizes the results of our findings in the recycled [³H]DNA challenged with nuclear DNA from normal and malignant tissues (25). Again, normal DNA is unable to form significant amounts of stable complexes (elution at 88° and above) with the [³H]DNA probes. In all instances, the lymphoma [³H]DNAs hybridized in stable complexes to the nuclear DNA of the original types from which the particles were obtained and used to generate the labeled DNA. Further, with only one exception, all of the Burkitt's and Hodgkin's disease [³H]DNAs cross hybridize with each other's DNA.

In summary, several features emerged from this study of the lymphomas. The particle-related sequences found in Burkitt's and Hodgkin's lymphomas possess sequences in common, an observation in accord with our earlier findings (7, 20,

Table VI: Hybridization of Recycled [³H]DNA Probes Synthesized with Human Lymphoma Particles with Nuclear DNA from Normal and Tumor Tissues

Origin of [³H]DNA recycled probe	Nuclear DNA	No. tested positive total	Percent positives
Burkitt's lymphomas	Burkitt's	7/7	100
	Hodgkin's	2/2	100
	Normal (spleen)	0/4	0
	IM* (spleen)	0/1	0
	IM* (cell)	0/1	0
Hodgkin's disease	Hodgkin's	3/3	100
	Burkitt's	2/3	67
	Normal (spleen)	0/3	0

* IM = infectious mononucleosis

21, 26), that Hodgkin's and Burkitt's particles both share sequences with the Rauscher murine leukemia agent. Further, in view of the previous association of the Epstein-Barr virus with Burkitt's lymphoma (27, 28) and the non-neoplastic infectious mononucleosis (29, 30), it is revealing to note from Table VI that the leukocyte DNA of patients with infectious mononucleosis was devoid of the Burkitt's sequences detected by the recycled [³H]DNA lymphoma probe, indicating that these latter sequences are specific for neoplastic tissues. The fact that the particle-related sequences in Hodgkin's and Burkitt's tumors are related to each other adds further weight to this conclusion. Finally, the observation that cells carrying multiple copies of the DNA of the Epstein-Barr virus do not complex with recycled [³H]DNA probes from either Hodgkin's or Burkitt's particles proves that these particle sequences have no detectable relation to the DNA of the Epstein-Barr virus.

IX. Evidence from Studies of Identical Twins

Although the comparison of leukemic patients with normal suggests that healthy individuals do not contain the leukemia-specific sequences, the data do not rule out the possibility that those who do come down with the disease do so because they in fact inherit the required information in their germ line. One way to resolve this issue is to study the situation in identical twins. Since identical twins are monozygous, i. e., derive their genomes from the same fertilized egg, any chromosomally transmitted information must be present in both. It had already been shown by Goh and his colleagues (31, 32) in the case of chronic myelogenous leukemia that only the leukemic member of each of two identical twin pairs contained the marker Philadelphia chromosome. It was of obvious interest to examine this situation for the leukemia-specific sequences. If the leukemic member of the pair contains the particle-related DNA sequences, and does so because he inherited them through his germ line, then these same sequences must be found in the leukocyte DNA of his healthy sibling. To perform the experiment, it was necessary to locate identical twins with completely convincing evidence for mono-zygosity and where only one of them was leukemic. Further, the twins had to be of adult age since at least a unit of whole blood is required to provide enough leukocyte DNA to carry out the required hybridization.

Two sets of identical twins satisfying all these requirements were found and an experiment similar to the one outlined above was performed with each pair (33). In each instance, particles containing the reverse transcriptase and 70S RNA were again isolated from the leukocytes of the leukemic members and used to generate the [³H]DNA endogenously. The [³H]DNA was purified and sequences shared with normal DNA removed by exhaustive hybridization in the presence of a vast excess of normal DNA from random healthy blood donors. This was then followed by hydroxyapatite chromatography to separate paired from unpaired [³H]DNA. It is important to emphasize that in the recycling step, the normal DNA used came from the leukocytes of healthy, random blood donors and not from the normal twin. To have used the latter would have obviously confused the issue. The residue of the tritiated DNA that did not pair with the normal DNA was then used to test for the presence of a sequence in the leukocyte DNA of the patient and that of his healthy sibling.

The results obtained with the two sets of twins are described in Fig. 7, and it is evident that the same situation holds between the members of the twin pairs as was observed in the comparison of unrelated leukemic patients and random nor-mals (Fig. 5 and Table V). The leukemic twin contains particle-related sequences that cannot be detected in the leukocytes of his healthy sibling.

The fact that we could establish a sequence difference between identical twins implies that the additional information found in the DNA of the leukemic mem-bers was inserted after zygote formation. This finding argues against the applica-bility of the virogene hypothesis to this disease since it would demand that the leukemia-specific sequences found in the DNA of the individual with the disease must surely also exist in the genome of his identical twin. These results are also inconsistent with the possibility that individuals who succumb to leukemia do so because they inherit the complete viral genome.

X. Implications of the Unique DNA Sequences in Leukemias and Lymphomas

The data we have summarized on the existence of viral lateral-related sequences unique to the DNA of human malignant cells imply that they are inserted in somatic DNA, a process known to occur with RNA tumor viruses in animal cells in tissue cultures (34) and in whole animals (35). The fact that these viral sequences can be incorporated into somatic DNA suggests that this could also occur in early embryogenesis and thus involve a cell destined to differentiate into the germ line. An event of this nature would be selected for in any attempts at developing inbred strains characterized by high frequency of cancer.

Indeed this seems to have occurred in the course of producing the AKR mouse, a strain in which spontaneous leukemia occurs with virual certainty. It has been shown (36) that the DNA of the AKR mouse contains murine leukemia virus sequences that are not present in the DNA of the NIH Swiss mouse. These se-

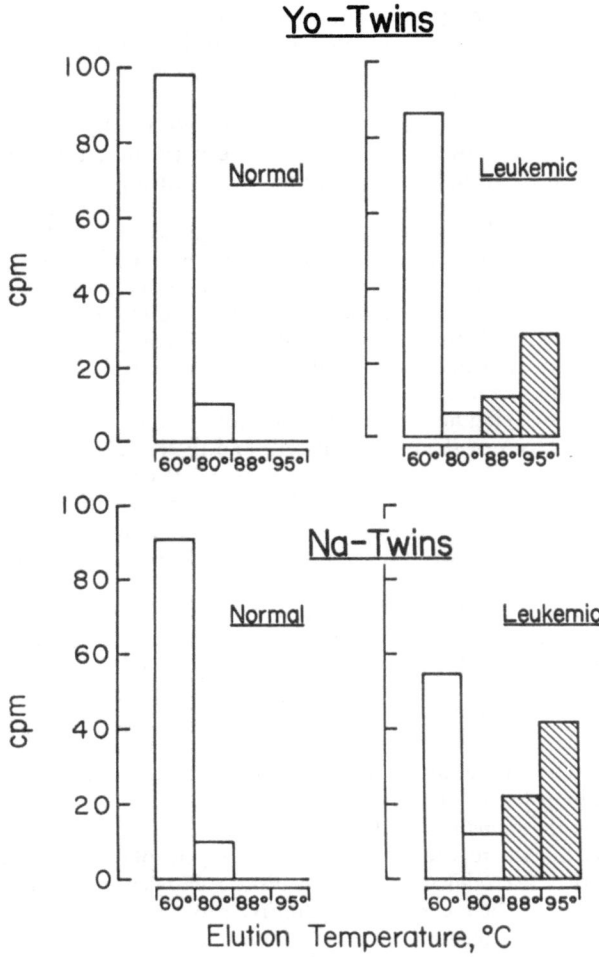

Fig. 7: Hydroxyapatite elution profile of a hybridization reaction of the recycled leukemic twin [^{3}H]DNA probe to nuclear DNA from normal leukocytes, normal twin leukocytes, and leukocytes from the same leukemic twin. The annealing reaction mixtures contained 20 A$_{260}$ units of cellular DNA, 0.004 pmol of [^{3}H]DNA, and 15 µmol NaH$_2$PO$_4$ (pH 7.2) in a final vol of 0.01 ml. The reaction was brought to 98° for 60 sec and 0.04 mmol of NaCl was added. The reaction mixture was then incubated at 60° X 50 hr. The reaction was stopped by the addition of 1 ml of 0.05 M NaHPO$_4$ (pH 6.8). The sample was then passed over a column of hydroxyapatite of 20-ml-bed vol at 60°. The column was washed with 40 ml of 0.15 M NaHPO$_4$ (pH 6.8) at 60°, 80°, 88°, and 95°. Fractions of 4 ml were collected, the A$_{260}$ of each fraction was read, and the DNA was precipitated with 2 µg/ml of carrier yeast RNA and 10 per cent trichloroacetic acid. The precipitate was collected on Millipore filters, which were dried and counted. In all cases, greater than 80 per cent of the nuclear DNA reannealed. A background count of 8 cpm was subracted in all instances (33).

quences were localized by genetic and molecular hybridization, and it was found that they are either identical to or closely linked to the Akv-1 locus.

The case of the AKR mouse was very likely an inadvertent result of its selection. An even more remarkable instance is the deliberate insertion of viral sequences into the germ line (37). This was accomplished by infection of preimplantation mouse embryos at the 4–8 cell stage with the murine leukemia virus (MuLV) followed by reimplantation in the uteri of surrogate mothers. Of 15 such animals born, one developed lymphatic leukemia at 8 weeks of age. Molecular hybridizations revealed leukemia-specific viral sequences in the DNA of all eight different organs examined, whether they were of mesenchymal origin or not. In agreement with our earlier findings (35), these sequences were not found in normal mesenchymal tissue nor were they detected in the DNA of non-target tissues in animals made leukemic by injection of virus after birth.

In summary, except for strains deliberately inbred for high spontaneous occurrence of disease, the mesenchymal neoplasias of mice and men would appear to have a similar underlying mechanism. In both instances new viral-related sequences are found in the DNA of the malignant cells and these are not found in the DNA of uninvolved tissues. They are therefore not germinal unless one wishes to invoke a rather unlikely specific elimination in the course of the differentiation of every cell but the malignant one. Despite its implausibility, this possibility should be exploited by testing for the leukemic-specific sequences in the germ line DNA (sperm) of leukemic individuals.

It must be emphasized that conclusions as to the validity of the virogene-oncogene hypothesis are only relevant to the particular instances examined and cannot be generalized to any other viral-related cancers even in the same animal, let alone to other species. In any event, it is evident that our findings with respect to the human mesenchymal tumors suggest more optimistic pathways for the control of these diseases than would be available if the total information were already in the genome. The data imply that we may not be forced to master the control of our own genes in order to cope with these neoplasias.

The fact that the human particles possess sequences homologous to those found in viral agents known to cause the corresponding neoplasias in mice encourages the hope that they are relevant to human disease. However, despite the considerable progress that can be recorded, no definitive proof exists at the present writing that the virus-like particles found in the human neoplasias are either viruses or etiologic agents of the cancers in which they are found. Proof will ultimately come when it proves possible to produce the relevant malignancy in a susceptible animal by injection of the particles purified from human tumors. It should, however, be noted that we have known of the mouse mammary tumor virus for more than 35 years and no one has yet succeeded in producing mammary tumors with this agent in any animal other than the mouse.

Under the circumstances, it would seem prudent not to wait for the definitive experiment with the human particles, but rather to proceed with attempts at further exploration of their significance and possible clinical usefulness.

We should like to list a few areas of possible exploitation and then turn our attention to a brief description of what has been accomplished along these lines.

1. The existence of the leukemia-specific sequences can provide the clinician with

a hitherto unsuspected parameter that could potentially be a useful adjunct in monitoring therapy.

2. One could attempt to grow the human particles in tissue culture in order to provide a more accessible source of these particles for further biochemical characterization with the ultimate hope of generating useful reagents for diagnostic, therapeutic or monitoring purposes.

3. Another, less ambitious approach is to purify one of the protein sub-components from the human particles for further characterization. This could then be used for the production of a monospecific antiserum that might be clinically useful.

XI. Particulate Reverse Transcriptase in the Leukocytes of Leukemic Patients in Remission

We have already noted (Table V) that positive simultaneous detection tests, indicating the presence of particles containing reverse transcriptase and the 70S RNA template, were obtained in more than 99 % of the leukemic patients examined. It was of obvious interest to see whether these particles could be detected in the leukocytes of leukemic patients who are in good clinical remission.

Peripheral blood leukocytes were obtained from patients at the Baltimore Cancer Research Center and from the M. D. Anderson Hospital. The leukocytes from some of the leukemic patients were obtained by leukophoresis and immediately stored at $-7°$ until used. The clinical statuses of the patients at the time of leukophoresis are summarized in Table VII. A complete remission was defined as the absence of symptoms related to the disease, normal results on physical examination, a hemoglobin of greater than 10 g/100 ml, leukocyte count greater than 3000/mm³, platelet count greater than 100,000/mm³, no blasts in the peripheral blood smear, and less than 5 % blasts in the bone marrow.

Table VIII summarizes the results of simultaneous detection assays for high molecular weight RNA and reverse transcriptase in the leukocytes from the patients examined. Outcomes are designated as positive only when the peaks of tritiated DNA found in the 70S and 35S regions were eliminated by prior treatment with ribonuclease, a feature establishing that the [³H]DNA is complexed to a large RNA molecule. If the peaks are not removed subsequent to RNase digestion, the reaction is scored as a negative outcome. In the present study two untreated leukemic patients were available for testing prior to remission induction and both were positive at that time. Three of the nine patients in complete remission demonstrated a 70S or 35S peak of acid-precipitable radioactivity that was abolished by RNase treatment. The "negatives" were subjected to a simultaneous detection assay via a cesium sulphate gradient, a procedure that obviates the problem generated by fragmentations of the RNA template during manipulation.

It will be noted from Table IX that samples from the untreated patients were all positive. The [³H]DNA-RNA hybrids were detected in nine out of eleven patients in complete remission. In this group, six of seven AML patients and two of three acute lymphocytic leukemia (ALL) patients demonstrated a positive reaction. In five of the patients, the simultaneous detection tests were negative by velocity sedimentation analysis but were positive when analyzed in the cesium

Table VII:

Patient	Age	Sex	Diagnosis[+]	Clinical[*] status	Remission duration at time of sample (days)	Total remission duration (days)
1-A	62	F	AML	UN	–	–
1-B	"	"	"	CR	7	64
2-A	42	M	AML	UN	–	–
2-B	"	"	"	CR	45	96
2-C	"	"	"	REL	–	–
3-A	40	F	AML	UN	–	–
3-B	"	"	"	CR	7	32
4-A	54	F	AML	UN	–	–
4-B	"	"	"	CR	7	218+
5	34	F	AML	CR	42	109
6	53	M	AML	CR	7	87
7	53	F	AML	CR	100	112
8	40	M	ALL	CR	1214	1600+
9	42	M	ALL	CR	1062	1662+
10	35	M	ALL	CR	1149	1735+
11	42	M	AML	CR	1051	1590+

[+] AML = acute myelogenous leukemia; ALL = acute lymphocytic leukemia
[*] UN = untreated; CR = complete remission; REL = relapse
Clinical status of leukemic patients when leukophoresis was performed for enzyme studies.

Table VIII:

Patient	Clinical status	CPM 70S	CPM 35S	Reaction
1B	CR	0		–
2A	UN	400		+
2B	CR	224		+
2C	REL		475	+
4A	UN	320		+
4B	CR	0		–
6	CR	975		+
7	CR	0		–
8	CR	0		–
9	CR	0		–
10	CR	0		–
11	CR	120		+

Test for 70S and 35S RNA-[^{3}H]DNA in leukocytes from leukemic patients. CPM in 70S or 35S represents acid-precipitable radioactivity that was removed from the 70S and 35S by prior treatment with ribonuclease A and T_1.

Table IX:

Patient	Clinical Status	RNA Region CPM	RNA Region % Total	Reaction
1A	UN	459	26	+
1B	CR	293	43	+
2A	UN	869	39	+
2B	CR	346	31	+
2C	REL	829	90	+
3A	UN	129	33	+
3B	CR	210	30	+
3C	CR	216	40	+
5	CR	248	30	+
6	CR	236	32	+
7	CR	187	29	+
8	CR	296	12	+
9	CR	0	0	−
10	CR	503	61	+
11	CR	52	32	−

Cesium sulfate analysis of RNA[³H]DNA in leukocytes from leukemic patients. The CPM in the RNA or RNA-DNA hybrid region and the percent of the total CPM applied to the gradient are enumerated. A positive reaction represents heat and ribonuclease-sensitive acid-precipitable radioactivity in the RNA or hybrid region of the gradient as described in the text. The [³H]DNA found in the hybrid density regions is hybridized to smaller DNA-RNA complexes, which would result from fragmentation of the larger 70S and 35S RNA molecules.

sulphate gradients. Hybrids of small molecular size would not be identified as 70S with 35S complexes, but can be detected as complexes in the hybrid region of the cesium sulphate gradient. Only one of the patients (#9) was negative by both glycerol and cesium sulphate gradient analyses. This patient did not appear to differ clinically at the time of the examination from the other remission patients exhibiting positive reactions. In the course of these studies we also examined by cesium sulphate analysis two pooled, normal white blood cell samples and five non-neoplastic spleens for the presence of particles capable of yielding RNA-tritiated DNA hybrids in an endogenous reaction and all were negative, as had been true in our previous studies (Table V).

It is obvious that finding the leukemia characteristic particles in the white blood cells of patients in remission is disappointing and does not accord with the generally accepted assumption that there is a normal and a leukemic population of leukocytes in acute leukemia (38). The goal of contemporary chemotherapy and immunotherapy is to reduce the size of the leukemic component (to zero if possible) to allow the bone marrow and the peripheral blood to repopulate with non-neoplastic cells. A number of clinical observations suggest that remission leukocytes are in fact normal cells. First, the prolongation of life is directly proportional to the duration of the remission. Secondly, a small but increasing number of patients

413

with acute lymphoblastic leukemia in long-term remission appear to go on to cure, indicating a permanent extinction of the leukemic cell population (39).

The morphology and functional properties of remission leukocytes have been studied by a number of techniques. These include karyotype analysis (40–45), ability to form colonies in agar (46–49), and the detection of leukemia-related antigens (50, 51). In general, these studies have supported the concept that remission leukocytes represent the return of a population of normal cells. Also, relapses are usually heralded by the detection of the abnormality associated with leukemic cells, and a number of these techniques have been suggested as ancillary tools in following the response of patients to chemotherapy. However, there have been instances in the above reports of patients in well-consolidated remissions whose peripheral leukocytes or bone marrow cells demonstrated persistence of aneuploidy, leukemia-related antigens, or abnormal colony formations in agar; these abnormalities appear unrelated to the effects of maintenance of chemotherapy. In this connection, mention should be made of Killmann's deductions (52) based on the demonstrated capacity of leukemic cells to differentiate; on these grounds he questions whether the normal-looking cells observed in the bone marrow of AML patients in remission are in fact derived from non-leukemic ancestor cells.

The data presented indicate that with regard to certain biochemical markers, which may be virus-related, remission leukocytes may more closely resemble the leukemic cells than normal cells. Quite surprisingly, two of the three ALL patients in long-term remission still had evidence of particles in their peripheral leukocytes. Further, the enzyme was detected in seven of eight patients with AML in remission. We are unable to determine if all or a fraction of the peripheral white cells studied possessed the leukemic characteristics. Thus we cannot directly answer the question whether one or two white cell populations are present.

Mak and his colleagues (53, 54) have described particulate activity in the supernatants of short-term cultures derived from bone marrow of leukemic patients in remission. The activity of the cultures from remission patients equaled, and in some instances exceeded, that detected in the cultures derived from patients in relapse.

There are a number of plausible explanations for the persistence of the particulate enzyme and its associated template in the remission leukocytes. The normal cell found in remission could be infected with a non-oncogenic C-type virus or conversely the remission leukocyte could have acquired resistance to transformation whereas susceptibility to infection was unaltered. Second, as a result of chemotherapy, a portion of the leukemic clone could have evolved into a non-neoplastic clone still capable of expressing some viral function. There are a number of *in vitro* models for the latter phenomenon. Thus, it has been shown that cells transformed with a murine sarcoma virus can spontaneously, or after exposure to antimetabolites, revert to a normal morphology. Certain clones of these morphological revertants behave in a non-malignant manner, yet some viral functions are expressed or can be induced (55).

A more direct method for examining such questions is to use the molecular hybridization to answer the following questions: 1) Do remission cells have leukemia-specific DNA nucleotide sequences? 2) If present, are some leukemia-specific DNA sequences not expressed or are critical DNA sequences deleted? These areas are presently under investigation.

414

XII. Attempts to Produce Human RNA Tumor Particles in Cell Cultures

All would agree that an important advance would result from the establishment of particle-producing cells in short, or preferably long-term culture. An alternative but equally useful outcome could be obtained by the successful infection of established cell lines with the human virus-like particles. Although not yet achieved, a number of recent reports suggest that this desirable situation may eventually be obtained. Thus, McGrath et al. (56) describe a human breast carcinoma cell line that may ultimately be converted into a source of breast cancer particles. Kotler et al. (57) have succeeded in using arginine starvation to induce the release of virus-like particles from human leukemic cells. We have already noted that short-term cultures of leukemia bone marrow aspirates in a conditioned medium has led to the production of particles recoverable from the culture supernatants (53, 54).

Probably the most interesting recent announcement along these lines came from Gallo and his colleagues (58, 59, 60) who reported the isolation of a C-type virus (HL23V) from cultured peripheral white blood cells derived from a patient with acute myelogenous leukemia. The reverse transcriptase of this putative human oncornavirus was found to be antigenically related to the reverse transcriptase of the simian sarcoma virus type-1 (SSV-1) and to the gibbon ape lymphoma virus (GALV). The spontaneously released viruses from the human leukemia cells were successfully transmitted to A204, a human rhabdomyosarcoma cell line. The infected A204 (HL23V) culture was an excellent producer, yielding virus in sufficient quantities to permit biochemical and immunological characterization.

The potential implications of these observations made it mandatory to undertake the task of identifying the nature of the virus particles released. We will here briefly summarize our efforts along these lines.

The A204 (HL23V) culture produced high titers of particles that were found by [³H]-uridine labeling to possess the characteristic buoyant density (1.16 g/ml) of oncornavirus. Simultaneous detection assays (15) of the culture supernatants demonstrated that the particles encapsulated 70S RNA and reverse transcriptase.

The reverse transcriptase from A204 (HL23V) culture supernatants was examined for relatedness to the SSV enzyme. Figure 8 shows that the antiserum prepared against the SSV reverse transcriptase was capable of inactivating the reverse transcriptase activity of HL23V particles only to about 60 %. The partial inhibition of enzyme activities suggested the possible presence of a second virus containing an antigenically unrelated enzyme.

To identify the unknown component in the HL23V particles, a search was instituted amongst known oncornaviruses using immunologic and molecular hybridization techniques. Probable candidates were quickly narrowed down to the RD-114/CCC baboon endogenous virus group. Figures 9A and 9B show hydroxyapatite temperature elution profiles of viral (SSV and BV-M7) cDNA annealed to the total RNA from HL23V particles. The extent of the hybridization and the thermal stability indicate that the HL23V particles contain the complete information of both the simian sarcoma virus (SSV) and the baboon endogenous virus (BV-M7).

To determine whether all of the genetic information of HL23V can be accounted for by these two viruses, the reciprocal hybridization was performed. In these

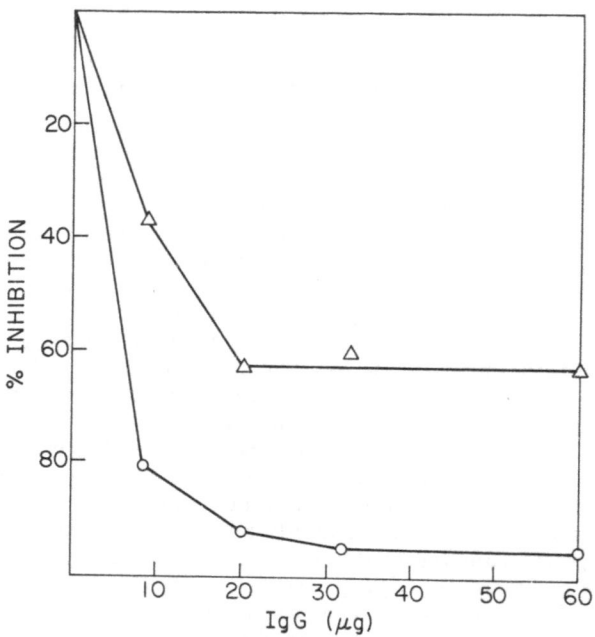

Fig. 8: Effects of anti-SSV reverse transcriptase IgG on HL23 reverse transcriptase activity. Increasing amounts of IgG purified from normal goat serum and from goat antiserum directed against SSV reverse transcriptase were mixed with NP-40-disrupted HL23, incubated for 15 min at 37° and then assayed for reverse transcriptase. SSV was similarly treated and assayed. Both HL23 and SSV input were standardized to incorporate 10 pmoles of [³H]-TP in a synthetic template assay. The reverse transcriptase reactions (100 µl) contained the following in µmoles: Tris-HCl (pH 8.0), 5; MnCl₂, 0.02; KCl, 4; dithiothreitol, 0.04; 0.02 each of dGTP and [³H]-dGTP (500 cpm/pmole) and oligo dG₁₂: poly Cm at 4 µg/ml. After incubation at 37° for 30 min, the reactions were terminated and assayed for acid-precipitable radioactivity. Using incorporations at identical inputs of normal IgG as control, the percent inhibition of the SSV and HL23 polymerase activity by the increasing levels of immune IgG were computed. 0 = V; △ HL23 virus.
the increasing levels of immune IgG were computed. 0 = SSV; △ = HL23 virus.

experiments, cDNA probe synthesized endogenously with HL23V particles, was annealed to RNAs from SSV-1 or BV-M7 or both. Figure 10 shows that the HL23V-cDNA hybridized 37 % and 44 % to the RNAs of BV-M7 and SSV-1, respectively. These individual hybridizations were additive as demonstrated by the complete complexing of HL23V-cDNA to a mixture of BV-M7 and SSV-1 RNAs. These data indicate that the genetic information of HL23V virions is completely accounted for, within the limits of the sensitivity of the molecular hybridization technique used, by the complete genomes of both SSV-1 and BV-M7.

To supplement and confirm these findings by an independent method, competition molecular hybridizations were performed using cDNA synthesized from SSV. Viral RNA from SSV was labeled with ¹²⁵I. SSV-cDNA can protect this ¹²⁵I-SSV-RNA more than 79 % from ribonuclease digestion at molar ratios of 5:1 (cDNA:RNA). Table X shows that when unlabeled viral RNAs were added in vast excess to compete this homologous reaction, both SSV and HL23V RNA

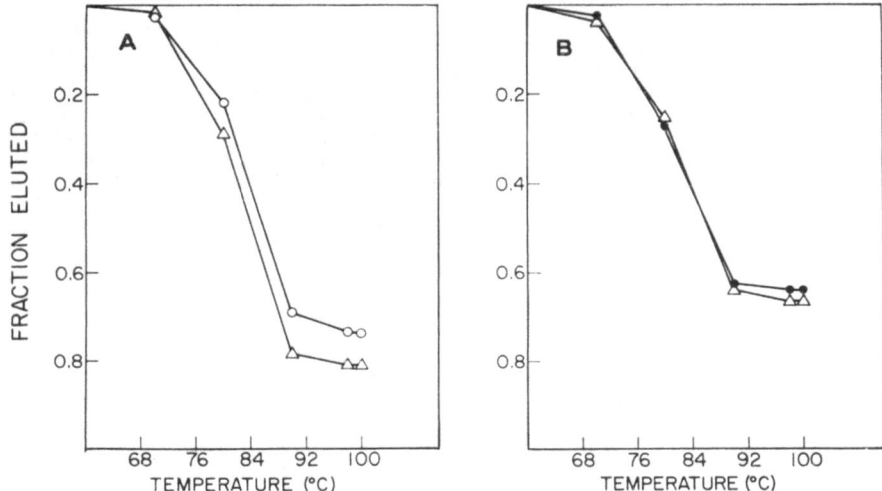

Fig. 9: Hybridization of [³H]-DNA transcripts of (A) SSV-1 and (B) BV (M7 isolate) to HL 23 viral RNA. SSV-1 and BV-M7 were obtained from Pfizer, Inc. (Maywood, N. J.) and were derived from sucrose density gradient-banded tissue-culture supernatants of a chronically infected human lymphoblastoid cell line (NC-37) and baboon kidney-canine thymus coculture (BKCT), respectively. HL23 virus was prepared from high-speed pellets of 2-day old media from HL23 virus-infected human rhabdomyosarcoma cell cultures. [³H]-DNA probes for each of the viruses were isolated from the 60–70S RNA:DNA hybrids of standard large-scale simultaneous detection assays. Hybridization reactions were set up between the various probes (500–1000 cpm/assay) and viral RNAs (0.2–1.0 μg) in 20 μl volumes in sealed siliconized glass tubes in 0.8 M phosphate buffer, pH 6.8, 0.1 % SDS and 10 mM EDTA. After heating at 100 °C for 1 min, the reactions were incubated at 68 °C for 20 h (Cot ≥ 2). The reactions were anlyzed by thermal elution hydroxyap-atite chromatography. Fractions of the total radioactivity eluted above 60 °C were plotted as a function of temperature. 0 = SSV-1 RNA, ● = BV-M7 RNA, △ = HL23V RNA.

Table X: Analysis of HL23V for SSV Genomic Content by Competition Hybri-dization

Competing RNA	*Competing RNA* ¹²⁵I-SSV RNA	% Resistance of ¹²⁵I-SSV RNA
None	–	72
SSV-1	1500	3
GALV	1200	15
MuLV-R	1800	75
Mouse 18S + 20S	450	74
HL23V	2300	6

Hybridization reactions (5.5 μl) were performed as described in Fig. 9 and contained 0.11 ng ¹²⁵I-SSV RNA (1.2 X 10⁸ cpm/μg), 0.68 ng [³H]-SSV cDNA (2 X 10³ cpm/μg) and 0.5–0.25 μg of the indicated competing RNA. Following incubation at 68° for 48 h, the reactions were diluted with 0.01 M Tris-HCl, pH 8.0, 0.4 M NaCl, 0.01 M EDTA and divided into four equal aliquots. Ribonuclease A (25 units/ml) and ribonuclease T₁ (5 units/

417

ml) were added to two aliquots and the samples incubated at 37° for 1 h. Nuclease resistance was the ratio of acid-precipitable ^{125}I in the samples with and without ribonuclease. Recovery of input acid-precipitable ^{125}I was greater than 90 %. SSV RNA was isolated from virions by disruption with SDS, Pronase treatment, rate sedimentation in a sucrose-SDS gradient and equilibrium density gradient centrifugation in potassium iodide. Viral RNAs from GALV-1 and MuLV-R were isolated by similar procedures excepting the KI gradient. HL23V RNA was total RNA from purified virus and the mouse 18S and 20S RNAs were extracted from purified ribosomal subunits from NIH/3T3 tissue culture cells. [^{3}H]-SSV cDNA was synthesized from SSV RNA and oligo dT with AMV DNA polymerase in the presence of 0.1 mg/µl actinomyc in D and 0.5 mg/ml distamycin A. The reaction contained TTP, dATP and dGTP at 1 mM each and [^{3}H]-dCTP (25 Ci/mMole) at 0.05 mM. This SSV cDNA protected ^{125}I-SSV RNA 33 %, 75 % and 87 % from ribonuclease digestion at molar input ratios of 0.4, 3 and 15, respectively (cDNA:RNA).

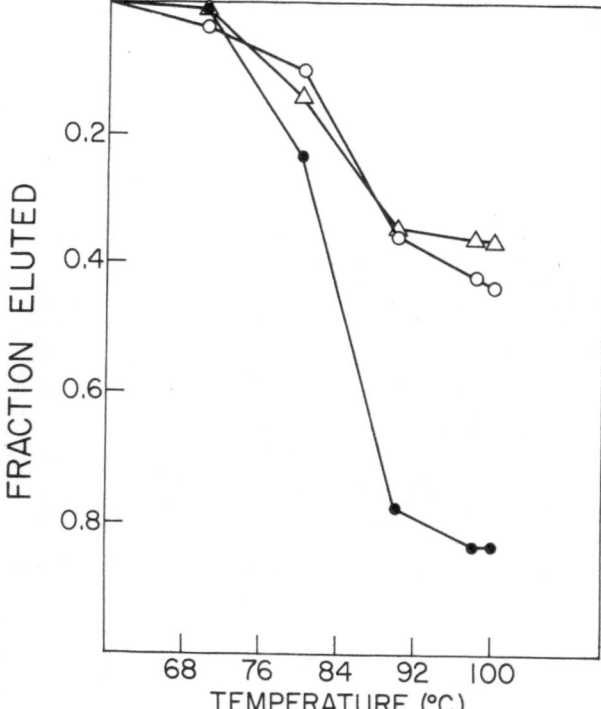

Fig. 10: Reconstruction hybridizations. HL23V [^{3}H]-DNA probe was hybridized to SSV and BV-M7 RNAs individually and in combination.
0 = SSV RNA, △ = BV-M7 RNA,
● = SSV and BV-M7 RNAs.

rendered the ^{125}I-SSV completely digestible. The GALV competed less successfully, illustrating the sensitivity of this technique for detecting the small sequence differences known to exist between GALV and SSV.

HL23V was further tested for its immunological similarity to SSV and BV-M7. The virus was concentrated by ultracentrifugation from culture supernatants of A204 (HL23V) and used as competing antigens in radioimmune assays for the p30 and gp45 of SSV grown in NC-37. As shown in fig. 11, the extent of competition of HL23V in both of these radioimmune assays was indistinguishable from SSV. Further, an immunodiffusion analysis of HL23V was made with antisera

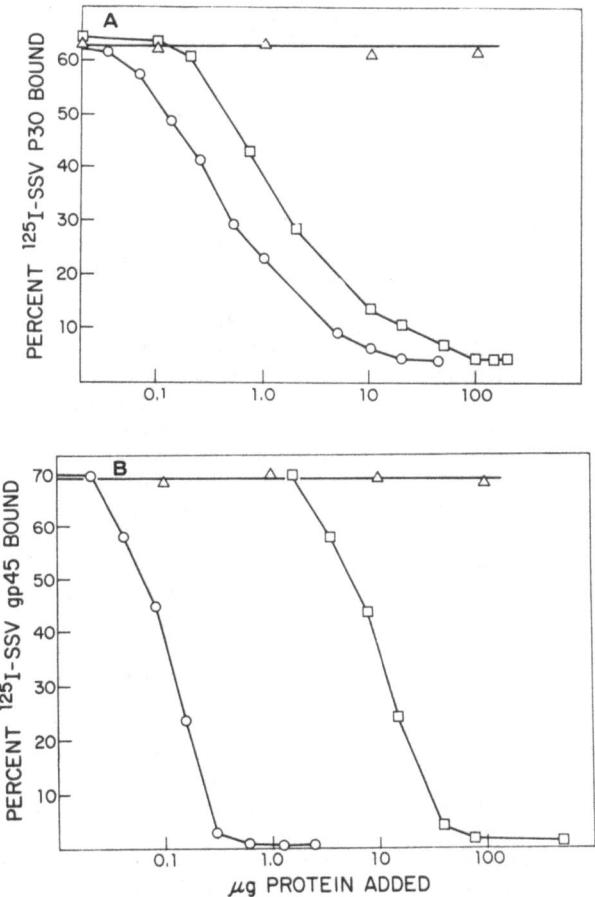

Fig. 11: Competition radioimmunoassays. HL23V was assayed for the presence of proteins antigenically related to the p30 (A) and gp45 (B) of NC-37 grown SSV-1. Antisera used for the studies with SSV-p30 were prepared by immunizing rabbits with the purified p30. An NC-37 absorbed rabbit antiserum prepared by inoculation of disrupted virions and used for the studies with SSV-gp45 was kindly supplied by Dr. D. Larson (Pfizer, Maywood, N. J.). The p30 protein of SSV-1 was purified from sonicated virus, followed by phospho-cellulose and Sephadex G75 column chromatography and isoelectric focusing. It was iodin-ated and repurified and the iodinated p30 antigen preparations obtained had specific activities of 6 X 10⁶ cpm/µg. The gp45 protein of NC-37 grown SSV was purified from sonic-disrupted virus by column chromatography on agarose 5M in guanidium hydro-chloride. Analysis of the preparations by 5 % sodium dodecyl sulfate polyacrylamide gel electrophoresis and isoelectric focusing indicated homogeneity of the 45,000-dalton antigen. Succinimidyl-3-(4-hydroxphenyl) propionate (ICN Pharmaceuticals, Inc.) was first labeled with ¹²⁵I and purified. The purified gp45 was then labeled by conjugation with the ¹²⁵I-labeled ester and chromatographed on a Sephadex G-25 column. Titrations of the antisera were performed in 200 µl reactions that included 0.2 % bovine serum albumin (BSA) in saline, 5000 cpm of ¹²⁵I-antigen and dilutions of antibody. After 1 h incubation at 37 °C,

100 μg of normal rabbit carrier IgG and a titered amount of goat anti-rabbit IgG were added. The reaction was incubated for 15 h at 4 °C. The samples were centrifuged and both precipitates and supernatants were counted in a Searle Autogamma counter model 1185. The results are expressed as percent cpm precipitated. Greater than 80 % of the labeled antigen could be bound by specific antisera. Competition assays were performed in a similar manner, except that unlabeled competing antigen was added to the original incubation mixture. The unlabeled competing antigens were SSV = (0), HL23V = (□), SSV-gp45 = (●) and MPMV = (△).

prepared against the major and internal structure of proteins of the woolly monkey (p30) and of the baboon virus (p28). The lines of identity obtained with BV-M7 and SSV indicate that, by these criteria, aga in HL23V cannot be differentiated from a mixture of these two agents.

In summary, immunologic and hybridization analyses indicate that the particles produced by A204 (HL23V) consist of a mixture of two viruses that are indistinguishable immunologically and by nucleotide sequence from two known non-human primate viruses, the baboon endogenous virus M-7 (61) and the woolly monkey virus SSV-1 (62). It will be noted that our conclusions and results (63) are in complete agreement with those of Gilden and his collaborators (64) whose experiments, complementary to ours, involved hybridizations to the cytoplasmic RNA of various cell lines infected with HL23V and antigenic analysis of the type-specific p12 and p15 antigens.

Any attempts to establish productive long-term cultures are always exposed to the all pervasive danger of laboratory contamination with animal oncornaviruses. Because of this, any evidence that agents produced in tissue cultures are either identical or even similar to a known animal oncornavirus has been accepted as sufficient evidence to condemn the culture and its particles as irrelevant to the human disease. It is important to recognize, however, that this is not a logically compelling argument. For example, it could well be true that some animal viruses originated from a human source. It is even less certain to conclude that an agent is human if it cannot be identified either by base sequence or by antigenic properties with a known animal virus. This line of reasoning makes the untenable assumption that our catalogue of all tumor viruses is complete.

The clinically relevant question for any putative human candidate particle is not necessarily its origin but its relation to the human disease. Are there at present any criteria that can be used usefully to decide whether a given tissue culture virus (e. g., HL23V) is in fact relevant to human neoplasia? A possible resolution can be achieved by answering the following two questions: (1) Can one provide evidence at the level of protein and/or nucleotide sequence for the presence of the putative agent in the *original tumor material* from which the tissue culture was established? (2) Can one provide evidence at the level of protein and/or nucleotide sequence for the persence of the putative agent in the malignant cells of other patients with the same disease?

A positive answer to the first question in the form of evidence for their presence in the original tumor cells would serve to eliminate the trivial explanation that the particles arose in the culture by laboratory contamination. The answer to the second question will decide the general relevance of the observation to human leukemia. Unless a positive response is obtained in a major portion of the patients examined, no basis exists for identifying the HL23V particles as clinically significant agents of human leukemia. We have examined leukemic cells of 13 patients for the presence of p30 and gp45 of SSV by radioimmune assays. When these are carried out under conditions that eliminate nonimmunologic interference, no evidence for the presence of these antigens could be detected. This failure would appear to limit the usefulness of the SSV-p30 as a clinical tool or as a serious etiologic candidate.

XIII. Purification of Reverse Transcriptase from Human leukemic Spleens

We have already mentioned the biologic and logistic difficulties that have attended attempts at obtaining whole human viral particles for characterization. At the present writing there exists no tissue culture source of authentic human RNA tumor viruses for use in biochemical and immunological investigations. One way to obviate these problems is to forego temporarily the more ambitious goal of characterizing the whole particle and focus rather on individual protein components of the human particles. Of these, one of the most accessible is the reverse transcriptase since its activity can be followed during fractionation.

The human leukemic reverse transcriptase has been partially purified from fresh peripheral blood cells obtained from patients with acute myelogenous leukemia (65, 66). However, the very large amounts of white blood cells required precluded definitive isolation of the enzyme in amounts that would establish its purity by gel analysis and thus permit an unambiguous characterization of its biophysical and biochemical properties. One way out of this dilemma was to explore the use of spleens as a source of leukemic enzyme. In addition to providing a possible solution of the logistic problem, such experiments would provide useful information on the relation between diseased tissue and the presence of the virus-like particles. Leukemias often involve the spleen, and splenectomies are occasionally performed therapeutically in instances of massive spleen enlargement or persistent platelet destruction.

We first worked out the technology of enzyme isolation from leukemic spleens using the murine Rauscher leukemia model. It was found that isopycnic separation of virus particles and their conversion to cores by non-ionic detergents (67, 68) provided material suitably enriched for enzyme. Usually in such experiments 70 grams of chronic lymphocytic spleens were used. After thawing, mincing and resuspension, and homogenization, the extracts were clarified by low speed centrifugation to remove nuclei and mitochondria. The remaining particulate elements were then recovered by high speed centrifugation at 80,000 X g for 90 min. Particles were concentrated by isopycnic centrifugation in sucrose gradients and converted to cores as described previously (67, 68). After recovery, the cores were disrupted with 1 % NP-40 and 0.7 M KC1 and then subjected to column fractionations on DEAE cellulose, phosphocellulose, and agarose gels with results as described in Fig. 12. One main peak of activity is observed on the DEAE column (Fig. 12A) containing 5 % of the input and greater than 90 % of the enzyme, yielding a 19-fold enrichment. When the active fractions of the DEAE cellulose columns are pooled and then chromatographed on phosphocellulose (Fig. 12B), about 25 % of the protein contains the enzyme activity, with a recovery of 71 % and an increase in specific activity of 2.8-fold.

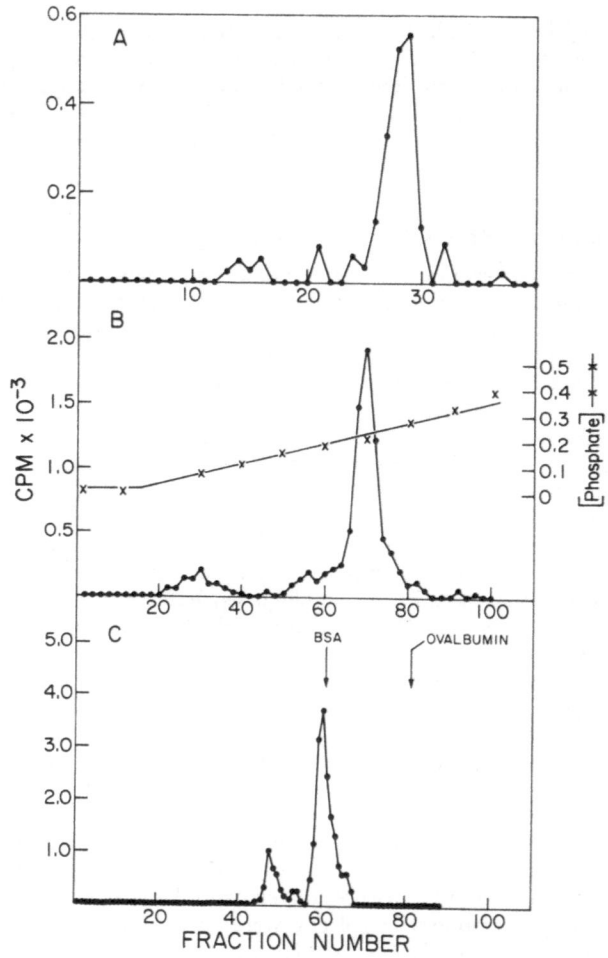

Fig. 12: (A) DEAE-cellulose chromatography of leukemic spleen enzyme. Core-like particles isolated from a leukemic spleen were treated with 1 % Nonidet P-40 and 0.7 M KCl, and the solubilized enzyme activity was chromatographed on a 16.5 cm X 2.5 cm column. Elution was with 0.4 potassium phosphate. 10 µl of each fraction (3.2 ml) were assayed using on oligo dT-poly rA template.

(B) Phosphocellulose chromatography of leukemic spleen enzyme. The fractions from the pooled DEAE-cellulose peak activity were diluted and chromatographed on a 17 cm X 1.5 cm column. Elution was with 160 ml of an 0.01 M-0.05 M potassium phosphate gradient; 1.6 ml fractions were collected and 10 µl aliquots assayed for oligo dT-poly rA-templated activity.

(C) Agarose gel filtration of leukemic spleen enzyme. The peak of activity eluted from phosphocellulose was subjected to gel filtration on a 50 cm X 0.9 cm agarose column. The elution rate was 4 ml/hr and 0.4 ml fractions were collected. Aliquots of 4 µl were assayed for enzyme activity with an oligo dT-poly rA template.

The concentrated phosphocellulose enzyme is then passed through a 0.5 M agarose column on which one routinely observes two peaks of activity (fig. 12C). If the first peak of activity is rechromatographed on the same type of column, a shift of most of the activity to the position of the second peak occurs. Thus, the first peak would appear to be an aggregate (possibly a dimer) of the enzyme. A summary of the column fractionations in terms of recoveries and specific activities is recorded in Table XI.

Table XI: Purification of RNA-dependent DNA Polymerase from a Viral Core Fraction of Human Leukemic Spleen

Fraction	Total Protein (mg)	Total Activity (pmoles)	Specific Activity (pmoles/mg)
1. Viral core region	3.90	2011	5.0×10^2
2. DEAE-cellulose pool	0.20	1949	9.7×10^3
3. Phosphocellulose pool	0.05	1400	2.8×10^4

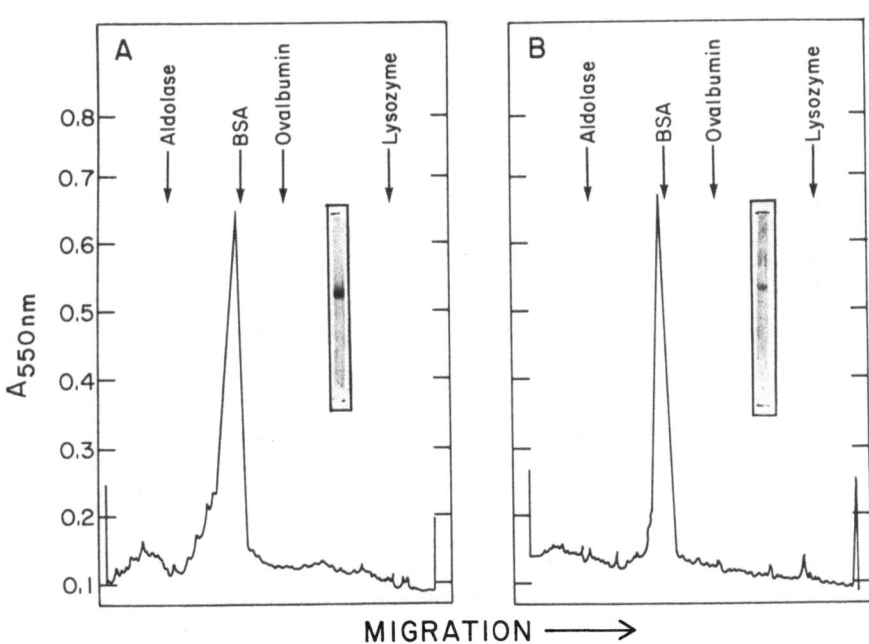

Fig. 13: Sodium dodecyl sulfate-polyacrylamide gel agarose enzymes. Fractions 48(A) and 60(B) of Fig. 12C were subjected to electrophoresis on sodium dodecyl sulfate polyacrylamide gels. After staining with Coomassie blue, the gels were scanned in a Gilford Model 2400 spectrophotometer. The stained gel of each fraction is also shown.

423

To examine the purity of the final enzyme preparation, portions of the two agarose peak fractions of Fig. 12C were electrophoresed on 5 % acrylamide gels in the presence of 0.1 % sodium dodecyl sulfate. Molecular weights of the separated polypeptides were determined using lysozyme, ovalbumin, bovine serum albumin and aldolase as molecular weight markers. As shown by the gel photographs and the scans of figures 12A and 12B, both agarose peaks yielded one major band corresponding to a molecular weight of 70,000 daltons, supporting the conclusion that the first agarose peak was in fact an aggregate of the second. A pool of the two agarose peaks constituted the final enzyme preparation.

Several parameters of the reverse transcriptase were examined. The reaction was found to proceed best at 37° and over a broad pH range from 7.0 to 8.2. The requirement for a divalent cation could be satisfied best by Mg^{++} (6 mM) although Mn^{++} was also effective over a very narrow range (0.5 to 1.2 mM), a feature also observed with the murine leukemic reverse transcriptases. In common with these, the purified leukemic spleen enzyme could utilize DNA but preferred RNA as a template. Further, the RNA templated activity was completely dependent on the presence of all four deoxyriboside triphosphates and exogenously added RNA (Table XII).

Table XII: **Deoxynucleoside Triphosphate and RNA Requirements of Leukemic RNA-dependent DNA Polymerase**

Reaction*	pmoles [^{3}H]dCMP polymerized**
1. Complete	4.6
2. -dATP	<0.024
3. -dGTP	0.076
4. -dTTP	<0.024
5. -dATP, dGTP, dTTP	<0.024
6. -RNA	0.032

* Incubation was for 20 min at 37° with 1.4 µg avian myeloblastosis virus RNA as template.
** [^{3}H]-dCTP was present at 1.04 X 10^4 cpm/pmole.

The critical diagnostic criterion of a putative reverse transcriptase is the ability to transcribe heteropolymeric RNA into a DNA complement. To test this, a reaction was run with the purified enzyme employing isolated AMV-RNA as the template. The product synthesized was purified, alkali-treated and hybridized either to AMV or RLV-RNA. An analysis on cesium sulfate gradient showed clearly that the tritiated product was complementary only to AMV-RNA. Thus, the enzyme purified from the human leukemic particles satisfied this operational definition of a reverse transcriptase.

The results (69) we have just described represent the first instance of a human reverse transcriptase isolated to the purity required for complete characterization. In addition, the procedure provides enough protein to generate monospecific antisera for ultimate use as detecting devices.

XIV. Present Status and Future Prospects

The application of nucleic acid hybridization and the other techniques of molecular biology have permitted us to illuminate some of the issues of human cancer noted in the questions listed in the introductory paragraphs. The answers obtained may be summarized in the following statements:

(1) Human neoplasias do contain RNA molecules possessing detectable homologies to the RNA of tumor viruses known to cause similar cancers in animal systems.

(2) The RNA molecules indentified in the human tumors possess the size and physical association with reverse transcriptase that characterizes the RNA of the animal oncornaviruses.

(3) Further, the tumor-specific RNA is encapsulated in a particle possessing the size and density of the RNA tumor viruses.

(4) The RNA of the human tumor particles possess homology to the RNA of the viruses causing the corresponding diseases in animals.

(5) Viral-related sequences are unique to the DNA of tumor cells, are inserted postzygotically, and are therefore not resident in the germ line.

The availability of the mesenchymal and mammary tumor animal model systems provided us with the viral agents that generated the radioactive DNA probes used to search for and find the homologous sequences in the particulate fractions of the corresponding human neoplasias. Our invention and perfection of the "simultaneous detection test" enabled us to characterize the size and particulate nature of the RNA detected in the human tumors. Beyond this, it evolved into an important technical advance since it permitted us to bypass the restriction of being forced to start with a known animal viral agent. Thus, we were able to extend our investigations beyond breast cancer and the mesenchymal tumors to other clinically important human neoplasias. The use of the simultaneous detection test established that a variety of human carcinomas contained particles having the diagnostic criteria associated with the oncornavirus-like particles. The neoplasias examined included a variety of cancers of brain (70), the gastrointestinal tract and lung (71), and skin (72).

Having found these particles in the human tumors, where does one go from there? An obvious need is to characterize them more fully biochemically and immunologically so that they can be compared with the similar agents found in the animal systems. However, here we are faced with a logistical problem that has thus far interposed serious obstacles. The amount of tumor material available and its particle content are such that it is difficult to isolate particles in sufficient quantity and purity to perform the desired biochemical examinations. Adequate characterizations will not be readily feasible until these particles are obtainable in suitable yield from established cell lines. To date this desideratum has not been achieved. Nevertheless, it may still prove possible to exploit some of the implications derivable from certain of their features. In particular, at least a portion of the RNA sequences found in the particles associated with each primary tumor site appears to be unique. As we have already noted, the particles found in human breast cancer share no sequences in common with those found in the mesenchymal tumors. These differences appear to extend to the particles found in other sorts or primary tumors. Thus, we have been able to distinguish by cross hybridization the sequences found in particles from stomach cancers from those found in the colon. Similarly, the sequences found in lung cancer particles were easily differentiated from those found in other tumor sites tested. It would appear from our survey that the sequences found in these particles are histogenically specific.

These results suggest the possibility of developing a novel pathway for specific tumor detection. From the outset, it was evident that the nucleic acid hybridization technology we had developed and used to provide fundamental information of the molecular basis of the cancer cell was not likely to be useful in a clinical setting. In the first place, it has thus far been successfully applied only to tumor cells, and there is little likelihood that there would be enough circulating tumor-specific nucleic acids to be useful for diagnostic purposes. Further, the hybridization procedure is too sophisticated, too laborious, and too expensive to be introduced into the clinical pathology laboratory.

It seems clear that one must find a way of translating the sequence differences of the tumor particles into a parameter that would be more amenable to detection by the devices more commonly used in the clinical laboratory. One approach would depend upon the plausible expectation that the sequence differences observed in the different particles would be reflected in proteins that might be distinguishable antigenically. Were this realized, one could immediately hope to use the very sensitive and less restrictive methods of immunology. These are not only very sensitive, but they are in routine use in clinical laboratories.

To exploit this approach and obviate the logistic and other difficulties attending attempts to study the whole particles, one might focus rather on isolating and characterizing individual protein components. Of these, one of the most amenable is the reverse transcriptase since it can be followed during fractionation by means of its enzyme activity. As we have shown here, this approach has led to the successful isolation and purification of the reverse transcriptase of the particles found in leukemic spleens. These same methodologies can be and have been applied to other human neoplastic tissue. With these specific proteins available, monospecific antisera can be generated that could hopefully be used for detection in the body fluids of tumor-bearing individuals. The potential value of providing a useable specific assay for the presence of tumor cells has been even further enhanced by the recent advances in adjuvant chemotherapy. Efforts along these lines could convert what has thus far been an exercise in molecular biology into a potentially powerful clinical tool.

Acknowledgments

Supported by grant CA-02332 from the U.S. Public Health Service and by Virus Cancer Program contract NO1-6-1010 with the National Cancer Institute.

References:

1. Hall, B. D., and Spiegelman, S. (1961) Proc. Nat. Acad. Sci. USA 47, 137–146.
2. Axel, R., Schlom, J. and Spiegelman, S. (1972) Nature 235, 32–36.

3. Axel, R., Schlom, J. and Spiegelman, S. (1972) Proc. Nat. Acad. Sci. USA *69*, 535–538.
4. Schlom, J., Spiegelman, S. and Moore, D. H. (1971) Nature *231*, 97–100.
5. Hehlmann, R., Kufe, D. and Spiegelman, S. (1972) Proc. Nat. Acad. Sci. USA *69*, 435–439.
6. Kufe, D., Hehlmann, R., and Spiegelman, S. (1972) Science *175*, 182–185.
7. Hehlmann, R., Kufe, D. and Spiegelman, S. (1972) Proc. Nat. Acad. Sci. USA *69*, 1727–1731.
8. Gallo, R. C., Miller, N. R., Saxinger, W. C. and Gillespie, D. (1973) Proc. Nat. Acad. Sci. USA *70*, 3219–3224.
9. Vaidya, A. B., Black, M. M., Dion, A. S. and Moore, D. H. (1974) Nature *249*, 565–567.
10. Baltimore, D. (1970) Nature *226*, 1209–1211.
11. Temin, H. M., and Mizutani, S. (1970) Nature *226*, 1211–1213.
12. Spiegelman, S., Hall, B. D. and Storck, R. (1961) Proc. Nat. Acad. Sci. USA *47*, 1135–1141.
13. Rokutanda, M., Rokutanda, H., Green, M., Fujinaga, K., Ray, R. K. and Gurgo, C. (1970) Nature *227*, 1026–1029.
14. Spiegelman, S., Burny, A., Das, M. R., Keydar, J., Schlom, J., Travnicek, M. and Watson, K. (1970) Nature *227*, 563–567.
15. Schlom, J., and Spiegelman, S. (1971) Science *174*, 840–843.
16. Schlom, J., Spiegelman, S. and Moore, D. H. (1972) Science *175*, 542–544.
17. Gulati, S. C., Axel, R. and Spiegelman, S. (1972) Proc. Nat. Acad. Sci. USA *69*, 2020–2024.
18. Axel, R., Gulati, S. C. and Spiegelman, S. (1972) Proc. Nat. Acad. Sci. USA *69*, 3133–3137.
19. Baxt, W., Hehlmann, R. and Spiegelman, S. (1972) Nature New Biol. *240*, 72–75.
20. Spiegelman, S., Kufe, D., Hehlmann, R. and Peters, W. P. (1973) Cancer Research *33*, 1515–1526.
21. Kufe, D., Margrath, I. T., Ziegler, J. L. and Spiegelman, S. (1973) Proc. Nat. Acad. Sci. USA *70*, 737–741.
22. Todaro, G. J. and Huebner, R. J. (1972) Proc. Nat. Acad. Sci. USA *69*, 1009–1015.
23. Ruprecht, R. M., Goodman, N. C. and Spiegelman, S. (1973) Proc. Nat. Acad. Sci. USA *70*, 1437–1441.
24. Baxt, W. G. and Spiegelman, S. (1972) Proc. Nat. Acad. Sci. USA *69*, 3737–3741.
25. Kufe, D. W., Peters, W. P. and Spiegelman, S. (1973) Proc. Nat. Acad. Sci. USA *70*, 3810–3814.
26. Kufe, D., Hehlmann, R. and Spiegelman, S. (1973) Proc. Nat. Acad. Sci. USA *70*, 5–9.
27. Henle, G., Henle, W., Clifford, P., Diehl, V., Kafuko, G., Kirya, B., Klein, G. Morrow, R., Munube, G., Pike, P., Tukel, P. and Ziegler, J. (1969) J. Nat. Cancer Inst. *43*, 1147–1157.
28. zur Hausen, H., Schulte-Holthausen, H., Klein, G., Henle, W., Henle, G., Clifford, P. and Santesson, L. (1970) Nature *228*, 1056–1058.

29. Henle, G., Henle, W. and Diehl, V. (1967) Proc. Nat. Acad. Sci. USA 59, 94–101.
30. Niederman, J. C., Evans, A. S., Subrahmanyan, L. and McCollum, R. W. (1970) New Eng. J. Med. 282, 361–365.
31. Geh, K. and Swisher, S. N. (1965) Arch. Int. Med. 115, 475–478.
32. Geh, K., Swisher, S. N. and Herman, E. C., Jr. (1967) Arch. Int. Med. 120, 214–219.
33. Baxt, W., Yates, J. W., Wallace, H. J., Jr., Holland, J. F. and Spiegelman, S. (1973) Proc. Nat. Acad. Sci. USA 70, 2629–2632.
34. Goodman, N. C., Ruprecht, R. M., Sweet, R. W., Massey, R., Deinhardt, F. and Spiegelman, S. (1973) Int. Jour. Cancer 12, 752–760.
35. Sweet, R. W., Goodman, N. C., Cho, J.-R., Ruprecht, R. M., Redfield, R., R. and Spiegelman, S. (1974) Proc. Nat. Acad. Sci. USA 71, 1705–1709.
36. Chattopadhyay, S. K., Rowe, W. P., Teich, N. M. and Lowy, D. R. (1975) Proc. Nat. Acad. Sci. USA 72, 906–910.
37. Jaenisch, R., Fan, H. and Croker, B. (1975) Proc. Nat. Acad. Sci. USA 72, 4008–4012.
38. Frei, E. and Freireich, E. J. (1965) Adv. in Chemotherapy 2, 269–298.
39. Simone, J., Aur, R. J., Hustu, H. O. et al. (1972) Cancer 30, 1488–1494.
40. Reisman, L. E., Zuelzer, W. W. and Thompson, R. I. (1964) Cancer Res. 1448–1460.
41. Sandberg, A. A., Takaaki, J., Kikuchi, Y. et al. (1964) Ann. N. Y. Acad. Sci. 113, 663–716.
42. Whang-Peng, J., Freireich, E. J., Oppenheim, J. J. et al. (1969) J. Nat. Cancer Inst. 42, 881–897.
43. Trujillo, J. M., Cork, A., Hart, J. S. et al. (1974) Cancer 33, 824–833.
44. Duttera, M. J., Whang-Peng, J., Bull, J. M. C. et al. (1972) Lancet 1, 715–717.
45. Craddock, C. G. and Crandall, B. F. (1973) Blood 42, 1013.
46. Greenberg, P. L., Nichols, W. C. and Schrier, S. L. (1971) New Eng. J. Med. 284, 1225–1232.
47. Harris, J. and Freireich, E. J. (1970) Blood 35, 61–63.
48. Moore, M. A. S., Williams, N. and Metcalf, D. (1973) J. Nat. Cancer Inst. 50, 603–623.
49. Bull, J. M., Duttera, M. J., Stashick, E. D. et al. (1973) Blood 42, 679–676.
50. Gutterman, J. U., Mavligit, G., Burgess, M. A. et al. (1974) J. Nat. Cancer Inst. 53, 389–392.
51. Halterman, R. H., Leventhal, B. and Mann, D. L. (1972) New Eng. J. Med. 287, 1272–1274.
52. Killmann, S. A. (1968) Ser Haemat 1, 103–128.
53. Mak, T. W., Aye, M. T., Messner, H. et al. (1974) Brit. J. Cancer 29, 433–437.
54. Mak, T. W., Manaster, J., Howotson, A. F. et al. (1974) Proc. Nat. Acad. Sci. USA 71, 4336–4340.
55. Fischinger, P. J., Nomura, S., Peebles, P. T. et al. (1972) Science 176, 1033–1035.
56. McGrath, C. M., Grant, P. M., Soule, H. D., Glancy, T. and Rich, M. A. (1974) Nature 252, 247–250.
57. Kotler, M., Weinberg, E., Haspel, O., Olshevshy, U. and Becker, Y. (1973)

Nature New Biol. *244*, 197.

58. Gallagher, R. E. and Gallo, R. C. (1975) Science *187*, 350–353.
59. Teich, N. M., Weiss, R. A., Salahuddin, S. Z., Gallagher, R. E., Gillespie, D. H. and Gallo, R. C. (1975) Nature *256*, 551–555.
60. Gallo, R. C., Gallagher, R. E., Miller, N. R., Mondal, H., Saxinger, W. C., Mayer, R. J., Smith, R. G. and Gillespie, D. H. (1974) Cold Spring Harbor Symposium on Quantitative Biology *XXXIX*, 933–961.
61. Benveniste, R. E., Lieber, M. M., Livingston, D. M., Sherr, C. J. and Todaro, G. J. (1974) Nature *248*, 17–20.
62. Theilen, G. H., Gould, D., Fowler, M. and Dungworth, D. L. (1971) J. Nat. Cancer Inst. *47*, 881–889.
63. Chan, E., Peters, W. P., Sweet, R. W., Ohno, T., Kufe, D. W., Spiegelman, S., Gallo, R. C. and Gallagher, R. E. (1976) Nature *260*, 266–268.
64. Okabe, H., Gilden, R. V., Hatanaka, M., Stephenson, J. R., Gallagher, R. E., Gallo, R. C., Tronick, S. R. and Aaronson, S. A. (1976) Nature *260*, 264–266.
65. Sarngadharan, M. G., Sarin, P. S., Reitz, M. S. and Gallo, R. C. (1972) Nature New Biol. *240*, 67–72.
66. Mondal, H., Gallagher, R. E. and Gallo, R. C. (1975) Proc. Nat. Acad. Sci. USA *72*, 1194–1198.
67. Feldman, S. P., Schlom, J. and Spiegelman, S. (1973) Proc. Nat. Acad. Sci. USA *70*, 1976–1980.
68. Michalides, R., Spiegelman, S. and Schlom, J. (1975) Cancer Res. *35*, 1003–1008.
69. Witkin, S., Ohno, T. and Spiegelman, S. (1975) Proc. Nat. Acad. Sci. USA *72*, 4133–4136.
70. Cuatico, W., Cho, J.-R. and Spiegelman, S. (1973) Proc. Nat. Acad. Sci. USA *70*, 2789–2793.
71. Cuatico, W., Cho, J.-R. and Spiegelman, S. (1974) Proc. Nat. Acad. Sci. USA *71*, 3304–3308.
72. Balda, B.-R., Hehlmann, R., Cho, J.-R. and Spiegelman, S. (1975) Proc. Nat. Acad. Sci. USA *72*, 3697–3700.

RNA Tumor Viruses and Leukemia: Evaluation of Present Results Supporting their Presence in Human Leukemias

Robert C. Gallo, M. D.
Laboratory of Tumor Cell Biology
National Cancer Institute
Bethesda, Maryland 20014

RNA Tumor Viruses and Leukemia: Evaluation of Present Results Supporting their Presence in Human Leukemias

I. Introduction

Type-C RNA viruses have been isolated from many species. In several, they have been often associated with leukemia and shown to reproduce the disease on inoculation into recipient animals. In a few species the data appear now to be conclusive that they are the major cause of the natural disease. Two major difficulties in verifying results that the virus causes the disease in some animal systems have been: (1) the long latent period for evident disease, and (2) the fact that many type-C viruses are apparently not oncogenic. Regarding the latter, we have argued for a major subdivision of these viruses based on a molecular hybridization assay (see below).

II. Class 1 and Class 2 Viruses

We isolate RNA from the virus and make it radiolabeled and then hybridize it to excess DNA purified from uninfected normal tissues of the animal believed to be the natural host (1, 2). By this assay, the RNA of some viruses hybridizes virtually completely to the cell DNA and the quality of the hybrids are good (judged by measuring the temperature required to dissociate the RNA-DNA complex). We call these viruses class 1 (1). There is usually data (besides the hybridization results) which indicates that these viruses are really normal cell gene products. We believe that they carry out some normal function, probably during development (3–6). In addition, it is possible that they play an important evolutionary role in transmitting information horizontally between different species, information which may subsequently be of advantage to the recipient species and become transmitted vertically (parent to progeny) in the germ line of that species. In this case, it becomes part of the normal genetic elements of the recipient. In this respect, Todaro and his colleagues have provided evidence for interspecies transfer of virus from a

431

primate to certain cats (7; and see Todaro elsewhere in this workshop). This is now the feline endogenous virus, RD114.

Examples of class 1 viruses include: RAV_0 of chickens; the guinea pig endogenous virus; the xenotropic endogenous viruses of mice; RD114, the endogenous virus of cats; and the only isolate to date of an endogenous virus from primates, the baboon endogenous virus (BaEV) (see next section).

The RNA of other type-C viruses show only limited hybridization to the DNA of uninfected normal cells of the persumed host. These we call class 2 (1). As a rule they are oncogenic. Examples of these are: avian myeloblastosis (AMV) and sarcoma viruses of chickens (AvSV); the leukemia and sarcoma viruses of mice (MuLV, MSV); the leukemia and sarcoma viruses of cats (FeLV, FSV); and the leukemia-sarcoma viruses isolated from primates, the gibbon ape leukemia virus (GalV) and the woolly monkey (simian) sarcoma virus (SSV). I think it is because of the genetic differences of these viruses compared to their host combined with their ability to add this *new* information to the DNA of the host, that gives them their oncogenic capacity. Although it is not yet known, I suspect the bovine leukemia virus (See A. Burny elsewhere in this workshop) will also be a class 2 virus.

Most of the class 2 viruses are infectious for the species they produce neoplasias under natural conditions. The exact route of infection is not clearly known, but in the case of AMV the leukemia is thought to occur most commonly from congenital infection (8), while in cats it appears to by contact between animals and possibly by congenital infection (9). It is important to note that many *normal* animals may contain class 2 viruses. This has given rise to mouch confusion. It does not mean the virus is endogenous in the genetic or molecular sence. For instance, many normal cats get infected and do not get disease. It must depend on other factors, e. g., genetic resistance or susceptibility to activation, immune response, or possibly fine variation in the genetic composition of the virus.

If class 1 viruses are gene products, what is the origin of class 2 viruses? We believe class 2 viruses are derived from class 1 viruses by genetic change in the class 1 viruses when the latter escape host control. This can occur when it becomes infectious for its own host and by processes not understood undergoes genetic change. The "new" virus is different from the original and on its way to becoming class 2 (see Fig. 1). In this case, a class 1 and class 2 virus will be related (by antigenic tests of their proteins and by nucleic acid hybridization). Thus, AMV is related to RAV_0 and MuLV and MSV are related to the xenotropic murine endogenous viruses. In these cases then we think the class 2 viruses evolved from the class 1 viruses. In contrast, in cats FeLV and FSV are not related to RD114, yet there is considerable (20–40 %) of the information in FeLV which is related to normal cat DNA (10). In this case, I suspect that FeLV evolved from *another* class 1 virus of cats, different from RD114. In the case of primates, like in cats, the class 2 viruses (GalV and SSV) are not related to the class 1 virus, the endogenous virus of baboons (BaEV). However, unlike the situation with FeLV, FSV, there is almost no hybridization of the RNA of GalV and SSV to DNA from normal primates (11). We suspect that GalV and SSV were derived from another species, and Todaro and his colleagues (12) and our laboratory (11) have provided evidence that these viruses originated from a mouse (see dashed line pathway, Fig. 2). This is analogous to the above mentioned acquisition of RD114 by certain cats from a primate

432

(see solid line pathway in Fig. 2). However, apparently in the case of SSV and GaLV there has not been integration into the germ line of primates. Instead, the virus has become a horizontally moving infectious agent of primates (see next section). In contrast, in the case of RD114 after acquisition from a primate estimated to have occurred in the distant past (7), the virus apparently integrated into the germ line and became part of the normal genome of certain cats (class 1). Thus, it appears that if a class 1 virus escapes host control and enters a new species, it can become either an infections agent for the recipient species (a class 2 virus) or it can become endogenous to the recipient species (class 1) (see Figs. 1 and 2).

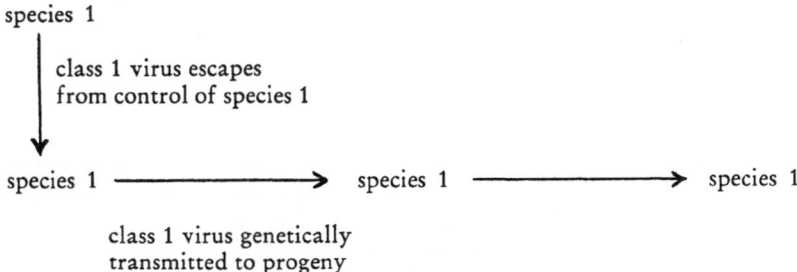

Fig. 1: Schematic illustration of the transmission of a truely endogenous type-C virus (Class 1 virus) from one animal to another animal of the same species. Normally, the class 1 virus is under host control and is vertically transmitted in the germ line. Somehow the virus has escaped from this control, and it is transmitted to other animals. How it escaped control is not known. Perhaps this involves minor genetic change in host in virus, or in both. Once it becomes transmitted horizontally it undergoes some slight genetic change.

Infects only same species, but by mechanisms not understood some genetic change in viral genes occur, and virus becomes a class 2 virus for species 1, although still highly related to its class 1 precursor virus, differences exist. Example: AMV from RAV_0; MuLV from murine xenotropic endogenous virus.

A second mechanism for formation of a class 2 virus might be by direct genetic alteration of the endogenous class 1 virogene followed by expression and formation of virus with new genetic components. For instance one can envision the class 1 virogene of the normal animal as a "hot spot" for mutation by chemicals or radiation or a "hot spot" for receiving new information as when a DNA virus infects a cell. This is the so called "Virus Hot-Spot" proposal outlined in more detail at this workshop in 1973 (4). In this case, the virus did not cause the disease, but it was a pruduct of the disease. However, once formed, it could transmit the oncogenic information to other cells in the same animal. If it escapes host control it might be transmitted to other animals of the same species or to another species, and in these instances it can become a primary cause of the natural disease. Some of these concepts are summarized in Fig. 3.

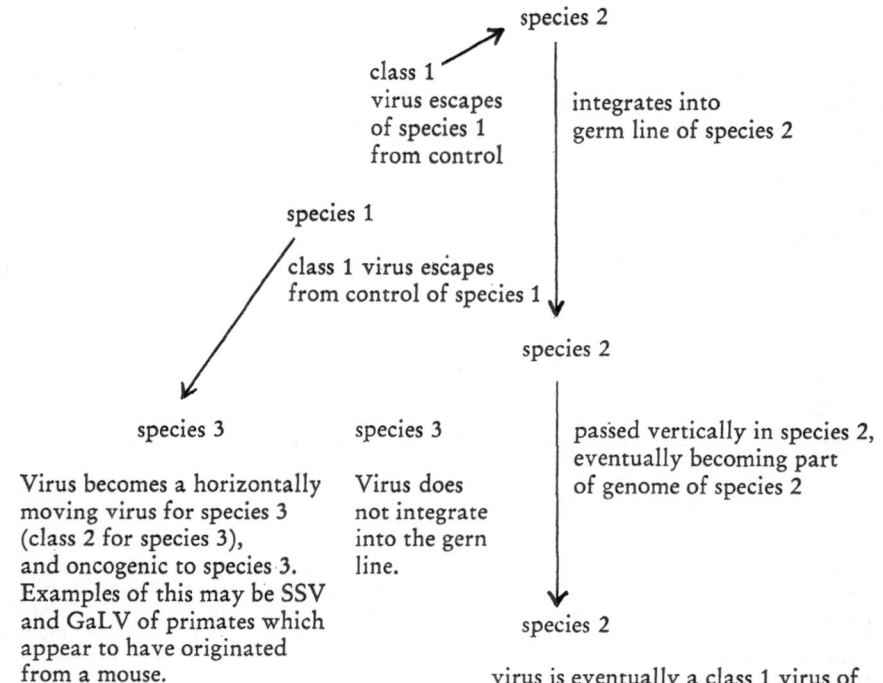

Fig. 2: Interspecies transmission of type-C virus. There is now evidence that type-C viruses can be transmitted from one species to another. As illustrated, in some instances a class 1 virus of one species (here called species 1) escapes from host control, enters a new species and becomes integrated into the germ line of the new species (here called species 2). Presumably, it offers a selective advantage to species 2 because it is maintained and eventually becomes part of the normal cellular genome of species 2. In this example, the virus was initially class 1 for species 1 and class 2 for species 2, but it eventually becomes a class 1 virus of species 2. Todaro and colleagues have provided the first example of this in providing data for transmission of a primate type-C class 1 virus to cats. This virus apparently became the endogenous cat virus known as RD114. Alternatively, the class 1 virus of species 1 may not integrate into the germ line and not be maintained in the new species (here called species 3) but instead persists as a class 2 infectious virus horizontally transmitted from species 1 to species 3 and between members of species 3. This may be the origin of the primate type-C infectious class 2 viruses, SSV and GaLV which appear to be capable of moving horizontally among some primates and which may have originated from a rodent.

PROPOSED MECHANISM FOR FORMATION OF
CLASS II ONCOGENIC RNA VIRUSES

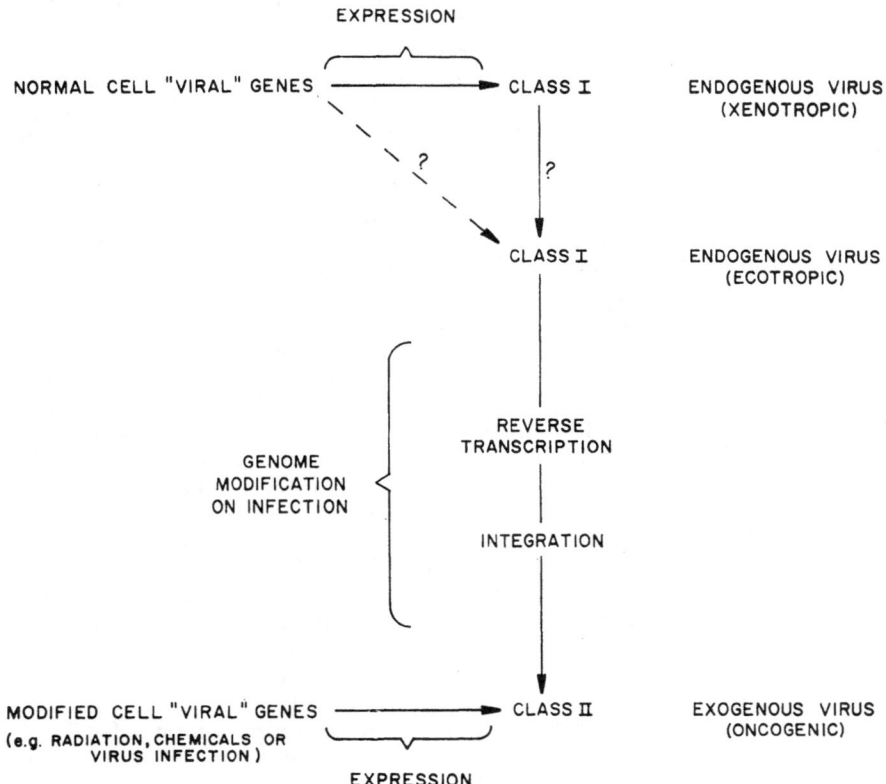

Fig. 3: Hypothetical scheme for origin of a class 2 virus. The model like other theories proposes that type-C viruses originate from normal cell genes. Complete expression leads to formation of the class 1 endogenous virus which is not able to infect most or all cells of the host it originates from (xenotropic virus). Other endogenous viruses are ecotropic, i.e., they can infect cells of their host. I believe these viruses evolved from the xenotropic class 1 viruses by minor genetic change. Once they become infectious more substantial genetic change may occur leading to the formation of a class 2 virus which is often oncogenic. An alternative route for formation of a class 2 virus is by direct mutation (e.g. by chemicals or radiation) of a "hot spot" within the class 1 viral genes of the normal cells. If this occurs and it is followed at some later stage by complete expression, the consequence should be creation of a class 2 virus, i.e., a virus with at least some genetic difference from the normal host. This hypothesis "virus-hot spot" theory has been discussed in more detail previously (4).

435

III. The Primate Type-C RNA Tumor Viruses

As discussed above, type-C viruses have been isolated in recent years for the first time in primates. The first was isolated (13) from a woolly monkey, a household pet of a woman living in California. The animal developed a spontaneous fibrosarcoma of the neck which yielded the virus. To this date there is only *one* isolate of the "woolly monkey" virus which has become known as the simian sarcoma virus (SSV). Almost simultaneously viruses were isolated from gibbon apes with various hematopoietic neoplasms, especially myelogenous and lymphoid leukemias (14). Of great interest, these isolates first came from a colony of 195 gibbons, 103 of whom were *injected with blood from humans with malaria.* The control group of 92 animals were not inoculated (15). *All 10 neoplasms developed in the inoculated animals.* Virus was isolated only from the animals with neoplasms. Recently, 3 isolates of the gibbon ape leukemia virus (GaLV) were obtained from brain extracts from "normal gibbons", but 2 of the 3 came from animals injected with extracts of brains from humans with Kuru (16), and the 3rd was a cage-mate of the other two. There have been a few isolates from gibbons not injected with human material, but *all* had close contact with man. It was surprising that despite the fact that SSV came from a new world monkey and the gibbon isolates from an old world ape, the various GaLV isolated and SSV ere extremely closely related.

When injected into some recipient primates SSV has produced sarcomas and malignant brain tumors (13, 17). Injection of GaLV into young gibbons has produced in some instances myelogenous leukemia (18). More importantly, apparently GaLV can spread horizontally among gibbon cage-mates and produce leukemia in animals that do not develop a sufficient immune response (18).

I believe that the above studies are of unusual importance: *first* because they are the first isolates of type-C viruses from any primate; *second,* because the viruses are proven oncogenic; *third,* because they provide the closest model of animal neplasias for man we have; and *fourth,* because I strongly suspect that these repeated relationships to man are not mere coincidences. Although the origin of these viruses may have been from mice (12, 11), it is clear that now they have become infectious agents among primates. For the reasons descibed above, combined with results I will describe below, I believe that these viruses form a family of closely related class 2 type-C viruses infectious for primates, including man, and capable of inducing neoplasias among them.

IV. Assays for Type-C Virus Markers in Human Leukemia and Evaluation of Results

Although the earliest evidence for type-C virus in human leukemia came from pioneering electron microscopic studies, particularly by Dmochowski and his associates (e. g., see references 19 and 20 for reviews by Dmochowski, it is clear that if viruses are involved in the leukemias of man, fully formed, released, and infectious virus must be a very rare event. Virus if present, must be at a very low level, or defective (i. e. unable to replicate and therefore not generally detectable by microscopy or bioassays) or be suppressed (i. e., full provirus is present in at least some cells but is not fully expressed). For these reasons we turned to molecular biological and immunological approaches to determine if markers of type-C virus could be detected in human leukemias. There are 5 viral related molecules or structures which have been described in some human leukemic cells: (1) reverse transcirptase; (2) viral related nucleic acids; (3) p30 protein; (4) membrane protein related to gp 70; (5) cytoplasmic particles with similarities to intracytoplasmic virus.

Reverse transcriptase (RT). Evidence for a DNA polymerase in some human leukemic cells with properties like the viral enzyme began in 1970 with a report by Gallo *et al.* (21) describing this activity in 3 patients with acute leukemia. Later this enzyme was partially purified, shown to be biochemically distinct from the major 3 DNA polymerases of uninfected cells (22–26), and localized to a cytoplasmic particulate fraction of the cell (22–26). Also during this period, the properties of viral RT became known in detail, and it was possible to set up certain criteria for calling samples positive for RT. Table 1 lists those criteria used in our

Table I: Criteria for Reverse Transcriptase in Human Leukemic Cells

1. found in cytoplasmic particulate fraction.
2. carries out endogenous RNase sensitive, actinomycin D resistant DNA synthesis.
3. in some cases it can be shown that the DNA is covalently attached to an RNA primer and hydrogen bonded to an RNA template.
4. after partial purification (and if free from significant contamination with cellular DNA polymerases) RT will show strong preference for poly A·oligo dT compared to poly dA·oligo dT as template-primer.
5. utilizes poly C·oligo dG as template-primer efficiently and this is a relatively specific template-primer for RT.
6. the molecular weight is about 70,000.
7. immunologically closely related to RT from wooly monkey (simian) sarcoma virus and gibbon ape leukemia virus.

laboratory. The detailed assays will not be described here since they have been included in recent reviews from our laboratory (26). Detection and characterization of this polymerase in extracellular viruses is simple, but it is very difficult to detect small amounts of RT in cells. This is due to the presence of proteases, nucleases, and most importantly, interference and confusion in the assay by the presence of the much greater amounts of the cellular DNA polymerases, DNA polymerases α, β, γ and the mitochondrial DNA polymerase (27). In my judgement, there is no really simple assay for RT in cells which gives confidence that one is actually measuring RT. The most sensitive and simplest assay I know of is the "simultaneous detection" assay for RT and high molecular weight RNA developed by Spiegelman and his group (see ref. 28 and Spiegelman in this volume for details of this assay). In this approach after isolation of the cytoplasmic particulate fraction from the cell, DNA is synthesized from nucleic acids native to the same fraction by simply incubating this fraction (containing nucleic acids and polymerase) in the presence of the substrate nucleotides (dATP, TTP, dCTP, dGTP), one or more of which are radiolabeled, in the presence of appropriate buffers. The reaction is shown to be at least partially sensitive to RNase and resistant to actinomycin D. Product analysis is then performed, and the newly synthesized DNA is shown to be joined to a large RNA molecule. These results, taken together, suggest that the template is a high molecular weight RNA (hence viral-like) and the reaction RNA directed (hence like reverse transcriptase). Using this assay, the results indicate that most and perhaps all leukemie cells contain this complex. This has been confirmed by our laboratory (29) and by Mak *et al.* (30). An additional factor supporting the conclusion that this assay detects reverse transcriptase and viral-like RNA is the failute by Spiegelman's group to detect positives in normal human tissues (28, 31). The strengths of this approach are its sensitivity, simplicity and capacity for application of relatively small quantities of tissue. Its weakness is the possibility of giving false positive results.

Greater assurance that the enzyme is, in fact, RT comes only from purification and biochemical characterization of the polymerase (22, 25, 32), followed by immunological (32, 24, 25, 33) comparisons to known RT from animal RNA tumor viruses. This is the approach used in our laboratory, and by this approach our positive samples are limited to about 20 % of patients with leukemia. Moreover, our samples with patients in remission have uniformly been negative. In the case of adult AML and to date *only* in this patient population, when RT was found and purified, in every case it was antigenically closely related (possibly identical) to RT from SSV. We now have 8 cases of AML where this has been demonstrated (32, 24, 25, 33), but even in adult AML we have found this in a fraction of the patients studied.

The advantage of this approach, of course, is that when a positive is scored, one has assurance it scores for viral reverse transcriptase. The disadvantages are its complexity, time, requirement for larger amount of tissue, and the greater likelihood of false negatives. We think to detect and verify RT in leukemic cells that it is essential to utilize the cytoplasmic particulate function. Essentially, this is a microsomal-membrane fraction but it includes some mitochondria. In our experience, it is almost essential to use fresh cells. For details the reader is referred to four recent papers from our laboratory (25, 24, 32, 33) and recent method reviews (34). *Viral Related Nucleic Acids.* Three characteristics have been used for determining a nucleic acid found in leukemic cells is viral related: (1) size; (2) in the case of some RNA molecules, their association with (RT; (3) nucleotide sequence composition. The latter has been estimated by the technique of molecular hybridization. We have already touched on the first two. Viral-like size is high molecular weight, i. e., about 35S or a 70S complex. This was first demonstrated by Spiegelman's group in leukemic cells by the indirect simultaneous detection assay described above (31) and confirmed by us in a few patients (29, 35). Subsequently, Mak *et al.*, provided evidence for 70S RNA by pulsing cells with ^{3}H-uridine and isolating cytoplasmic particles released into the media in short term culture containing labeled 70S RNA (30).

Association of the RNA with RT is shown by assaying the endogenous RT reaction of the cytoplasmic particulate fraction and determining that the DNA synthesized is associated with a large RNA molecule (31, 29, 30, 35).

The last characteristic, nucleotide sequence composition, is perhaps the most important. It is designed to determine if a given nucleic acid in the cell contains sequences related to a known type-C RNA tumor virus. The approaches that have been used to obtain this information are listed in Table 2. The advantage and disadvantage of each will be discussed separately, and the results summarized.

1) *Viral cDNA to Cell RNA.* In this approach viral cDNA labeled probes are prepared by carrying out endogenous DNA synthesis with disrupted virus. The virus may be any test animal RNA tumor virus. The cDNA represents a transcript of the viral genomic RNA. The cDNA is radiolabeled because one or more of the deoxyribonucleoside triphosphate substrates are radiolabeled. The cDNA is then hybridized to RNA purified from the leukemic cell. Various hybridization assays may be employed, e. g., analysis of hybrids by cesium sulfate centrifugation or by S1 nuclease digestion (a nuclease specific for single stranded nucleic acids, leaving undigested and hence TCA precipitable the hybrid molecules). Details of these procedures have been summarized in a recent review (36). The advantages of this technique are its simplicity, speed, and capacity to generate high specific activity probes. The disadvantages are that the cDNA made are small (4S or smaller), and although it is possible to make cDNA which represents the entire viral RNA genome, it is generally a very unbalanced copy. In other words much of the cDNA is only from a small fraction of the viral RNA. Therefore, it is a limited probe. Another disadvantage is that it only looks at the cell RNA. A negative result does not mean that the viral information is not present; it only suggests that it is not detectably expressed. It may ba present in the cell DNA but remain unexpressed.

Hehlman *et al.* used this approach to detect sequences in most or all human leukemic cells related to RLV (37, 28). They found none related to AML or MMTV. Thus, there was some specifity. They did not find these in the normal cells they examined. However, the amount of hybridization was low. Questions arise concerning the interpretation of these results. Are they really viral or simply sequences in cells related to viral sequences? Therefore, the specifity pattern (i. e., to which virus) becomes very important. The negative data with AMV are really not so helpful since on evolutionary basis we expect more sequences in human cells related to mouse than to birds. Regarding, the negatives in normals, again as mentioned above, this approach does not mean they are not there. It means only they were not expressed at a level detectable by the assay. In this regard, using the same approach, we have found RLV related sequences in normal PHA stimulated human lymphocytes (38). A. Tavitian elsewhere in this workshop has used this approach with MuSV and SSV (39). He finds hybridization with the cDNA from SSV and with cDNA from the murine virus to leukemic cell RNA (39).

In summary, unless a major degree of hybridization is obtained with a given viral cDNA probe and cell RNA and good quality hybrids are obtained, results of this kind can not prove the presence of added viral information. They do show that viral related sequences are present; they are at least consistent with the viewpoint that virus is present; and as the simplest and earliest approach used, they provided impetus for further experiments.

2) *Viral cDNA to Cell DNA.* The probe (labeled viral cDNA) is the same as that described above. However, instead of cell RNA, cell DNA is used. This, of course, examines not only what is expressed, but unexpressed genetic information. To my knowledge, there are no published reports using this approach with human leukemic cells. Recently G. Aulakh in our laboratory did apply this with cDNA from RLV, and he has detected DNA sequences *distally* related to RLV 70S RNA

in human leukemic cells (40). However, neither these nor any published results mean that leukemic cells are infected by RLV. They indicate only that leukemic cells contain some nucleic acids with some nucleotide sequences of RLV.

3) *Viral 70S RNA to Cell DNA.* With this method the entire 70S RNA genome of the virus is radiolabeled. The RNA can be radiolabeled by pulsing virus infected and growing cells with ^{3}H-uridine and isolating the labeled 70S RNA from the released virions. This technique and the subsequent hybridization of the 70S RNA to excess cell DNA has been most extensively employed by M. Baluda and his colleagues with AMV and avian leukemia. The advantages of the technique stem mainly from the use of the whole genome which theoretically, of course, is a much more complete probe than the cDNA methods. The disadvantages are that some of the RNA degrades, and it is difficult to prepare the RNA with sufficiently high specific activity as is often needed. The latter difficulty has been circumvented by another labeling technique. In collaboration with W. Prensky at Sloan Kettering, D. Gillespie and C. Saxinger in our group have isolated unlabeled 70S RNA from virus and labeled it *in vitro* with I^{125}. This results in a probe of higher specific activity. We have used this 70S RNA from different viruses to hybridize to human leukemic cell DNA (24). Using this method, we initially did not find extensive hybridization of the RNA of any virus to leukemic cell DNA (24)* (see note added in proof).

4) *cDNA From Human Leukemic Cell Cytoplasmic "Particles" to Viral 70S RNA.* This approach merits special discussion, *first,* because it has been employed in only a few laboratories; *second,* because as the newest method it is not generally understood; and *third,* because unexpectedly, it has given the most interesting positive results, albeit not always easy to interpret. While examining leukemic cells for reverse transcriptase we discovered that the enzyme was located in a cytoplasmic particulate fraction (22–25, 32, 33, 35). Before the enzyme is purified, it is associated with RNA in the "particle" (35). This particulate fraction can be purified and the "particles" treated as if they were virions in the sense that an endogenous DNA synthesizing system can be detected and utilized. Surprisingly these particulate fractions frequently exhibit biophysical characteristics of mature type-C virions (24). This includes apparent morphological integrity in repeated banding in sucrose gradients, size, and density (24, 35). We employed the "particle" isolation approach to obtain reverse transcriptase while Baxt *et al.* first used them to prepare labeled DNA probes (cDNA complementary to RNA in the "particles"). These cDNA probes were tested to see if they contained nucleotide sequences homologous to RNA of some animal tumor viruses. Again, positive results were obtained with RLV but not with AMV or MMTV, Baxt, *et al.* then used this cDNA to provide evidence that leukemic cells contain nucleotide sequences not present in normal leukocytes (41). This was done by hybridizing this cDNA to excess normal cell DNA and finding that a very small portion did not hybridize to leukemic cell DNA. Baxt has subsequently claimed that the extra sequences are related to the RNA of RLV (42). These observations have major implications, but they have not yet been confirmed. It should be emphasized again that these results do not mean that human leukemia is due to infection by RLV. They do argue that extra information is present, most likely the result of addition by a virus which appears to have at least some sequences in common with RLV. We also used this cDNA synthesized from the endogenous reaction of the cytoplasmic

"particles" from fresh human leukemic blood cells (35, 43). Our approach was to hybridize this DNA to RNA from many RNA tumor viruses to determine if there was an "affinity pattern", i. e., did the cDNA probe hybridize to RNA of various viruses in some particular manner? Would it be qualitatively like any of the known viruses? We found: (1) that in the case of myelogenous leukemias the cDNA hybridized significantly more to the RNA of SSV than to any other virus, and (2) the hybridization to RNA from other viruses followed a pattern like SSV, i. e., cDNA from SSV hybridized to RNA from the other viruses with the same relative pattern as the cDNA from the leukemic cells (i. e. to SSV>MuSV >FSV>MuLV>RD114 >FeLV >AMV) (35, 43). These results were confirmed by Mak *et al.* (30).

5) *cDNA from Cytoplasmic Particles of Human Leukemic Cells to DNA of Virus Infected Cells.* This approach uses the labeled cDNA described above (#4) to hybridize to the DNA provirus from tissue culture cells infected with different viruses. We have recently initiated this type of study, and our preliminary results with one patient indicate positive hybridization to cells infected with SSV and more so to cells infected with the baboon endogenous virus.

P30 Protein. This viral internal structural protein is assayed for in cells by several approaches. One method, the complement fixation assay, is thought by some to be the more definitive (R. Gilden, personal communication), but it is not as sensitive as some others. A radioimmune assay (see Todaro elsewhere in this workshop) has been recently widely employed. One approach is to find in cells a protein of approximately 30,000 molecular weight (p30) which will compete in the assay of a known viral p30 and labeled antibody to the test viral p30. It is imperative with this method to show specifity since proteases of molecular weights of approximately 30,000 could give false positive reactions by hydrolyzing the labeled antibody. This appears to have been the case with some suggestions of detection of the p30 of RLV in human leukemia.

Strand and August (43) and Sherr and Todaro (44) have reported detection of a p30 protein related and possibly identical to the p30 protein of the baboon endogenous type-C virus in a variety of human tissues. Since there is now evidence for endogenous (class 1) viral genes in many vertebrate species and since the baboon virus is the only endogenous virus isolated so far from primates, these results were taken to indicate detection of partial expression of a human endogenous type-C virus, i. e., that the p30 protein was a gene product of a putative human class 1 virogene (44, 45). An alternate interpretation in my mind is that they may have found the p30 of the baboon endogenous virus itself, as a consequence of infection of man by this baboon virus (see later section on isolates of primate type-C viruses from human tissues and also note added in proof).

In addition to these results Sherr and Todaro (46) have reported detection of a p30 protein in fresh blood leukocytes of 5 patients with acute leukemia related or identical to the p30 of SSV. Very careful controls were carried out to show specifity. Strand and August have reported similar results but believe this protein to be present more widely in the human population (44). To date Sherr and Todaro have not reported detection of the p30 related or identical to SSV in normal human tissues, but as indicated above Strand and August believe they can detect it in some (44). If they are correct, it suggests rather wide-spread infection of the human population with a virus related or identical to SSV.

Cell Surface Proteins Related to Viral Envelope Proteins. A few groups are examining leukemic cell membrane proteins to determine if any related or identical to envelope proteins (particularly the glycoprotein 70) of specific type-C viruses. Two general approaches are used. (1) Using human sera to determine if there are antibodies directed specifically against a membrane protein of human leukemic cells, and then determining if the antibody also reacts with viral envelope proteins. (2) Purifying viral envelop proteins and determining if antibodies raised against these proteins react specifically with a human leukemic cell membrane protein. Some approaches like these have been used by Metzgar and Bolognesi. They have preliminary data which indicate detection of such proteins on leukemic cells related in some cases to the friend leukemia virus and in others to the primate class 2 type-C viruses (the GaLV-SSV viruses) (47).

Specificity of Viral Markers Found in Fresh Leukemic Blood Cells to SSV and to Baboon Virus. It is clear from the studies described in the preceding sections that many laboratories now with many techniques have found evidence for viral markers (proteins and nucleic acids) in leukemic cells. The problem now is one of interpretation. Do these findings represent detection of normal cell gene products which are leated to viral gene products but have nothing to do with virus? If they represent virus are they only products of an endogenous (class 1 virus) present in all cells (normal or leukemic) in all members of the species and not involved in the disease? What is the meaning of finding markers related to RLV in some laboratories while others find markers related to other viruses? My interpretation of these data is as follows. Type-C viruses of most mammalian species are at least somewhat related by some tests, e. g., it would not be surprising if the genome of RLV contained some nucleotide sequences related or even identical to some in the primate viruses. This is, in fact, known to be the case. No one has published finding markers related to AMV. AMV is not related to the mammalian type-C viruses. If the data are taken together, they strongly imply that it is markers primarily related to the primate type-C viruses which are being found in man, both the SSV-GaLV group and the baboon virus. If SSV-GaLV markers also are detected in some normal tissues of some people, the data are no less significant, if indeed, the findings really represent markers of these viruses rather than related proteins and nucleic acids which are really not viral. As noted earlier the SSV-GaLV group are not endogenous to man in the genetic sense. If they really are in some normal tissues, it must mean that like EBV the virus is widespread in man. This could mean that the situation is somewhat analogous to feline leukemia where the virus, FeLV, infects many cats but produces leukemia in only a fraction (9).

Induction of Exponential Growth of Blood Leukocytes from Patients with Myelogenous Leukemia and Isolation of Type-C Viruses.
Studies with many animal cells indicate that DNA synthesis and cell replication are important for production of type-C virus. Other studies, e. g., with Friend leukemia, indicate that differentiation may also be helpful. In this respect, human AML blood cells are characteristically retarded both in their replication and in their ability to differentiate (4, 5). Hence, when we recently identified a source of conditioned medium (CM) which was produced by a fibroblast strain of a cultured whole human embryo which stimulated prolonged exponential growth of myelogenous leukemia cells in suspension culture (48, 49), we were hopeful that this would

result in the production of detectable *complete* type-C virus by the cultured AML cells. The factor(s) in the CM is heat stable (56 °C for 1 hour) and differs from typical colony stimulating activity (CSA) by many criteria. These include: a) induction of *prolonged* growth in suspension culture; b) growth is exponential; c) it has no effect in the soft agar system, i. e., it does not promote colony formation; d) it is specific for myelogenous leukemic cells having no effect on normal bone marrow cells, CLL cells or ALL cells (49, 50).

We initially treated cells (blood or bone marrow) from 16 patients with myelogenous leukemia. These included 2 remission patients with no detectable (by morphology) leukemic cells. All responded to the CM factor (50). In those with a marker chromosome the marker persisted in culture. These results provide derect evidence for the following conclusions: (1) intrinsic differences exist between normal and leukemic cells in recognition and/or response to some growth promoting factors; (2) similar differences exist between myelogenous and lymphoid cells; (3) myelogenous leukemia cells can be grown *in vitro*; (4) some remission myelogenous cells must still be different from normal myelogenous cells; (5) some myelogenous leukemic cells can be induced to differentiate confirming previous suggestions for this by several groups (e. g., see ref. 57 for review by Sachs).

Cells from several patients (5 of 16) expressed readily detectable viral markers (proteins and/or leukemic cells) specifically related to SSV (50), and cells from one patient (patient A. S. or HL-23) released classical budding type-C virus (48, 49, 51). This virus was transmitted to several secondary cell lines for larger production (51). It is infectious and oncogenic for at least some primates (52). Most importantly, the fresh blood (uncultured) cells of this patient contained RT related to SSV (33), and we and our colleagues have been able to reisolate this virus from the same patient. The original isolate came from passage 10 of her myelogenous leukemic cells obtained from her (pre-treatment) first hospitalization in October, 1973 (see Table 3). Subsequently, virus was isolated in our laboratory and also by G. Todaro from earlier passages of these cells which were kept frozen and later put into culture. These were from passages 5 and 7. We also went back to this original blood sample kept in liquid nitrogen and again isolated the virus (49, 51). In addition, we subcultured the first blood sample at *passage* 1 and isolated the virus again from the subculture (49).

Fourteen months later (December, 1974) when she was in partial remission we received a bone marrow specimen. After only a few passages in culture virus was again identified (by electron microscopy and by reverse transcriptase) (49) and subsequently again isolated by N. Teich and R. Weiss by co-cultivation with a normal human embryonic fibroblast line (51). Finally, a blood sample obtained in December, 1973 (2 months after the first blood sample (now also appears to be releasing virus (unpublished results of P. Markham and F. Ruscetti). See Table 2 for a summary of the isolations.

Type-C viruses related or identical to SSV have now also been isolated twice from a child with lymphosarcoma leukemia by Nooter *et al.* (ref. 53 and see elsewhere in this workshop), by Gabelman *et al.* from a patient with CLL and lung cancer (54), and from a few different human embryos by Panem *et al.* (55).

It should be noted that now there are several reports of isolates of SSV (or an SSV related virus) from man and only one from a woolly monkey (see Table 4).

Labeled Probe	Unlabeled Test Nucleic Acid	Reference for example	Comments
(1) Viral cDNA	cell RNA	28	viral cDNA is from the endogenous RT reaction of virions
(2) Viral cDNA	cell DNA	40	viral cDNA is from the endogenous RT reaction of virions
(3) Viral 70S RNA	cell DNA	24	viral 70S RNA is prepared by pulse labeling virus infected cells with ^{3}H-uridine and then isolating labeled viral RNA or by labeling purified 70S RNA *in vitro* with I^{125}.
(4) cDNA from cytoplasmic particles from leukemic cells	viral RNA	31, 35, 43	This cDNA is a product of the endogenous RT reaction of human leukemic cells.
(5) cDNA from cytoplasmic particles from leukemic cells	DNA of infected cells	42, 38	This DNA of infected cells includes the DNA provirus

* For more details see text.

Some of our isolates in addition to the SSV component also contain a virus related or identical to the baboon endogenous virus. Thus, the virus isolate appears to be a mixture of both types of primate type-C viruses. We have recently learned that the virus isolated from human embryos by Panem et al. (56) in addition to having a component related or identical to SSV also has one related or identical to the baboon virus (S. Panem and W. Kirsten, unpublished results).

Although molecular hybridization experiments fail to detect *complete provirus* related to SSV or to our isolates in the fresh cells of this or other patients with AML (23, 37), we have been able to find in her fresh uncultured blood cells the following viral related markers: (1) 35S and 70S RNA (38); (2) reverse transcriptase related to reverse transcriptase of SSV and hence to RT from the viruses we isolated (33, 48); (3) cytoplasmic viral-like particles containing 70S, 35S RNA and the RT (38); (4) cDNA probe synthesized from the endogenous RT reaction of the cytoplasmic particles hybridized to the RNA of SSV, to the RNA of the baboon endogenous type-C virus, to DNA from baboon virus infected human cells but significantly less to DNA from normal human cells (38).

Reasons for Confidence that Virus came from Patient HL-23 not as a Contaminant

Table III: Cell specimens from HL23 and Virus isolates

Cell specimen	Date received	Nature of specimen	Extracellular virus detected by[a]		Comments
			RT	EM	
HL23–1[b]	10/16/73	peripheral blood	pass 5	pass 10	virus = HL23V-1 transmitted to secondary cells
HL23–2	10/16/73	peripheral blood[b]	pass 3	pass 3	same original blood sample as specimen 1
HL23–3	10/02/74	peripheral blood	NT	NT	cells not viable
HL23–4	12/13/74	peripheral blood	pass 8	neg.	virums may be detected by direct cocultivation
HL23–5	12/13/74	bone marrow	pass 5	pass 5	virus = HL23V-5, transmitted to secondary cells (N. Teich and R. Weiss, personal communication)
HL23–6	01/25/75	peripheral blood	neg.	NT	cells grew poorly
HL23–7	01/25/75	bone marrow	neg	NT	cells grew poorly
HL23–8	01/25/75	bone marrow	NT	NT	used for cocultivation only; results neg.

a RT = reverse transcriptase, EM = electron miscroscopy, pass = passage number at a split ratio of 1 : 2, neg. = negative, NT = not tested.
b Cell specimens 1 and 2 were from one fresh blood sample. Specimen 1 was cultured immediately after receipt; specimen 2 was cultured beginning 10/01/74 from an ampoule of cells frozen on 10/16/73. Virus now isolated from passage 5, 7, and 10 of specimen 1. Original results *all* on pass. 10 isolate.

It is important to emphasize certain facts about these virus isolates in regards to the possibility that they might represent contaminaion with SSV. Our reasons for believing these isolates are not contaminants are as follows. (1) The fresh uncultured cells of the patient contained proteins (33, 48) and nucleic acid (38) related to the virus isolates as have several (but not all) other patients. (2) The same virus was isolated several times from different specimens from the same patient (see Table 3) after only short term passages in culture. A contaminant would have occurred with the same virus several times with the same patient and only this patient. (3) Other laboratories have independently isolated the same or a very related viruses from human tissues.

Table IV: Reported isolations of Virus of the »Woolly Monkey« (Simian) Sarcoma Virus (SSV)

Source of Isolate	Species and History	Reference
1. fibrosarcoma	woolly monkey pet of a woman	Wolfe, L., Deinhardt, F., Theilen, G., Kawakami, T., and Bustad, L., *J. Nat. Can. Inst.* 47:1115, 1971.
† 2. acute myelogenous leukemia blood cells	Human. classical AML of a woman. Cells treated with growth factor	Gallagher, R. and Gallo, R., *Science.* 187:350, 1975.
† 3. acute myelogenous leukemic bone marrow	Human. Same patient as #2. Cells treated with growth factor	Teich, N., Weiss, R., Salahuddin, Z., Gallagher, R., Gillespie, Gallo, R., *Nature.* 256:551, 1975. Gallagher, R., Salahuddin, Z., Hall, W., McCredie, K. and Gallo, R., *PNAS* (72:4137,
† 4. normal lung fibroblasts	Human. embryo, 8 weeks gestation	Panem, S., Prochownik, E. V., Reale, F. R., and Kirsten, W. H., *Science.* 189:297, 1975.
5. normal lung fibroblasts	Human. embryo 16 weeks gestation	Panem, S. (as above)
† 6. lung carcinoma cells co-cultivated with XC cells	Human. chronic lymphocytic leukemia and lung cancer	Gabelman, N., Waxman, S., Smith, W., Douglas, S. D., *Int. J. Cancer.* 16: 1, 1975.
* 7. lymphosarcoma leukemia bone marrow cells	Human. cells co-cultivated with XC cells	Nooter, K., Aarsen, A. M., Bentvelzen, P., de Groot, F. G., van Pelt, F. G., *Nature* 256:595, 1975.
* 8. lymphosarcoma leukemia blood cells	Human. cells co-cultivated with human embryonic fibroblasts	Nooter, K., (as above)
* 9. acute myelogenous blood cells	Human. Same patient as #2 and #3. Different sample	Markham, P. (unpublished)

* With these isolates data is not complete to say with certainty that virus belongs to "SSV family."
† In several instances with human isolates (those marked with symbol †) virus highly related to the baboon type-C virus was also present with the woolly monkey related virus.

Conclusions

We believe human myelogenous leukemia blood cells do not frequently permit *complete* expression of type-C viral information, but this information is at least partially present in many and perhaps all AML patients. This is in contrast to the case of some animals like cats where most animals with leukemia actively produce virus. On the other hand, even with cats there is variation. The occasional (or rare) infected animal does not completely express virus (M. Essex, personal communication). Conversely, patient A. S. (HL-23) may be the unusual or rare human, who after appropriate growth stimulation of her leukemic cells, expresses completely and releases whole virus. One difficulty with our interpretation is our inability to detect the complete provirus.* This results in a paradox revolving around the question – how do human leukemic cells become transformed and how can they release virus if they lack the complete genetic information apparently essential in animal model systems for transformation and virus production? We think that generally the integrated complete provirus may be in only a small number of cells, perhaps not even the leukemic cell precursors. Release of fragments of the provirus by the infected cells may be sufficient, in some instances, to transform leukocyte precursors. This model is compatible with the existing data on human leukemia, including the detection of extra sequences in human leukemic DNA by Spiegelman and associates (41). At least one tissue or cell population should contain cells with complete provirus. *Portions* of this provirus may integrate into leukocyte progenitors, a necessary prelude to leukemic transformation. On occasion complete provirus may integrate into some leukocyte precursors, the necessary event for the rare complete virus production. We suggest that the site of integration for fragments or whole provirus is the "hot spot" region discussed before at this workshop (4) and that this may alter gene expression by a mechanism called "paraprocessing" (1) which in turn leads to transformation. If this speculation is correct, detection of the complete provirus as the proof for the involvement of these viruses in man will be extremely difficult.* Other approaches will be necessary such as additional virus isolates from other laboratories and/or a clear seroepidemiological studies.

---

* *Note added in proof*
Recently, we have for the first time been able to identify a DNA provirus in humans. We have found the provirus of a virus highly related or identical to the baboon endogenous type-C virus in the DNA of uncultured tissues from several but not all patients with leukemia (F. Wong-Staal, D. Gillespie, and R. Gallo, *Nature*, July 1976). We believe these results conclusively demonstrate that humans are infected by type-C virus. The results suggest an interspecies transfer of virus from baboon to man in the past. Whether the virus now spreads by way of an intermediary vector or directly – human to human is not known. There is no proof that this acquired viral information is causatively involved in leukemia although we naturally suspect that it may be. Since a major component of the repeated isolates of HL23 virus from a patient with AML is highly related to the baboon endogenous type-C virus, the new results clearly indicate that these isolates are from the patient not from laboratory contamination.

References

1. Gillespie, D., and Gallo. R. C.: *Science 188:* 802, 1975.
2. Gillespie, D., Sexinger, W. C., and Gallo, R. C.: Information Transfer in Cells Infected by RNA Tumor Viruses and Extension to Human Neoplasia. *In,* Progress in Nucleic Acid Research and Molecular Biology, Vol 15, Ed. by J. N. Davidson and Waldo E. Cohn (Academic Press, New York, 1975), 1.
3. Huebner, R. J. and Todaro, G. J.: *Proc. Nat. Acad. Sci. USA 64:* 1087, 1975.
4. Gallo, R. C.: On the Origin of Human Acute Myeloblastic Leukemia: Virus "Hot Spot" Hypothesis. *In,* Modern Trends in Human Leukemia, Ed. by R. Neth, R. C. Gallo, S. Spiegelman, and F. Stohlman (J. F. Lehmanns Verlag, Munich, 1974), 227.
5. Gallo. R. C.: On the Etiology of Human Acute Leukemia. *Medical Clinics of North America 57:* 343, 1973.
6. Mayer, R. J., Smith, R. G., and Gallo, R. C.: *Science 185:* 864, 1974.
7. Todaro, G. J., Benveniste, R. E., Callahan, R., *et al.:* Endogenous Primate and Feline Type-C Viruses In, Cold Spring Harbor Symposium on Quantitative Biology: Tumor Viruses, Volume 39, (The Cold Spring Harbor Laboratory, Cold Spring Harbor, New York 1975), 1159.
8. Weiss, R. A.: *In,* Analytical and Experimental Epidemiology of Cancer. Ed. by W. Nakahara, T. Hirayama, K. Nishioka, and H. Sugano (University Park Press, Baltimore, 1973), p. 201.
9. Essex, M.: *Advances in Cancer Res. 21:* 175, 1975.
10. Gillespie, D., Gillespie, S., Gallo, R. C., East, J. L., and Dmochowski, L.: *Nature New Biol. 244:* 51, 1973.
11. Wong-Staal, F., Gallo, R. C., Gillespie, D.: *Nature 256:* 670, 1975.
12. Lieber, M., Sherr, C., Todaro, G., Benveniste, R., Callahan, R., and Coon, H.: *Proc. Nat. Acad. Sci. USA* (in press).
13. Wolfe, L., Deinhardt, F., Theilen, G., Kawakami, T., and Bustad, L.: *J. Nat. Can. Inst. 47:* 1115, 1971.
14. Kawakami, T. G., Huff, S. D., Buckley, P. M., *et al., Nature New Biology 235:* 170, 1972.
15. DePaoli, A., Johnsen, D. O., and Noll, W. W.: *J. Amer. Vet. Med. Assoc. 163:* 624, 1973.
16. Todaro, G., Lieber, M., Benveniste, R., Sherr, C., Gibbs, C., and Gajdusek, D. C.: *Virology* (in press).
17. Johnson, L., Wolfe, L., Whisler, W., Norton, T., Thakkar, B., and Deinhardt, F.: *Proc. Amer. Assoc. Cancer Res.* , 1975.
18. Kawakami, T. (Personal Communication).
19. Dmochowski, L., and Bowen, J.: *Seventh National Cancer Conference Proceedings* (J. B. Lippincott, Philadelphia 1973), 697.
20. Dmochowski, L., Yumoto, T., Grey, C. E., Hales, R. L., Langford, P. L., Taylor, H., Freireich, E. J., Shullenberger, C. D., Shively, J. A., and Howe, C. D.: *Cancer 20:* 760, 1967.
21. Gallo, R. C., Yang, S. S., and Ting, R. C.: *Nature 228:* 927, 1970.
22. Sarngadharan, M. G., Sarin, P. S., Reitz, M. S., and Gallo, R. C.: *Nature New Biology 240:* 67, 1972.

23. Gallo, R. C., Sarin, P. S., Smith, R. G., Bobrow, S. N., Sarngadharan, M. G., Reitz, M. S., Jr., and Abrell, J. W.: *In,* DNA Synthesis *In Vitro* (Proceedings of the 2nd Annual Steenbock Symposium), (University Park Press, Baltimore, 1972), 251.
24. Gallo, R. C., Gallagher, R. E., Miller, N. R., Mondal, H., Syxinger, W. C., Mayer, R. J., Smith, R. G., and Gillespie, D. H.: *In,* Cold Spring Harbor Symposium on Quantitative Biology: Tumor Viruses, Vol 29, 1975, 933.
25. Gallagher, R. E., Todaro, G. J., Smith, R. G., Livingston, D. M., and Gallo, R. C.: *Proc. Nat. Acad. Sci. USA 71:* 1309, 1974.
26. Sarin, P. S., and Gallo, R. C.: *In,* International Review of Science, Chapter 8, Vol 6, (Butterworth and Medical and Technical Publishing Co., Oxford, 1974), 219.
27. Lewis, B. J., Abrell, J. W., Smith, R. G., and Gallo, R. C.: *Biochim. Biophys. Acta 349:* 148, 1974.
28. Hehlman, R., and Spiegelman, S.: *In,* Modern Trends in Human Leukemia, Ed. by R. Neth, R. C. Gallo, S. Spiegelman, and F. Stohlman (J. F. Lehmanns Verlag, Munich, 1974), 157.
29. Gallagher, R. E., Mondal, H., Miller, D. P., Todaro, G. J., Gillespie, D. H., and Gallo, R. C.: *In,* Modern Trends in Human Leukemia, Ed. by R. Neth, R. C. Gallo, S. Spiegelman, and F. Stohlman, (J. F. Lehmanns Verlag, Munich, 1974), 185.
30. Mak, T. W., Kurtz, S., Manaster, J., et al.: *Proc. Nat. Acad. Sci. USA 72:* 623, 1975.
31. Baxt, W., Hehlman, R., and Spiegelman, S.: *Nature New Biol. 244:* 72, 1974.
32. Todaro, G. J., Gallo, R. C.: *Nature 244:* 206, 1973.
33. Mondal, H., Gallagher, R. E., and Gallo, R. C.: *Proc. Nat. Acad. Sci. USA 74:* 1194, 1975.
34. Allaudeen, H. S., Sarngadharan, M. G., Gallo, R. C.: *In,* Methods of Cancer Research, Ed. by Harris Bush (Academic Press, New York, in press), Vol 12.
35. Gallo, R. C., Miller, N. R., Saxinger, W. C., and Gillespie, D.: *Proc. Nat. Acad. Sci. USA 70:* 3219, 1973.
36. Gillespie, D., Gillespie, S., and Wong-Staal, F.: *In,* Methods of Cancer Research, Ed. by Harris Bush (Academic Press, New York, in press), Vol 11.
37. Hehlmann, R., Kufe, D., and Spiegelman, S.: *Proc. Nat. Acad. Sci. USA 69:* 435, 1972.
38. Reitz, M., Miller, N., Wong-Staal, F., Gallo, R., and Gillespie, D., *Proc. Nat. Acad. Sci. 733:* 1976.
39. Tavitian, A. (This symposium).
40. Aulakh, G., Gillespie, D., and Gallo, R. C., (In preparation).
41. Baxt, W. G., and Spiegelman, S.: *Proc. Nat. Acad. Sci. USA 69:* 3741, 1972.
42. Baxt, W.: *Proe. Nat. Acad. Sci. USA 71:* 2853, 1974.
43. Miller, N. R., Saxinger, W. C., Reitz, M. S., Gallagher, R. E., Wu, A. M., Gallo, R. C., and Gillespie, D.: *Proc. Nat. Acad. Sci. USA 71:* 3177, 1974.
44. Strand, M., and August, J. T.: *J. Virology 14:* 1584, 1974.
45. Sherr, C. J., Todaro, G. J.: *Proc. Nat. Acad. Sci. USA 71:* 4703, 1974.
46. Sherr, C. J. and Todaro, G. J.: *Science 197:* 850, 1975.
47. Bolognesi, D., (Personal Communication).

48. Gallagher, R. E., and Gallo, R. C.: *Science 187:* 350, 1975.
49. Gallagher, R. E., Salahuddin, S. Z., Hall, W. T., McCredie, K. B., Gallo, R. C.: *Proc. Nat. Acad. Sci. USA* 72:4137, 1975.
50. Gallagher, R. E., and Gallo, R. C.: *In,* Proceedings of the IInd International Congress on Pathological Physiology, Prague, Czechoslovakia 1975 (in press).
51. Teich, N. M., Weiss, R. A., Salahuddin, S. Z., Gallagher, R. E., Gillespie, D., and Gallo. R. C.: *Nature 256:* 551, 1975.
52. Deinhardt, F., (Personal Communication).
53. Nooter, K., Aarssen, A. M., Bentvelzen, P., deGroot, F. G., van Pelt, F. G.: *Nature 256:* 595,1975.
54. Gabelman, N., Waxman, S., Smith, W., Douglas, S. D.: *Int. J. of Cancer,* in press.
55. Panem, S., Prochownik, E. V., Reale, F. R., Kirsten, W. H.: *Science 189:* 297, 1975.
56. Panem, (Personal Communication).
57. Sachs, L., Harvey Lectures, Series 68, (Academic Press, New York, 1974), 1.

Murine and Simian C-Type Viruses:
Sequences Detected in the RNA of
Human Leukemic Cells by the c-DNA Probes

A. Tavitian, C. J. Larsen, R. Hamelin & M. Boiron.

Laboratoire d'Hématologie Expérimentale, Hôpital Saint-Louis
75010 – Paris – France

Introduction

The detection of viral-related RNA sequences in human leukemic, human breast cancer, and other human cancer cells has been facilitated in recent years by molecular hybridization techniques of human ribonucleic acid to the complementary DNA (c-DNA) synthesized in-vitro by animal type – cRNA tumor viruses (1–5). Our laboratory has been interested in the search for such sequences in the nucleic acids of various types of acute and chronic human leukemias. The approach was based essentially upon the evaluation of the annealing rate of single stranded c-DNA to cellular RNA and DNA.

We report some of the annealing experiments we performed in the search for virus-like sequences in the nucleic acids of human acute and chronic leukemias with the aid of two synthetic c-DNA probes synthesized with the murine sarcoma-leukemia viruses (Moloney Isolate) (M-MSV-MLV) produced continously by the transformed rat cell line 78 A-1 and a simian probe synthesized with the simian (Wooly Monkey) sarcoma and simian sarcoma-associated viruses (SSV) produced by the Normal Rat Kidney NRK cell line.

Methods and Results

Both c-DNA probes were synthesized and prepared as described previously and represented extensive complementary copies of their respective 70S RNA genomes (6). However, the SSV probe seemed less uniform in terms of complementarity to its 70S viral RNA genome in that a 8 to 10-fold excesss of c-DNA was necessary to render the 70S RNA resistant to RNAase digestion in high salt (as compared to 2–3 fold excess in the case of M-MSV MLV).

Annealing reactions between the tritium labelled c-DNA of both viruses and the RNA of leukemic cells were performed as described previously (7) (or at higher temperatures : 68° in 4 x SSC). The rate of annealing was estimated by the S_1 nuclease assay (7). The percentage of hybridization was expressed by normalizing against the values given by the RNA of the respective virus producing cells (78 A_1 or NRK) taken as 100 percent, and after substraction of the background obtained by the blanks of c-DNAs processed without RNA.

Hybridization reactions with RNA from human leukemic and "normal" cells.

In previous experiments it was shown that hybrids of M-MSV(MLV)-c-DNA and human RNA were found in 22 out of 46 leukemias whereas none of the 10 controls tested (including material obtained from bone marrow cells, buffy coats and continuous human cell lines) was positive (8).

We report here the results obtained in 12 leukemias and 4 controls which were available for concomitent study with both the simian and the murine probes. Table I summarizes the results of this type of study. It can be seen that there is

Table I: Hybridization to human cellular RNAs of the c-DNAs of M-MSV (MLV) and SSV

Origin of cellular RNA		Hybridization rates	
		with M-MSV-MLV c-DNA	with SSV c-DNA
Normal human leucocytes I		1.1 %	1.75 %
Normal human leucocytes II		1.3 %	1.25 %
Human spleen I		1.0 %	2.0 %
Human spleen II		1.2 %	1.6 %
N° 31	CML	2.9 %	4.75 %
N° 47	ALL	1.4 %	1.8 %
N° 45	ALL	3.5 %	1.7 %
N° 53	ALL	0 %	14.5 %
N° 60	ALL	5.5 %	6 %
N° 64	AML	0 %	4.5 %
N° 78	AML	0 %	2 %
N° 82	ALL	2.9 %	4 %
N° 83	AML	0 %	1.75 %
N° 85	CML	0 %	1.8 %
N° 86	ALL	4.8 %	2 %
N° 89	ALL	43 %	11.5 %

a certain but not absolute correlation between the two probes with regard to the positivity or the negativity of the hybridization test. For instance, the acute myeloblastic leukemia N°64 which revealed a negative cellular RNA hybridization with the murine M-MSV(MLV) c-DNA probe showed a positive annealing of its RNA with the SSV c-DNA probe; and this was the case also with one acute lymphoblastic leukemia N°53 which in fact gave the highest rate of hybridization with the SSV probe whereas there was no positive hybridization with the murine probe. On the contrary leukemia N°86 appeared completely negative when SSV c-DNA was used as a probe and was slightly positive with the M-MSV (MLV) probe.

Unrelatedness of the sequences detected in human RNA by each c-DNA probe.

Since there was not an absolute corroboration in the results obtained by hybridizing human leukemic RNAs with the c-DNA of SSV and M-MSV(MLV), it seemed of interest to compare the homology existing between the probes by cross hybridization experiments. Each c-DNA probe was therefore annealed with its homologous 70S RNA genome as well as with the heterogenous counterpart. Fig. 1 represents the results of this experiment and shows that there is at most 10 % homology between the two viruses. The c-DNA which is common to both viral genome was isolated after alkaline digestion of the hybrids; we failed to hybridize this c-DNA to the RNA of the acute lymphoblastic leukemia N°89 which was scored as highly positive when the entire c-DNA probes of both SSV and M-MSV(MLV) were used for the annealing tests.

Host cell information in the murine and simian viruses.

Table II shows the association rates of the simian and murine c-DNA to sheared cellular DNA of various origin. It can be seen that the SSV virus produced in

Figure 1: Cross hybridization of the nucleic acids (c-DNA and 70S RNA) of SSV and M-MSV (MLV) viruses.

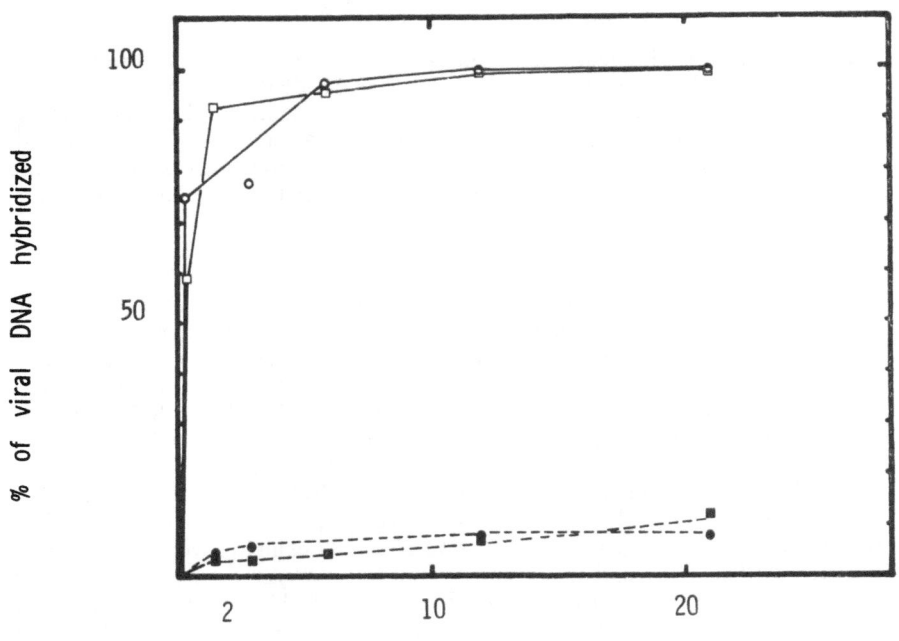

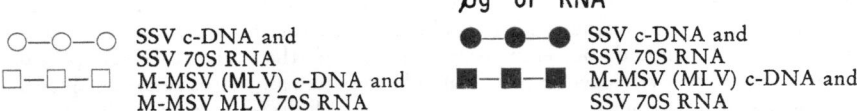

○—○—○ SSV c-DNA and SSV 70S RNA ●—●—● SSV c-DNA and SSV 70S RNA
□—□—□ M-MSV (MLV) c-DNA and M-MSV MLV 70S RNA ■—■—■ M-MSV (MLV) c-DNA and SSV 70S RNA

Constant amount of c-DNA (1 500 cpm) were hybridized with the indicated amounts of 70S RNA for 70 hours at 68° in 4 x SSC.

453

Table II: Association rate of c-DNAs to cellular DNAs

Original of cellular DNA	Associated c-DNA (%)	
	MSV M (MLV)	SSV
Salmon sperm	2.2 %	3.4 %
78 A$_1$	100 %	93 %
SSV/NRK	15.3 %	100 %
Human spleen	11.0 %	9.2 %
Rat embryo	15.7 %	85.7 %
Mouse embryo	44 %	41.7 %

The c-DNA synthesized on M-MSV-MLV and SSV-1 virus were annealed to cellular DNAS during 70 hours at 68° in 4 x SSC. The rate of the H^3-labelled associated c-DNA was determined by S$_1$ Nuclease Assay.

NRK cells contained a much higher percentage of rat sequences as compared to the percentage of rat sequences (15,3 %) in the M-MSV(MLV) viruses that are produced in the 78 A-1 rat fibroblast cell line. In contrast, the proportion of human (10 %) and mouse (42–44 %) sequences are quite comparable in both viruses. It is likely however that the mouse sequences present in both viruses are not the same since there exists only 9 to 10 % homology between those virus stocks.

Discussion

Many authors advanced that some viral sequences are present in leukemic cells and that these sequences are not expressed in normal non leukemic cells (1 – 5). Corolarry results were found by Gallo and associates who reported that the c-DNA synthesized endogenously by RNA dependent-DNA polymerase in virus like particles from human acute leukemic cells was hybridizable to SSV and Kirsten sarcoma viral RNA to a higher extent than to murine leukemia viruses (8). However it was not established by these authors whether the sequences that were detected by their hybridization procedure were identical when using different viral RNA genomes. It was already observed two years ago by Benveniste and Todaro that the endogenous type C viruses of several species exhibited very little, if any, nucleic acid homology and that, among the infectious type-C viruses of different species existed a very small degree of relatedness with the noticeable exception of Kirsten mouse leukemia virus and simian sarcoma (Wooly-Monkey) or gibbon ape viruses (9). Our own experiments show clearly that the sequences detected in human ribonucleic acid from leukemic fresh cells are completely different if the simian c-DNA probe or the murine c-DNA probe are used for the molecular hybridization studies. It should be emphasized moreover than the c-DNA portion homologous to both virus genomes was unable to detect any virus related sequences in the RNA of leukemic cells, even though it was able to form stable hybrids with rat cellular DNA.

References

1. Axel, R., Schlom, J. & Spiegelman, S. (1972) Nature *235*, 32–36.
2. Helmann, R., Kufe, D. & Spiegelman, S. (1972) Proc. Nat. Acad. Sci. USA *69*, 435–439.
3. Kufe, D., Helmann, R. & Spiegelman, S. (1972) Science *175*, 182–185.
4. Helmann, R., Kufe, D. & Spiegelman, S. (1972) Proc. Nat. Acad. Sci. USA *69*, 1727–1731.
5. Gallo, R. C. & Gallagher, R. E. (1974) Ser. Haematol VII, 224, 273.
6. Tavitian, A., Hamelin, R., Tchen, P., Olofsson, B. & Boiron, M. (1974) Proc. Nat. Acad. Sci. USA *71*, 755–759.
7. Larsen, C. J., Marty, M., Hamelin, R., Peries, J., Boiron, M. & Tavitian, A. (1975) Proc. Nat. Acad. Sci. USA 72, 4900–4904.
8. Gallo, R. C., Miller, N. R., Saxinger, W. C. & Gillespie, D. (1973) Proc. Nat. Acad. Sci. USA *70*, 3219–3224.
9. Benveniste, R. E. & Todaro, G. J. (1973) Proc. Nat. Acad. Sci. USA *70*, 3316–3320.

Prevention of Herpes-Associated Malignancies in Primates: Problems and Prospects[1]

Laufs, R. and Steinke, H.

Hygiene-Institut der Universität Göttingen

Herpesviruses are known to induce carcinoma, leukemia or malignant lymphoma in different animal species. Herpesviruses are also suspected as being causal agents in human malignant neoplasia. In particular the Epstein-Barr virus (EBV) stands first among candidate human cancer agents (1). The present knowledge indicates an aetiological relationship between EBV and two human malignant tumors: Burkitt's lymphoma and nasopharyngeal carcinoma (2, 3). Herpesviruses are transmitted horizontally and hence are subject to immunologic intervention, specifically by vaccines that stimulate immunity and prevent or limit proliferation of the naturally acquired virus on subsequent infection (4).

The first example of a naturally occurring malignant tumor to be controlled in this way was the herpesvirus induced Marek's lymphoma. A live attenuated herpesvirus almost completely prevents this neoplastic disease of chickens (5). Live virus vaccines in general induce higher level and longer lasting immunity than killed vaccines and require only a small dose of virus to immunize. However, there are no reliable in vitro markers for the oncogenicity of live attenuated herpesviruses that might apply to man. The applicability of live attenuated vaccines derived from potentially oncogenic herpesviruses seems slight.

Therefore killed vaccines derived from the oncogenic herpesviruses have to be developed. At the present level of knowledge only killed cancer virus vaccines seem to be administerable to man. For the control of those human cancers suspected of having a herpesvirus cause a killed vaccine completely free of viral DNA would be desirable, since traces of the viral DNA in such a preparation might be able of bringing about malignant transformation (6). Chickens can be significantly protected against Marek's lymphoma by killed vaccines free of virus nucleic acid (7). A viral nucleic acid-free vaccine for EBV could be prepared by purification of plasma membranes from human lymphoid cells which do have EBV-determined membrane antigens expressed on the cell surface. Antibodies to these antigens also have virus neutralising activity (8).

The preparation of nucleic acid-free herpesvirus vaccines would probably solve the safety problems. But a vaccine has not only to be safe, it also has to be efficient against the natural occuring infection. Even if an EBV vaccine free of nucleic acid is available the efficacy of the killed herpesvirus vaccine in man remains to be determined. Killed whole herpesvirus types 1 and 2 vaccines prepared for preventing or treating primary or recurrent acute episodes of herpesvirus infection in man, have not been highly encouraging in terms of effectiveness. Because of the

[1] Supported by the Deutsche Forschungsgemeinschaft, D-53 Bad Godesberg, West Germany.

anticipated long incubation period for herpesvirus cancer in man, it may be a long time before the protective efficacy of a killed EBV vaccine can be measured in terms of cancer prevention (4).

Since the oncogenic herpesviruses isolated from nonhuman primates, H.saimiri (HVS) and H.ateles (HVA) regularely induce malignant lymphoma in nonhuman primates within 1–2 months after infection (9, 10) we used these viruses in animals phylogenetically related to man to study the safety and efficacy of killed herpesvirus vaccines. The work with the primate model system offers a wider range of experimental possibilities and the questions in respect to the efficacy of killed vaccines against herpesvirus induced cancer can be answered within a short period of time.

The vaccines were prepared by inactivation of HVS (strain S.295C, friendly supplied by Dr. L. V. Meléndez) and HVA (isolate No. 810, friendly supplied by Dr. L. V. Meléndez) with heat (56 °C for 4 hours) and formaldehyde (100 µg HCHO/ml for 6 days) as recently described (11). The 100-fold concentrates of the virussuspensions which were free of serum and cells, were used as vaccines. The virus specific antigenicity of the vaccines was determined by the complement fixation (CF) test. The DF titers ranged between 1:32 and 1:64. For immunisation four to six intramuscular inoculations of the vaccine adsorbed on to Aluminium-hydroxydgel as adjuvant were given to each monkey within 12 weeks (11).

The killed vaccines proved to be safe in 121 vaccinated monkeys of four different species (S.oedipus, C.jacchus, A.trivirgatus and C.aethiops) (12, 13, 14). Several of these monkeys have now been under observation for two years without any sign of a clinical disease. The vaccines induced high titers of neutralising and complement fixing antibodies in all vaccinated monkeys. Even 9 vaccinations given to a monkey did not induce any kind of incompatibility. The killed herpesvirus vaccines were not only free of infectivity and immunogenic but proved also to be non oncogenic. In spite of the fact that the vaccines are not free of viral nucleic acid, none of the 121 vaccinated monkeys developed a tumor. In contrast to the tumor bearing monkeys and to the latently infected monkeys HVS and HVA could not be isolated from fresh peripheral white blood cells from the vaccinated monkeys. In all our in vivo experiments infectivity and oncogenicity of HVS and HVA are very closely correlated. One single infectious particle was able to induce a tumor and we never found a tumor which did not produce complete virus particles after cocultivation in vitro. The survival curve of HVS in vitro is multicomponental after treatment with heat as well as after treatment with formaldehyde. The inactivation of the oncogenicity followed that of the infectivity.

The vaccinated monkeys (S.oedipus and C.jacchus) were resistant against the intramuscular challenge with 200–300 LD_{50} of cell-free oncogenic herpesvirus (12, 13). The challenged animals remained clinically well without signs of an infection and have now been under observation for 1–2 years while the non-vaccinated control monkeys died of malignant lymphoma 34–52 days after inoculation. The resistance against the oropharyngeal route of infection remains to be determined. This experiment seems of great importance since the natural route of infection is different from that used in the challenge experiments described. Therefore the oropharyngeal route of infection has to be used for future challenge experiments.

In certain virus infections, e.g. measles, infectious hepatitis, German measles, the passive immunisation by administration of specific serum antibodies during the incubation period may result in prevention or modification of the clinical disease. We investigated if in analogy to these virus infections a state of relative temporary insusceptibility to the oncogenic HVS can be induced in nonhuman primates (S.oedipus) by the administration of antibodies against HVS which have been formed in another host. The passive immunisation with hyperimmune serum against HVS obtained from tumor bearing animals as well as hyperimmune serum obtained from the vaccinated monkeys protected against malignant lymphoma when the monkeys were challenged with 30–40 LD_{50} of cell-free HVS 24 hours after the administration of the specific serum antibodies (15).

The vaccination with the killed oncogenic herpesviruses did not prevent but delayed tumor development after tumor cell transplantation (14). Humoral antibodies do not protect against the cullular transmission of herpesviruses (16). We could demonstrate that the killed HVS vaccine induces a specific cellular immunity in marmoset monkeys (S.oedipus) as well as in C.aethiops monkeys. However, in freshly prepared tumor cells HVS specific antigens could not be demonstrated so far.

The fact that the killed HVS and HVA vaccines were not capable of bringing about malignant transformation in 121 monkeys vaccinated within 1–2 years does not justify the use of an EBV vaccine prepared in the same way in man. A similar prepared EBV vaccine, however, could be used to study the efficacy of a killed EBV vaccine in nonhuman primates. Such studies are now possible since it was shown that EBV induces malignant lymphoma in S.oedipus and A.trivirgatus (17, 18).

We applied the method developed for the production of the killed HVS and HVA vaccines to EBV. For vaccine production the EBV producing human lymphoid cell line P3 HR 1K (1) and the EBV producing marmoset lymphoid cell line B 95-8 (19) were used. The CF titers of the killed vaccines were considerably lower than those obtained with HVS and HVA and ranged between 1:1 and 1:16. The killed EBV vaccines were used for the immunisation of 10 C.jacchus monkeys. The monkeys received 5 inoculations within 10 weeks. As yet all of the animals remained clinically well. The killed vaccines induced specific humoral antibodies against EBV.

We are working at a cell membrane vaccine against EBV which is free of viral DNA and which could be used in man. Preliminary experiments indicate, however, that it is difficult to prepare membrane vaccines which contain enough EBV specific antigenicity to induce a potent immune response. It seems doubtful if such a membrane preparation will ever be economically practical for vaccines. Further the immunologic response can sometimes enhance as well as prevent or suppress tumor. A membrane vaccine enhanced tumor growth in mice induced by the mouse mammary tumor virus (20).

The killed EBV vaccines prepared by the same procedure as the HVS and HVA vaccines as well as DNA free membrane vaccines tested in the nonhuman primate system might be expected to yield a great amount of data on safety, efficacy, and regimen that can be extrapolated to a human vaccine. However, it seems still questionable if a killed EBV vaccine will be efficient against the human tumor suspected of having a herpesvirus cause.

459

References

1. Klein, G.: The Epstein-Barr virus. In: The Herpesviruses, edit. by Kaplan, A. S., pp. 521–555 (Academic Press, New York and London, 1973).
2. Miller, G.: The oncogenicity of Epstein-Barr vius. J. Inf. Dis. 130; 187–205 (1974).
3. Epstein, M. A., and Achong, B. G.: The EB virus. Rev. Microbiol. 27: 413–435 (1973).
4. Hilleman, M. R.: Herpes simplex vaccines: Prospects and problems. Cancer Res., 36: 856–858 (1976).
5. Churchill, A. E., Payne, L. N., and Chubb, R. C.: Immunization against Marek's disease using a live attenuated virus. Nature 221: 744–747 (1969).
6. Epstein, M. A.: Towards an anti-viral vaccine for a human cancer. Nature 253: 6 (1975).
7. Kaaden, O. R., Dietzschold, B., and Überschär, S.: Vaccination against Marek's disease: Immunizing effect of purified turkey herpes virus and cellular membranes from infected cells. Med. Microbiol. Immunol., 159: 261–269 (1974).
8. Epstein, M. A.: Implications of a vaccine for the prevention of EBV infection: Ethical and logistic considerations. Cancer Res., 36: 711–714 (1976).
9. Laufs, R., and Meléndez, L. V.: Oncogenicity of herpesvirus ateles in monkeys. J. Natl. Cancer Inst. 51: 599–608 (1973).
10. Laufs, R., and Fleckenstein, B.: Susceptibility to herpesvirus saimiri and antibody development in Old and New World monkeys. Med. Microbiol. Immunol. 158: 227–236 (1973).
11. Laufs, R.: Immunisation of marmoset monkeys with a killed oncogenic herpesvirus. Nature 249: 571–572 (1974).
12. Laufs, R., and Steinke, H.: Vaccination of nonhuman primates against malignant lymphoma. Nature 253: 71–72 (1975).
13. Laufs, R., and Steinke, H.: A killed vaccine derived from the oncogenic herpesvirus ateles. J. Natl. Cancer Inst., 55: 649–651 (1975).
14. Laufs, R., and Steinke, H.: Vaccination of nonhuman primates with killed oncogenic herpesviruses. Cancer Res., 36: 704–706 (1976).
15. Laufs, R., and Steinke, H.: Passive immunisation of marmoset monkeys against neoplasia induced by a herpesvirus. Nature 255: 226–228 (1975).
16. Lodmell, D. L., Niva, A., Hayashi, K., and Notkins, A. L.: Prevention of cell-to-cell spread of herpes simplex virus by leukocytes. J. Exp. Med. 137: 706–720 (1973).
17. Shope, T., Dechairo, D., and Miller, G.: Malignant lymphoma in cottontop mormosets after inoculation with Epstein-Barr virus. Proc. Natl. Acad. Sci. U.S.A. 70: 2487–2491 (1973).
18. Epstein, M. A., Hunt, R. D., and Rabin, H.: Pilot experiments with EB virus in owl monkeys (Aotus trivirgatus). I. Reticuloproliferative disease in an inoculated animal. Int. J. Cancer 12: 309–318 (1973).
19. Miller, G., Shope, T., Lisco, H., Stitt, D., and Lipman, M.: Epstein-Barr virus: transformation, cytophathic changes, and viral antigens in squirrel monkey and marmoset leukocytes. Proc. Natl. Acad. Sci. U.S.A. 69:383–387 1972).
20. Stutman, O.: Correlation of in vitro and in vivo studies of antigens relevant to the control of murine breast cancer. Cancer Res. 36: 739–747 (1976).

New Properties of Mammalian Cells Transformed by Herpes Simplex and Cytomegaloviruses

Fred Rapp, Ph. D.

Department of Microbiology
The Milton S. Hershey Medical Center
The Pennsylvania State University
College of Medicine
Hershey, Pennsylvania 17033

New properties of nammalian cells transformed by herpes simplex and cytome-galoviruses by Fred Rapp, Ph. D.

The relationship of herpes simplex viruses (HSV) and cytomegaloviruses (CMV) to human neoplasia has been difficult to assess. On the basis of seroepidemiological evidence, HSV type 2 has been associated with the etiology of squamous cervical carcinoma (1–5). Women with cervical carcinoma have increased frequency of antibodies to HSV-2 than do controls matched for race, age, and socioeconomic level. The percentages vary considerably from study to study, but this may be due to the use of different serological techniques (a very serious and confusing problem) in determining antibody titers.

Herpesvirus particles have been reported in one case of prostate carcinoma cells as demonstrated by electron microscopy (6). This observation is in need of confirmation and its value is questionable, since the same group of workers previously alleged that 15 percent of men from 15 years of age harbor HSV-2 without symptoms in the prostate and vas deferens and pass this virus venereally (7). Women do tend to experience acute infections with this virus, with recurrent infection an almost certain manifestation. Virus is not readily isolated, however, from the female genital tract during latent stages nor from biopsies of cervical carcinoma. Tumor biopsies have repeatedly failed to exhibit virus antigens, but HSV-2 antigens have reportedly been observed by immunofluorescence in the cytoplasm of exfoliated cervical carcinoma cells (8–10). Furthermore, one culture of tumor cells was induced to produce HSV-2 particles under the stress of high pH (11). As with many other such reports, this observation has not been extended by the investigators submitting the original work.

One cervical tumor was found by hybridization experiments to contain 39 % of HSV-2 DNA in up to 3.5 fragments per cell and these were linked to host cell DNA (12). The tumor cells also contained small amounts of RNA transcripts which were complementary to virus DNA. These results may point to the requirement of a repressed virus genome in the maintenance of malignant transformation, and clearly suggest that less than the total genome may be involved. However, at this point the evidence is insufficient for further discussion.

461

It therefore became obvious that additional reproducible evidence was needed to demonstrate the oncogenic potential of HSV. We thus turned to an examination of the ability of this virus to transform mammalian cells *in vitro*.

Transformation by Herpes Simplex Virus In Vitro

It was well known that direct inoculation of HSV into newborn animals (specifically rodents) leads to death of the animal in most cases. Attempts to transform cells *in vitro* were also hampered by the cytopathology induced by the virus. These problems have now been resolved by the use of various methods to inactivate the infectivity of the virus, while boosting its transforming ability by introducing defective particles into the virus population.

Ultraviolet (UV) light was the first method of inactivation employed; it had previously been used to destroy virus infectivity while augmenting transforming potential of known tumor viruses (12–15). UV-irradiation of HSV-1 and HSV-2 with subsequent inoculation onto mouse L cells deficient in the enzyme thymidine kinase (TK), biochemically transformed these cells into thymidine kinase positive cells (16, 17). This phenomenon, involving the new synthesis of a virus-specific enzyme, was demonstrated to be a heritable change of the cells. The significance of this experiment lies in the fact that this was the first evidence that genetic information of HSV could be maintained and expressed in established mammalian cells.

Duff and Rapp (18–20), in experiments carried out simultaneously, extended the usefulness of UV-irradiation to demonstrate transformation by numerous strains of HSV-1 and 2. Inactivated virus was able to transform hamster embryo cells *in vitro* into continuous cell lines with morphological and growth characteristics differing from those of the parental cells.

The continued presence of the virus in the transformed cells has been demonstrated by the presence of herpes-specific antigens in the cytoplasm of approximately 5–30 % of the cells and on the membranes of approximately 60 % of the cells (18–20). CP-1 antigen (a partially purified virus antigen of HSV) was found by immunological techniques on the membranes of the HSV-1-transformed cells (21). Furthermore, one of the original HSV-2 hamster cell lines (333–8–9) has been found to contain virus RNA transcripts hybridizing to both HSV-1 and HSV-2 DNA (22). This result is not surprising since HSV-1 and HSV-2 DNA share base sequences (23, 24). It is significant to note that only a small percentage of the viral genome is transcribed in the transformed cells (22). In more recent experiments with a variety of HSV-2-transformed hamster cells, approximately 8–38 % of the virus genome has been detected by reassociation kinetics (Frenkel, Roizman and Rapp, unpublished experiments).

The oncogenic potential of the transformed hamster cell lines was evaluated by inoculation into newborn hamsters (18, 20). Some of these cell lines have been shown to induce primary tumors with extensive metastases. Both fibrosarcomas and adenocarcinomas have been induced by the cells tested (the former by fibroblastoid cultures and the latter by epithelioid cultures). The tumor-bearing hamsters developed neutralizing antibody to HSV inversely proportional to the latent period and, therefore, to the oncogenicity of the cell line (20). Pre-immunization of these animals with HSV-1 led to increased metastases.

Type C particles were not seen in either the transformed or tumor cell lines (25), and neither type C-specific virus RNA nor gs antigens were found in the transformed cells (26).

The HSV-2-transformed hamster cells were resistant to superinfection by HSV-1 and HSV-2 when low multiplicities of infection were used (27). This suggests the possible existence of a cellular repressor capable of inhibiting virus replication in the transformed cells.

The transforming potential of UV-irradiated HSV was substantiated by Kutinová et al. (28). These investigators exposed a weakly oncogenic hamster cell line to UV-irradiated HSV-2; injection of the resultant cells into hamsters revealed acquisition of increased oncogenic potential. These "supertransformed" cells demonstrated herpes-specific antigens.

More recently, we have developed a quantitative transformation assay using Swiss mouse 3T3 fibroblasts and UV-irradiated HSV-1 and HSV-2 (29). Morphological transformation was indicated by loss of contact inhibition, and the number of foci were proportional to the dose of irradiation. The transformed colonies were of two morphological types: fibroblastoid or epithelioid. HSV antigens were observed by the indirect immunofluorescence test in both types of cells.

This system has been extended using a TK⁻ subline of the 3T3 cells (Buss and Rapp, unpublished experiments). This enables the use of the selective medium, HAT, to eliminate those cells without the ability to synthesize the enzyme, thymidine kinase (Fig. 1). Under the conditions employed, only cells transformed by HSV and given the ability to synthesize this enzyme by the virus genome can

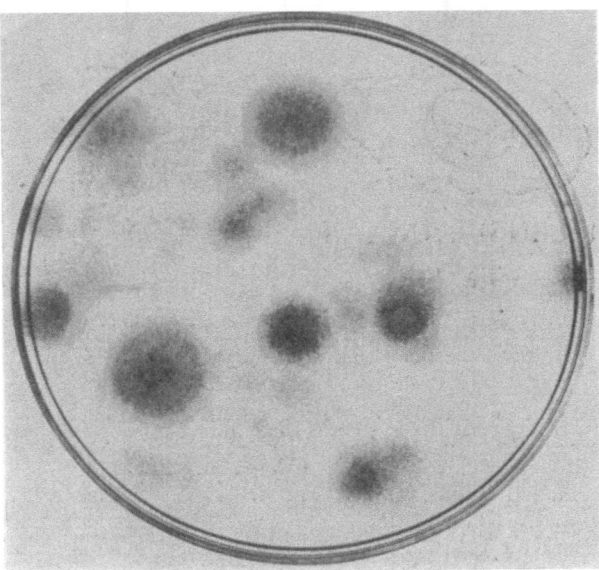

Fig. 2: Foci of 3T3 cells in HAT selective medium after exposure of TK⁻ cells to irradiated herpes simplex virus type 2.

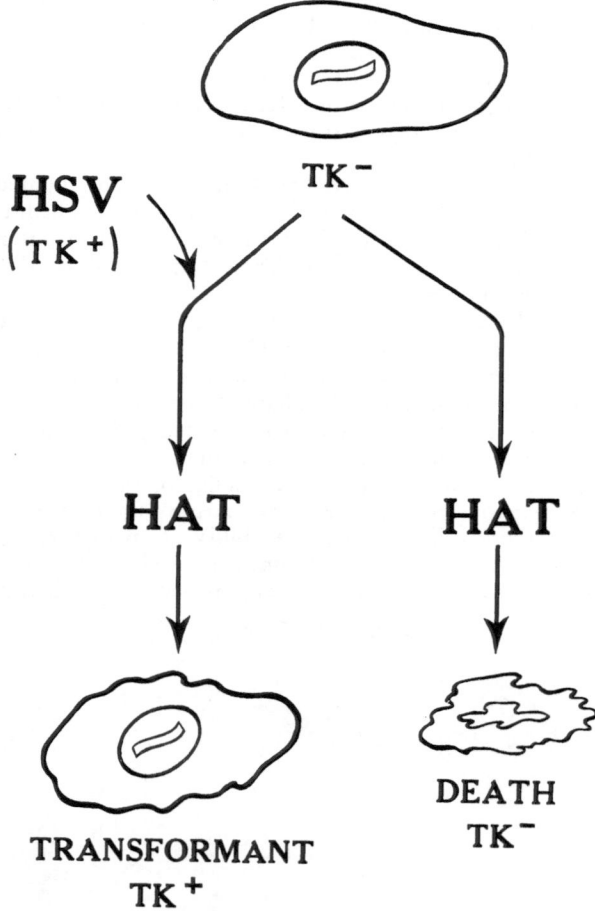

Fig. 1: Use of selective HAT medium to measure transformation of 3T3 cells by herpes simplex virus. Only those cells acquiring the ability to synthesize thymidine kinase can replicate.

replicate. The advantage of this system is the elimination of background foci which allows standardization of the technique. The foci observed (Fig. 2) can be counted and differences in virus isolates or strains quantitated (Fig. 3).

Photodynamic inactivation can also reduce infectivity of viruses (30, 31). Photodynamically inactivated HSV-1, HSV-2 and SV40 can transform hamster embryo fibroblasts (32) and the transformed clones exhibit loss of contact inhibition and morphological alterations. The SV 40-transformed cells consistently synthesized the T antigen, while only 8–10 % of the HSV-1 and HSV-2 cell lines showed diffuse cytoplasmic HSV antigens by immunofluorescence assays. No gs antigens of on-

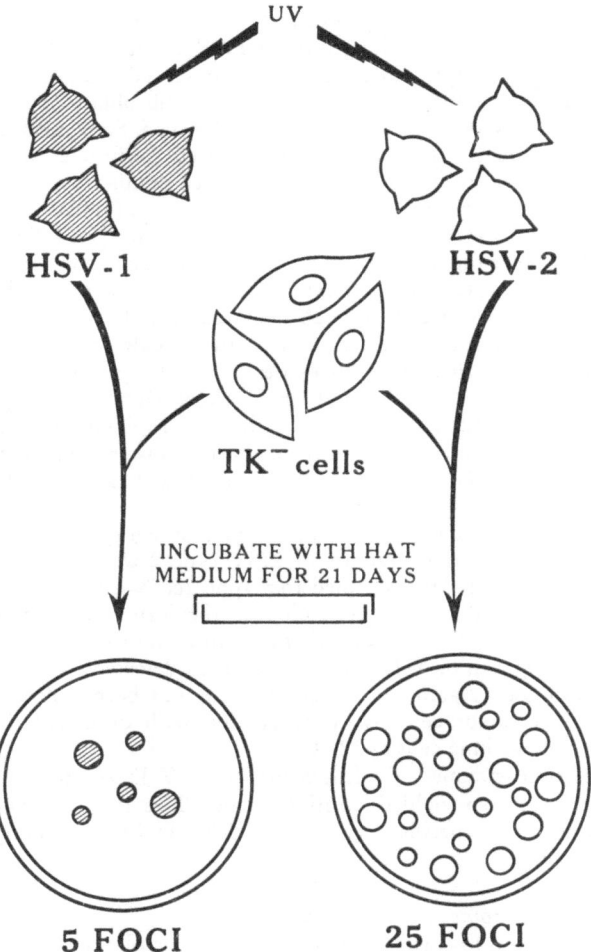

Fig. 3: Schematic representation of strain differences observed for HSV-1 and HSV-2 in ability to transform 3T3 cells.

cornaviruses were detected in these cell lines. The three transformed cell lines established have since been inoculated subcutaneously into syngeneic hosts, i. e. newborn hamsters, and though they differ in relative oncogenic potential, primary metastatic tumors have developed (33). Explanted tumor cells synthesized virus-specific cytoplasmic antigens. Tumor-bearing hamster sera also reacted with infected and transformed cells but no neutralizing activity could be detected in these sera. These data indicate that though photodynamic treatment, like UV, may inactivate viruses such as HSV, it may also potentiate their transforming ability.

In vitro transformation of cells by non-inactivated virus particles would be useful because virus rescue would then be a theoretical possibility. Darai and Munk (34) exposed human embryonic lung cells to HSV-1 strains at high temperatures (42 °C) to inhibit the lytic infection. They observed transformed cells with epithelioid morphology, differing from the original fibroblastoid lung cells. Syncytia formation and cytoplasmic antigens were observed. Some resistance to superinfection was also noted. These data have not been confirmed and it is possible that the original lines were derived from HeLa cell contamination.

Macnab (35), using temperature-sensitive mutants of HSV-2 and wild-type HSV-1 and 2, transformed rat embryo cells. Transformed cell lines were either epithelioid or fibroblastoid initially, but occasionally changed to mixed morphological types upon passage. Indirect immunofluorescence tests revealed virus-specific antigens in the transformed cells, though no virus particles were seen by electron microscopy. Rescue of infectious herpesvirus by co-cultivation with susceptible cells proved futile and there was no evidence for the presence of RNA tumor viruses. This investigator also repeated the work of Duff and Rapp (18, 19) by transforming hamster embryo fibroblasts with UV-irradiated HSV-2. These cells were tumorigenic after inoculation into newborn hamsters, where fibrosarcomas were induced. The oncogenicity of the HSV-transformed rat cells has not yet been reported.

Takahashi and Yamanishi (36) transformed human embryo and hamster embryo cells by temperature-sensitive mutants of HSV type 2 at restrictive temperature (38.5 °C). Morphologically transformed foci appeared 3–4 weeks after virus inoculation. The transformed hamster cells induced the formation of tumors in newborn and adult hamsters. Both species of transformed cells contained HSV-specific antigens in the cytoplasm of 5–10 % of the cells, as detected by indirect immunofluorescence techniques. Again, no infectious virus has been isolated from either the transformed or tumor cells by co-cultivation with or inoculation onto permissive human embryo lung cells at 32 °C.

Use of restriction enzymes and fragments of HSV DNA in transforming experiments (37) have also yielded positive results. This type of experiment may soon reveal whether a specific fragment of HSV DNA is responsible for the transforming event.

Transformation by Cytomegalovirus In Vitro

Support for the theory that CMV may induce neoplasia is seen in the data presented by St. Jeor et al. (38, 39). These observations indicate that CMV can stimulate host cell DNA synthesis under permissive (human embryo lung cells) and restrictive (human embryonic kidney cells and monkey Vero cells) conditions. Heat-treated virus and UV-irradiated virus were unable to induce this stimulation. Therefore, it seems plausible that some virus function(s) is necessary for elevation of cell DNA synthesis.

Other investigators have subsequently reported the stimulation of host cell cytoplasmic RNA in human fibroblast cells (WI-38) after infection with CMV (40). This induction was postulated to require an early virus-specific protein. Stimulation of host cell DNA was not observed in this system. However, these same investigators subsequently reported the induction of both host-cell DNA and ribosomal-RNA synthesis in guinea pig cells abortively infected with CMV (41).

Again, virus inactivated by heat or UV-irradiation did not cause stimulation of macromolecular synthesis.

In general, these results are similar to those already obtained with SV40 (42, 43), polyoma (44, 45) and adenoviruses (46–48), all established tumor viruses. In addition, this stimulation of DNA synthesis was seen in human leukocytes infected with EBV (49).

Strengthening the case, Albrecht and Rapp (50) exposed hamster embryo fibroblasts to UV-irradiated CMV and obtained morphologically transformed foci. Virus-specific antigens were detected in the cytoplasm of 0.5 % of the cells while 47 % yielded bright membrane fluorescence. Mixed hemagglutination assays and ^{125}I-labeled anti-globulin tests revealed that the virus-specific membrane antigen(s) present in transformed cells are similar to antigens found in CMV-infected human cells (51).

The CMV-transformed cells were oncogenic on transplantation to animals, inducing fibrosarcomas. Tumor-bearing hamster sera did not contain neutralizing antibody to CMV, but did react with CMV-infected, transformed and tumor cell antigens in fluorescent antibody tests. Microcytotoxicity tests performed with spleen cells from tumor-bearing hosts revealed that these animals have a cell-mediated immune response to the homologous tumor cells (52).

Lang et al. (53) have also indicated that human diploid fibroblasts can grow for generations in agarose after infection with human CMV. Eventually, however, cytopathology and cell lysis resulted and cell lines could not be established.

The most recent finding concerns the possible transformation of human cells by CMV (54). Normal human prostate cells, obtained from a 3-year-old male donor, yielded infectious virus upon early passages of in vitro culture, revealing the carrier state of these cells. Subsequent passage of these prostate cells led to virus latency and persistence of the virus genome. Virus-specific antigens were observed both in the cytoplasm and on the membrane, and the frequency of virus positive cells increased with IUdR pretreatment. Other evidence for the presence of CMV genetic material was ascertained indirectly by the observation that splenic lymphocytes from hamsters with CMV-specific tumors were cytotoxic for the transformed human prostate cells and directly by molecular hybridization which demonstrated 10–15 genome equivalents of CMV per transformed cell. All attempts to rescue virus were unsuccessful. Long term cultures have now been established; these have maintained the diploid human karyotype and preliminary results suggest they may be oncogenic when transplanted into athymic (nude) mice. This observation of in vitro transformation of human cells by CMV requires extension but should open new pathways for further study of the interaction of CMV with mammalian cells.

Discussion

Herpesviruses, now including EBV, HSV and CMV, have clearly demonstrated the ability to induce transformation of a variety of cell types. Cells from tumors caused by herpesvirus-transformed cells have been grown in culture and yield cell types morphologically similar to the original transformed cells. Markers of virus presence are evident in both transformed and homologous tumor cells. Virus-

467

specific antigens (cytoplasmic, nuclear and membrane), virus-coded enzymes and glycoproteins and the virus genome have been detected in most of the transformants. However, infectious virus particles have been isolated only rarely and only from EBV-transformed lines.

It has been established that herpesviruses can induce chromosomal aberrations and breaks (55–58). It is possible that one of the early proteins specified by the virus aids in the association and, perhaps, integration of the virus genome into the cellular genetic material where breaks have occurred. This could occur during the repair process.

Following transformation, some of the virus-specific glycoproteins are incorporated into host cell membranes. This should affect cell-cell relationships, possibly leading to loss of contact inhibition. In addition, the immunogenicity of the new surface glycoproteins will greatly influence the oncogenic potential of these virus-transformed cells.

The data presented thus far clearly demonstrate the *in vitro* transforming ability of three human herpesviruses, EBV, HSV and CMV. The relationship of cell culture studies to naturally occurring neoplasias is obviously in need of further investigation.

Acknowledgements

This work was supported by Contract No. NO1 CP53516 within The Virus Cancer Program of the National Cancer Institute, NIH, PHS.

This review rests heavily on work carried out by many collaborators, including Drs. Albrecht, Duff, Geder, Glaser, Lausch and St. Jeor, and graduate students Ms. Buss, Li and Reed.

References

1. Rawls, W. E., Tompkins, W. A., and Melnick, J. L. 1969. Am. J. Epidemiol. *89*: 547.
2. Rawls, W. E., Iwamoto, K., Adam, E., Melnick, J. L., and Green, G. H. 1970. Lancet *2*: 1142.
3. Nahmias, A. J., Josey, W. E., Naib, Z. M., Luce, C. F., and Guest, B. 1970. Am. J. Epidemiol. *91*: 547.
4. Royston, I., and Aurelian, L. 1970. Am. J. Epidemiol. *91*: 531.
5. Adam, E., Kaufman, R. H., Melnick, J. L., Levy, A. H., and Rawls, W. E. 1972. Am. J. Epidemiol. *96*: 427.
6. Centifanto, Y. M., Kaufman, H. E., Zam, Z., Drylie, D. M., and Deardourff, S. L. 1973. J. Virol. *12*: 1608.
7. Centifanto, Y. M., Drylie, D. M., Deardourff, S. L., and Kaufman, H. E. 1972. Science *178*: 318.
8. Royston, I., and Aurelian, L. 1970. Proc. Nat. Acad. Sci. USA *67*: 204.
9. Aurelian, L., Strandberg, J. D., and Davis, H. J. 1972. Proc. Soc. Exp. Biol. Med. *140*: 404.
10. Hollinshead, A. C., Lee, O., Chretien, P. B., Tarpley, J. L., Rawls, W. E., and Adam, E. 1973. Science *182*: 713.

11. Aurelian, L., Strandberg, J. D., Meléndez, L. V., and Johnson. L. A. 1971. Science *174*: 704.
12. Frenkel, N., Roizman, B., Cassai, E., and Nahmias, A. 1972. Proc. Nat. Acad. Sci. USA *69*: 3784.
13. Defendi, V., and Jensen, F. 1967. Science *157*: 703.
14. Latarjet, R., Cramer, R., Goldé, A., and Montagnier, L. 1967. *In* Carcinogenesis: A Broad Critique (Williams and Wilkins, Baltimore, Maryland), pp. 677–695.
15. Duff, R., Knight, P., and Rapp, F. 1972. Virology. *47:* 849.
16. Munyon, W., Kraiselburd, E., Davis, D., and Mann, J. 1971. J. Virol. *7*: 813.
17. Davis, D. B., Munyon, W., Buchsbaum, R., and Chawda, R. 1974. J. Virol. *13:* 140.
18. Duff, R., and Rapp, F. 1971. Nature (New Biol.) *233*: 48.
19. Duff, R., and Rapp, F. 1971. J. Virol. *8*: 469.
20. Duff, R., and Rapp, F. 1973. J. Virol. *12*: 209.
21. Reed, C., Cohen, G., and Rapp, F. 1975. J. Virol. *15*: 668.
22. Collard, W., Thornton, H., and Green, M. 1973. Nature (New Biol.) *243*: 264.
23. Kieff, B. D., Hoyes, B., Bachenheimer, J., and Roizman, B. 1972. J. Virol. *9:* 738.
24. Ludwig, H. O., Biswal, N., and Benyesh-Melnick, M. 1972. Virology *49*: 95.
25. Glaser, R., Duff, R., and Rapp, F. 1972. Cancer Res. *32*: 2803.
26. Rapp, F., Conner, R., Glaser, R., and Duff, R. 1972. J. Virol. *9*: 1059.
27. Doller, E., Duff, R., and Rapp, F. 1973. Intervirology *1*: 154.
28. Kutinová, L., Vonka, V., and Brouček, J. 1973. J. Natl. Cancer Inst. *50:* 759.
29. Duff, R., and Rapp, F. 1975. J. Virol. *15*: 490.
30. Wallis, C., and Melnick, J. L. 1964. Virology *23*: 520.
31. Wallis, C., and Melnick, J. L. 1965. Photochem. Photobiol. *4*: 159.
32. Rapp, F., Li, J. H., and Jerkofsky, M. 1973. Virology *55*: 339.
33. Li, J. H., Jerkofsky, M., and Rapp, F. 1975. Int. J. Cancer *15*: 190.
34. Darai, G., and Munk, K. 1973. Nature (New Biol.) *241*: 268.
35. Macnab, J. C. M. 1974. J. Gen. Virol. *24:* 143.
36. Takahashi, M., and Yamanishi, K. 1974. Virology *61*: 306.
37. Wilkie, N. M., Clements, J. B., Macnab, J. C. M., and Subak-Sharpe, J. H. 1974. Cold Spring Harbor Symp. Quant. Biol. *39*: 657–666.
38. St. Jeor, S., and Rapp, F. 1973. Science *181*: 1060.
39. St. Jeor, S., Albrecht, T. B., Funk, F. D., and Rapp, F. 1974. J. Virol. *13*: 353.
40. Tanaka, S., Furukawa, T., and Plotkin, S. A. 1975. J. Virol. *15*: 297.
41. Furukawa, T., Tanaka, S., and Plotkin, S. A. 1975. Proc. Soc. Exp. Biol. Med. *148*: 211.
42. Kit, S., de Torres, R. A., Dubbs, D. R., and Salvi, M. L. 1967. J. Virol. *1*: 738.
43. Gershon, D., Sachs, L., and Winocour, E. 1966. Proc. Nat. Acad. Sci. USA *56:* 918.
44. Dulbecco, R., Hartwell, L. H., and Vogt, M. 1965. Proc. Natl. Acad. Sci. USA *53*: 403.
45. Gershon, D., Hausen, P., Sachs, L., and Winocour, E. 1965. Proc. Natl. Acad. Sci. USA *54*: 1584.

46. Takahashi, M., van Hoosier, G. L., Jr., and Trentin, J. J. 1966. Proc. Soc. Exp. Biol. Med. *122*: 740.
47. Ledinko, N. 1967. Cancer Res. *27*: 1459.
48. Zimmermann, J. E., Jr., Raška, K., Jr., and Strohl, W. A. 1970. Virology *42:* 1147.
49. Gerber, P., and Hoyer, B. H. 1971. Nature (London) *231*: 46.
50. Albrecht, T., and Rapp, F. 1973. Virology *55*: 53.
51. Lausch, R. N., Murasko, D. M., Albrecht, T., and Rapp, F. 1974. J. Immunol. *112*: 1680.
52. Murasko, D. M., and Lausch, R. N. 1974. Int. J. Cancer *14*: 451.
53. Lang, D. J., Montagnier, L., and Latarjet, R. 1974. J. Virol. *14*: 327.
54. Rapp, F., Geder, L., Murasko, D., Lausch, R., Ladda, R., Huang, E., and Webber, M. 1975. J. Virol. *16:* 982.
55. Hampar, B., and Ellison, S. A. 1973. Proc. Natl. Acad. Sci. USA *49:* 474.
56. Stich, H. F., Hsu, T. C., and Rapp, F. 1964. Virology *22*: 439.
57. Rapp, F., and Hsu, T. C. 1965. Virology *25*: 401.
58. O'Neill, F. J., and Rapp, F. 1971. J. Virol. *7*: 692.

Failure to Immortalize Human "Null" Cells by Epstein Barr Virus (EBV) "In Vitro"

V. Diehl, H. H. Peter, F. Knoop, D. Hille, J. R. Kalden

Section of Hematology and Section of Clinical Immunology, Medizinische Hochschule Hannover, West-Germany

It es now well established that Epstein Barr Virus (EBV) specifically immortalizes B lymphocytes 'in vitro' to continously growing lymphobalstoid cultures (1, 2, 3). The same virus failed to induce T lymphocytes into longterm lymphoblastoid cell cultures suggesting that T cells lack EBV specific receptors (1, 2). We would like to report on experiments in which we failed to immortalize a subpopulation of human 'Null' cells in the presence of EBV. This subpopulation is detectable in lymphocyte preparations isolated by IgG-anti-IgG columns.

Peripheral blood lymphocytes were isolated from 13 healthy persons and 14 patients with malignant melanomas by a four step purification procedure (4). All donors were EBV sero-reactive with a mean VCA titer of less than 1:20. From 100 ml of defibrinated blood, first a crude lymphocyte preparation was prepared by Ficoll-Urografin density gradient centrifugation *(fraction F)*.

In a second and third step fraction F lymphocytes were depleted of iron phagocytosing macrophages and cells adhering to plastic surface. The remaining non-phagocytic, non-adherent lymphocyte population was referred to as *fraction FFF*, while the plastic adherent cells were termed *fraction AD*. The final purification step consisted of a passage of FFF lymphocytes over IgG-anti-IgG columns (5). By this procedure all B cells and the majority of Fc-Receptor carrying lymphocytes ('K' cells) were removed, leaving in the post-column fraction FFF-C approximately 70 % T cells and a subpopulation of 'Null' cells with low affinity for IgG-anti-IgG columns. A small proportion of these 'Null' cells formed EA-rosettes, whereas EACrosettes ranged below 1.0 %. Table 1 summarizes the cell composition of the different lymphocyte fractions. Since there was no significant difference between melanoma patients and control persons the results of both groups were presented together.

'K' cell activity was measured in whole blood and lymphocyte fractions F, FFF and FFF-C by an antibody dependent cellular cytotoxicity reaction (ADCC) utilizing as target cells a human melanoma cell line (IGR3), sensitized with rabbit anti-melanoma IgG (4). The results obtained with three leukocyte target cell ratios are shown in Table 1; details are presented elsewhere (4, 6). It can be seen that the B cell free lymphocyte fraction FFF-C retained significant ADCC activity, although it was strongly reduced compared to the activities measureable in fractions F and FFF. Furthermore, when lymphocytes of fraction FFF-C were separated into E-rosettes forming lymphocytes (T cells) and 'Null' cells, ADCC activity was only found in the 'Null' cell population. These results, together with the immunological and morphological criteria, suggested that the 'Null' cell

Morphological and immunological characteristics of purified human peripheral lymphocytes, ADCC activity and rate of establishment of lymphoblastoid cell cultures in the presence of EBV

| | Lymphocyte Fractions | | | |
	F	FFF	AD	FFF-C
Lymphocytes	93,1 ± 1,8[a]) (11)	96,1 ± 1,2 (23)	38,3 ± 3,2 (17)	99,2 ± 0,4 (23)
Monocytes	2,6 ± 1,0 (11)	2,1 ± 0,9 (23)	45,4 ± 3,2 (17)	0,6 ± 0,3 (23)
Granulocytes	4,2 ± 1,0 (11)	1,7 ± 0,3 (23)	15,5 ± 2,5 (17)	0.5 (23)
E-Rosettes	54,8 ± 3,6 (20)	54,1 ± 4,1 (20)	n. t.	69,9 ± 3,3 (17)
EA-Rosettes	12,2 ± 3,0 (10)	12,3 ± 2,2 (10)	n. t.	1,5 ± 0,7 (9)
EAC-Rosettes	10,0 ± 1,6 (10)	8,3 ± 1,7 (10)	n. t.	1.0 (10)
Surface Ig Pos.	10,0 ± 0,8 (18)	4,0 ± 0,4 (27)	27,3 ± 1,5 (10)	0 (27)
ADCC[b]) 12:1	46,6 ± 1,6 (7)	53,0 ± 8,0 (14)	n. t.	11,7 ± 2,1 (12)
25:1	51,2 ± 6,5 (7)	65,0 ± 7,9 (14)	n. t.	15,0 ± 4,8 (12)
50:1	63,5 ± 5,8 (7)	72,8 ± 7,4 (14)	n. t.	26,5 ± 4,3 (12)
Cultures				
without EBV	0/11[c])	0/15	0/17	0/18
with EBV	3/11 (27 %)	2/15 (13 %)	11/17 (65 %)	0/18

a) Percentage of total cell population; mean ± standard error (n).
b) ADCC = antibody-dependent cellular cytotoxicity against 51 Cr labeled IGR 3 melanoma cells, tested at 3 leukocyte to target cell ratios.
c) Cultures established/cultures started.

compartment in our post column fraction FFF-C represents a subpopulation of 'K' cells with low affinity FC-receptors.

The question, whether this cell type would be susceptible to EBV induced blast formation, was investigated by setting up 18 cultures of fraction FFF-C, together wirth a total of 56 cultures of the other lymphocyte fractions, in the presence of EBV. The initial cell inoculum was 2 x 10^6 cells per culture vial (25 ml Falcon plastic screw cap bottles) in 5 ml RPMI-1640 medium supplemented with 20 % fetal calf serum, penicillin and streptomycin.

EBV was derived from supernatants of B-95-8 cultures (marmoset lymphoblasts) (7) and added to the cultures in a final concentration of 1:10. The results are summarized in the lower part of Table 1. Without addition of exogenous

EBV no cultures were established from any one of the four fractions. By contrast, in the presence of EBV 3 out of 11 cultures with fraction F (27 %), 2 out of 15 cultures with fraction FFF (13 %) and 11 out of 17 cultures with fraction AD (65 %) gave rise to continously growing cell lines. None of 18 trials with cells of fraction FFF-C was successful. Irrespective of the presence or absence of exogenous EBV, lymphocytes of fraction FFF-C died within 10 days. A feeder-layer of allogeneic human embryonic fibroblasts prolonged the survival of FFF-C lymphocytes up to 2 months, but even under these conditions EBV induced blastoid transformation was not observed. Although the number of 'Null' cells present in fraction FFF-C was small (10–30 %), the prolonged survival by means of a feeder layer should have provided sufficient time to allow a virus – 'Null' cell – interaction to take place. However, the preliminary experiments do not exclude the possibility that through a decreased EBV receptor affinity 'Null' cell immortalization would need a higher EBV multiplicity or increased numbers of 'Null' cells. To exclude a mere threshold sensitivity for EBV, experiments are now in progress to increase the number of 'Null' cells in fraction FFF-C before exposure to EBV (8).

References

1. Jondal, M., Klein, G., J. Exp. Med. *138*, 1365, 1973.
2. Pattengale, P. K., Smith, R. W., Gerber, P., J. Natl. Canc. Inst. *52*, 1081, 1974.
3. Schneider, U., zur Hausen, H., Inst. J. Cancer *15*, 59, 1975.
4. Peter, H. H., Pavie-Fischer, J., Fridman, W. H., Aubert, C., Cesarini, J. P., Roubin, R., Kourilsky, F. M., J. Immunology, 115, 539, 1975.
5. Wigzell, H., Sundquist, K. G., Yoshida, T. O., Scand. J. Immunol., *1*, 75, 1972.
6. Peter, H. H., Knoop, F., Kalden, J. R., Z. f. Immunitätsforschung, in press.
7. Miller, G., Lipman, M., Proc. Nat. Ac. Sci. USA, *70*, 190, 1973.
8. Diehl, V., Peter, H. H., Kalden, J. R. and Hille, D. In preparation.

This work was supported by the Deutsche Forschungsgemeinschaft, Bad Godesberg, W.-Germany (Di-184-4).

The Role of Viruses in Human Leukemia
A Summary

Harald zur Hausen

Institut für Klinische Virologie
852 Erlangen, Loschgestrasse 7
Federal Republic of Germany

It is certainly a hard task to summarize discussions dealing with virological aspects of human leukemia. The diverging views, the different approaches render it almost impossible to review comprehensively the data presented. It is unavoidable, in addition, that the biased views of the author are applied to the issues raised at this meeting.

Is there any progress visible as compared to the last meeting 2 years ago at this very place? Progress in the elucidation of the role of viruses in human leukemia? Progress in our understanding of the mechanisms leading to virus-induced leukemia in general?

It appears to be easier to start with the second question first: many elegant studies were reported dealing with virus-induced leukemogenesis in avian as well as in mammalian systems. BALUDA pointed out the importance of the target cell for a specific response in terms of cell transformation and stressed the acquisition of new DNA sequences in transformed cells (1). Nontransformed cells contain DNA which reveals 60 % of homology with avian myeloblastosis virus (AMV) sequences only. His data were somewhat contrasted by GRAF's studies who presented evidence for the cell specificity of various AMV strains, each of them transforming different target cells (2). Based on his experiments GRAF claims that the different types of tumors observed in BALUDA's studies are due to a mixture of different AMV strains present within the original inoculum.

In this respect it was interesting to learn that the helper RAV-virus, present in preparations of defective erythroblastosis virus (2), induces by itself severe anemia in chicken, but no erythroblastosis. This may have some relevance for human leukemias, where (as stressed by MOLONEY) refractory anemia or even pancytopenia frequently is a preceding disorder.

The avian systems was also investigated in DUESBERG's studies in order to identify the localization of transforming sequences within the avian sarcoma virus genome (3). Sarcomavirus-specific sequences were identified in 3 different strains of sarcoma viruses by selecting specific fragments of partially degraded viral genomes and subjecting them to fingerprinting after further partial digestion. These studies come close to experiments reported by BISHOP's group in isolating sarcoma-specific sequences by hybridization techniques (4). I hesitate to agree to call such sequences "oncogene" since transformation of lymphatic cells occurs naturally by leukosis viruses which appear to lack the respective sequence.

BAUER and HOFSCHNEIDER reported the isolation of a new particle from the allantoic fluid of embryonic eggs (5). It seems to differ from known avian leukosis viruses in that it does not share antigens with AMV. It also reveals distinct properties of its RNA-dependent DNA polymerase.

Turning now to the mammalian systems, the situation becomes increasingly complex: many of the newly isolated mammalian oncornaviruses offer the fascinating possibility to study their evolution across the species-barrier. As explained by TODARO, endogenous viruses of baboons are also found in a number of cat species (6) and permit a rough calculation when an infectious process took place from the baboon to the cat or vice versa. This as well as similar systems may provide us with an entirely new approach to study the evolution of certain species. It should not be overlooked, at the same time, that most of these studies are performed with material derived from laboratory animals. It is abvious, therefore, that the possibility of inadvertent contaminants has to be excluded.

JAENISCH presented extremely interesting data on genetic control of oncornavirus information in the mouse system (7). He studied the infection of embryos at the 4–8 cell stage and looked into the presence of virus-specific DNA within the germ line as well as within somatic cells at later stages of development. This seems to offer a new approach in the regulation of virus-specific information in mammals. It was interesting to learn at this occasion that cells at very early stages of embryonic development are non-permissive for those viruses he tested (murine leukemia viruses and SV 40). One wonders whether there exists a specific mechanism which protects such cells and possibly also germ line cells against early genetic damage.

Studies on the role of FRIEND leukemia virus in the differentation of mouse pluripotential stem cells into erythroblasts were reported by OSTERTAG. HARDESTY also alluded to this question (8). The ingenious cell separator used by OSTERTAG, based on laser-beam scanning and computer-directed deflection of drops, appears to represent an elegant and important tool in the elucidation of cell differentation. This was also convincingly demonstrated by GREAVES (9) experiments. OSTERTAG's statements on the possible role of DMSO in the induction of viral and globin messengers RNA-synthesis by affecting repressor binding within the cell may deserve further studies.

Transfection experiments revealing the existence of DNA proviruses were rather briefly discussed at this meeting. BENTVELZEN made the interesting observation that DNA from spleens of Rauscher virus leukemic mice transfects and transforms efficiently when applied under appropriate conditions. In this respect it seems interesting to note that similar studies have not yet been reported with human leukemic cell DNA. One could imagine that similar events may take place in tissue culture or by transfecting cells of primates in vivo with DNA originating from human leukemia cells.

Interesting new aspects were contributed by BURNY in his studies on the viral etiology of bovine lymphosarcoma (11). The epidemiology of this disease resembles the spread of feline leukemias which were, unfortunately, not discussed at this meeting. It is of interest to note that 100 % of animals developing disease revealed antibodies to viral antigens. This in part to such an extent that they can be measured by relatively insensitive immunoprecipitation methods. This appears to contrast markedly the situation in human leukemia, where the demonstration of even leukemia-specific antigens, as pointed out by GREAVES (9), is presently either impossible or requires difficult manipulations.

The presence of bovine oncornaviruses in commercially available batches of calf serum, as observed by BURNY (11). should be another word of caution in claims of new oncornaviruses from tissue culture cells maintained with such reagents.

Turning now to human leukemia and lymphosarcoma, isolates from human disease naturally require special attention. Two claims of successful oncornavirus isolations were reported at this meeting (12) and others are found in the literature (13, 14, 15). GALLO described extensively the successful isolation of such viruses from a patient with acute myelogenous leukemia (12). According to his studies the agent appears not to be an endogenous virus of man or certain primates. It shares many characteristics with the simian sarcoma virus and it is not yet entirely clear whether it can be differentiated at all from this agent. Although repeatedly isolated from the same patient, there are some disturbing observations which are difficult to reconcile with a role of this virus in human myelogenous leukemia:

(i) recent studies reveal the presence of two different oncornaviruses in these isolates. One of them appears to be idential with simian sarcoma virus, the other shares features with baboon endogenous virus (16).

(ii) no convincing levels of antibodies directed against these isolates can be demonstrated in the patient, nor in other individuals suffering from the same disease, or in healthy control persons (17).

(iii) DNA-sequences related to these agents have not been demonstrated in the DNA derived from spleen cells of the patient from whom the viruses were recovered.

Thus, there remains the possibility, as remote as it may be, of a laboratory contamination. Further studies appear to be essential to clarify the origin of the isolated agents. The second isolate was reported by NOOTER. It has been obtained from a child with lymphosarcoma. This virus has not yet been further characterized. Although the data seem to be intriguing, the use of rat XC-cells for plaquing this agent raises some questions. Endogenous rat oncornaviruses have recently been found in XC-cells.

The third group isolating putative human oncornaviruses was not represented at this meeting. KIRSTEN and PANEM were able to recover a simian sarcoma virus-like agent from human embryonic lung fibroblasts (13).

It is obvious that each of these isolations requires great interest. It appears to be a long way to clarify whether they indeed represent human viruses. If so, it will be an even longer way before they can be implicated in human leukemic disease.

SPIEGELMAN reported the presence of specific DNA sequences, as determined in his endogenous reaction, in almost every kind of human tumors (18). The significance of these findings should be further elucidated, since they are also found in two human malignancies most probably induced by a DNA containing virus (19).

The various isolations of oncornaviruses from primates should support attempts to recover similar agents from human leukemias and lymphomas. It is of particular interest that oncornaviruses have been isolated from acute myelogenous leukemias in gibbons.

There are, however, certain features of most human leukemias which are presently difficult to reconcile with an oncornavirus-induction. Although anologies to animal leukemias sponsor intensively the current interest in oncornaviruses, it may be worthwhile to consider some of the diverging aspect:

(i) In contrast to most animal oncornavirus-induced tumors it appears to be extremely difficult to demonstrate any kind of oncornavirus-specific molecules in human leukemic cells. This is also shown in GREAVE's study on antigens specific for acute lymphatic leukemia (9).

(ii) Sera derived from leukemic patients appear to lack antibody-activities against known oncornaviruses. This certainly includes the woolly monkey isolate. In regard to all known naturally occurring oncornavirus-induced leukemias and lymphomas it would be exceptional if man would respond without antibody production.

(iii) Human leukemias and lymphomas represent, at least in their vast majority, monoclonal diseases. Thus, the continuous production of transforming particles appears to be somewhat unlikely.

(iv) The failure to demonstrate viral particles in human leukemic cells certainly contrasts the situation in animal systems.

In this respect it was somewhat surprising that the only virus known to be oncogenic in man and consistently associated with specific lymphatic diseases, the Epstein-Barr virus (EBV), played a minor role at this meeting. This DNA-containing herpes group virus was briefly discussed by DIEHL showing that NULL cells apparently lack receptors for EBV-infection (20). It has to be remembered that EBV is found in virtually 100 % of African Burkitt's lymphoma cells, as well as in very few cases of similar histology outside of the African tumor belt; that it infects and transforms specifically B-lymphocytes, but is also found in every epithelial tumor cell of human nasopharyngeal carcinoma (19). This virus induces lymphoproliferative disease in marmosets and transforms and "immortalizes" human lymphocytes efficiently (19).

The most potent and effective leukemogenic agent in primates, herpesvirus saimiri, was also discussed in one presentation only (21). LAUFS reported on prevention of saimiri-induced oncogenesis by prior inoculation of heat- and formaline-inactivated vaccines. It should be noted that herpesvirus saimiri induces lymphomas or acute lymphatic leukemias after short incubation periods in 100 % of inoculated marmosets (22).

Returning to human leukemias, there is presently no good reason to speculate that these diseases are herpesvirus-induced. In such case it would be, most probably, not too difficult to detect virus-specific antigens within the transformed cell or on their surface. The entire lack of these "footprints" in human leukemic cells remains a puzzle in regard to their suspected viral etiology. It could be relevant in this respect that there exists a group of transforming viruses which are most difficult to trace within their transformed host cells, the human papilloma or wart viruses (23). In spite of numerous attempts it has not yet been possible to detect papilloma virus-specific T-or surface antigens within their transformed host cells. Recent results reveal that there exist several types of human papilloma viruses which can be differentiated by biochemical methods (zur Hausen and Gissmann, unpublished results). There may be other candidate viruses along these lines and it appears to me to be a good bet that at least some forms of human leukemias (if they do have a viral etiology at all) should be due to non-enveloped viruses.

I am stating this because it is my feeling that our intensive search for human analogies to well established laboratory system in animals may misguide us. Most probably it will be worthwhile to persue also different avenues in our search for a viral etiology of human leukemia. If the intensive search for human oncorna-viruses fails to provide conclusive evidence we should be prepared to look as well into the role of other agents in the induction of this malignant disease.

References

1. Baluda, M. A., et al. this volume.
2. Graf, T., et al. this volume.
3. Duesberg, P., et al. this volume.
4. Stehelin, D., Varmus, H. E., and Bishop, J. M., Detection of nucleotide sequences associated with transformation by avian sarcoma viruses. VIIth Int. Symp. Comp. Leukemia Res., Oct. 13–17, 1975, Copenhagen, in print.
5. Bauer, G., et al. this volume.
6. Todaro, G., this volume.
7. Jaenisch, R., et al. this volume.
8. Hardesty, B., et al. this volume.
9. Greaves, M. F., et al. this volume.
10. Nooter et al. this volume.
11. Kettmann et al. this volume.
12. Gallo, R. C., this volume.
13. Kirsten, W., and Panem, S., Kinetics of type-C virus induction from normal diploid human fibroblast cell strains. VIIth Int. Symp. Comp. Leukemia Res. Oct. 13–17, 1975, Copenhagen, in print.
14. Gabelman, N., Waxman, S., Smith, W., and Douglas, S. D., Appearance of C-type virus-like particles after co-cultivation of a human tumor-cell line rat (XC) cells. Int. J. Cancer 16, 355—369, 1975.
15. Vosika, G. J., Krivit, W., Gerrard, J. M., Coccia, P. F., Nesbit, M. N., Coalson, J. J., and Kennedy, B. J., Oncornavirus-like particles from cultured bone marrow cells preceding leukemia and malignant histiocytosis. Proc. Nat. Acad. Sci. 72, 2804–2808, 1975.
16. Gillespie, D. H., and Gallo, R. C., Concepts concerning the origin of RNA tumor virus markers in human leukemic cells. VIIth Int. Symp. Comp. Leukemia Res., Oct. 13–17, 1975, Copenhagen, in print.
17. Kurth, R., Discussion at VIIth Int. Symp. Comp. Leukemia Res., Oct. 13–17, 1975, Copenhagen, in print.
18. Spiegelman, S., this volume.
19. zur Hausen, H., Oncogenic herpesviruses, Biophys. Biochem. Acta 417; 25–53, 1975.
20. Diehl, V., this volume.
21. Laufs, R., and Steinke, this volume.

22. Melendez, L. V. (ed.), Symposium on viruses of South American monkeys: importance of these viruses in oncogenic studies. J. Nat. Cancer Inst. 49, 209–294, 1972.
23. zur Hausen, H., Gissmann, L., Steiner, H., Dippold, W., and Dreger, I., Papilloma viruses and human cancer. VIIth Int. Symp. Comp. Leukemia Res., Oct. 13–17, 1975, in print.

IS-Elements in Bacteria

by
P. Starlinger

Institut für Genetik
der Universität zu Köln
5 Köln 41, Weyertal 121

The first extrachromosomal genetic elements discovered in bacteria were temperate bacteriophages, which can exist either as extracellular virus, as chromosomes replicating autonomously within cells or integrated into the bacterial chromosome. Integration of viruses into host chromosomes has subsequently attracted considerable attention by tumor virologists. This may justify the discussion of other types of genetic elements in bacteria in a meeting on human leucaemia.

In addition to temperate bacteriophages, there are other extrachromosomal genetic elements in bacteria. Some of them are called plasmids. They lack the extracellular state, but exist either autonomously within the bacterial cytoplasm or integrated into the bacterial chromosome.

A third class of genetic elements has been described in recent years. It apparently lacks the ability to multiply autonomously and exists only integrated into the bacterial chromosome. Within this chromosome, however, it can be transposed to various positions. At present, three such elements, called IS1, (= insertion sequence) IS2 and IS3 are known. Their length is 0.8, 1.4 and 1.25 kilobases, respectively (1–5).

The presence of these elements can be detected by various effects which they show at the point of insertion:

1) Integration into the continuity of the gene causes the loss of gene function (6,7).
2) Insertion into a gene within an operon causes severe polar effects on genes distal to the mutated gene (6, 7, 8).
3) At least one representative of class IS2 carries a promoter. Genes linked to this promoter are expressed constitutively (9).
4) If two circular chromosomes, e. g. the E. coli chromosome and the F-factor, share an IS-element, e. g. IS2 or IS3, recombination within the IS-elements leads to the fusion of these two chromosomes. This mechanism accounts, at least in some instances, for the integration of the F-factor into the E. coli chromosome upon formation of Hfr strains or for the joining and disjoining of parts of bacterial R-factors (10, 11).
5) Two copies of the same IS-element, inserted in inverted position relative to each other and bordering between them a certain gene may form a transposon (12). The gene for tetracyclin resistance, carried on plasmid R6–5 and also on phage P22 may serve as an example, in which the IS-element is IS3 (13, 14).

The physical and biochemical characterization of IS-elements has been possible in bacteria, due to the relative ease with which bacterial and especially bacteriophage

DNA can be handled. However, elements with very similar properties have been characterized by genetic methods in higher organisms also. Most notable are the controlling elements in maize and mutable genes in Drosophila (15, 16). Should it turn out that similar elements have a more widespread occurrence, even among vertebrates, they may well deserve also the attention of those interested in the genesis of malignant tumors.

Acknowledgement

Work done in the author's laboratory was supported by the Deutsche Forschungsgemeinschaft through Sonderforschungsbereich 74.

References

1. E. Jordan, H. Saedler and P. Starlinger: 0°- and Strong Polar Mutations in the gal Operon are Insertions. Molec. Gen. Genetics *102*: 353 (1968).
2. J. A. Shapiro: Mutations caused by the Insertion of Genetic Material into the Galactose Operon of Escherichia coli. J. Mol. Biol. *40*: 93 (1969).
3. P. Starlinger and H. Saedler: Insertion Mutations in Microorganism. Biochemie *54*: 177 (1972).
4. H. J. Hirsch, P. Starlinger and P. Brachet: Two Kinds of Insertions in Bacterial Genes. Molec. Gen. Genetics *119*: 191 (1972).
5. M. Fiandt, W. Szybalski and M. H. Malamy: Polar Mutations in lac, gal and phage consist of a few DNA Sequences inserted with either Orientation. Molec. Gen. Genetics *119*: 223 (1972).
6. E. Jordan, H. Saedler and P. Starlinger: Strong-Polar Mutations in the Transferase Gene of the Galactose Operon in E. Coli. Molec. Gen. Genetics *100*: 296 (1967).
7. S. L. Adhya and J. A. Shapiro: The Galactose Operon of E. Coli K12. I. Structural and Pleiotropic Mutations of the Operon. Genetics *62:* 231 (1969).
8. M. H. Malamy: Some Properties of Insertion Mutations in the lac Operon. In: The Lactose Operon, ed. J. R. Beckwith and D. Zipser, Cold Spring Harbor Laboratory 1970.
9. H. Saedler and H. J. Reif: IS2, A Genetic Element for Turn-off and Turn-on of Gene Acticity in E. coli. Molec. Gen. Genetics *132*: 265 (1974).
10. S. Hu, E. Ohtsubo, N. Davidson and H. Saedler: Electron Microscope Heteroduplex Studies of Sequence Relations among Bacterial Plasmids: Identification and Mapping of the Insertion Sequences IS1 and IS2 and R-Plasmids. J. Bacteriol. *122*: 764 (1975).
11. S. Hu, E. Ohtsubo and N. Davidson: Electron Microscope Heteroduplex Studies of Sequence Relations among Plasmids of E. coli: Structure of F13 and Related F-Primes. J. Bacteriol *122*: 749 (1975).
12. R. W. Hedges and A. E. Jacob: Transposition of Ampillicin Resistance from RP4 to Other Replicons. Molec. Gen. Geneteics *132*: 31 (1974).
13. K. Ptashne and S. N. Cohen: Occurrence of Insertion Sequence Regions on Plasmid Deoxyribonucleic Acid as Direct and Inverted Nucleotide Sequence Duplications. J. Bacteriol. *122*: 776 (1975).

14. B. Tye, K. Russel, Chan and D. Botstein: Packaging of an Oversize Transducing Genome Phage P22. J. Mol. Biol. *85*: 485 (1974).
15. J. R. S. Fincham and G. R. K. Sastry: Controlling Elements in Maize. Annual Rev. Genetics 8: 15 (1974).
16. B. Rasmuson, M. M. Green and B. M. Karlsson: Genetic Instability in Drosophila melanogaster: Evidence for Insertion Mutations. Molec. Gen. Genetics *133*: 237 (1974).

Circadian Variation of α- Amanitine Sensitive RNA-Synthesis in Normal Human Lymphocytes

R. Mertelsmann
H. W. Heitbrock
I. Medizinische Universitätsklinik

M. Garbrecht
II. Medizinische Universitätsklinik
Hamburg, Bundesrepublik Deutschland

A major aspect of successful cancer chemotherapy is the dose-time schedule of application of cytostatic drugs. Clinical trials have proven the superiority of intermittent high-dose combination chemotherapy, the intervals between administrations being of paramount importance. In spite of a number of studies in animal models demonstrating the additional importance of the day-time of application[1, 2], these aspects have not been taken into account for human cancer chemotherapy so far. Since RNA synthesis by DNA-dependent RNA polymerases is one of the sites of action of cytostatic drugs, e. g. Actinomycin D, we have studied RNA synthesis by α-amanitine sensitive RNA polymerase B in isolated nuclei from human normal and chronic lymphocytic leukemia (CLL) lymphocytes over a 48 h period of observation.

All patients (8 controls, 2 CLL patients) were hospitalized and obeyed to a constant pattern of life (sleep from 22.00 to 6.30 h, meals at 8.00, 12.00, and 18.00 h). Plasma cortisol concentrations were determined every 6 hours in 4 patients proving the regularity of this important body rhythm. No medical treatment was given during and at least two weeks prior to the investigation. 20 ml of citrated venous blood were taken every 6 hours (00.00, 6.00, 12.00, 18.00 h) and lymphocytes isolated using a modified standard procedure[3] (cf. Legend to Fig. 1). Contamination by non-lymphoid cells was less than 3 % in all patients studied as determined by cytochemical criteria[4].

Nuclei were prepared according to Wiegers and Hilz[5] and assayed for RNA polymerase activity after sonication (for incubation conditions see legend to Fig. 1)[6]. Absolute lymphocyte counts in all 8 normal patients exhibited diurnal variations following a rhythm of approximately 24 h, as described by Sharp[7]. Data were fitted to a cosine function using Fast Fourier Transformation[8]. The computed mean cosine function was

$$f(t) = 3081 + 760 \cos(\omega t - 20.7)$$

(t = time in hours, ω = angular frequency fixed at 15 °/h) with the acrophase at 01.23 h and lowest values at 13.23 h (Fig. 1). Differences between lymphocyte counts at 00.00 and 12.00 h are highly significant (p < 0.01).

Variance analyses as well as trend analyses proved the high significance of the fitted cosine function. A definite rhythm of RNA polymerase B activities, i. e.

Fig. 1: Absolute lymphocyte counts in peripheral blood in normals and in patients with chronic lymphocytic leukemia (CLL)

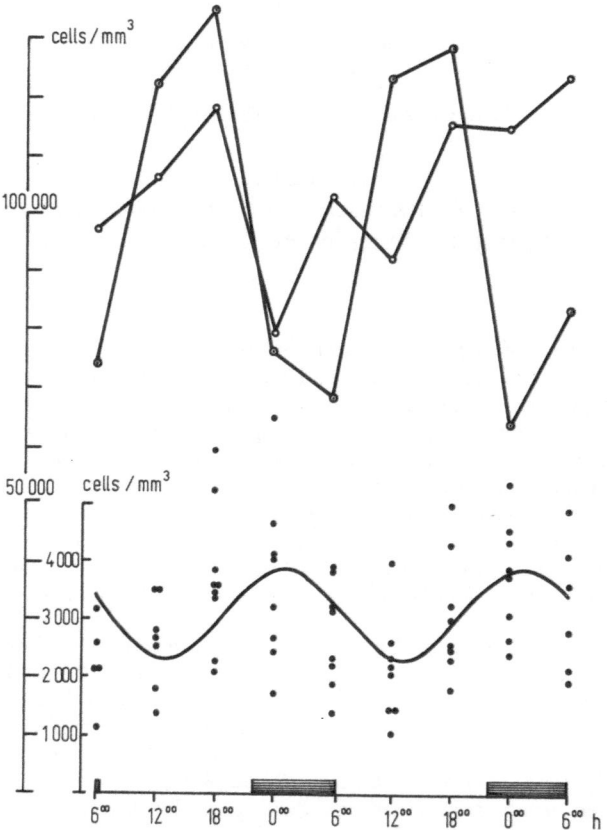

Fig. 1: *Absolute lymphocyte counts in peripheral blood in normals and in patients with chronic lymphocytic leukemia (CLL).*
Absolute cell counts were determined using a NEUBAUER counting chamber and differential counts of stained blood smears.
Lymphocyte counts (.) of 8 normal subjects and their fitted cosine function (-) are represented in the lower graph.
The upper graph contains the data from 2 patients with CLL. The computative acro-phase of the regular curve was 15.00 h.

α-amanitine sensitive incorporation of ³H-UMP into acid precipitable material, was observed in all normal subjects during the period of investigation. These variations followed a regular 24 hour rhythm in 6 of 8 normal subjects with maximum acitivty at 00.00 h and minimum incorporation of ³H-UMP at 12.00 h (Fig. 2). Differences between enzyme activities at 00.00 and 12.00 h are highly significant (p <0.001). The mean level of activity was 42.2 pmoles (³H) UMP in-

Fig. 2: Activities of RNA polymerase B (α-amanitin sensitive) in normal and leukemic lymphocytes during a period of 48 hours

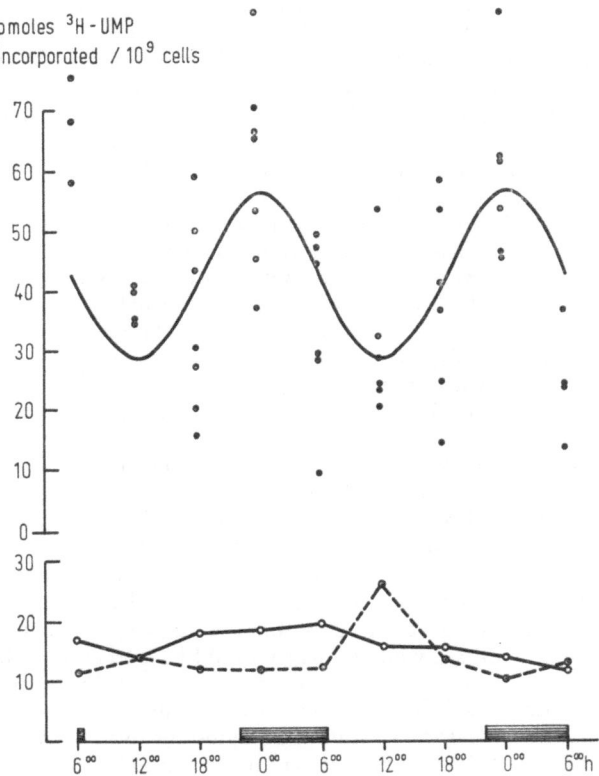

Fig. 2: *Activities of RNA polymerase B (α-amanitine sensitive) in normal and leukemic lymphocytes during a period of 48 hours.*

Lymphocytes were prepared using a modified standard procedure[3]. Citrated venous blood was layered on top of a Ronpacon[R]-Ficoll-mixture (10 % Ronpacon w/v, 6.4 % Ficoll w/v) and centrifuged for 20 minutes at 1200g at room temperature. Lymphocytes were removed from the interphase, resuspended in isotonic buffer and sedimented at 175g for 20 minutes. RNA polymerase activity was determined by incubation of 50 µl of enzyme solution (sonicated nuclei[6]) in a final volume of 100 µl under the following conditions:

ATP, CTP, GTP 1 mM each, 1 µM (^{3}H) UTP (specific activity 10 or 49 Ci/mmole). 225 mM Tris HCl pH 8.5, 0.12 M $(NH_4)_2SO_4$, 2.5 mM $MgCl_2$, 2.5 mM $MnCL_2$, 50 mM K-EDTA, 3 mM ß-mercaptoethanol, 2 µg of denatured calf thymus DNA, 15 % glycerol (v/v). After incubation for 30 minutes at 37 °C the reaction was terminated by pipetting duplicate aliquots of 30 µl on Whatman GF/FA filter discs, followed by TCE precipitation[6].

RNA polymerase activity is expressed in pmoles (^{3}H)-UMP incorporated per 10^9 cells. The values from 6 normal subjects are shown in the upper part of the figure. The data obtained from 2 patients with chronic lymphocytic leukemia are represented in the lower part of the figure. No significant circadian variation of the enzyme activity could be demonstrated in CLL.

corporated /10^9 nuclei (range 32.9–50.0) with an amplitude of 14.3 (range 5.5–27.0). Single cosine functions were computed for each subject, computative acrophases being between 22.26 and 02.58 h. The mean cosine function was

$$f(t) = 42.2 + 14.3 \cos(\omega\tau - 6.1)$$

with the acrophase at 00.24 h (Fig. 2). Statistical analysis (variance analyses, trend analyses) proved the high significance of fitted cosine functions.

Variation of RNA polymerase B activities of two normal subjects were not compatible with a circadian rhythm, in spite of the regular circadian variation exhibited by these patients' lymphocyte counts. Mathematical analysis demonstrated an ultradian rhythm (2 periods/24 h) in one and a reversed rhythm (lowest values at 00.00 h) in the other. In two patients with CLL, no rhythmicity of α-amanitine sensitive RNA synthesis could be detected. Mean values of RNA polymerase B acitivty were 16.2 and 13.9 pmoles (^{3}H) UMP incorporated/10^9 nuclei, being significantly lower as compared to normal controls (p <0.05). In contrast to the constant RNA polymerase activity, white blood cell counts exhibited extreme variations, 79,400–123,800/mm^3 in one and 62,00–135,000/mm^3 in the other. The patient with the more stable disease, requiring no specific therapy, exhibited a remarkably regular circadian rhythm of peripheral blood lymphocyte counts (Fig. 1).

Comparing our results with the circadian variation of RNA contents of total human white blood cells described by Kohler et al.[9], an inverse relationship with the amount of total RNA as well as of 5S-RNA is observed, while 4S-RNA contents follow a pattern similar to that of RNA polymerase B. Provided that activity of RNA polymerase B, the enzyme responsible for heterogenous nuclear RNA (pre mRNA) synthesis, is representative of overall RNA synthetic activity[6] of the cell, 5S-RNA would be a fraction of slow turnover accumulating at times of even low RNA synthesis, while 4S-RNA would be a fraction of high turnover. It has to be taken into account, however, that RNA synthesis is only one facet of RNA metabolism. No definite conclusions can be drawn from our observations for a dose-time schedule for application of cytostatic drugs. The existence of a circadian rhythm of RNA polymerase activity in normal and its absence in CLL lymphocytes, however, allows a rational approach towards a chronotherapy. Taking into account pharmacokinetic aspects, drugs, which exert their effect via inhibition of RNA synthesis, certainly should not have their maximum cytostatic activity during the time when the host's lymphocytes are most actively synthesizing RNA, a probable prerequisite for immunological defence mechanisms.

A more detailed report will be published elsewhere. This work was supported by grants of the Deutsche Forschungsgemeinschaft. We thank Mrs. Marianne Helmrich for excellent technical assistance and are indebted to Mr. W. Rehpenning for carrying out variance and trend analyses (Abt. Medizin. Dokumentation and Statistik, Universität Hamburg).

References

1. Davies, G. J., MacDonald, J., Halberg, F., and Simpson, H. W., Lancet 779 (1974, II).
2. Haus, E., Halberg, F., Scheving, L. E., Pauly, J. E., Cardoso, S., Kühl, F. W., Sothern, R. B., Shiotsuka, R., and Hwang, D. S., Science 177, 80–82 (1972).

3. Böyum, A., Scand. Journ. Lab. Clin. Invest., Suppl. 21, 77–89 (1968).
4. Löffler, H., Klin. Wschr. 39, 1220–1222 (1961).
5. Wiegers, U., and Hilz, H., Febs Letters 23, 77–79 (1972).
6. Garbrecht, M., Mertelsmann, R., and Schöch, G., Klin. Wschr. 51, 730–734 (1973).
7. Sharp, G. W. G., J. Endocrinology, 21, 107–114 (1960).
8. Halberg, F., Haus, E., Cardoso, S. S., Scheving, L. E., Kühl, J. F. W., Shiotsuka, R., Rosene, G., Pauly, J. E., Runge, W., Spalding, J. F., Lee, J. K. and Good, R. A., Experientia 29, 909–1044 (1973).
9. Kohler, W. C., Karacan, I., and Rennert, O. M., Nature 238, 94—96 (1972).

Terminal Deoxynucleotidyl Transferase as a Biological Marker for Human Leukemia

P. S. Sarin and R. C. Gallo

Laboratory of Tumor Cell Biology
National Cancer Institute
National Institutes of Health
Bethesda, Maryland 20014

Abstract

High levels of terminal deoxynucleotidyl transferase have been observed in leukocytes of 7 out of 20 patients with chronic myelogenous leukemia in acute blast phase of the disease. These levels are comparable to the levels observed in human and calf thymus gland and cell lines with some T cell characteristics (Molt 4 and 8402). Negligible levels of this activity were observed in chronic myelogenous leukemia not in an acute blast phase of the disease, chronic lymphocytic leukemia, human B cells, mature T cells, and the mixed population of lymphocytes present in normal human blood. The detection of this enzyme in some patients with chronic myelogenous leukemia in acute blast phase of the disease suggests that the blast proliferation may involve primitive stem cells which have more lymphoid than myelogenous characteristics. This enzyme assay may be of use as a biological marker for following patients during treatment and in remission.

Introduction

Terminal deoxynucleotidyl transferase, an enzyme that catalyzes the polymerization of deoxyribonucleotides onto the 3'-OH ends of oligo or polydeoxynucleotide initiators in the absence of a template was initially considered to be specific for the thymus gland (1). Recently, this enzyme has been detected in various forms of human leukemia (2–7) including acute lymphocytic leukemia (ALL) (2, 6, 7), acute myelomonocytic leukemia (AMML) (3), and chronic myelogenous leukemia (CML) in acute blast phase of the disease (5, 6, 7). High levels of this enzyme have also been observed in cell lines with T-cell characteristics (Molt 4 and 8402) derived from cells of patient with acute lymphoblastic leukemia (8, 9). The presence of high levels of this enzyme in cells from patients with chronic myelogenous leukemia in acute blast phase of the disease and its absence in the chronic phase of the disease (6, 7) suggest that this enzyme can be useful as a biological marker for following patients during treatment and in remission.

In this report we present a comparison of the levels of this enzyme in leukocytes of patients with chronic myelogenous leukemia in acute blast phase with the levels present in leukocytes from patients with CML not in acute blast phase, ALL, chronic lymphocytic leukemia (CLL), normal blood lymphocytes, human and calf thymus gland and cell lines with B and T cell characteristics. In addition, we show that in leukocytes of a CML patient in remission, levels of this enzyme returned to the level present in normal leukocytes.

Materials and Methods

Materials: Tritium labeled deoxyribonucleoside triphosphates were obtained from Schwarz-Mann. Unlabeled deoxyribonucleoside triphosphates were obtained from P. L. Biochemicals. Oligo- and poly-ribo and deoxyribo-nucleotides were obtained from Miles Laboratories and P. L. Biochemicals.

Terminal transferase assays: Terminal transferase activity was assayed at 37° for 1 hr as described earlier (5, 6, 8) in a standard reaction mixture (0.05ml) which contained 50 mM Tris HCl (pH7.5), 50 mM KCl, 0.1 mM $MnCl_2$, 5 mM dithiothreitol (DTT), 100 µM of the labeled deoxyribonucleoside triphosphate, 2.5 µg of poly(dA) as a primer, and 5 µl of the enzyme fraction. The specific activity of the labeled deoxyribonucleoside triphosphates used was [³H] dGTP (1500 cpm/pmole) and [³H]dTTP (2200 cpm/pmole). The reaction was arrested by the addition of 50 µg of yeast tRNA and 2 ml of 10 % trichloracetic acid, collected on Millipore filters and counted in a scintillation counter (10).

Source of cells: White blood cells from leukemic patients were collected by the use of an IBM white cell separator (11). Lymphoblast cell lines (Molt 4 and 8402) with T cell characteristics, established in tissue culture were originally derived from peripheral blood of patients with ALL (12). All these cell lines were obtained from Hem Research Associates, Bethesda, Maryland. Another B cell line (NC37) was derived from human normal blood lymphocytes (13) and was obtained from J. L. Smith Memorial for Cancer Research, Pfizer, Inc., Maywood, New Jersey. Fresh human blood lymphocytes were obtained by phlebotomy from normal subjects purified from other blood components, and stimulated with phytophemagglutinin for 72 hrs. as described earlier (14). Fresh human thymus, obtained from children undergoing cardiac surgery, and calf thymus were obtained from Hem Research Associates, Bethesda, Maryland.

Cytogenetic studies on the cells of patients with chronic myelogenous leukemia in chronic and acute blast phase showed the presence of philadelphia chromosome (Ph_1).

Cell extractions: All cell extractions were carried our at 0–4 °C. Cells were washed with phosphate buffered saline (pH 7.4) twice, and suspended in 5 volumes of buffer A (10mM Tris.HCl (pH 7.4), 10 mM KCl and 1.5 mM Mg^{2+}) and allowed to swell for 10 min. The cells were manually disrupted in a tight fitting stainless steel homogenizer and mixed with equal volume of buffer B (50 mM Tris.HCl (pH 7.5), 5 mM DTT, 1 M KCl, 1 % triton X100, 20 % glycerol) and stirred in ice for 2 hrs. The soluble extract was removed, dialyzed against buffer C (50 mM Tris. HCl (pH 7.5), 5 mM DTT, 20 % glycerol) containing 0.5M KCl and subsequently against buffer C. Human and calf thymus gland was processed according to an earlier procedure (6).

Enzyme purification: Terminal transferase was purified by successive chromatography on DEAE cellulose, phosphocellulose and hydroxyapatite as described earlier (5, 6, 8).

Results

Terminal transferase levels in various cells. High levels of terminal transferase were observed in cells of some patients with chronic myelogenous leukemia in acute blast phase of the disease. These levels are comparable to the levels of terminal transferase observed in lymphoid cell lines with T cell characteristics such as Molt 4 and 8402 (6, 8, 9) and human and calf thymus gland (Table 1). Insignificant levels of terminal transferase were observed in B cell lines (NC37, SB and 8392), PHA stimulated normal human blood lymphocytes, chronic myelogenous leukemia not in an acute blast phase, chronic lymphocytic leukemia and acute myelogenous leukemia, except one AML patient whose cells contained low but definite terminal transferase activity (Table 1). Table 2 summarizes our results on the detection of terminal transferase in the cells of a number of leukemic patients. As shown in this table, we have observed high levels of terminal transferase in 7 out of 20 patients with chronic myelogenous leukemia in acute

Table I: Terminal transferase activity in normal and malignant cells*

Source of Cells	Diagnosis	Incorporation of [^{3}H]dGMP (nmoles per hr per 10^8 cells)
1. Peripheral blood leukocytes from patient:		
#1–7	CML (Blast Crisis)	18–27
#8–20	CML	0.01–0.03
#21	AML	0.2
#22–28	AML	0.03–0.04
#29–33	ALL	4–10
#34–37	CLL	0.05–0.09
2. Normal pheripheral human blood lymphocytes	PHA stimulated (T Cells)	0.03–0.05
3. B-Cells		
NC 37	Normal	0.07
8392	ALL	0.1
SB	ALL	0.01
4. Cell Lines with T-Cell features		
Molt-4	ALL	26
8402	ALL	29
5. Thymus gland		
Human		18
Calf		21

* Terminal transferase assays were carried out at 37° for 1 hr in the presence of 0.1 mM Mn^{2+} in a standard reaction mixture as described in Materials and Methods.

blast phase and in 5 out of 5 patients with acute lymphocytic leukemia. Cells from four patients with chronic lymphocytic leukemia and 7 patients with acute myelogenous leukemia were negative for terminal transferase. Cells from one patient with acute myelogenous leukemia, however, showed definite but low levels of terminal transferase acitivity.

Table II: Terminal transferase in human leukemic cells

Diagnosis	Number of Cases Tested	Number Positive for TdT
1. Chronic Myelogenous Leukemia		
Acute Blast Phase	20	7
Chronic Phase	13	0
2. Acute Myelogenous Leukemia	8	1
3. Acute Lymphocytic Leukemia	5	5
4. Chronic Lymphocytic Leukemia	4	0

The distribution of terminal transferase acitivity on a sucrose gradient (5–20 %) from extracts of Molt-4 cells and cells from two CML patients in acute blast phase of the disease is shown in figure 1. The levels of activity observed in patient #1 and a T cell line (Molt 4) are similar.

Terminal transferase levels in remission: We also analyzed the cells of a CML patient whose cells had high levels of terminal transferase in the acute blast phase, after chemotherapy and induction of remission. Cells were obtained from this patient when he was in complete hematological remission and examined for the presence of terminal transferase. As shown in Table 3, the level of terminal transferase returned to the negligible levels characteristic of normal blood lymphocytes and B cell lines.

Table III: Terminal transferase in CML cells*

Diagnosis	Incorporated of [^{3}H]dGMP (nmoles per hr per 10^8 cells)
Chronic Myelogenous Leukemia	
1. Acute Blast Phase	27
2. Remission	0.1

* Terminal transferase assays were carried out at 37° for 1 hr as described in Materials and Methods.

Properties of purified terminal transferase: Terminal transferase was purified from CML cells (patient #1) by successive chromatography on DEAE cellulose, phosphocellulose and hydroxyapatite columns (5, 6, 8). Terminal transferase and DNA polymerase β were eluted together from DEAE cellulose in 0.05 M KCI

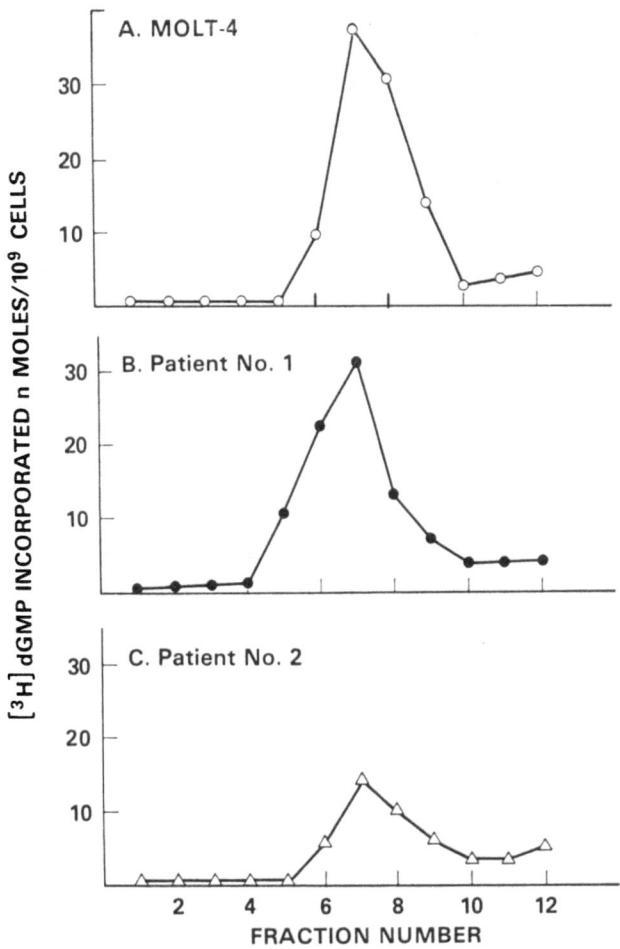

Fig. 1: *Sucrose gradient analysis of terminal transferase:* An aliquot (0.2 ml) of the cell extract was layered on top of a 4.5 ml sucrose gradient (5–20 %) made in 50 mM Tris-HCl, pH 7.5, 1 mM dithiothreitol, 0.5 M KCl and 0.1 mg/ml bovine serum albumin and centrifuged for 16 hrs. at 189,000 xg in a spinco SW 50.1 rotor. Fractions were collected from the bottom of the tube and an aliquot (10 µl) was assayed for terminal transferase as described in *Materials and Methods.* (A) Molt-4, O—O; (B) Patient #1, ●—●; (C) Patient #2, △—△.

wash (5, 6, 8). The DEAE cellulose pool was subsequently chromatographed on a phosphocellulose column. Figure 2A shows the elution of terminal transferase around 0.2M KCl, whereas DNA polymerase β is eluted at 0.34 M KCl. A second minor peak of terminal transferase observed around 0.25 M KCl is a column artifact, and it is produced by the sudden increase in the salt concentration

495

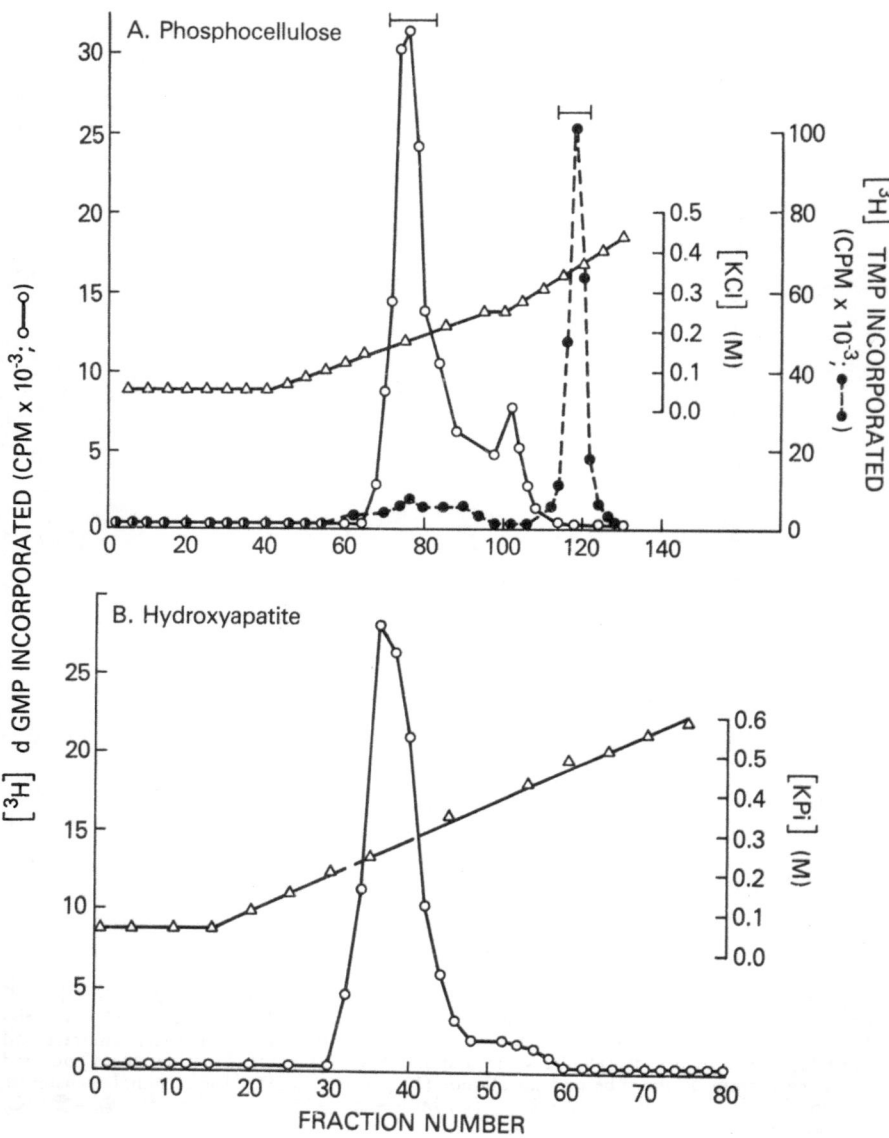

Fig. 2: A. *Chromatography of terminal transferase on phosphocellulose:* The DEAE cellulose (0.05 M KCl wash) pool containing the terminal transferase activity was adsorbed on a phosphocellulose column (Whatman P-11) (4 x 1.4 cm) equilibrated with buffer C. After washing the column with buffer C (50 ml), the column was developed with 50 ml linear gradient of KCl between 0.05 and 0.7 M. Fractions (0.5 ml) were collected and assayed for terminal transferase as described in *Materials and Methods.* DNA polymerase

assays to detect DNA polymerase β in the column fractions were carried out in a standard reaction mixture which contained (dT)$_{15}$·poly (dA) as the template-primer and [³H]dTTP as the labelled substrate under conditions described in *Materials and Methods*. Poly(dA), (○—○); dT$_{15}$·poly(dA), (●—●).

B. *Chromatography of terminal transferase on hydroxyapatite:* The phosphocellulose fractions containing the terminal transferase activity were pooled and dialyzed before adsorption on a hydroxyapatite column (4 x 1.4 cm) equilibrated with buffer D. The column was washed with 20 ml buffer D, and then developed with 50 ml linear gradient of buffer D and 0.8 M phosphate buffer (pH 7.5) containing 1 mM DTT, 0.05 % triton X-100 and 20 % glycerol. Fractions (0.5 ml) were collected and assayed for terminal transferase as described in Materials and Methods with poly(dA) as the initiator (○—○).

of the gradient. The enzyme from the phosphocellulose column was further purified by chromatography on a hydroxapatite column. It was eluted from this column with 0.25 M phosphate buffer (figure 2B). The enzyme at this step was approximately 1000 fold purified and was used for the experiments described below.

The effect of the addition of unlabeled deoxyribonucleoside triphosphates on the activity of terminal transferase in the presence of Mn^{2+} is summarized in table 4. As shown in this table, the polymerization of one deoxyribonucleoside triphosphate is affected by the addition of other deoxyribonucleoside triphosphates, a property characteristic of terminal transferase. DNA polymerases on the other hand require all four deoxyribonucleoside triphosphates for optimum DNA synthesis.

Table IV: Effect of the Addition of Deoxyribonucleoside Triphosphates on the Polymerization of [³H] dGTP Catalyzed by Terminal Deoxynucleotidyl transferase from CML cells

Substrate	[³H] dGMP Incorporated per reaction*	
	pmoles	%
[H³] dGTP	44	100
[H³] dGTP + dATP	4.0	9
[H³] dGTP + dATP + dCTP	2.8	6
[H³] dGTP + dATP + dCTP + dTTP	2.0	5

* Terminal transferase assays were carried out at 37° for 30 min. in the presence of 0.1 mM Mn^{2+} in a standard reaction mixture as described in Materials and Methods. Activated salmon sperm DNA was used as the initiator at a final concentration of 50 µg/ml. 20 µM of [³H] dGTP and 80 µM of the unlabeled deoxyribonucleoside triphosphates were used where indicated.

As shown in table 5 terminal transferase purified from CML cells, cell line 8402, and calf thymus gland efficiently utilizes oligo and polydeoxyribonucleotides as initiators. Oligo (dA) and poly (dA) are the most effective initiators for this enzyme whereas oligo and polyribonucleotides are very inefficient (1, 5, 6, 8).

The purified enzyme has a Mn^{2+} optimum of 0.1 mM, Mg^{2+} optimum of 7 mM (figure 3), and a pH optimum of 7.5 (figure 4). Terminal transferase activity

Table V: Comparison of response of terminal transferase from Human Leukemic cells, Calf Thymus and of the 8402 cell line to various DNA and RNA initiators

Initiator	pmoles [^{3}H] dGMP incorporated per reaction*		
	CML	Calf Thymus	8402
1. Deoxyribonucleotide			
$(dA)_{15}$	730	2500	850
$(dC)_{15}$	250	650	380
$(dT)_{15}$	80	200	180
$(dA)_n$	200	2300	730
$(dC)_n$	15	70	70
$(dT)_n$	130	400	290
2. Ribonucleotide			
$(A)_4$	5	2	9
$(A)_n$	7	2	7
$(U)_n$	3	2	4

* Terminal transferase assays were carried out at 37° for 30 min., as described in Materials and Methods, in the presence of 0.1 mM Mn^{2+}. The initiator concentration used for the assays was 50 µg/ml. $(dN)_{15}$ represents an average chain length of 15 derived from oligodeoxyribonucleotides of chain length from 12 to 18.

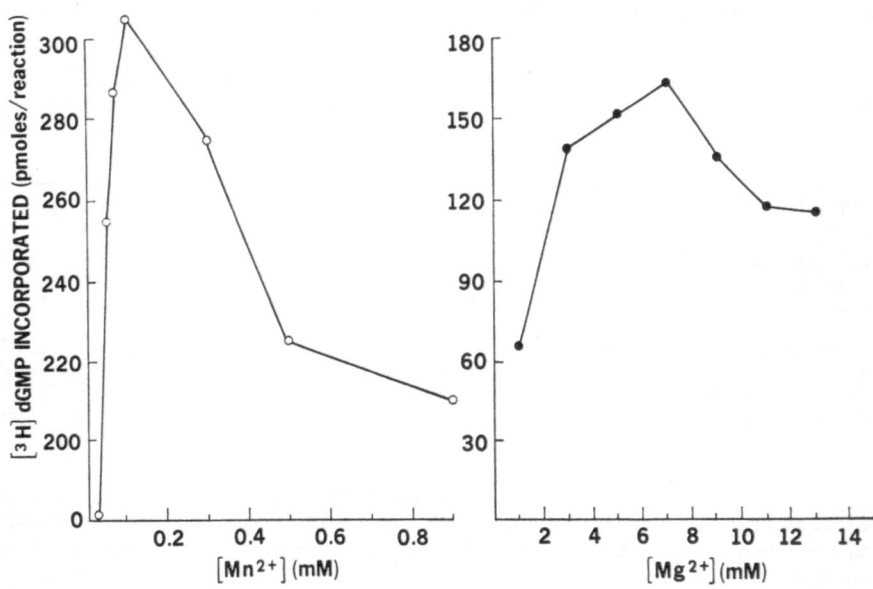

Fig. 3: Effect of divalent cation concentration on poly(dA) initiated [^{3}H]dGMP incorporation by terminal transferase. (A) Mn^{2+} (O—O); (B) Mg^{2+} (●—●).

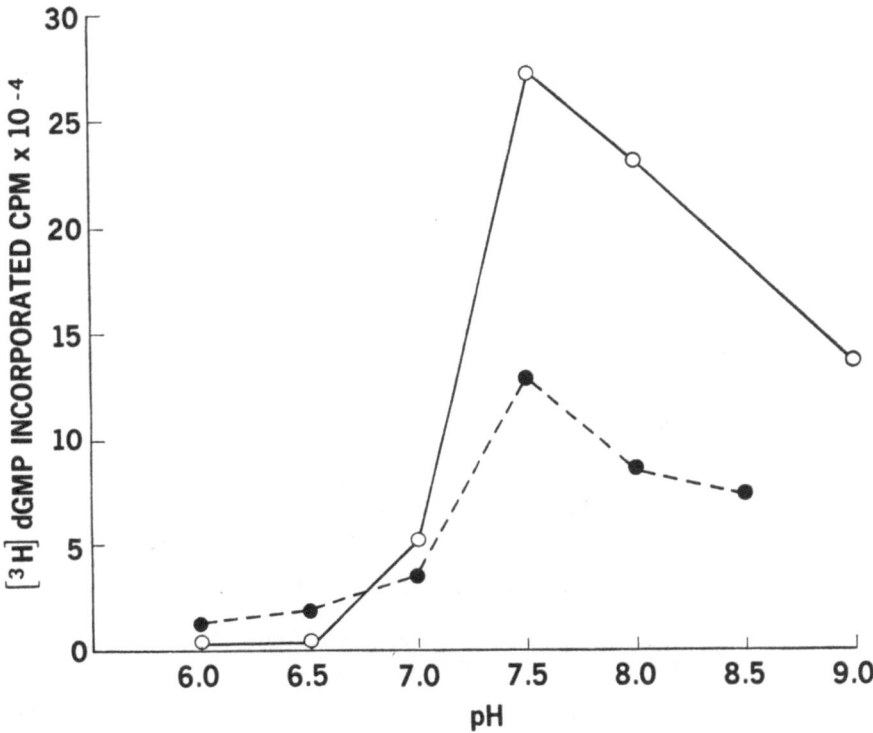

Fig. 4: Effect of pH on poly dA initiated [³H]dGMP incorporation by terminal transferase. Mn^{2+} (O—O); Mg^{2+} (●—●).

was inhibited by N-ethylmalemide and sodium pyrophosphate as shown in figure 5. DNA polymerase β, on the other hand, is only inhibited by N-ethylmalemide at high concentrations (15). The purified enzyme has a sedimentation value of 3.4S as estimated by sucrose density gradient centrifugation (16) with ovalbumin as a marker (figure 6). This value is similar to the value reported for terminal transferase from thymus gland and from cell lines with T cell characteristics (1, 5, 6, 8).

Discussion

Terminal transferase, an enzyme first isolated from calf thymus was considered to be specific for thymus tissue since it was not detected in bone marrow, liver, lungs, lymph nodes and spleen (17). Recent studies have shown that this enzyme is also present in peripheral blood from many patients with acute lymphocytic leukemia (2, 6, 7) and in some patients with acute myelomonocytic leukemia (3) or chronic myelogenous leukemia in acute "blast" phase of the disease (5, 6, 7). Low levels of terminal transferase have also been reported in normal bone marrow

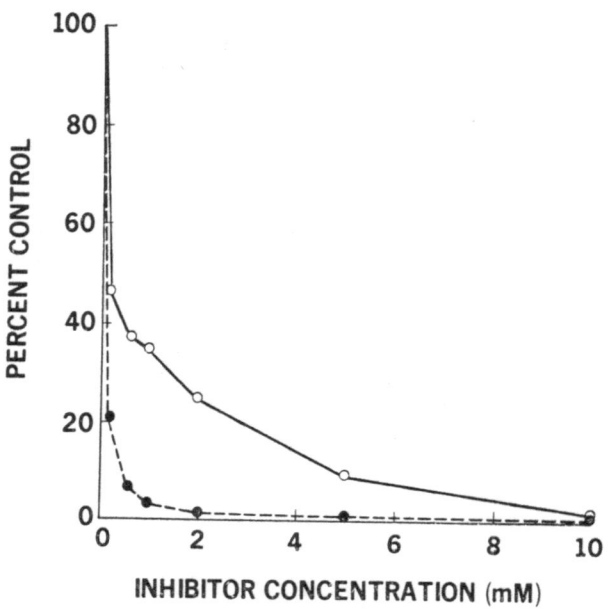

Fig. 5: Effect of inhibitor concentration on terminal transferase activity (A) N-Ethylmaleimide (O—O); (B) Sodium pyrophosphate, (●—●).

(3, 7). Based on the detection of terminal transferase in acute lymphocytic leukemia cells, McCaffrey et al. (2, 7) suggested that these cells were of thymus related lineage.

In this report and elsewhere (5, 6) we have shown that high levels of terminal transferase are present in leukocytes of some patients with chronic myelogenous leukemia in acute blast phase of the disease. Similar results have recently been reported (7). These levels are comparable to the levels of activity observed in human and calf thymus tissue and in cell lines with T cell characteristics (Molt 4 and 8402). Insignificant levels of this activity are detected in normal cells, B cell lines, CLL and AML cells. Cells from one patient with AML, however, contained definite but low levels of terminal transferase activity. In addition we find that high levels of terminal transferase detected in the leukocytes of a CML patient in acute "blast" phase of the disease returned to levels present in normal cells after hematological remission. These results suggest that in some CML patients in acute blast phase of the disease, there is an induction of terminal transferase which returns to negligible levels (observed in normal cells) after hematological remission. It may, therefore, be possible to use terminal transferase as a sensitive biological marker to follow these patients during treatment and in remission.

In our studies so far, we have observed high levels of terminal transferase in 7 out of 20 patients with chronic myelogenous leukemia in acute blast phase of the disease, demonstrating that this enzyme is not present in all CML cells in blast phase. All of the patients with acute lymphocytic leukemia, on the other hand,

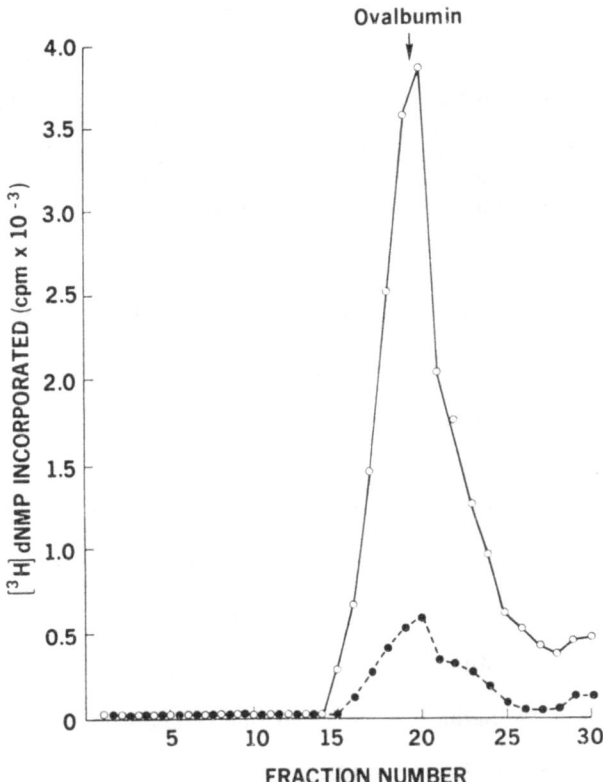

Fig. 6: *Sedimentation analysis of terminal transferase:* An aliquot (0.2 ml) of the purified enzyme was layered on top of a 4.5 ml sucrose gradient (5–20 %) made in 50 mM Tris-HCl, pH 7.5, 1 mM DTT, 0.5 M KCl, and centrifuged for 16 hrs. at 189,000 xg in spinco SW 50.1 rotor. Ovalbumin as a marker protein was centrifuged on a parallel gradient. Fractions (0.15 ml) were collected from the bottom of the tube and an aliquot (10 μl) was assayed for terminal transferase as described in Materials and Methods. [³H]dGMP incorporation with (dA)₁₅ as initiator (O—O). [³H]dTMP incorporation with (dT)₁₅·poly (dA) as initiator (●--●).

contained terminal transferase. These results point to the possibility that in some CML in acute blast phase, undifferentiated lymphoblasts (which may be precursor to T cells) rather than myeloblasts may be the cells which proliferate. The possibility of lymphoblastic conversion in CML has recently been suggested (7, 18, 19). If lymphoblastic conversion occurs in some cases of CML as it appears, then terminal transferase levels may also be useful as a diagnostic marker to predict the type of CML patients that may respond to treatment with predisone and Vincristine.

Acknowledgement

We thank Dr. Bayard Clarkson, Dr. Timothy Gee and Dr. Yashar Hirshaut, Sloan Kettering Institute; Dr. Kenneth McCredie, M. D. Anderson Hospital; Dr. Martin Oken, University of Minnesota; Dr. Bruce Chabner, National Cancer Institute; and Dr. George Canellos, Harvard Medical School for Leukemic Cells. We thank Bong Hee Ro for expert technical assistance.

References

1. Bollum, F. J.: *In, The Enzymes,* Boyer, P. D. (ed.), Academic Press, vol. X: 145–171, 1974.
2. McCaffrey, R., Smoler, D. F., and Baltimore, D.: *Proc. U.S. Nat. Acad. Sci., 70:* 521–525, 1973.
3. Coleman, M. S., Hutton, J. J., Simone, P. D., and Bollum, F. J.: *Proc. U.S. Nat. Acad. Sci., 71:* 4404–4408, 1974.
4. Srivastava, B.: *Cancer Research, 34:* 1015–1026, 1974.
5. Sarin, P. S. and Gallo, R. C.: *J. Biol. Chem., 249:* 8051–8053, 1974.
6. Sarin, P. S., Anderson, P. N., and Gallo. R. C.: *Blood,* 11–20, 1976.
7. McCaffrey, R., Harrison, T., Parkman, R., and Baltimore, P.: *N. Engl. J. Med., 292:* 775–780 1975.
8. Sarin, P. S. and Gallo, R. C.: *Biochem. Biophys. Res. Communs., 65:* 673–682, 1975.
9. Srivastava, B. and Minowada, J.: *Biochem. Biophys. Res. Communs., 51:* 529–535, 1973.
10. Sarngadharan, M., Sarin, P. S., Reitz, M. and Gallo, R. C.: *Nature New Biol., 240:* 67–72, 1972.
11. Jones, A. L.: *Transfusion,* 8: 94–103, 1968.
12. Huang, C., Hou, Y., Woods, L., Moore, G., and Minowada, J.: *J. Nat. Cancer Inst., 53:* 655–660, 1974.
13. Durr, F. E., Monroe, J. H., Schmitter, R., Traul, K. A., and Hirshaut, Y.: *Int. J. Cancer, 6:* 436–449, 1970.
14. Gallo, R. C. and Whang-Peng, J.: *In, Biological effects of polynucleotides,* Beers, R. and Braun, W. (eds.) Springer-Verlag, New York: 303–334, 1971.
15. Smith, R. and Gallo, R.: *Proc. U.S. Nat. Acad. Sci., 69:* 2879–2884, 1972.
16. Martin, R. C. and Ames, B. N.: *J. Biol. Chem., 236:* 1372–1379, 1960.
17. Chang, L. M. S.: *Biochem. Biophys. Res. Communs., 44:* 124–131, 1971.
18. Boggs, D. R.: *Blood,* 44: 449–453, 1974.
19. Gallo, R. C.: *N. Engl. J. Med., 292:* 804–805, 1975.

Terminal Deoxynucleotidyl Transferase in Normal and Neoplastic Hematopoietic Cells

Ronald McCaffrey, Thomas A. Harrison,
Patrick C. Kung, Robertson Parkman,
Allen E. Silverstone, and David Baltimore

From the Center for Cancer Research and the Department of Biology, Massachusetts Institute of Technology, Cambridge, Massachusetts, the Division of Hematology-Oncology, and Immunology of the Department of Medicine, Children's Hospital Medical Center, the Sidney Farber Cancer Center, and the Department of Pediatrics, Harvard Medical School, Boston, Massachusetts.

Introduction

In 1973 we first reported our finding of terminal deoxynucleotidyl transferase (TdT) in the circulating leukemic cells of a child with acute lymphoblastic leukemia (1). Until that time this unique DNA synthetic enzyme had been thought to be a special biochemical property of cells undergoing maturation in the thymus (2). Its presence in circulating lymphoblastic leukemia cells suggested that the thymus might play a role in the pathogenesis of this disease in man, analogous to the central position it plays in the pathogenesis of lymphoblastic leukemia in the AKR mouse (3, 4, 5). In addition, it appeared to have potential clinical utility as a new biochemical leukemia cell marker (1, 6).

We have now accumulated extensive data on the expression of this unusual enzyme in leukemia cells from a large number of patients. We have, in addition, been able to identify TdT in both human and murine bone marrow, and have partially characterized the TdT-positive normal marrow cells. Several new facts have emerged from this work which allow for new insight into the cellular origins of leukemia cells in various clinical entities.

Enzyme Extraction and Identification

The preparation of cells and tissues for TdT assays is as previously described (1, 6, 7, 8) with some recent modifications. Immediatley before homogenization phenylmethylsulfonylfluoride, a serine protease inhibitor, and ethanol are added to a concentration of 20 mM and 5 % respectively, in order to inhibit proteolytic degradation of TdT when samples containing cells rich in proteolytic activity (e. g. phagocytic cells in normal bone marrow, or chronic myelogenous leukemia) are studied. After detergent treatment, the crude homogenate is extracted with high salt which results in more efficient enzyme solubilization (8). TdT activity is then identified following phosphocellulose chromatography of the crude homogenate.

The assay involves providing the enzyme source with a radio-labeled deoxynucleotide triphosphate (usually ^{3}H-dGTP) and a pre-formed DNA primer molecule (usually a short polymer of deoxyadenylic acid, oligo(dA)$_{14}$) onto whose 3'-OH terminus deoxynucleotide monophosphates can be polymerized from deoxynucleotide triphosphate substrates (7, 8).

TdT in leukemia cells

Leukemic cells from almost every patient with acute lymphoblastic leukemia (ALL) contain TdT as part of their biochemical phenotype. The phosphocellulose elution pattern of TdT from the circulating blast cells of a typical patient with ALL is shown in Figure 1. This phosphocellulose elution profile shows two discrete peaks of TdT activity which (Fig. 1B and 1C) maintain their separateness after

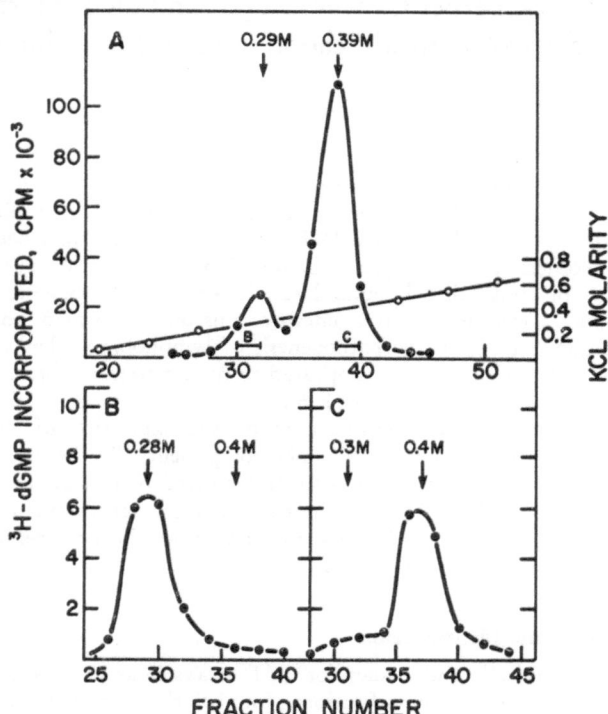

Fig. 1: TdT activity from peripheral blood of a patient with acute lymphoblastic leukemia.
Panel A: Activity recovered on initial phosphocellulose chromatography. Panels B and C: activities recovered after rechromatography on phosphocellulose of pooled fractions from initial column (indicated as "B" and "C" in panel A), after dialysis and passage through a DEAE cellulose column.

chromatography on DEAE, followed by rechromatography on a second phosphocellulose column. The relative ratios shown on initial phosphocellulose chromatography of the early eluting (peak I) to late eluting (peak II) peak are fairly
constant. In a few patients virtually all the TdT activity was confined to the
peak II region, with the peak I region reduced to a "shoulder."

The phosphocellulose pattern shown in Figure 1 is typical of newly diagnosed
patients with ALL using leukemic cells from either peripheral blood or bone
marrow. However, in 4 (out of 4 studied) bone marrow samples taken from ALL
patients with acute, unexpected bone marrow relapse the pattern shown in Figure 2
was seen. Here peak I predominates, with peak II reduced to a shoulder.

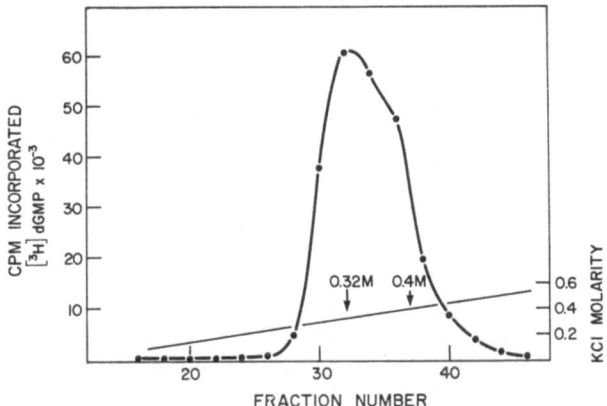

Fig. 2: TdT activity from bone marrow of a patient with acute unexpected bone marrow
relapse.

The significance of these patterns has not been established. It is not known
whether these peaks exist in separate cell types, whose ratio varies in different
stages of the disease, or whether their relative ratios represent molecular
phenomena within a single cell population.

We have identified TdT activity in leukemic cells from 32 of 36 patients
clinically considered to have ALL. A wide spectrum of patients was sampled, both
children and adults, representing both T-cell and null-cell disease. However, as
shown in Table 1 it is now evident that TdT is not confined to leukemic cells from
patients who are considered to have ALL by the usuall clinical and morphological
criteria. As shown in this table, 8 of 22 patients with blast crisis chronic
myelogenous leukemia had TdT positive cells. Only 3 of these 8 enzyme-positive
samples were felt to have lymphoblastic morphology by their physicians. Some
patients with undifferentiated leukemic cell morphology and monomyelocytic leukemia also had TdT positive cells. The TdT activities observed in these non-ALL
samples were similar, in terms of chromatographic pattern, to the ALL samples.

In a later section we will propose that this commonality of TdT activity in cells
from diverse clinical syndromes implies a biologic relatedness in terms of the

cellular origin of these diseases (the papers by Greaves et al. and Sarin et al. in this volume should also be consulted in this regard).

Terminal transferase in human leukemia cells

Cells Positive		
Acute lymphoblastic leukemia	32 of 36	patients
Blast crisis chronic myelogenous leukemia	8 of 22	"
Acute undifferentiated leukemia	3 of 4	"
Acute monomyeloblastic leukemia	1 of 2	"
Cells Negative		
Acute myeloblastic leukemia	9 of 9	patients
Stable phase chronic myelogenous leukemia	6 of 6	"
Chronic lymphatic leukemia	6 of 6	"
Sezary syndrome	2 of 2	"
Lymphosarcoma cell leukemia	3 of 3	"

TdT in normal cells

THYMOCYTES

The phosphocellulose elution pattern of TdT from human thymocytes is quite similar to leukemia cell TdT. (Compare Figure 1 and Figure 3 below). When thymocytes are further separated on a discontinuous bovine serum albumin (BSA) gradient and assayed for TdT (7), the enzyme activity is maximally expressed in cells from gradient layers 3, 4 and 5 (Fig. 4). When thymocytes from such a BSA gradient are studied for other characteristics, only cells from layers 2 and 3 are found to respond to phytohemagglutinin and allogeneic lymphocytes (9). TdT is therefore maximally expressed in thymocytes which are distinct from those thymocytes which are capable of mature T-lymphocyte immunologic reactivity. In the mouse thymus, TdT is also maximally expressed in cells of medium density as determined by BSA gradient analysis (8).

The ratio of peak I to peak II TdT acitivity varies from layer to layer in BSA gradients of both human and murine thymocytes. Medium density thymocytes contain predominantly peak II, whereas peak I predominates in low density thymocytes. In the murine thymus, during the repopulation period which follows cortisone-induced involution, the ratio of peak I to peak II changes dramatically (Fig. 5). In the first few days following cortisone shock, peak I containing cells predominate. The pre-cortisone ratios are gradually reachieved around day 6.

This fluctuation in peak I/peak II ratios is reminiscent of the variant patterns described above for relapse versus well established disease in ALL. One possible interpretation of these results is that peak I may exist in a more primitive (precursor type) cell, which accumulates during acute "explosive" events, such as thymic repopulation following cortisone shock, or acute leukemia relapse.

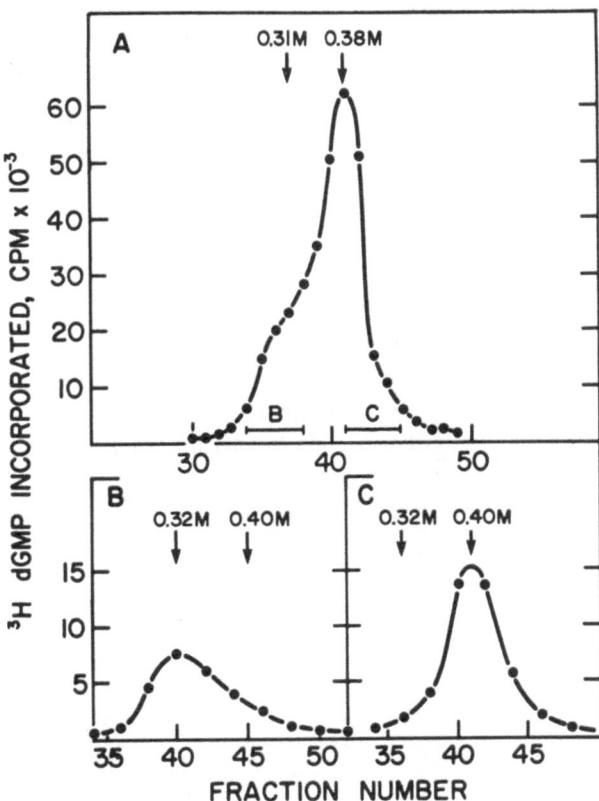

Fig. 3: TdT acitivity from normal human thymocytes.
Panel A: Activity recovered on initial phosphocellulose chromatography. Panels B and C: activities recovered after rechromatography on phosphocellulose of pooled fractions from initial column (indicated as "B" and "C" in pael A), after dialysis and passage through a DEAE cellulose column.

BONE MARROW

It is now clear that there exists in normal bone marrow a population of cells which expresses TdT activity (7, 8, 10). In man, the phosphocellulose chromatographic pattern is a broad peak, eluting between peak I and II positions (Fig. 6). It is similar to the pattern observed when bone marrow cells from ALL patients with acute bone marrow relapse are analyzed (Fig. 6). In the mouse, the normal bone marrow enzyme chromatographs in the thymocyte peak I position, with a small peak in the peak II position, similar to that seen in low density thymocytes. Biochemically the marrow activity from either species is indistinguishable from the thymocyte or leukemic cell activity of the same species.

Some information is available on the nature of the normal marrow cell population(s) which contains TdT. TdT-positive cells can be eliminated from normal

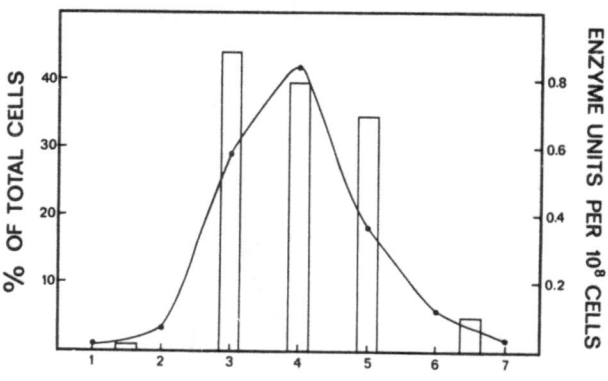

FRACTION NUMBER

Fig. 4: TdT activity in normal thymocytes fractionated on a 17 to 33 per cent discontinuous bovine serum albumin gradient.

Fractions are numbered from the top of the gradient (17 per cent BSA). The number of cells at each interface, expressed as a per cent of the total number of cells recovered, is shown as closed circles. Enzyme units per 10^8 cells are represented by vertical bars. Bars between fraction numbers refer to assays on pooled cells.

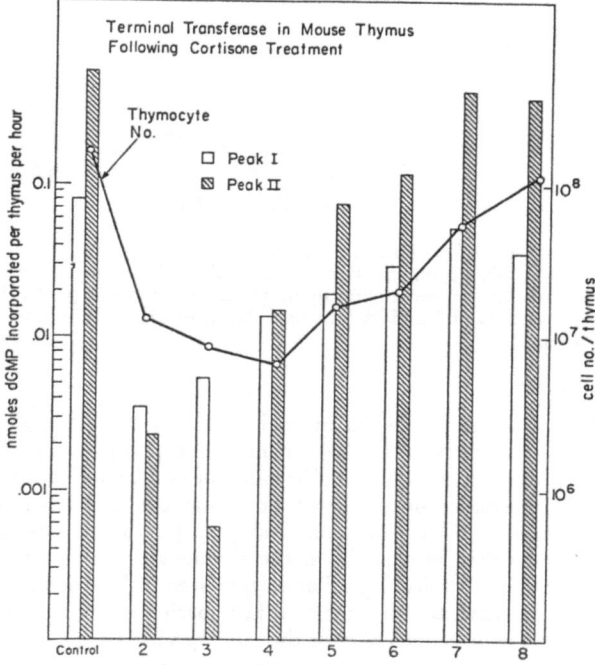

Fig. 5: Effect of cortisone treatment on number of cells and TdT activity in murine thymus.

A single 150 mg/kg dose of cortisone acetate was given to C57Bl/6J mice on day 0. The number of cells per thymus and TdT activity per thymus were determined sequentially thereafter.

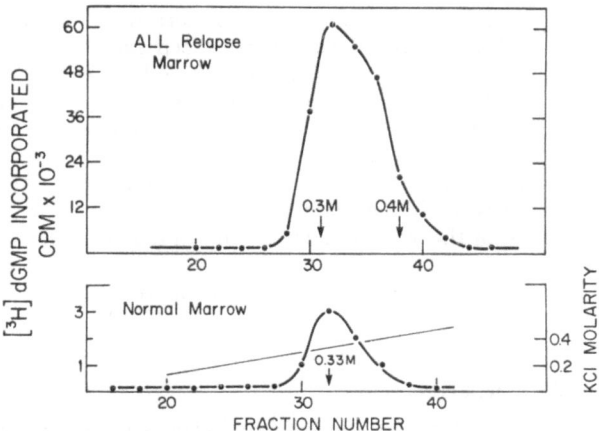

Fig. 6: Chromatographic profiles of TdT activity in acute unexpected bone marrow relapse and normal bone marrow.

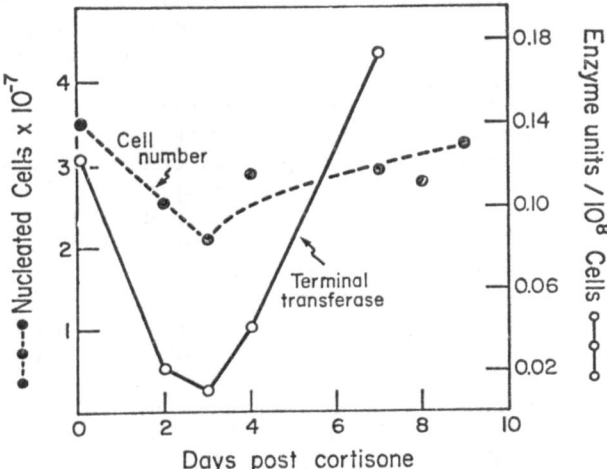

Fig. 7: Effect of cortisone treatment on number of cells and TdT activity in murine bone marrow.
TdT and cell number in the femur and tibia bone marrow were determined as a function of time after a single 150 mg/kg dose of cortisone acetate was given to C57Bl/6J mice on day 0.

mouse marrow by cortisone administration (Fig. 7). Cell losses from the marrow compartment following such perturbation are due to a combination of *in situ* destruction, and redistribution to other sites (thymus, spleen, nodes, peripheral blood) and involve predominately marrow lymphocytes (11, 12). The almost total loss of marrow TdT following cortisone administration suggests a lymphoid nature of the TdT-positive cells.

509

This impression is supported by independent studies with the thymic hormone thymopoietin (13). When normal murine marrow cell suspensions are incubated with thymopoietin, a certain fraction of marrow lymphocytes can be induced to express thymocyte surface markers. These marrow thymopoietin-responsive cells are believed to be prothymocytes (14). In preliminary studies (Silverstone, Cantor, Boyse, Goldstein and Scheid) the induction of Thy 1 antigen in murine marrow cells, followed by the specific elimination of such cells by cytotoxic treatment with anti-Thy 1 antibody, has resulted in the loss of 50–70 % of marrow TdT activity. This suggests that most of the marrow TdT activity in the mouse resides in marrow prothymocytes.

The precise identification of the enzyme-positive marrow population(s) will be of major interest.

Significance of TdT in leukemia cells

The finding of a normal marker on neoplastic cells is generally taken to mean that the tumor cells are related, in a derivative sense, to the cell line which normally expresses the marker in question. Thus, lymphoid malignancies are frequently classified on this basis, using T-lymphocyte and B-lymphocyte surface properties as markers (15). Although there are limitations to the use of such cell phenotypes to construct the ontogeny of neoplastic differentiation (16), it can provide a substrate for useful working hypotheses.

We have analyzed and interpreted the observation of TdT in leukemic cells in the light of its restricted distribution in normal animals (2, 7, 8, 10, 17). We have taken its presence in leukemic cells to mean that such cells are of the same lineage as those normal marrow or thymus cells which also express TdT. In the thymus it is maximally expressed in thymocytes which can be considered "primitive" in that they lack the functional properties associated with mature T-lymphocytes (7, 8, 9). In the marrow, the majority of the TdT-positive cells are cortisone-sensitive and thymopoietin-responsive and may be thymic precursor cells (prothymocytes). In our view, leukemic cells with this enzyme would derive from either TdT-positive thymic lymphocytes or TdT-positive marrow cells and therefore be lymphoid in nature.

We are aware that this sort of biochemical re-classification of leukemic cells does violence to traditional clinical and morphological concepts. The established categories into which leukemic patients are now classified implies a homogeneity among members of specific categories which does not, in fact, exist. The papers in this volume by Moloney, DeSimone, Henderson, and Wiernik should be consulted in this regard. There is obvious diversity in clinical behavior, and response to therapy, among patients who are classified within a single category. There can be little argument about the need for a re-classification which results in more homogeneous grouping. Such attempts at reclassification are being made by Moore et al. (18) and by Dicke et al. (19) using in vitro growth patterns of leukemic cells, and by Greaves et al. (summarized in this volume) using cell surface markers, to categorize patients into meaningful groups.

The significance and utility in terms of clinical management, of a leukemia cell classification based on TdT positivity or negativity remains to be established. However, our postulation that TdT-positive leukemic cells are lymphoblastic in nature, irrespective of their conventional morphological classification, is testable clinically. The combination of the drugs vincristine and prednisone results in high remission rates in ALL, but low rates in non-lymphoblastic leukemia (20). Prospective studies are underway to determine whether the presence of TdT in leukemic cells from diverse clinical syndromes augurs for responsiveness to classic anti-ALL therapy.

Our inability at this time to distinguish, either biochemically or chromatographically, between the enzyme activity observed in normal bone marrow and that present in samples from patients with early bone marrow relapse prevents TdT from being a useful tool in monitoring remission or predicting relapse. However, further enzyme purification and/or the development of a fluorescent antibody assay may discriminate between normal marrow and leukemia-associated TdT, and permit such a use.

On a biological level, the isolation and characterization of the normal bone marrow and thymus cell populations which express TdT should provide important defined cell populations for a variety of fundamental studies. Comparisons between these normal TdT-positive cells, and TdT-positive leukemia cells should be helpful in determining the specificity of particular leukemia cell characteristics. TdT-positive normal cells should also be fruitful populations for studies involving leukemogenic agents or events, particularly if they can be propagated in *in vitro* culture systems.

Acknowledgements

We are indebted to Drs. William C. Moloney, David S. Rosenthal, Joel M. Rappeport, John Truman, Norman Jaffe, Demetrius Traggis, Bruce Camitta, Audrey Evans, Jonathan Glass, Robert McAllister, W. H. Churchill, Willy Piessens, Gerard Price, Dane Boggs, George Sartiano, Edwin Foreman, Bayard Clarkson and Mortimer Greenberg for providing us with some of the clinical samples used in this study, to the late Dr. Frederick Stohlman, Jr., for both clinical samples and much stimulating discussion of this work in progress and to Drs. David G. Nathan and Fred S. Rosen for support and encouragement. This work was supported by grants AM 05581, CA 13472, CA 14051, CA 18662, AI05877 and FR-128 from the National Institutes of Health and a contract with the Virus Cancer Program of the National Cancer Institute. Dr. McCaffrey is a recipient of Research Career Development Award no. CA 00099. Dr. Kung is a postdoctoral fellow of the Jane Coffin Childs Memorial Fund for Medical Research. Dr. Parkman is a scholar of the Leukemia Society of America, Inc. Dr. Silverstone is a postdoctoral fellow of the American Cancer Society, Massachusetts Division. Dr. Baltimore is an American Cancer Society professor of microbiology.

References

1. McCaffrey, R., Smoler, D. F. and Baltimore, D. Terminal deoxynucleotidyl transferase in a case of childhood acute lymphoblastic leukemia. *Proc. Nat. Acad. Sci. USA* (1973) 70: 521–525.
2. Chang, L. M. S. Development of terminal deoxynucleotidyl transferase activity

in embryonic calf thymus gland. *Biochem. Biophys. Res. Commun.* (1971) 44: 124–131.

3. Siegler, R. Pathology of Murine Leukemias. In *Experimental Leukemia,* M. A. Rich, editor, Appleton-Century-Crofts (1968) New York, pp. 51–95.

4. Nagaya, H. Thymus function in spontaneous lymphoid leukemia 1. Premature leukemogenesis in "young" thymectomized mice bearing "old" thymus grafts. *J. Immun.* (1973) 111: 1048–1051.

5. Nagaya, H. Thymus function in spontaneous lymphoid leukemia II. *In vitro* response of "preleukemic" and leukemic thymus cells to mitogens. *J. Immun.* (1973) 111: 1052–1060.

6. McCaffrey, R., Smoler, D. F., Harrison, T. A. and Baltimore, D. A thymus specific enzyme in acute lymphoblastic leukemia cells. In *Advances in the Biosciences,* vol. 14, T. M. Fliedner and S. Perry, editors. Pergamon Press (1974), New York, pp. 527—534.

7. McCaffrey, R., Harrison, T. A., Parkman, R. and Baltimore, D. Terminal deoxynucleotidyl transferase acitivity in human leukemic cells and in normal human thymocytes. *New Eng. J. Med.* (1975) 292: 775–780.

8. Kung, P. C., Silverstone, A. E., McCaffrey, R. P. and Baltimore, D. Murine terminal deoxynucleotidyl transferase: cellular distribution and response to cortisone. *J. Exp. Med.* (1975) 141: 855–865.

9. Parkman, R. and Merler, E. Discontinuous density gradient analysis of the developing human thymus. *Cell Immunol.* (1973) 8: 328–331.

10. Coleman, M. S., Hutton, J. J., DeSimone, P. and Bollum, F. J. Terminal deoxynucleotidyl transferase in human leukemia. *Proc. Nat. Acad. Sci. USA* (1974) 71: 4404–4408.

11. Blomgren, H. and Anderson, B. Characteristics of the immunocompetent cells in the mouse thymus: cell population changes during cortisone induced atrophy and subsequent regeneration. *Cell Immun.* (1971) 1: 545–560.

12. Clayman, H. N. Corticosteroids and lymphoid cells. *New Eng. J. Med.* (1972) 287: 388–397.

13. Goldstein, G. Isolation of bovine thymin: a polypeptide hormone of the thymus. *Nature* (1974) 247: 11–14.

14. Boyse, E. A. and Abbott, J. Surface reorganization as an initial inductive event in the differentiation of prothymocytes to thymocytes. *Fed. Proc.* (1975) 34: 24–27.

15. Seligmann, M., Preud'Homme, J. L., and Brouet J. C. B and T Cell markers in human proliferative blood diseases and primary immunodeficiencies, with special reference to membrane bound immunoglobulins. *Transplant. Rev.* (1973) 16: 85–113.

16. Greaves, M. F., Brow, G., Capellaro, D., Janossy, C. and Revesz, T. Immunologic approaches to the identification of leukemic cells (1975) *Eur. J. Cancer,* in press.

17. Bollum, F. J. Terminal deoxynucleotidyl transferase, In *The Enzymes,* vol. 10, R. D. Boyer, editor, Academic Press (1974), New York, pp. 145—171.

18. Moore, M. A. S. Marrow culture: a new approach to classification of leukemia. In *Blood Cells,* vol. 1, M. Bessis, Editor, Pergamon Press, New York, in press.

19. Dicke, K. A., Spitzer, G. and Ahearn, M. J. Colony formation *in vitro* by leukemic cells in acute myelogenous leukemia with phytohemagglutinin as stimulating factor. *Nature* (1976) 259: 129–130.
20. Perry, S. Human leukemia – An overview (1974 In *Modern Trends in Human Leukemia*. R. Neth, R. C. Gallo, S. Spiegelman and F. Stohlman, editors, J. F. Lehmans Verlag, Munchen, Germany, pp. 6–19.

A New, not Virus Related Reverse Transcriptase in the Chicken System

G. Bauer, G. Jilek and P. H. Hofschneider

Max-Planck-Institut für Biochemie, Martinsried bei München

We thank Drs. K. Moelling, J. Beard, R. C. Gallo and S. Spiegelman for generous gifts of REV, AMV and IgG against AMV reverse transcriptase, and Drs. R. Friis and A. Vaheri for their kind help in performing the described virological controls and radio-immune assays. We also thank Miss Terttu Jelve for her continuous help in purifying the particles. The work was supported by the Deutsche Forschungsgemeinschaft and by Dr. E. Vielitz, Lohmann Tierzucht Cuxhaven, who supplied leukosis virus-free eggs.

Materials and Methods

Labelled deoxyribonucleoside triphosphates were products of Amersham/Buchler and Schwarz Mann. Unlabelled deoxyribonucleoside triphosphates and PolyA $(dT)_{12}$ were obtained from Boehringer, Mannheim. All other templates used were products of P. L. Biochemicals, Milwaukee. Bovine Serum Albumin (A grade) was from Calbiochem.

AMV was generously supplied by Dr. J. Beard.

Purified REV, strain T, was kindly provided by Dr. K. Moelling and Dr. R. Friis, University of Giessen.

Anti-IgG was a generous gift of the laboratories of Dr. Gallo and Dr. Spiegelman.

Most of the experiments were performed with allantoic fluid of eggs from SPF-VALO chickens. The eggs were generously supplied, to the greater part, by Dr. E. Vielitz, Lohmann Tierzucht, Cuxhaven.

Standardpolymerase assay: The concentrations were 10 mM MgAcetat, 20 mM KCl, 50 mM Tris - HCl, pH 8.3, 10 mM DTE, 1 mM ATP. The usual assays of 100 µl volume contained 5 µCi labelled deoxynucleoside triphosphate (8 Ci/mMol) and 1 µg of template-primer complex. For the test of particles the assay contained NP 40 in final concentration of 0.1 %. Tests of purified enzyme contained 50 µg bovine serum albumin in 100 µl reaction mix.

When heteropolymeric nucleic acid was used as template, the unlabelled deoxynucleoside triphosphates were each at a concentration of 0.3 mM.

To get optimal activity with pC(dG), one has to use extremely clean reagents and has to heat the template-primer to 80 °C for 5–10 minutes before using it.

The reaction mix was incubated at 37 °C and the reaction was stopped by adding 10 % TCA, containing 1 % pyrophosphate. The acid-insoluble radioactivity was collected by filtering the samples through Millipore nitrocellulose filters (pore size of 0.6 μ).

Purification of the polymerases from particles, AMV and REV was as described by Markus et al. (11).

Sedimentation gradients of the enzymes in glycerol was as described by Markus et al. (11).

The IgG-inhibition test of purified polymerases was as described by Watson et al. (15), except that the preincubation of enzyme together with IgG was at 0–4 °C for 12 hours instead of 15 min at 37 °C.

Introduction

In the past years reverse transcription was not only discussed as an unique step in RNA virus-related transformation but also as a possible mechanism involved in transfer of genetic information in normal cells, uninfected with virus. For this reason studies have been performed to detect, in addition to viral reverse transcriptase, corresponding cellular enzymes. However, all enzymes studied could be either related to viruses (1) or do not have the typical template specificity of "true" reverse transcriptase (2, 3, 4): i. e. more efficient utilization of $pA(dT)_{12}$ than of $pdA(dT)_{12}$, high activity with $pC(dG)_{12}$ and the ability to synthesize DNA complementary to natural heteropolymeric RNA (5, 6, 7). As ist was not possible till now, to isolate a cell-specific enzyme with these characteristics from normal cells, the demonstration of reverse transcriptase is often taken as an unmistakable viral footprint. Thus in looking for early diagnostic signals, indicating tumor formation in human tissue, reverse transcriptase has been regarded as a serious candidate. Here we describe the isolation of a reverse transcriptase from particles in the allantoic fluid of embryonated chicken eggs. This enzyme could not be related to Avian Leukosis Viruses/Avian Sarcoma Viruses (ALV/ASV) or Reticuloendotheliosis Viruses (REV), the only chicken viruses known to contain reverse transcriptase, and so is very likely of cellular origin.

Results

Detection and purification of enzyme-containing particles. The allantoic fluid of ten day-old embryonated chicken eggs was collected, cleaned from cells and cell debris and subjected to ultracentrifugation, as for the collection of enveloped RNA viruses. The first pellet was resuspended in buffer and centrifuged through the 20 % sucrose step of a discontinuous gradient onto a cushion, consisting of 50 % sucrose. The material above the 50 % cushion was tested for its ability to use ribohomopolymers and deoxyribohomopolymers as templates for DNA synthesis. The result is shown in Table 1. As can be seen from the table, the ribohomopolymers pC and pA, as well as the deoxyribohomopolymer pdA are quite efficient templates for the isolated activity. As the activity exhibited some of the template characteristics of reverse transcriptase (use of $pC(dG)_{12}$) as well as of cellular DNA polymerase (preference of $pA(dT)_{12}$ over $pdA(dT)_{12}$) we expected to have a mixture of different enzyme activities.

In the next step the material was fractionated on a linear sucrose gradient, and

Table I: Homopolymer-directed DNA synthesis by the crude particle fraction obtained after centrifugation of the allantoic fluid and subsequent discontinuous sucrose gradient centrifugation

Template-primer complex	labelled dNTP	cpm ^{3}H-dNMP incorporated
pC (dG)$_{12-18}$	^{3}H-dGTP	16 629
pA (dT)$_{12}$	^{3}H-dTTP	8 648
pdA (dT)$_{12}$	^{3}H-dTTP	55 159

Legend to Table 1: The allantoic fluid of leukosis virus-free eggs, embryonated for ten days, was cleaned of cells and cell debris. It was then subjected to ultracentrifugation in a fixed-angle rotor (Rotor 30 Beckman) at 27,000 RPM for 45 minutes at 4 °C. The pellets were resuspended in STE buffer (0.1 M NaCl, 0.01 M Tris – HCl pH 8, 0.001 M EDTA) and layered on a discontinuous sucrose gradient in a Beckman SW 27.1 Rotor. The material was centrifuged through 20 % sucrose onto a 50 % cushion (26,000 RPM, 2.5 hours). The material above the 50 % sucrose was collected and diluted to a protein concentration of 0.9 mg/ml. 9 µg of material were incubated under standard polymerase assay conditions, as described in materials and methods, using different template-primer complexes at a concentration of 1 µg/100 µl. The mixture contained NP 40 to a final concentration of 0.1 % and 5 µCi of the respective ^{3}H-deoxynucleoside triphosphate (8 Ci/mMol) in a total volume of 100 µl. Incubation was at 37 °C for 60 minutes. The reaction was stopped by the addition of TCA and the acidinsoluble radioactivity of the total volumes was determined.

Table II: Homopolymer-directed DNA synthesis by purified particles, obtained after velocity sedimentation and sucrose density gradient centrifugation

Template-primer	labelled dNTP	reaction conditions	cpm ^{3}H-dNMP incorporated
pC	dGTP	complete	159
(dG)$_{12-18}$	dGTP	complete	0
pC (dG)$_{12-18}$	dGTP	– NP 40	104
pC (dG)$_{12-18}$	dGTP	– particles	0
pC (dG)$_{12-18}$	dGTP	– Mg^{++}	0
pC (dG)$_{12-18}$	dGTP	complete	17 179
pC (dG)$_{12-18}$	dTTP	complete	0
pdC (dG)$_{12-18}$	dGTP	complete	4 100
pA (dT)$_{12}$	dTTP	complete	5 168
pdA (dT)$_{12}$	dTTP	complete	720

Legend to Table 2: 0.4 µg of particles, which had been purified as described in Figure 1 and 2 were incubated under standard polymerase assay conditions as described in Materials and Methods, in the presence of different Template/Primer complexes as indicated. Conditions were as described in the legend to Table 1.

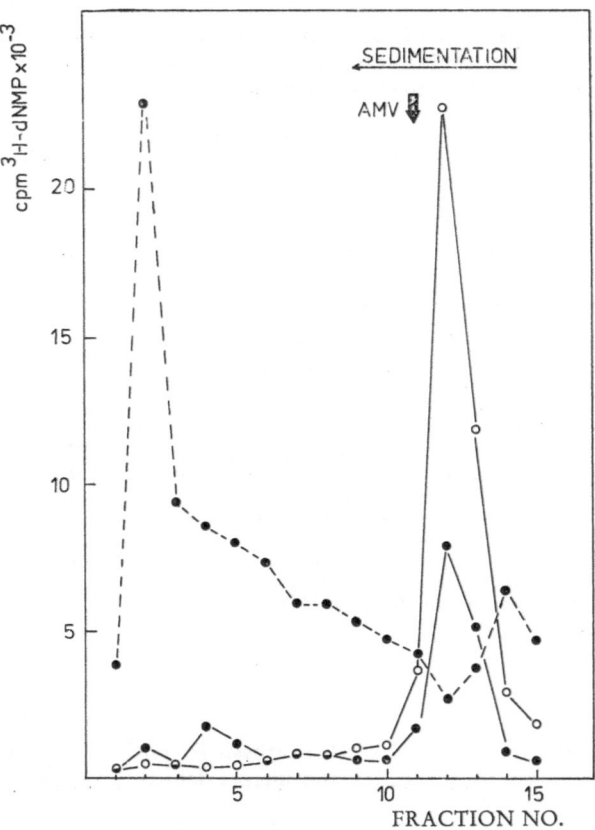

Legend to Fig. 1: Velocity gradient of the sediment from allantoic fluid. The material, after being handled as described in the legend of Table 1, was layered on a continuous sucrose gradient, ranging from 20 to 35 % sucrose w/w (in STE buffer) and centrifuged in a Rotor SW 27.1 in a Spinco ultracentrifuge at 26,000 RPM for 50 minutes. The material was collected from the bottom and the fractions were tested with the template/primers pC (dG) (○—), pA(dT) (●—●), and pdA(dT) (●- - -●) under standard conditions for 1 hour. The acid insoluble radioactivity from the 100 μl reaction mixture was estimated.

the response to the set of templates, as used in the experiment of Table 1, was tested with each fraction. The result is seen in figure 1. Two different enzyme activities can be separated: a pdA-dependent activity, sedimenting to the bottom of the tube, and a slower sedimenting activity, utilizing pA, pC and pdA in the ratio expected for reverse transcriptase. Comparison with AMV, sedimented in a parallel gradient under identical conditions, showed that the material carrying the pC- and pA-directed DNA polymerase sediments slightly slower than AMV. From this and from the fact that the presence of nonionic detergent (NP 40) was requisite for the detection of the pC- and pA-directed DNA polymerase activity, we conclude that the polymerase is particle-bound.

518

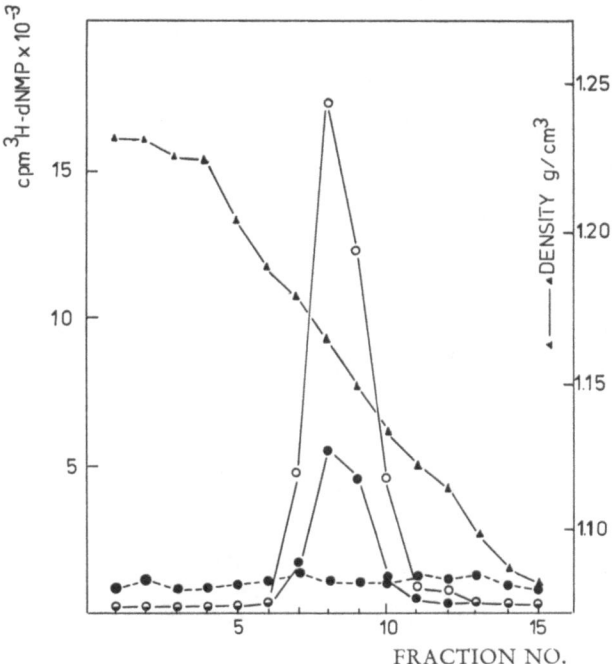

Legend to Fig. 2: Sucrose density gradient of the particles containing polymerase. Fraction 12 and 13 from the gradient described in figure 1 were diluted with STE buffer and layered on a continuous sucrose gradient, ranging from 20 to 50 % sucrose w/w. It was centrifuged in a Rotor SW 41 at 30,000 for 16 hours. The material was collected from the bottom and tested as described in Figure 1. The density of the fractions was calculated by measuring the refractive index. The activity is expressed as cpm of ^{3}H-dNMP incorporated into acid insoluble material within 60 minutes in a volume of 100 μl. (O—O pC·dG, ●—● pA·dT, ●– –● pdA·dT dependent activities).

The fractions with the best response to pC and pA (fraction 12 and 13) were further analyzed by sucrose density gradient centrifugation. The fractionated density gradient was again tested with the same set of templates as before. As seen in figure 2, only one activity peak can be observed in response to the ribohomopolymer templates. The weak pdA-directed activity is distributed all over the gradient.

For the further characterization of the activity, the particles from the peak fraction of the density gradient were tested with an extended set of template-primer complexes (Table 2). The enzyme reaction is dependent on the presence of nonionic detergent, Mg^{++}, primer, template and corresponding deoxynucleoside triphosphate. Template or primer alone do not allow the reaction, and therefore terminal deoxynucleotidyltransferase (8) can be excluded. Furthermore, the efficient utilization of $pC(dG)_{12}$ excludes that R-DNA polymerase (polymerase γ) (9, 10) activity is being tested. The high preference of this template-primer complex and of $pA(dT)_{12}$ over $pdA(dT)_{12}$ clearly differentiates the particle-bound enzyme from the normal cellular DNA polymerases (5, 7) and is typical for reverse transcriptase.

Characterization of the purified enzyme

For final characterization of the enzyme, particles were disrupted by NP 40 in the presence of high salt and the enzyme was further purified by affinity chromatography on polycytidylate-sepharose (11). The adsorbed and then eluted material, which contained too little protein to measure, was tested with homopolymeric (Table 3) and heteropolymeric templates (Table 4). The enzyme exhibits no activity

Table III: Homopolymer-directed DNA synthesis by purified reverse transcriptases from particles and AMV

Template-primer	labelled dNMP	cpm ^{3}H-dNMP incorporated by enzyme isolated from	
		Particles	AMV
$(dG)_{12-18}$	dGTP	0	0
pC $(dG)_{12-18}$	dGTP	28 417	149 651
pdC $(dG)_{12-18}$	dGTP	14 525	80 658
pA $(dT)_{12}$	dTTP	6 679	32 940
pdA $(dT)_{12}$	dTTP	813	639

Legend to Table 3: Reverse transcriptase was purified from concentrated, disrupted particles or AMV by affinity chromatography on polycytidylate-sepharose, as described by Markus et al. (11). After washing the column, the enzymes were eluted by 0.4 M KCl. One of the active fractions was tested under standard polymerase assay conditions, using different template-primer complexes. The activity is expressed as incorporation of radioactivity into acid insoluble material in 100 µl per 90 minutes. In each case the values were obtained from linear kinetics.

with $(dG)_{12}$ alone, which proves that no polycytidylic acid is eluted from the column, i. e. the enzyme is template-free.

The template characteristics of the purified enzyme are identical with those shown for the particle-bound enzyme in Table 2. When the purified enzyme is compared with AMV reverse transcriptase, the template characteristics and the relative utilization of the templates are almost identical. This result clearly distinguishes the particle enzyme from an enzyme, which was purified by Kang and Temin (3) from a fraction from uninfected chicken cells, exhibiting endogenous RNA-directed DNA polymerase activity. When they tested the isolated activity with synthetic templates, they found a preference for pdA over pA, which is typical for normal cellular DNA polymerases. In contrast, the enzyme purified by us shows just the opposite template preference, which is typical for (viral) reverse transcriptase.

To demonstrate that the enzyme could use heteropolymeric RNA, we used globin mRNA as a template for reverse transcription, having added $(dT)_{12}$ as primer (12). To be sure of measuring reverse transcription of the heteropolymeric

Table IV: Response of reverse transcriptases from particles or AMV to natural, heteropolymeric RNA

Template	Primer	Reaction conditions	cpm ^{3}H-dGMP incorporated by	
			particle enzyme	AMV enzyme
globin mRNA	$(dT)_{12}$	complete	3 299	3 800
globin mRNA	$(dT)_{12}$	complete + Act. D	2 866	
globin mRNA	$(dT)_{12}$	complete + RNAse	0	
globin mRNA	–	complete	866	
globin mRNA	$(dT)_{12}$	– dCTP	880	
–	$(dT)_{12}$	complete	0	
pC	$(dG)_{12-18}$	complete	100 883	96 200

Legend to Table 4: Aliquots of the purified enzymes were incubated in the presence of 2.5 µg rabbit globin mRNA and 1 µg $(dT)_{12}$ per 100 µl in the complete system. The conditions were as described for the standard polymerase assay in materials and methods, with the addition of (unlabelled) dATP, dCTP, dTTP to a final concentration of 0.6 mM respectively. The only labelled deoxynucleoside triphosphate was ^{3}H-dGTP (8 Ci/mMol) and was contained in a final concentration of 0.012 mM. Incubation at 37 °C was for 160 minutes in the case of particle enzyme and 40 minutes in the case of AMV enzyme. The acid insoluble radioactivity was determined from the total volume. For comparison an identical assay were run with $pC(dG)_{12-18}$ instead of globin mRNA as a template.

region of the mRNA, and not of the polyA-strand, ^{3}H-dGTP was used as labelled precursor. Table 4 shows the utilization of oligo dT · globin mRNA by the polymerase purified from particles. The full activity is dependent on the presence of template, primer, all four deoxynucleoside triphosphates, and can be completely inhibited by the presence of ribonuclease. Actinomycin D has no clear effect on the reaction, indicating that it does not proceed significantly further than hybrid synthesis. As can be seen from Table 4 as well, the utilization of globin mRNA in comparison to $pC(dG)_{12}$ is as efficient by the particle enzyme as by the AMV enzyme.

To prove that a faithful transcript had been synthesized by the particle enzyme, the reaction product was analyzed on CS_2SO_4 density gradients after different types of treatment. First the reaction product was purified and subjected to the centrifugation without further treatment. The radioacivity is then found in an intermediate position between RNA and DNA, demonstrating that the product is a RNA·DNA hybrid (figure 3A). After alkaline treatment the radioactivity is shifted to the region of DNA density, indicating that DNA had been synthesized by the enzyme (figure 3B). After incubation of the alkaline treated material under conditions suitable for hybridization and in the presence of excess newly-added globin mRNA the radioactivity is found near the RNA position of the density gradient (figure 3C). This demonstrates that the DNA product is in fact complementary to the messenger RNA originally used as template.

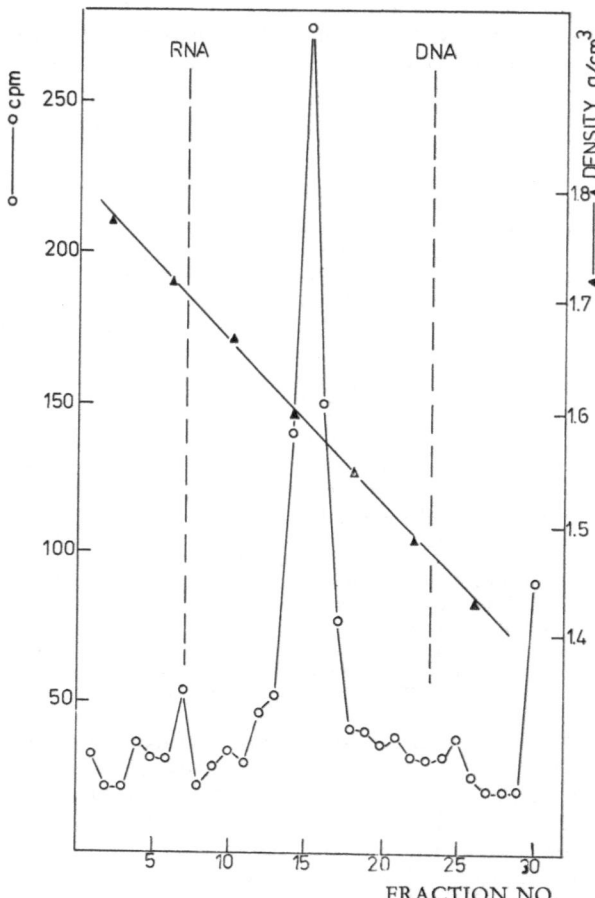

Fig.: 3 A
Legend to Figure 3A–C: Cs_2SO_4 density gradient analysis of ^{3}H-DNA, complementary to globin mRNA, synthesized by purified polymerase from particles. Reaction mixtures as described in the legend to Table 4 were incubated in the presence of oligo dT·globin mRNA, enzyme from particles and Actinomycin D (50 µg/ml) for 2 hours at 37 °C. The product was purified by two-fold phenolisation and subsequent alcohol precipitation. It was resuspended in 2X SSC buffer. The density of the product at this stage of treatment is shown in figure 3A. The product was further treated with 0.25 N KOH for 18 hours at room temperature and then again neutralized. The density of the product at this stage is seen in figure 3B. The alkaline treated product was incubated in a buffer containing 0.4 M NaCl, 2 mM EDTA, 10 mM Tris pH 7.4 and 50 % formamide together with 5 µg of globin messenger RNA at 37 °C for 20 hours. The density of this product is shown in figure 3C.

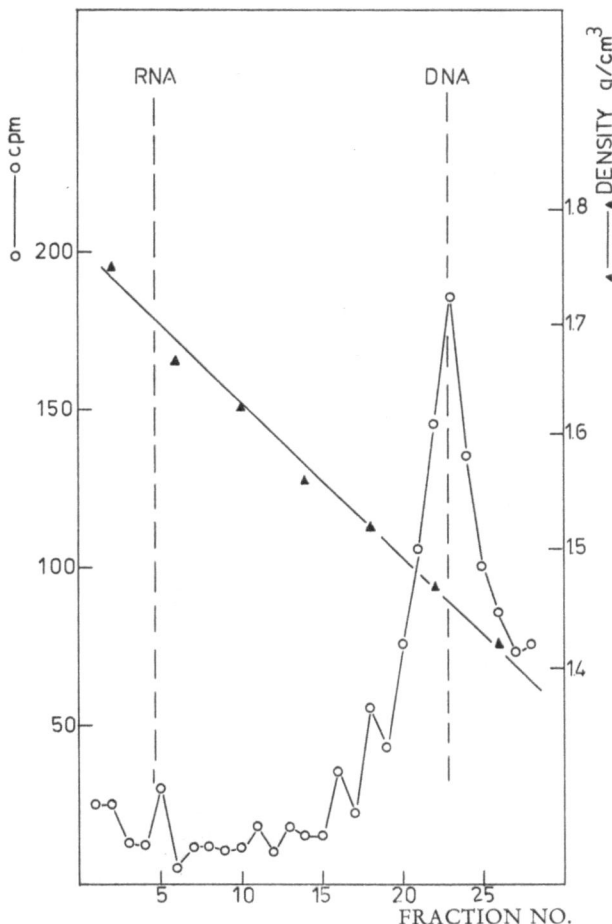

Fig.: 3 B
The density gradients were performed by mixing the products with Cs_2SO_4 at a density of 1.55 g/cm³ and centrifuging this mixture in a Rotor Ti 50 at 43,000 RPM, 15 °C for 60 hours. The gradients were fractionated from the bottom and the density measured via the refractive index. The fraction then were TCA-precipitated and the radioactivity measured.

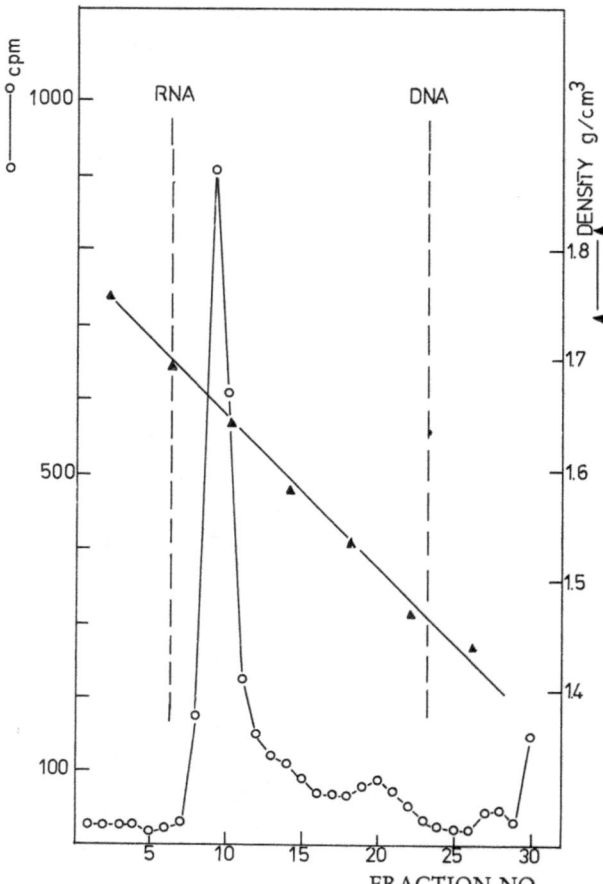

Fig.: 3 C

524

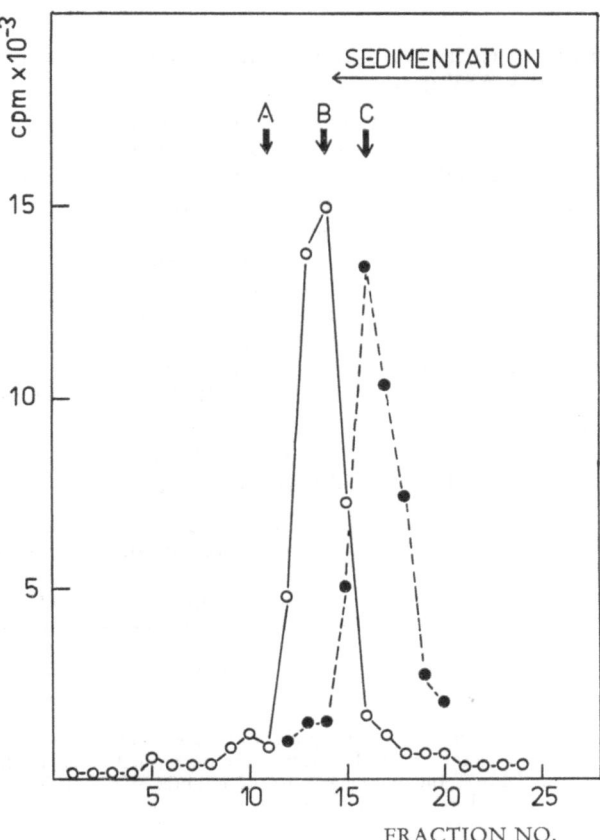

Legend to Fig. 4: Velocity sedimentation of reverse transcriptase from particles, REV and AMV.

Purified polymerases were sedimented in glycerol gradients, in the presence of 0.4 M KCl, as described by Markus et al. (8). The five gradients run under identical conditions contained particle polymerase, REV polymerase, AMV polymerase, aldolase and bovine serum albumin. After the run (17 hours) the gradients were fractionated from the bottom. The positions of the polymerases were found by standard polymerase tests with pC(dG) as template, the position, of the two marker proteins by measuring the protein concentration. The figure show the activity of the fractions, expressed as cpm ^{3}H-dGMP incorporated into acid insoluble material per hour in a reaction volume of 100 μl. ○—○ particle polymerase, ●—● REV polymerase, A = aldolase, B = AMV polymerase and C = bovine serum albumin.

Distinction of the »particle reverse transcriptase« from the reverse transcriptase of REV and the ALV/ASV group

As the enzyme had been shown to be a true reverse transcriptase by its template characteristics and its ability to synthesize a faithful transcript of heteropolymeric RNA, it was interesting and necessary to investigate whether the enzyme was related to or identical with the reverse transcriptase from chicken viruses. We first compared the reverse transcriptases from particles, REV and AMV in respect of their sedimentation constant. The enzymes and two marker proteins were sedimented in parallel gradients under identical conditions. The position of the enzymes was tested by activity tests of each fraction. As can be seen from figure 4, the particle enzyme sediments at the same rate as the AMV enzyme, but can be clearly distinguished from the REV enzyme with respect to sedimentation constant. As can be seen in Table 5, the particle enzyme and the REV enzyme can also be easily

Table V: Comparison of pC-directed DNA synthesis by reverse transcriptase from particles or REV with different divalent cations

Source of reverse transcriptase	cpm incorporated in the presence of		Relation of activities
	10 mM Mg^{++}	0.4 mM Mn^{++}	Mg^{++} : Mn^{++}
Particles	13 026	1 821	7.15
REV	468 000	1 082 820	0.43

Legend to Table 5: Purified reverse transcriptase was tested under standard conditions in the presence of pC(dG)$_{12-18}$ and ^{3}H-dGTP. Tests were performed either in the presence of 10 mM Mg^{++} or 0.4 mM Mn^{++}. Incubation was for 60 minutes at 37 °C. The acid insoluble radioactivity was determined in the total volume.

distinguished by their different preferences for divalent cations. Whereas the particle enzyme prefers Mg^{++} over Mn^{++}, the opposite is true for the REV enzyme.

As the antibody against AMV reverse transcriptase has been shown to inhibit the activity of all viruses of the ALV/ASV group, including the inducible ALV (13, 14), we used the antibody inhibition test to elucidate the relationship of the different enzymes. In particular the inhibition of particle and AMV enzyme by IgG against AMV reverse transcriptase was studied in parallel IgG dilution assays. The result is to be seen in figure 5 A and 5 B, where 5 B is just an enlargement of the region near the ordinate of figure 5 A. Whereas the AMV enzyme is inhibited very efficiently by small amounts of IgG, there is only a weak effect on the enzyme purified from the particles. An IgG concentration sufficient to neutralize AMV enzyme to 50 % does not show a significant effect on particle enzyme. The concentration has to be increased to about 70 fold, to obtain a 50 % inhibition. This clearly demonstrates that the particle reverse transcriptase is immunological different from the AMV enzyme.

Still more pronounced data have been obtained recently. Using another batch

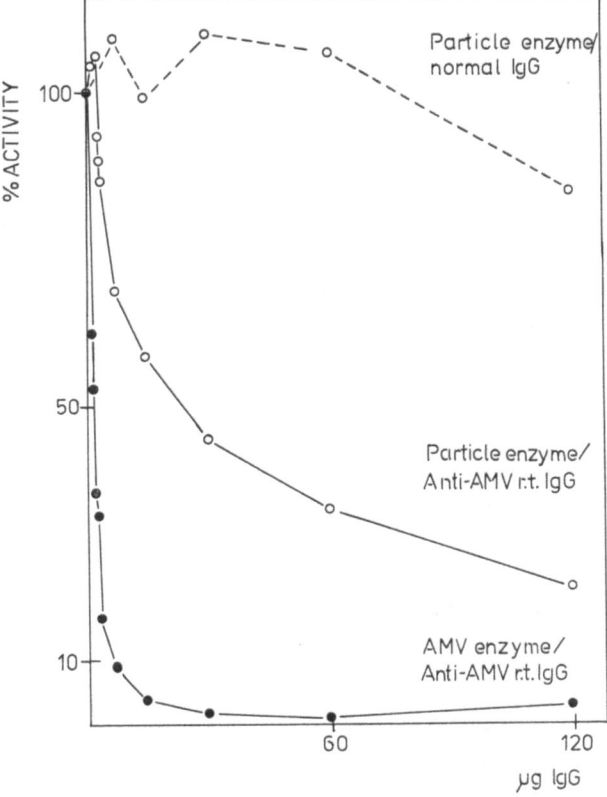

Legend to Fig. 5A and 5B: Comparative inhibition of particle and AMV reverse transcriptase by anti-AMV-enzyme IgG.
The inhibitory effect of various amounts of IgG directed against AMV reverse transcriptase and normal IgG on particle reverse transcriptase was compared to the effect on AMV reverse transcriptase. Constant amounts of enzyme were mixed with variable amounts, of IgG, in a reaction mixture of 50 µl, in the presence of 150 mM KCl, 50 µg BSA and 10 mM Tris-HCl, pH 8.2. Incubation was at 0–4 °C for 12 hours. Then each tube was brought to conditions for pC-dependent DNA synthesis and the remaining activity was measured in 1 hour incubation. 100 % activity was obtained from tests without added IgG, 100 % activity was about 15,000 cpm incorporated per hour in 100 µl reaction mix, for particle enzyme as well as for AMV enzyme. Parallel experiments ensured that under the conditions of the test the activity was proportional to the amount of enzyme and was linear within the time of the test.

of IgG, a comparatively much weaker effect on particle enzyme was found. This suggests that the observed inhibition by the antibody against AMV enzyme is due to antibodies against particle enzymes present in the used IgG preparations in small but different amounts. In any case, the particle enzyme is certainly not identical to the reverse transcriptase of the ALV/ASV group, and only weakly, if at all, related to them.

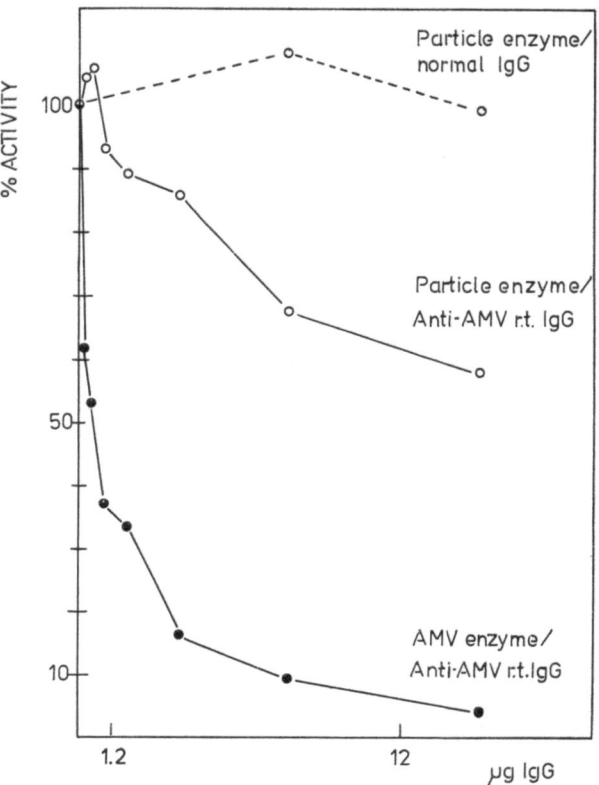

Fig.: 5 B

Conclusion

We were able to purify from particles from the allantoic fluid of ten day-old embryonated eggs an enzyme, which shows the biochemical characteristics of (viral) reverse transcriptase: preference for certain synthetic templates and the ability to synthesize DNA complementary to natural RNA. However the enzyme could be clearly differentiated from the reverse transcriptases of the known chicken RNA Tumor Viruses by several criteria:
1) the enzyme is different from the reverse transcriptase of REV in respect to sedimentation properties and ion-requirements.
2) the enzyme is only weakly, if at all, related to the reverse transcriptase of the viruses from the ALV/ASV group, which is known to be a single immunological species throughout the group.
3) enzymological comparison of particle enzyme to AMV enzyme, in recent experiments (data will be published elsewhere), has shown striking differences in the K_M-values for dGTP and dTTP.

As the enzyme has been proven not to be identical with the reverse transcriptase from the chicken viruses, and is completely different as well from the enzyme purified by Kang and Temin (3), we believe to have isolated a so far unknown chicken enzyme, which seems to be a good candidate for a cellular reverse transcriptase. As the enzyme could be detected in the eggs of all flocks of chicken tested (chicken from the bavarian countryside, from leukosis virus-free SPAFAS Inc., Norwich, Connecticut and from leukosis virus-free SPF-VALO chicken from Lohmann Tierzucht, Cuxhaven, West Germany), and could be isolated by separate purification from each one of 24 single eggs, we conclude that the enzyme might be ubiquitous and therefore has no obvious relation to the induction of malignancy. If this phenomenon is a more generalized one, demonstration of reverse transcriptase alone can not longer be taken as a solid proof for the presence of RNA tumor viruses.

Till now we only isolated the enzyme from particles from the allantoic fluid, and do not know the level of enzyme activity in the embryonic tissue. So it is very interesting and necessary to obtain more information about the nature of these particles. We are presently investigating this problem and know already that in spite of the similar density, particles can be clearly differentiated from Avian RNA tumor viruses in several respects:

1) the particles do not possess the biological properties of ALV/ASV, i.e. helper activity and interfering properties (these tests were kindly performed by Dr. R. Friis, University of Giessen).

2) the protein pattern of purified particles is completely different from the pattern of REV or ALV/ASV. This result could be very much strengthened by tests, kindly performed by Dr. A. Vaheri, University of Helsinki: he could not detect the major group specific antigen of ALV/ASV, the protein P 27 in preparations of particles when he applied a radioimmune assay for this protein.

Since the endogenous reaction is weak and very labile we were not yet able to study the nature of a nucleic acid possibly present as endogenous template. This question has to be answered, to be able to see whether the particles are a new group of endogenous viruses or cellular exclusions.

This problem and the search for intracellular enzyme are presently under investigation.

References

1. Mayer, R. J., R. G. Smith, and R. C. Gallo. 1974.
   Reverse Transcriptase in Normal Rhesus Monkey Placenta. Science *185*:864–867.
2. Bobrow, S. N., R. G. Smith, M. S. Reitz, and R. C. Gallo. 1972.
   Stimulated Normal Human Lymphocytes Contain a Ribonuclease-Sensitive DNA Polymerase Distinct from Viral RNA-Directed DNA polymerase. PNAS *69*:3228–3232.
3. Kang, Ch.-Y., and H. M. Temin. 1972.
   Endogenous RNA-Directed DNA Polymerase Activity in Uninfected Chicken Embryos. PNAS *69*: 1550–1554.
4. Scolnick, E. M., S. A. Aaronson, G. J. Todaro, and W. P. Parks. 1971.

RNA Dependent DNA Polymerase Activity in Mammalian Cells. Nature 229: 318–321.

5. Baltimore, D., and D. Smoler. 1971.
Primer Requirement and Template Specificity of the DNA Polymerase of RNA Tumor Viruses. PNAS 68: 1507–1511.

6. Gallagher, R. E., G. J. Todaro, R. G. Smith, D. M. Livingston, and R. C. Gallo. 1974.
Relationship between RNA-Directed DNA Polymerase (Reverse Transcriptase) from Human Acute Leukemia Blood Cells and Primate Type-C Virus. PNAS 71: 1309–1313.

7. Goodman, N. C., and S. Spiegelman. 1971.
Distinguishing Reverse Transcriptase of an RNA Tumor Virus from Other Known DNA Polymerases. PNAS 68: 2203–2206.

8. McCaffrey, R., D. F. Smoler, and D. Baltimore. 1973.
Terminal Deoxynucleotidyl Transferase in a Case of Childhood Acute Lympho-blastic Leukemia. PNAS 70: 521–525.

9. Bolden, A., M. Fry, R. Muller, R. Citerella, and A. Weissbach. 1972. The Presence of a Polyriboadenylic Acid-Dependent DNA Polymerase in Eukaryotic Cells. ABB 153: 26–33.

10. Weissbach, A., A. Bolden, R. Muller, H. Hanafusa, and T. Hanafusa. 1972.
Deoxyribonucleic Acid Polymerase Activities in Normal and Leukovirus-Infected Chicken Embryo Cells. J. Vir. 10: 321–327.

11. Markus, S. L., M. J. Modak, and L. F. Cavalieri. 1974. Purification of Avian Myeloblastosis Virus DNA Polymerase by Affinity Chromatography on Po-lycytidylate-Agarose. J. Vir. 14: 853–859.

12. Ross, J., H. Aviv, E. Scolnick, and P. Leder. 1972.
In Vitro Synthesis of DNA Complementary to Purified Rabbit Globin mRNA. PNAS 69: 264–268.

13. Nowinski, R. C., K. F. Watson, A. Yaniv, and S. Spiegelman. 1972. Serological Analysis of the Deoxyribonucleic Acid Polymerase of Avian Oncornaviruses. J. Vir. 10: 959–964.

14. Mizutani, S., and H. M. Temin. 1973.
Lack of Serological Relationship Among DNA Polymerases of Avian Leukosis-Sarcoma Viruses, Reticuloendotheliosis Virus, and Chicken Cells. J. Vir. 12: 440–448.

15. Watson, K. F., R. C. Nowinski, A. Yaniv, and S. Spiegelman. 1972.
Serological Analysis of the Deoxyribonucleic Acid Polymerase of Avian Oncornaviruses. J. Vir. 10: 951–958.

16. Moelling, K., H. Gelderblom, G. Pauli, R. Friis, and H. Bauer. 1975.
A Comparative Study of the Avian Reticuloendotheliosis Virus: Relationship to Murine Leukemia Virus and Viruses of the Avian Sarcoma-Leukosis Complex. Virology 65: 546–557.

Translation Level Control in Normal and Leukemic Cells

Boyd Hardesty, Gisela Kramer, Miguel Cimadevilla
Pairoh Pinphanichakarn and David Konecki

Clayton Foundation Biochemical Institute
Department of Chemistry
The University of Texas at Austin
Austin, Texas 78712

A useful model for consideration of the biochemical aspects of cancer holds the primary lesion to be a block in the normal processes of differentiation. Erythroleukemia induced in susceptible mice by Friend leukemia virus appears to fit this model which is illustrated in Figure 1. This virus blocks the differentiation of

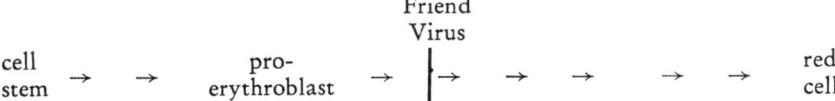

Fig. 1: Leukemia as a block in differentiation.

erythroid cells at the proerythroblast stage (1, 2) before any appreciable synthesis of hemoglobin takes place (3). Friend virus transformed proerythroblasts from leukemic mice can be carried as permanent lines and are easily propagated in suspension culture. Differentiation as reflected by hemoglobin synthesis may be induced *in vitro* by the simple expedient of adding certain aprotonic solvents, such as dimethylsulfoxide (DMSO), to the tissue culture nutrient in which the Friend leukemia cells (FLC) are grown (3–5). Thus, these cell lines provide an excellent system for the study of both transcriptional and translational control mechanisms involved in differentiation leading to the synthesis of hemoglobin. A better understanding of these controls eventually could lead to the manipulation of the regulatory elements involved in leukemia.

The ability of DMSO to overcome the viral induced block in hemoglobin synthesis is a salient feature of the Friend leukemia cell (FLC) system. Approximately 30 hr after the addition of DMSO, globin mRNA becomes detectable in FLC by hybridization with complementary globin DNA, and it reaches a maximal concentration 50–70 hrs after induction (6, 7). Ostertag and coworkers (8) have demonstrated that the rate of cytoplasmic globin mRNA synthesis reaches a maximum 24 hr after induction and decreases rapidly thereafter. Globin synthesis, on the other hand, as measured by the appearance of benzidine positive cells, is not apparent until the third day after induction and reaches a maximum around the fifth day (3, 6, 8). These results, in addition to those obtained by Paul and coworkers (9, 10), suggest the presence of posttranscriptional control elements in these cells. Harrison

531

et al. (10) have reported that one of their FLC lines, clone 707, contains the same amount of precursor nuclear globin mRNA before and after DMSO induction.

The reticulocyte hemin-controlled repressor

The rabbit reticulocyte system is one of the better characterized protein synthesizing systems and one in which translational level control is well estabished. Globin synthesis in both rabbit reticulocytes (11, 12) and their cell-free lysates (13, 14) is controlled by the availability of hemin. As shown in Figure 2, protein

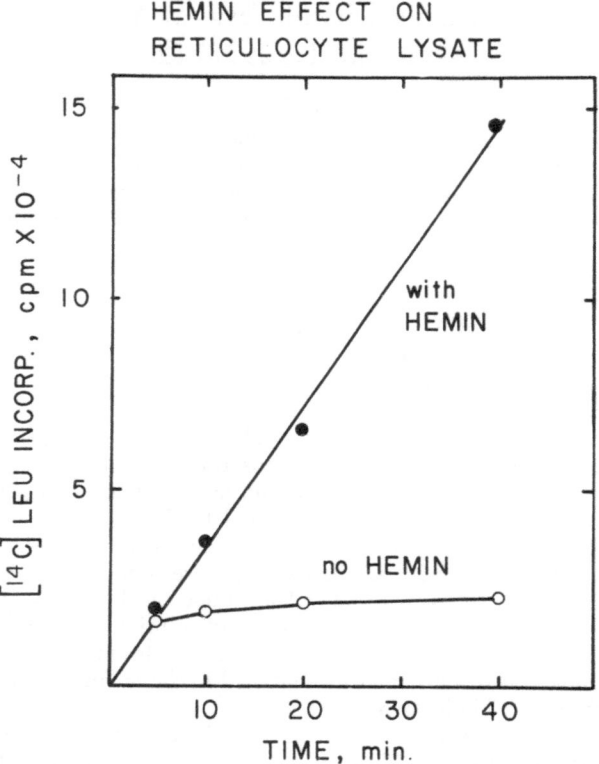

Fig. 2: Effect of hemin on protein synthesis in a rabbit reticulocyte lysate.
Protein synthesis in a reticulocyte lysate was measured in incubation mixtures containing the following in a final volume of 100 μl: 10 mM Tris-HCl (pH 7.5), 90 mM KCl, 1.5 mM MgCl₂, 5 mM dithioerythritol, 0.5 mM ATP, 0.2 mM GTP, 15 mM creatine phosphate, 26 units/ml creatine phosphokinase, 0.1 mM [^{14}C]leucine (40 Ci/mol), 0.1 mM all other [^{12}C] amino acids, 20 μl of rabbit reticulocyte lysate and, where indicated, 20 μg/ml of hemin (bovine, Type I). Incubation was carried out at 34° for the indicated periods of time. Reactions were stopped by diluting the incubation mixture with 0.40 ml of a cold solution containing 1 mM [^{12}C]leucine and 0.50 N NaOH. After incubation for 10 min at 37°, the samples were made 5 % in trichloroacetic acid an allowed to stand for 5 min at room temperature. The precipitate formed was collected on nitrocellulose

synthesis in a reticulocyte lysate ceases abruptly after incubation for 5 min at 34° unless hemin is added to the incubation mixture. In the latter case protein synthesis proceeds at a linear rate for at least 40 min. The cessation of protein synthesis observed in the absence of added hemin appears to be due to a block in initiation of new globin chains (13–17). Hemin enhances the synthesis of all proteins in reticulocyte lysates, including those programmed by exogenous mRNAs (18, 19), thus negating any specificity in its mode of action. It has been proposed that hemin either prevents the formation of an inhibitor of initiation (17, 20–22) or that it interacts with an initiation factor thus preventing its inactivation (23). Gross and Rabinovitz (21) have isolated an inhibitory protein from reticulocyte postribosomal supernatants incubated in the absence of hemin. This protein, which has been called a translational repressor or the hemin controlled repressor, HCR (21, 22), appears to inhibit protein synthesis by preventing the formation of a stable 40S ribosomal subunit·Met-tRNA$_f^{Met}$ initiation complex (22, 24, 25).

The FLC repressor

We have observed that hemin has a relatively low but detectable stimulatory effect on protein synthesis in lysates from uninduced FLC (26). The stimulation of protein synthesis by hemin is comparable to that observed in intact Krebs II ascites tumor cells or their lysates (27), but it is an order of magnitude lower than that observed in reticulocyte lysates (26). Moreover, mixing of equal volumes of reticulocyte and FLC lysates results in the less than additive synthesis of proteins. These results led us to examine the products formed in reticulocyte, FLC and mixed lysates by sodium dodecyl sulfate-polyacrylamide gel electrophoresis (28). As seen in Figure 3A, hemoglobin comprises approximately 90 % of the protein synthesized in the reticulocyte lysate as indicated by summating the counts in the portion of the gel within the limit bars. Authentic rabbit globin migrates into this portion of the gel under the conditions used. On the other hand, there is no detectable globin synthesis in lysates from uninduced FLC. Higher molecular weight proteins characteristic of FLC were synthesized (Figure 3B). As shown in Figure 3C, synthesis of rabbit globin is reduced by 60 % in the mixed lysate system while there appears to be no decrease in the synthesis of FLC proteins.

Subsequently we have purified partially by chromatography on DEAE-cellulose and Sephadex G-200 an inhibitory protein present in lysates from uninduced FLC which may be responsible for the differential inhibition of globin synthesis observed in the mixed lysate system. This repressor protein does not affect poly(U) directed synthesis of polyphenylalanine at a concentration twice as high as that necessary for maximal inhibition of reticulocyte mRNA translation (29), nor does it interfere with the completion and release of nascent globin chains initiated in intact reticulocytes (see Table I).

The FLC repressor, however, promotes the protein synthesis dependent breakdown of polysomes in a reticulocyte lysate. This is shown in Figure 4C. In the

filters (0.45 μm pore size, type HAWG, Millipore Corp., Bedford, MA), washed with three 5 ml portions of 5 % trichloroacetic acid and counted by liquid scintillation. (○) no hemin added; (●) hemin (20 μg/ml) added. [This figure is from (26)].

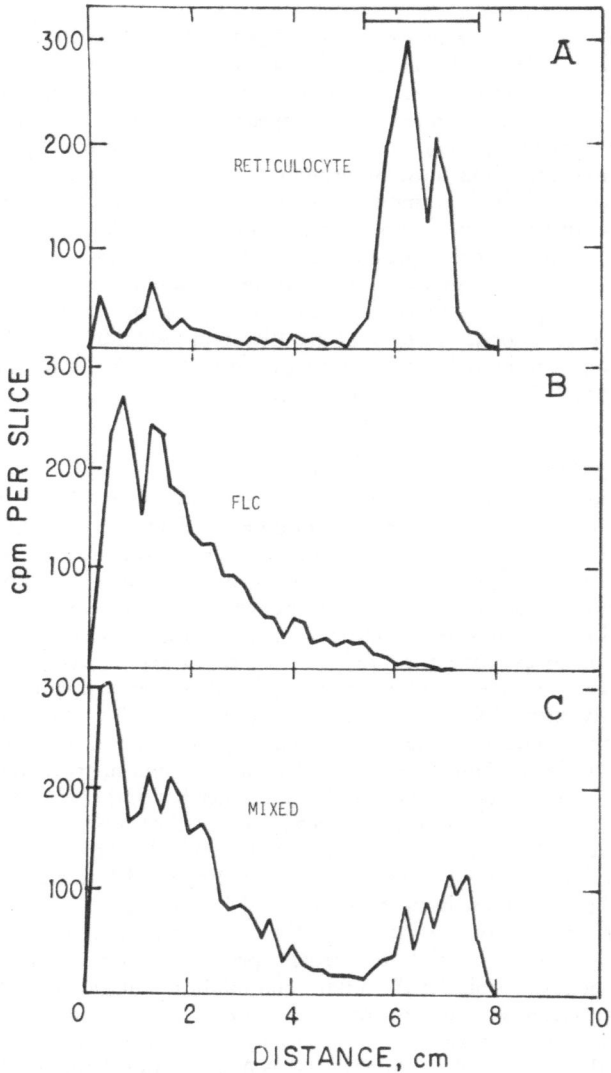

Fig. 3: Sodium dodecyl sulfate-polyacrylamide gel electrophoresis of the products synthesized in rabbit reticulocyte, FLC and mixed lysate systems. Incubation conditions were as described in Figure 2 except that [^{14}C]leucine (320 Ci/mol) was used and no hemin was added. Aliquots of 10 μl were analyzed under the conditions described by Weber and Osborn (28). After staining with Coomossie brilliant blue, the gels were destained electrophoretically, cut into 2 mm slices and counted by liquid scintillation in 10 ml of 10 % Biosolve (Beckman Instruments, Inc., Palo Alto, CA) in toluene counting fluid containing 5.0 g of 2,5 diphenyloxazole per liter of toluene. Counting efficiency was 14 %. The limit bars indicate the position of authentic rabbit globin. A, reticulocyte lysate; B, FLC lysate; C, mixed lysate system. [This figure is from (26).]

Table I: Effect of FLC Repressor on Release of Nascent Peptide Chains

| | [^{14}C]Leucine, cpm | | |
	Total	Ribosome-Free Fraction	Release %
Control, 0°	10,566	1,938	18
−FLC repressor	11,153	8,166	73
+FLC repressor	9,856	7,520	76

Table 1: Release of nascent chains labeled with [^{14}C]leucine in intact reticulocytes was measured in incubation mixtures containing the following in a final volume of 500 µl: 20 mM Tris-HCl (pH 7.5), 80 mM KCl, 2.5 mM MgCl$_2$, 5 mM reduced glutathione, 1 mM ATP, 0.4 mM GTP, 5 mM creatine phosphate, 9 units/ml creatine phosphokinase, 25 µg rabbit liver tRNA, 500 µg of the 40–70 % ammonium sulfate enzyme fraction from the postribosomal supernatant of rabbit reticulocytes, 0.1 mM all [^{12}C]amino acids and 1.0 mg of ribosomes containing [^{14}C]leucine labeled nascent peptides. Where indicated, FLC repressor (147 µg of protein) was added. Incubation was for 8 min at 37°. Samples of 200 µl were made 1 mM in cycloheximide and layered on top of 10–44 % (w/v) linear sucrose density gradients containing 50 mM Tris-HCl (pH 7.5), 100 mM KCl, 8 mM MgCl$_2$ and 0.1 mM cycloheximide. Centrifugation was for 90 min at 35,000 rpm in a SW 41 rotor (Spinco Division, Beckman Instruments, Inc., Palo Alto, CA). The gradients were fractionated from the top using an ISCO Model D density gradient fractionator and absorbance at 260 nm was recorded using an ISCO Model UA-2 ultraviolet analyzer. Fractions of 0.5 ml were collected and hot trichloroacetic acid precipitable radioactivity was determined. [This table is from (29).]

absence of the inhibitor (Figure 4B) the polysome profile obtained resembles that of the unincubated control (Figure 4A). These data suggest an effect of the FLC repressor on reattachment of ribosomes to mRNA during the initiation process.

The FLC repressor appears to block initiation of protein synthesis at a point before the NaF sensitive reaction of peptide initiation. This is shown in Figure 5. Ribosomes obtained from reticulocytes incubated with NaF are almost entirely monomeric and appear to be synchronized at a late stage of peptide initiation after attachment to mRNA (30). Edeine has been shown to inhibit protein synthesis on these ribosomes only after one round of translation has taken place, thus suggesting that the edeine sensitive step precedes the reaction inhibited by NaF (30). As can be seen in Figure 5, the kinetics of polypeptide synthesis in the presence of FLC translational repressor resemble those observed in the presence of edeine. Moreover, simultaneous addition of edeine and FLC repressor to the incubation mixture does not result in greater inhibition than that observed with edeine alone.

Comparison of HCR and FLC repressor

An obvious similarity between the HCR and the FLC repressor is that both inhibit natural mRNA translation at a step of peptide chain initiation. An obvious difference between these two repressors is that while formation of HCR in reticulocytes is controlled by the availability of hemin (17, 20–22), the FLC repressor does not appear to be controlled by this effector (26). Furthermore, functional differences clearly differentiate the HCR from the FLC repressor. The rabbit re-

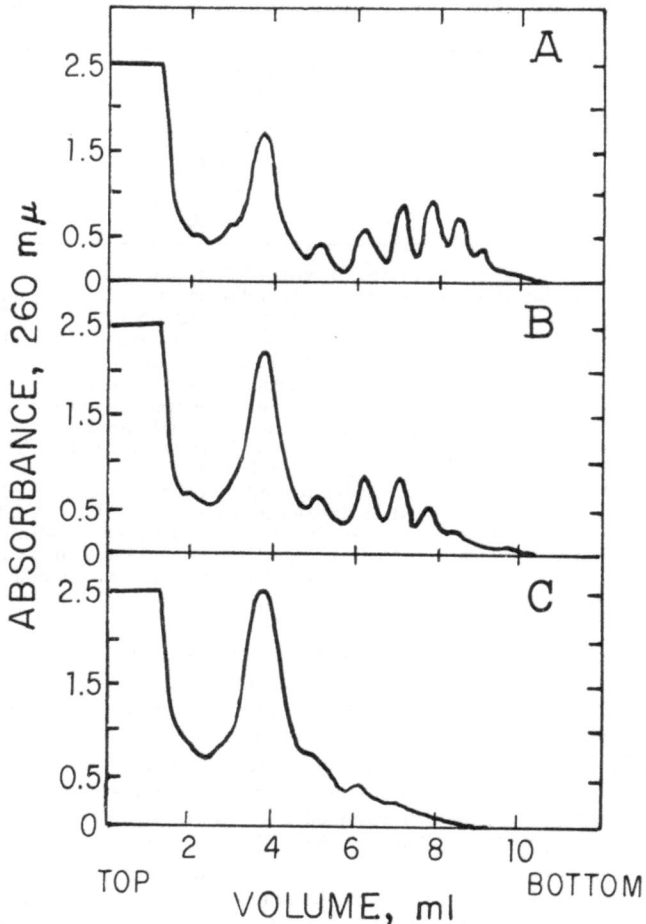

Fig. 4: Effect of FLC repressor on the polysome profile of rabbit reticulocyte lysates.
Reticulocyte lysates were incubated for 15 min at 34° in the presence of 20 μg/ml hemin under the conditions described in Figure 2. Reaction mixtures, 200 μl, were made 1 mM in cycloheximide and analyzed in 10–44 % (w/v) linear sucrose density gradients as described in Table I.

ticulocyte HCR has been shown to inhibit initiation factor dependent formation of methionylpuromycin with reticulocyte ribosomal subunits (25). As shown in Table II, the FLC repressor, unlike HCR or edeine, fails to inhibit methionylpuromycin synthesis even though it efficiently blocks globin mRNA-dependent synthesis of methionylvaline (29).

Also, it has been demonstrated that the inhibition of protein synthesis exerted by HCR in reticulocyte lysates may be overcome by an initiation factor which

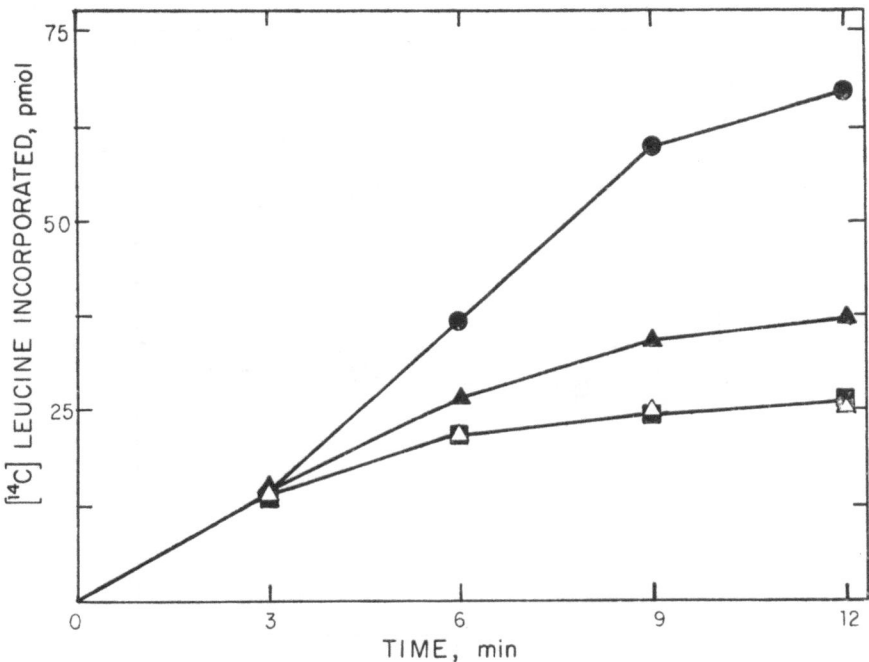

Fig. 5: Effect of FLC repressor and edeine on protein synthesis with NaF ribosomes. Peptide synthesis with unwashed ribosomes from rabbit reticulocytes previously incubated in the presence of NaF was measured in incubation mixtures containing the following in a final volume of 100 μl: 20 mM Tris-HCl (pH 7.5), 80 mM KCl, 2.5 mM MgCl₂, 5 mM reduced glutathione, 1 mM ATP, 0.4 mM GTP, 5 mM creatine phosphate, 9 units/ml creatine phosphokinase, 20 μM [¹⁴C]leucine (40 Ci/mol), 50 mM all other [¹²C]amino acids, 5 μg rabbit liver tRNA, 100 μg of protein of the 40–70 % postribosomal enzyme fraction from rabbit reticulocytes, and 100 μg of ribosomes. FLC repressor (147 μg of protein) and/or edeine (1 μM) were added as the first components of the mixture. Incubation was at 37° for the indicated periods of time. Reactions were terminated by the addition of 100 μl of 1.0 N NaOH and treated as described in Figure 2. (●) no inhibitor; (▲) FLC repressor; (■) edeine; (△) FLC repressor and edeine. [This figure is from (29).]

Table II: Effects of HCR and FLC Repressor on Methionylpuromycin Formation

Additions	Methionylpuromycin (pmol)
Control	2.72
+ HCR	1.36
+ FLC repressor	2.66
+ edeine	0.06

Table 2: Initiation factor dependent formation of methionyl-puromycin with reticulocyte ribosomal subunits was determined by a modification (29) of the stepwise incubation procedure described by Levin et al. (31).

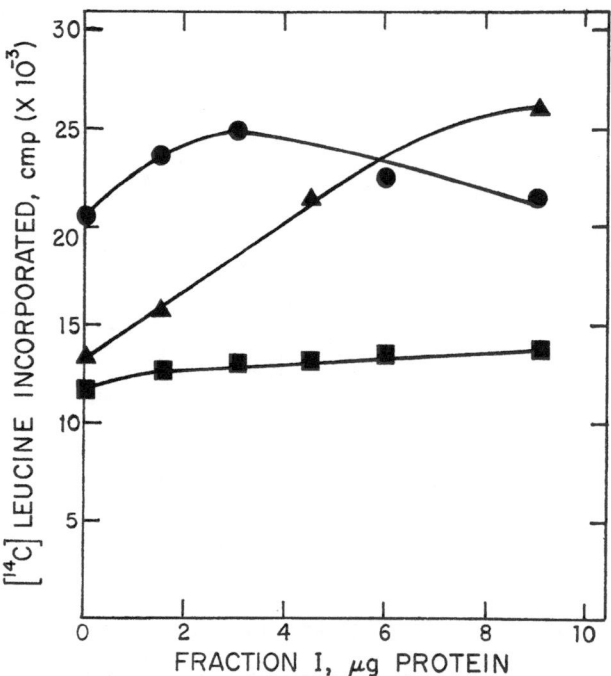

Fig. 6: Reversal of inhibition of protein synthesis by a rabbit reticulocyte initiation factor fraction.
Rabbit reticulocyte lysates were incubated under the conditions described in Figure 2. Where indicated, FLC repressor (147 μg of protein) or HCR (0.28 μg of protein) were added. The indicated amounts of protein of an initiation factor fraction obtained by chromatography of a reticulocyte ribosomal salt wash preparation on DEAE-cellulose, Fraction I (29), was added as indicated. (●) no inhibitor; (▲) HCR; (■) FLC repressor.

forms a ternary complex with GTP and Met-tRNA$_f^{Met}$ (25). Similar results are shown in Figure 6. Addition of increasing amounts of a protein fraction, obtained upon fractionation of the rabbit reticulocyte ribosomal salt wash fraction on DEAE-cellulose (29), that contains the ternary complex formation activity (Fraction I) results in the reversal of inhibition exerted by HCR. However, as seen also in this figure, the inhibition produced by the FLC repressor is impervious to increasing amounts of Fraction I.

Discussion

We have presented evidence for the presence of a translational repressor in lysates from uninduced FLC. Formation of this repressor, unlike formation of HCR in reticulocytes, is not controlled by the availability of hemin. Moreover, the FLC repressor appears to inhibit peptide chain initiation at a different step than HCR.
Paul and coworkers (in this volume) have described a lymphoma-FLC hybrid

cell line which may be induced by DMSO to synthesize globin mRNA without any detectable synthesis of hemoglobin. The data presented by these workers may reflect phenomena comparable to those involved in the inhibition of hemoglobin synthesis obtained in mixtures of lysates from FLC and reticulocytes. The existence of translational repressors in FLC suggests the possibility that virus-induced modification of translational control mechanisms might be involved in other leukemias. However, the relation of the FLC repressor to the primary biochemical lesion of this leukemia remains to be established.

Acknowledgements

The authors are grateful to M. Hardesty and J. Ybarra for their excellent technical assistance and to B. Anderson for her help in the preparation of the typescript. This work was supported in part by Grant CA-16608 from the National Cancer Institute and by Grant GB-30902 from the National Science Foundation. G. K. is a Fellow of the Deutsche Forschungsgemeinschaft and J. M. C. is the recipient of NIH National Research Service Award 1 F32 AM 05083–01 from the National Institute of Arthritis, Metabolism and Digestive Diseases.

References

1. Friend, C., Patuleia, M. C. and deHarven, E. (1966) Nat. Cancer Inst. Mono. 22, 505–522.
2. Patuleia, M. C. and Friend, C. (1967) Cancer Res. 27, 726–730.
3. Sato, T., Friend, C. and deHarven, E. (1971) Cancer Res. 31, 1402–1417.
4. Friend, C., Scher, W., Holland, J. G. and Sato, T. (1971) Proc. Nat. Acad. Sci. USA 68, 378–382.
5. Ostertag, W., Melderis, H., Steinheider, G., Kluge, N. and Dube, S. (1972) Nature New Biol. 239, 231–234.
6. Ross, J., Ikawa, Y and Leder, P. (1972) Proc. Nat. Acad. Sci. USA 69, 3620–3623.
7. Ross, J., Gielen, J., Packman, S., Ikawa, Y. and Leder, P. (1974) J. Mol. Biol. 87, 697–714.
8. Ostertag, W., Cole, T., Crozier, T., Gaedicke, G., Kind, J., Kluge, N. Krieg, J. C., Roesler, G., Steinheider, G., Weimann, B. J. and Dube, S. K. (1973) in Differentiation and Control of Malignancy of Tumor Cells (Nakahara, W., Ono, T., Sugimura, T. and Sugano, H., eds.) University of Tokyo Press, pp. 485–512.
9. Gilmour, R., Harrison, P., Wendass, J., Affara, N. and Paul, J. (1974) Cell Diff. 3, 9–22.
10. Harrison, P., Gilmour, R., Affara, N., Conkie, D., and Paul, J. (1974) Cell Diff. 3, 23–30.
11. Kruh, J. and Borsook, H. (1956) J. Biol. Chem. 220, 905–915.
12. Bruns, G. P. and London, I. M. (1965) Biochem. Biophys. Res. Commun. 18, 236–242.
13. Adamson, S. D., Herbert, E. and Godchaux, W. (1968) Arch. Biochem. Biophys. 125, 671–683.

14. Zucker, W. V. and Schulman, H. M. (1968) Proc. Nat. Acad. Sci. USA *59*, 582–589.
15. Grayzel, A. I., Hörcher, P. and London, I. M. (1966) Proc. Nat. Acad. Sci. USA *55*, 650–655.
16. Waxman, H. S. and Rabinovitz, M. (1966) Biochim. Biophys. Acta *129*, 369–379.
17. Howard, G. A., Adamson, S. D. and Herbert, E. (1970) Biochem. Biophys. Acta *213*, 237–243.
18. Lodish, H. F. and Desalu, O. (1973) J. Biol. Chem. *248*, 3520–3527.
19. Mathews, M. B., Hunt, T. and Brayley, A. (1973) Nature New Biol. *243*, 230–233.
20. Maxwell, C. R. and Rabinovitz, M. (1969) Biochem. Biophys. Res. Commun. *35*, 79–85.
21. Gross, M. and Rabinovitz, M. (1973) Biochem. Biophys. Res. Commun. *50*, 832–838.
22. Balkow, K., Mizuno, S. and Rabinovitz, M. (1973) Biochem. Biophys. Res. Commun. *54*, 315–323.
23. Raffel, C., Stein, S. and Kaempfer, R. (1974) Proc. Nat. Acad. Sci. USA *71*, 4020–4024.
24. Legon, S., Jackson, R. J. and Hunt, T. (1973) Nature New Biol. *241*, 150–152.
25. Ranu, R., Levin, D., Clemens, M., Cherbas, I. and London, I. M. (1975) Fed. Proc. *34*, 621.
26. Cimadevilla, J. M. and Hardesty, B. (1975) Biochem. Biophys. Res. Commun. *63*, 931–937.
27. Beuzard, Y., Rodvieu, R. and London, I. M. (1973) Proc. Nat. Acad. Sci. USA *70*, 1022–1026.
28. Weber, K. and Osborn, M. (1969) J. Biol. Chem. *244*, 4406–4412.
29. Cimadevilla, J. M., Kramer, G., Pinphanichakarn, P., Konecki, D. and Hardesty, B. (1975) Arch. Biochem. Biophys., *171*, 145–153.
30. Obrig, T., Irvin, J., Culp, W. and Hardesty, B. (1971) Eur. J. Biochem. *21*, 31–41.
31. Levin, D. H., Kyner, D. and Acs, G. (1973) J. Biol. Chem. *248*, 6416–6425.

Control of Peptide Chain Initiation in Uninfected and Virus Infected Cells by Membrane Mediated Events

Gebhard Koch, Hermann Oppermann, Patricia Bilello,
Friedrich Koch and Donald Nuss

Roche Institute of Molecular Biology
Nutley, New Jersey 07110

Abbreviations

MEM	Minimal Essential Medium
HIB	Hypertonic Initiation Block
VSV	Vesicular Stomatitis Virus
TPCK	L-1-Tosylamido-2-Phenylethyl Chloromethyl Ketone
DMSO	Dimethylsulfoxide
L	Immunoglobulin Light Chain
H	Immunoglobulin Heavy Chain
DEAE	Diethylaminoethyl-dextran
HEPES	N-2-hydroxyethylpiperazine-N'-2-ethanesulfonic acid

Summary

Initiation of protein synthesis in tissue culture cells is rapidly inhibited or blocked by addition of either DMSO, ethanol, TPCK, cytochalasin B, or sucrose to the growth medium. In contrast, these agents do not interfere with the initiation of protein synthesis in cell-free extracts to a comparable extent. These results support the hypothesis that protein synthesis in tissue culture cells can be influenced by membrane mediated events.

Translation of viral mRNA in RNA virus infected cells is resistant to a number of these inhibitors of peptide chain initiation and proceeds under conditions where translation of host mRNA is almost completely suppressed. It appears that viral mRNA possesses a greater ability than host mRNA to form mRNA-ribosome initiation complexes when the overall rate of peptide chain initiation is reduced. This observation has led to a number of predictions concerning the strategy of virus directed suppression of host mRNA translation.

Under optimal growth conditions protein synthesis appears to be regulated mainly, but not exclusively, by the amount of the mRNA available for translation. However, when cellular growth and/or the overall rate of peptide chain initiation is restricted, control of protein synthesis at the translational level becomes decisive with the translation of each mRNA species proceeding with its own characteristic efficiency, most probably as a result of inherent differential affinities of individual mRNA species for ribosomes.

Introduction

In spite of extensive studies, much remains to be determinded concerning mechanisms of translational control in tissue culture cells. We have previously suggested that this control can be exerted by membrane mediated events (Pong, Nuss and Koch, 1975).

An increase in the tonicity of the growth medium exerted by addition of either salt or sucrose (Oppermann, Saborio, Zarucki, and Koch, 1973) results in an immediate block in the initiation of protein synthesis (Saborio, Pong, and Koch, 1974), while elongation and termination of protein synthesis as well as processing, transport and secretion of proteins continue unabated. It is well known that infection of various tissue culture cell lines with a number of RNA or DNA viruses also results in an inhibition of cellular protein synthesis. This inhibition may result from competition between virus and host mRNAs for ribosome binding sites (Lawrence and Thach, 1974; Nuss, Oppermann and Koch, 1975) and/or a selective interference with host peptide chain initiation, perhaps due to the action of viral protein(s) (Matthews et la., 1973; Wright and Cooper, 1974; Racevskis, Kerwar and Koch, 1976). However, the identification of a factor which can selectively suppress the translation of host mRNA has not been forthcoming. Interestingly, a brief exposure of virus infected cells to hypertonic medium does result in a striking preferential inhibition of host mRNA translation (Nuss, Oppermann and Koch, 1975). This result suggests that the efficiency with which translation can be initiated must be greater for viral mRNA than for host mRNA. That is, viral mRNA might possess a stronger affinity for ribosomes than host mRNA, resulting in only a slight reduction in its translation when the overall rate of peptide chain initiation is reduced, and thus gaining a translation advantage. This interpretation could readily explain why infection of cells by isolated viral mRNA is promoted under experimental conditions that interfere with cellular protein synthesis (Koch, 1973). The observations that a brief exposure of virus infected cells to hypertonic conditions early in the infectious cycle results in a potentiation of virus directed suppression of host translation leads to the proposal that the latter process can be partially explained by an early indiscriminate reduction in the overall rate of peptide chain initiation. Indeed, this event, coupled with competition between host and viral mRNA for ribosome binding sites later in the infectious cycle when viral mRNA becomes more abundant, may adequately explain suppression of host translation directed by a number of RNA containing viruses (Nuss, Oppermann and Koch, 1975).

Initiation of protein synthesis in HeLa cells in vivo is inhibited by a number of agents in addition to medium hypertonicity (Saborio, Pong and Koch, 1974), including DMSO (Saborio and Koch, 1973); ethanol (Koch and Koch, 1974); TPCK (Pong, Nuss and Koch, 1975); and cytochalasin B (Koch and Oppermann, 1975). We have studied the effect of several of these experimental conditions on protein synthesis in uninfected and virus infected cells and on in vitro protein synthesis in cell-free extracts prepared from mammalian cells. The results support the proposal that under a number of natural and experimental conditions the rate of peptide chain initiation can be regulated by membrane mediated events.

Materials and Methods

Cells and Viruses

Cells were grown in suspension as described previously (Saborio, Pong and Koch, 1974; Nuss and Koch, 1976a) or in monolayers (Oppermann and Koch, 1976a). Infection of cells by poliovirus, Type 1, strain Mahoney or by VSV, serotype Indiana (Mudd and Summers, 1970) was performed as described (Nuss, Oppermann and Koch, 1975).

Experimental Conditions for Isotope Labeling

Cells were transferred to serum free MEM (Joklik-modified, Gibco F13) + 25 mM Hepes, pH 7.4, containing no, or 1/20 the normal concentration of methionine. The tonicity of the medium was adjusted by addition of appropriate aliquots of a 4 M NaCl solution. Cells were incubated for 15 min at 37 °C (to allow run-off of ribosomes from those mRNA molecules on which initiation of translation has been blocked) (Saborio, Pong and Koch, 1974), followed by an additional 15 min in the presence of [^{35}S]methionine (New England Nuclear, above 250 Ci/mM). After labeling, 50 μl aliquots were withdrawn and anlyzed according to Mans and Novelli (1961). The remainder of the cell suspensions was diluted 10 fold with ice cold chase-medium, containing 10 mM unlabeled methionine. The cells were centrifuged, resuspended in warm chase medium and incubated for another 15 min at 37 °C.

Lysis of Cells and SDS Polyacrylamide Gel Electrophoresis

Cytoplasmic extracts were prepared as previously described (Saborio, Pong and Koch, 1974; Nuss and Koch, 1976a), analyzed by polyacrylamide slab gel electrophoresis (Laemmli and Favre, 1973) and autoradiographed on medical X-ray film. Quantitation of [^{35}S]methionine incorporation into individual polypeptides was achieved in two ways; by measuring the area under the peaks on autoradiograph tracings or directly by excision and elution of individual peptide bands and determination of radioactivity by liquid scintillation spectrometry (Oppermann and Koch 1976 a).

Preparation of Cell-free extracts

Cell-free extracts were prepared from HeLa S$_3$ and mouse L cells according to the method of McDowell, et. al. (1972). The extracts were frozen in small aliquots in liquid N$_2$. An appropriate amount of extract was thawed immediately prior to use.

In vitro amino acid incorporation

The reaction mixtures (100 μl) contained 25 μl of cell-free extract, 1 mM ATP, 0.2 mM GTP, 220 μM creatine phosphate, 110 μg creatine phosphokinase, 25 mM HEPES-KOH, pH 7.6, 2.5 mM Mg acetate, 1 mM dithiotreitol, 2–10 μl [^{35}S]methionine (NEN), and 2–6 μg poly-A containing mRNA isolated from rabbit-peritoneal exudate cells (Koch, et. al., 1976). Incubation was at 25 °C. The reaction was terminated by spotting aliquots on Whatman No. 3 paper discs (2.3 cm) prewetted with 50 μl of an amino acid mixture containing 5 mM L-methionine. The discs were processed as described by Mans and Novelli (1961).

Results

Inhibitors of protein synthesis: Effect on Protein Synthesis In Vivo and In vitro

Protein synthesis in tissue culture cells is rapidly inhibited or blocked by an increase in the tonicity of the growth medium (Saborio, Pong and Koch, 1974), DMSO (Saborio and Koch, 1973), ethanol (Koch and Koch, 1974), cytochalasin B (Koch and Oppermann, 1975), and by TPCK (Pong, Nuss and Koch, 1975). An increase in the osmolarity of the medium results in a selective inhibition of peptide chain initiation (Saborio, Pong and Koch, 1974). This inhibition is independent of the solute used to raise the osmolarity in the medium (Oppermann, et al. 1973) and is completely reversible upon return to isotonic condition. Addition of DMSO, cytochalasin B, or TPCK also preferentially effects peptide Chain initiation. However, DMSO also triggers a premature release of nascent peptides (Saborio and Koch, 1973) and cytochalasin B inhibits overall protein synthesis by only 50 % (Koch and Oppermann, 1975). TPCK, although as selective als hypertonic condition in its inhibition of peptide chain initiation, is not reversible *in vivo* (Pong, Nuss and Koch, 1975).

We have analyzed the effect of various *in vivo* inhibitors of peptide chain initiation on the translation of mRNA in cell-free extracts (Table 1). The data

Table I: Inhibition of Protein Synthesis in vivo and in cell-free Extracts

Addition	Conc.	Exposure (min)	amino acid incorporation % of control in vivo	amino acid incorporation % of control in vitro	Reversible in vivo	References
Sucrose	0.2 M	5–10	5	100	+	1
DMSO	12 %	3	2	50	+	2
Polycations (DEAE-dextran)	160 μg	30	10	0	(+)	3
Ethanol	2 %	1	60	100	+	4
Ethanol	3 %	1	10	70	+	4
Cytochalasin B	20 μg	30	50	100	(+)	5
TPCK	30 μg	5–10	2	80	–	6
Trypsin	500 μg	20	5	0	+	7
Pronase	100 μg	30	5	0	+	7
Glycopeptides	5–100 μg	5–10	0–80	0–80	+	8

Table 1: Protein synthesis *in vivo* in suspended HeLa S3 or L cells was studied by following the incorporation of [35S]methionine or [3H]alanine into acid soluble proteins. The reversibility of the inhibition of protein synthesis *in vivo* was determined by sedimenting the cells and resuspension in fresh growth medium. Recovery of protein synthesis of better than 50 % (+) or 80 % + is listed in the second to last column in the table.

Protein synthesis *in vitro* was determined as described under Materials and Methods. The data on the inhibition of *in vivo* protein synthesis have been published in part previously (1. Oppermann, *et. al.*, 1973; 2. Saborio and Koch, 1973; 3. Saborio, Wiegers and Koch, 1975; 4. Koch and Koch, 1974; 5. Koch and Oppermann, 1974; 6. Pong, Nuss and Koch, 1975; 7. Koch, 1974; 8. Foch, Kubinski and Koch, 1974).

show that most of these agents inhibit protein synthesis to a much greater extent *in vivo* than *in vitro*. The different effects of these inhibitors on protein synthesis *in vivo* and *in vitro* have led to an inquiry as to whether the *in vivo* induced inhibition is a result of an indirect effect. That is, the primary action of these inhibitors might be exerted on the cell membrane, resulting in the activation and/or release of factor(s) which interfere with peptide chain initiation *in vivo*. This hypothesis is supported by the following observations: cell-free extracts, prepared from cells which had been exposed to either hypertonic conditions or TPCK *in vivo* for 15 min at 37 °C (the time required for complete run-off of ribosomes from polysomes) show no endogenous protein synthesis. Endogenous protein synthesis can be restored, however, by gel filtration over Sephadex G25 (Hoffman *et al.*, 1976) or by dialysis for 60 min at +4 °C, indicating that neither ribosomes nor mRNA are irreversibly inactivated by exposure of cells to TPCK or hypertonic conditions (McFarland and Koch, unpublished data).

Effect of inhibitors of peptide chain initiation and elongation on protein synthesis in various tissue culture cell lines and in virus infected cells

It was previously reported that one *in vivo* inhibitor of peptide chain initiation (excess NaCl) was less effective in inhibiting protein synthesis in poliovirus infected HeLa cells than in uninfected HeLa cells (Saborio, Pong and Koch, 1974; Nuss, Oppermann and Koch, 1975). This observstion has been extended and analyzed in detail in a number of uninfected and virus infected tissue culture cells (Nuss, Oppermann and Koch, 1975; Nuss and Koch, 1976a & b; Oppermann and Koch, 1976a & b). Although resistance of protein synthesis to hpertonic initiation block (HIB) varies from cell line to cell line and is higher when cells are grown in monolayer versus suspension (Oppermann and Koch, 1976a), a striking increase in resistance to HIB is observed following virus infection of cells (Fig. 1). Similar observations were obtained with other inhibitors of peptide chain initiation but not with inhibitors of peptide chain elongation such as puromycin and cycloheximide (Table 2). These results could be interpreted in several ways. Virus infection could result in changes in cell membrane structure, conferring a higher resistance of the synthesis of all proteins to HIB and other inhibitors of peptide chain initiation. Alternatively, viral mRNA translation selectively proceeds under conditions where host mRNA translation is severely inhibited resulting in the observed increased resistance.

Differential inhibition of mRNA translation by HIB

To further investigate the virus induced increase in resistance of protein synthesis to HIB, the synthesis of individual cellular proteins in uninfected cells and of host and viral proteins early in the replication cycle in several RNA and DNA virus infected cells was studied. Cells were pulse labeled under isotonic and hypertonic conditions and cytoplasmic extracts were subsequently analyzed by polyacrylamide gel electrophoresis (Nuss, Oppermann and Koch, 1975; Nuss and Koch, 1976a, b; Oppermann and Koch, 1976a, b). The results revealed that exposure of virus infected cells to appropriate hypertonic condition amplified the inhibition of host mRNA translation while viral mRNA translation was affected only slightly. We concluded therefore that viral mRNAs are more efficient messengers

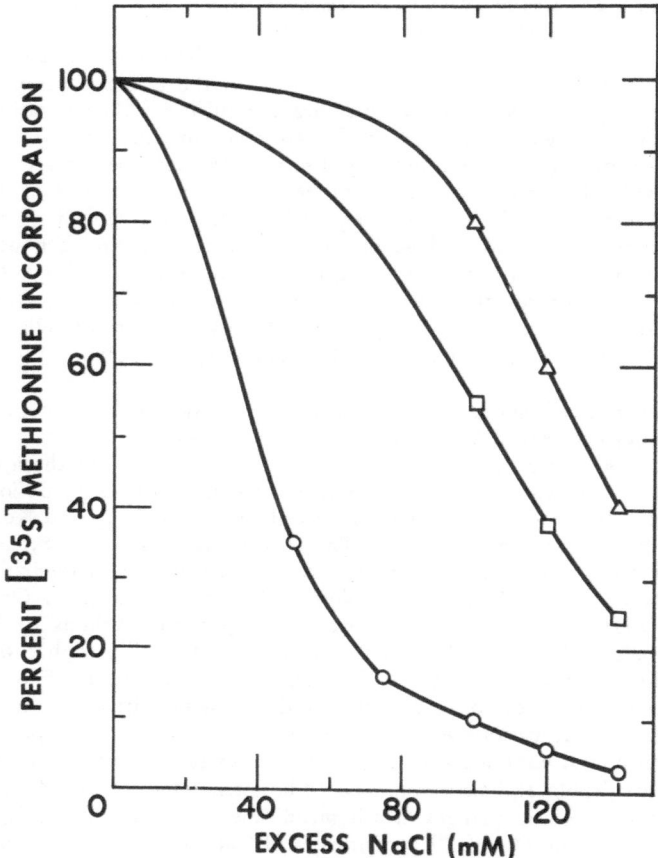

Fig. 1: Inhibition of protein synthesis in uninfected and virus infected HeLa cells by HIB.

    HeLa cells, uninfected (O—O), VSV infected (□—□) 300 min post infection or poliovirus infected (△—△) 180 min post infection were pulse labeled under isotonic or hypertonic conditions as described in the section on Materials and Methods.

than most host mRNAs and suggested that under conditions which result in a reduction in the overall rate of peptide chain initiation, each mRNA is translated with its own characteristic efficiency. To further investigate this hypothesis, the relative sensitivities of individual cellular mRNA translation to HIB were determined.

    The mouse plasmacytoma cell line MPC-11 synthesizes an immunoglobulin gamma heavy (H) chain of approximately 55,000 daltons and a 23,000 molecular weight kappa light (L) chain (Laskov and Scharff, 1970). The L and H chains are reported to account for as much as 20 % of the newly synthesized polypeptides (Laskov and Scharff, 1970). Since the synthesis of the two IgG polypeptides make

Table II: Inhibition of Protein Synthesis in uninfected and Poliovirus infected HeLa cells

Condition	amino acid incorporation % of control	
	uninfected	infected
Control	100	100
0.1 M NaCl excess	5	80
0.15 M NaCl excess	1	25
TPCK 30 μg/ml	2	30
50 μg/ml	1	20
ethanol 3 %	10	60
5 %	0	20
cytochalasin B 20 μg/ml	50	80
puromycin 10^{-3} M	10	10
cycloheximide 100 μg/ml	5	5

Table 2: HELa cells in suspension were infected with poliovirus or mockinfected and pulse labeled with [^{35}S]methionine 2.5 hrs post infection as described (Nuss, Oppermann and Koch, 1975) in the presence and absence of inhibitors of protein synthesis.

up a large proportion of the total protein synthesis and they can be easily identified and quantitated, MPC-11 cells provide a useful system to investigate the effect of HIB on the synthesis of several individual cellular polypeptides (Nuss and Koch, 1976a).

A comparison of the distribution of [^{35}S]methionine incorporation into MPC-11 polypeptides labeled under isotonic (panel A) and hypertonic (panel B) conditions is shown in Fig. 2. There is approximately a 3.5–4.0 fold increase in the relative incorporation into the L chain under hypertonic conditions (panel B) when compared to that observed under isotonic conditions (panel A). Likewise, there is an increase in the relative incorporation into the H chain polypeptide of approximately 1.5 fold. An estimation of the area under the curves for the L, H and total non-IgG proteins for this particular experiment reveals that the percent of total [^{35}S]methionine incorporation which is associated with the L chain, increases from a value of 6.9 % at isotonic conditions to a value of 27.2 % when cells are pulse labeled under hypertonic conditions. This value increases from 8.8 % to 12.8 % for the H protein. These results suggest that the mRNAs coding for the specialized IgG polypeptides are, as viral mRNA, efficient messengers relative to mRNA coding for other cellular proteins.

The experiment described in Fig. 2 was repeated with a number of other cell lines to compare the translational efficiencies of major mRNA species in different cells (Fig. 3). Inspection of the autoradiographs reveals several HIB resistant mRNA translation products: in MPC-11 cells (channels A & B), these include in addition to the L (23,000) and H (55,000) polypeptides, a peptide of 42,000 molecular weight and the histones (11,000 to 14,000). The translation of these non IgG mRNAs in other cell lines is also resistant to HIB, HeLa (channels D-F), L-929 (channels G-I) and BHK-21 (channels J-L). In contrast, the synthesis of two major cellular proteins, actin (41,000) and myosin (200,000) is highly sensitive to HIB.

547

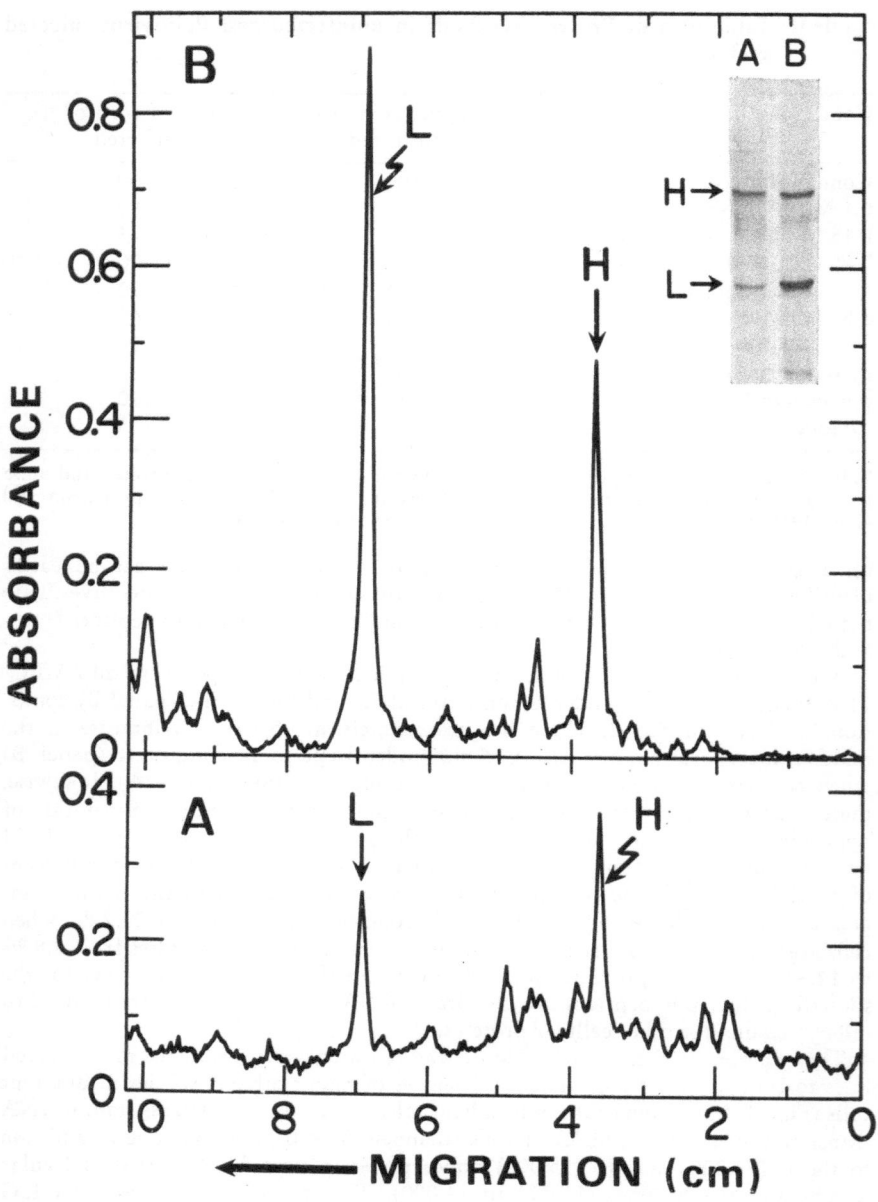

Fig. 2: Distribution of [^{35}S]methionine incorporation at isotonic and hypertonic conditions as revealed by absorbance scanning of gel autoradiographs.
An equal number of counts from the cytoplasmic extracts prepared from cells pulse

A further refinement of this technique will allow one to estimate the relative translational efficiencies of individual cellular mRNAs.

Comparison of the relative synthesis of IgG and non-IgG polypeptides under conditions of reduced rates of polypeptide chain initiation and of polypeptide chain elongation

As previously shown in Figs. 2 and 3, the distribution of amino acid incorporation into IgG and non-IgG polypeptides is significantly influenced by the rate of polypeptide chain initiation. Table 3 shows a more detailed analysis of the change in the relative synthesis of IgG L, H and non-IgG polypeptides with increasing concentration of excess NaCl or emetine (Lodish, 1971), an hinhibitor of peptide chain elongation. Notice that as the concentration of NaCl is increased, the overall incorporation of [^{35}S]methionine decreases while the percent of [^{35}S]methionine incorporation which is associated with the IgG polypeptides increases dramatically; similarly the ratio of L/H (after correction for the relative amounts of methionine residue in the two polypeptides) increases from 1.6 to 3.6 when protein synthesis is reduced by $\sim$95 %.

In contrast, the percent of [^{35}S]methionine incorporation which is IgG-specific, decreases when polypeptide chain elongation is reduced by exposure of cells to emetine. There is also a slight increase in the L/H ration (1.55–1.92) with increasing concentration of emetine. Under conditions where the elongation step in translation is rate limiting, the relative synthesis of individual polypeptides is thought to be proportional to the relative amounts of the mRNA coding for these peptides (Lodish, 1974; MacDonald and Gibbs, 1969). Accordingly, these results would indicate that this cell line contains twice the amount of message for L chain than for H chain. Thus, the value of 1.6–1.7 for the ratio of L/H at isotonic conditions indicates that L chain is synthesized under this condition at a lower rate than expected from the relative amounts of L and H mRNAs. This observation is in accord with several models proposed for the regulation of mRNA translation (MacDonald, Gibbs and Pipkin, 1968; MacDonald and Gibbs, 1969; Lodish, 1974), which predict that the translation of such mRNAs as the L chain mRNA which possesses a high rate constant for initiation is hindered in the elongation step by an increased density of ribosomes on the mRNA molecule under conditions where the overall rate of peptide chain initiation is high.

Comparison of the effects of HIB and virus infection on the relative synthesis of IgG and non-IgG proteins in myeloma cells

Virus induced suppression of host mRNA translation might be exerted by alterations of the protein synthesizing mechanism which allows ribosomes to specifically interact only with viral mRNA (Matthews *et al.*, 1973; Wright and Cooper, 1974). Alternatively, it was suggested that virus induced suppression of host mRNA translation, like HIB, acts at the level of peptide chain initiation (Liebowitz and Penman, 1971) and that an indiscriminate reduction in the rate of peptide chain initiation would provide a translational advantage for viral mRNA (Nuss,

labeled in isotonic (lower panel A) and hypertonic (140 mM excess NaCl) (upper panel B) medium were applied to the two gel channels. The actual autoradiographs are shown in the upper right hand corner of panel B.

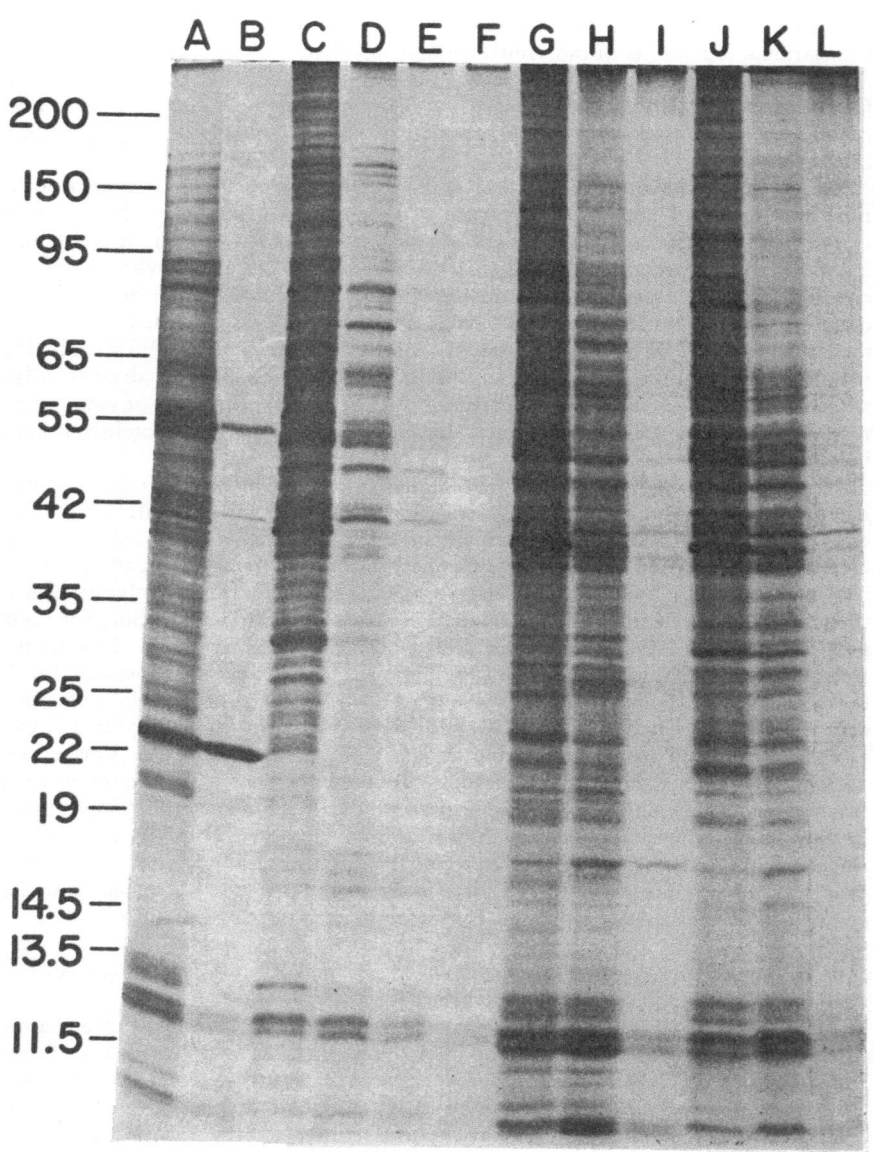

Fig. 3: HIB induced changes in the relative synthesis of individual cellular proteins.
Protein synthesis in various tissue culture cells was analyzed by isotope labeling and acrylamide gel electrophoresis under control and hypertonic conditions as described in Materials and Methods.
Myeloma cells, channel A and B, HeLa cells (C–F), L929 cells (G–I) and BHK21 cells

Table III: Effect of HIB and Emetine on the synthesis of IgG and non-IgG proteins in myeloma cells

| [35S]methionine incorporation % of Control | | HIB | | | | Emetine | | | |
HIB	Emetine	% of [35S] Protein as L+H	L	H	Ratio L/H	% of [35S] Protein as L+H	L	H	Ratio L/H
100	100	17.4	6.9	9.5	1.60	16.2	6.7	9.5	1.55
92		17.6	7.7	9.9	1.71				
	77					16.3	7.1	9.8	1.60
64	57	19.4	8.6	10.8	1.76	15.7	6.9	8.8	1.73
45	35	22.9	10.4	12.5	1.82	15.7	7.0	8.0	1.78
20	26	26.9	14.0	12.9	2.38	14.7	7.0	7.7	2.00
11	–	30.5	17.8	12.7	3.08	–	–	–	–
6	6	34.8	21.6	13.2	3.60	11.3	5.6	6.3	1.92

Table 3: MPC-11 plasmacytoma cells at a cell density of 3 x 10⁶ cells/ml in 3.8 ml of serum-free Joklik's MEM containing 1/20 the normal concentration of methionine plus 25 mM HEPES, pH 7.4 were incubated in the presence or absence of extra NaCl or emetine for 15 min at which time each sample received 100 μCi of [35S]methionine (NEN) and incubation was continued for an additional 15 min. After proper chase, cytoplasmic extracts were prepared and analyzed by polyacrylamide-SDS-gel electrophoresis as described previously (Nuss, Oppermann and Koch, 1975). The range of NaCl used to inhibit protein synthesis was from 0 to 140 mM excess while emetine was used at concentrations up to 400 ng/ml. As an indication of the levels of radioactivity measured in these experiments, approximately 170,000 cpm were recovered from the total control gel channel. The data are presented as the percent of total [35S]methionine incorporation which was found in the L and/or H bands and the ratio of radioactivity found in the L and H bands after correcting for the relative number of methionine residues in these respective polypeptides.

Oppermann and Koch, 1975). If this suggestion is correct, the synthesis of these cellular proteins which are resistant to HIB should also be resistant to virus-directed suppression. Since IgG synthesis in myeloma cells is relatively resistant to HIB, this cell system offers a special advantage for the analysis of the mode of inhibition of protein synthesis by virus infection. We, therefore, compared the effects ob HIB and virus infection on the relative synthesis of IgG and non-IgG proteins in myeloma cells.

(J–L). The first channels (A, C, G, and J) represent peptides labeled under isotonic conditions.

Extra NaCl was added to all other cell cultures in the following amounts 100 mM (D), 120 mM (E, H, K) and 140 mM (B, F, I and L). All cultures with extra NaCl received 2 X the amount of ³⁵S-methionine added to the isotonic control.

The electrophoretic mobilities of proteins was compared to the migration of proteins with known molecular weights: Muscle myosin, E. coli DNA dependent RNA polymerase subunits β, β', σ and α, bovine serum albumin, ovalbumin, myeloma IgG heavy (H) and light (L) chain, purified poliovirus coat proteins VP1, 2 and 3 and RNase. The migration of polypeptides in the discontinuous buffer systems does not accurately reflect their molecular weights. The assigned molecular weights serve merely for orientation on the autoradiographs.

Table IV: Effect of HIB and VSV infection on the synthesis of total protein and of IgG peptide chains in myeloma cells

[³⁵S]methionine incorporation % of Control		HIB		VSV	
HIB	VSV	% of [³⁵S] Protein as L	Ratio L/H	% of [³⁵S] Protein as L	Ratio L/H
100	100	6.9	1.60	6.4 ± 0.8	1.8 ± 0.1
64	50 ± 3	8.6	1.76	9.7 ± 0.0	2.3 ± 0.0
45	38 ± 1	10.4	1.82	10.9 ± 1.4	2.7 ± 0.3
20	17 ± 2	14.0	2.30	10.7 ± 1.6	3.0 ± 0.5
11	8	17.8	3.08	12.5	3.7

Table 4: This table shows the change in the percent of total ³⁵S-methionine incorporation associated with the L chain and the change in the L to H ratio in uninfected cells with increasing concentrations of excess NaCl (as in Table 3), and in VSV infected cells with time after infection at isotonic conditions. Adsorption of VSV, serotype Indiana (Mudd and Summers, 1970) was performed at room temperature for 20 min with MPC-11 cells suspended at a density of 1 x 10⁷ cells/ml in serum-free Dulbeco's MEM. Following adsorption, the cell suspension was diluted to a density of 1 x 10⁶ cells/ml in Dulbecco's MEM supplemented with 10 % horse serum and incubated at 37 °C in 250 ml tissue culture flasks (Falcone). The data presented in the column entitled VSV give the percent incorporation into host specific polypeptides at different time after infection (0 to 5 hrs). The data with infected cells represent the average of two experiments.

Infection of myeloma cells with VSV results in a rapid inhibition of total protein synthesis (Nuss and Koch, 1976a) and in alterations in the distribution of labeled amino acids into L, H and non-IgG polypeptides similar to that observed following exposure of uninfected cells to HIB (Table 4). These results support our proposal that a major event in the strategy of virus induced suppression of host mRNA translation is an indiscriminate reduction in the overall rate of peptide chain initiation (Nuss, Oppermann and Koch, 1975; Nuss and Koch, 1976a).

Discussion

Peptide chain initiation is inhibited selectively by an increase in the tonicity of the growth medium (Saborio, Pong and Koch, 1974). The application of this method to a study on protein synthesis in several RNA virus infected and uninfected cells has revealed that all viral mRNA species possess a greater ability to intitaiate translation than cellular mRNAs. Accordingly, viral protein synthesis can be unmasked from cellular protein synthesis by a brief exposure to the hypertonic initiation block (HIB) (Nuss, Oppermann and Koch, 1975). The translational efficiency for individual cellular mRNAs varies greatly. Inhibition of peptide chain initiation by HIB in myeloma cells increases the percent of [³⁵S] incorporation into L + H chains from, 17.5 % to 34.8 %, inhibition of peptide chain elongation by emetine reduces this percentage to 11.3 % (Table 3). These results indicate that translational control is operative in tissue culture cells also under standard growth conditions, however only to a limited extent.

Competition between viral and host mRNA for ribosomes in virus-infected cells is likely to have an impact on host protein synthesis. Competition alone may be sufficient to account for the shift from host to viral protein synthesis in virus infected cells where total protein synthesis remains constant during the virus replication cycle. In poliovirus infected HeLa cells (Nuss, Oppermann and Koch, 1975) and in VSV infected myeloma cells (Nuss and Koch, 1976c), however, total protein synthesis is inhibited at times prior to the detectable synthesis of viral RNA and viral proteins. The observation that the selective inhibition of peptide chain initiation by HIB results in the potentiation of the virus induced suppression of host protein synthesis at early times in the infectious cycle suggests that virus directed suppression may also be exerted at the level of peptide chain initiation.

Based on these observations, we would predict that the synthesis of those cellular proteins which show resistance to HIB should also be relatively resistant to virus directed suppression and those cellular proteins which are very sensitive to HIB should also be preferentially affected by virus infection. We tested this prediction in two virus-host cell systems a) in VSV infected myeloma cells, b) in poliovirus infected HeLa cells. The synthesis of IgG peptides, which make up 15 to 20 % of total protein synthesis in myeloma cells are relatively resistant to HIB, and also resistant to inhibition by VSV infection (Nuss and Koch, 1976c). The synthesis of actin in HeLa cells is considerably more sensitive to HIB and inhibition of protein synthesis exerted by infection with poliovirus than is the synthesis of other cellular proteins (Oppermann and Koch, unpublished results). These results support our previous proposal (Nuss, Opermann and Koch, 1975), that virus directed suppression of host protein synthesis need not involve virus specific or virus induced-factor(s) which possesses the capacity to actively discriminate between viral and host mRNA, but could perform its function by indiscriminately lowering the overall rate of peptide chain initiation for the translation of all mRNA.

Although the exact mechanism whereby virus infection or exposure of cells to excess NaCl inhibits peptide chain initiation is not clear, one straight forward explanation is that they both lower the rate of peptide chain initiation by interfering with the association of ribosomes and mRNA. In both instances this inhibition of peptide chain initiation might proceed by triggering existing cellular control mechanisms. It was previously suggested that protein synthesis in animal cells can be regulated by membrane mediated events (Pong, Nuss and Koch, 1975). This view is supported by the observation that several inhibitors of *in vivo* peptide chain initation such as increased medium osmolarity, TPCK, and cyto-chalasin B, show little effect on this process in cell-free extracts prepared from HeLa cells or L cells. The membrane-mediated regulation of protein synthesis may involve changes in cyclic nucleotides (Pong, Nuss and Koch, unpublished data) or changes in the membrane structure. Alterations in the structure of the cell membrane by exposure to proteolytic enzymes have been correlated with changes in surface adhesion of cells and in the growth rate of cells (Burger, 1970; Sefton and Rubin, 1970; Srere, 1974). Indeed, we observed that addition of protease-released membrane glycopeptides (10 to 100 µg/ml) to suspended HeLa cells results in a rapid inhibition of cellular protein synthesis (Koch, Kubinski and Koch, 1974). The protease-released membrane components also inhibit protein synthesis in cell-free extracts (Fisher and Koch, unpublished results).

Under optimal growth conditions, the relative synthesis of proteins in tissue culture cells appears to be regulated mainly, but not exclusively, by differential transcription of mRNA. However, under several natural (Fan and Penman, 1970) and experimental conditions which restrict growth and/or reduce the overall rate of peptide chain initiation, additional regulatory mechanisms on the translational level become decisive. We propose that control of protein synthesis on the translational level is amplified when the overall rate of complex formation between ribosomes and mRNA is indiscriminately lowered. When peptide chain initiation becomes rate limiting, then all mRNAs with high binding affinities to ribosomes are preferentially translated and every mRNA species exhibits a characteristic ability to initiate translation. Consistent with this interpretation is the recent observation that the binding affinities of synthetic oligonucleotides to ribosomal subunits depend on their nucleotide sequence composition, and their structure at the 5' end (G. Both, Y. Furuichi, S. Muthukrishnan, and A. Shatkin, manuscript in preparation). The differential affinities of individual mRNAs species for ribosomes might be a decisive factor in the regulation of the growth cycle. The techniques described here provide a suitable tool to investigate this possibility.

Infection by RNA-viruses is favored when the rate of peptide chain initiation is reduced (Koch, 1973). Since unfavorable growth conditions – especially amino acid starvation – result also in inhibition of peptide chain initiation, they are expected to sensitize cells for virus infection. This view is supported by the recent observation that infection of tissue culture cells by certain picornaviruses is severely inhibited by addition of nonessential amino acids to the growth medium (Verhagen, pers. commun.). Susceptibility to virus infection in animals and men might be influenced by similar mechanisms.

References

Burger, M. M. (1970). Nature *227*: 170–171.

Fan, H. and Penman, S. 61970). J. Mol. Biol. *50*: 655–670.

Hoffman, A., Bilello, P., Mittelstaedt, R., McFarland, E. and Koch, G. (1975). Arch. Biochem. Biophys. (submitted).

Koch, G. (1973). *In*, Current Topics in Microbiol. and Immunol. *62*: 89–138 (Braun, Wrand and Wecker eds.).

Koch, G. (1974). Biochem. Biophys. Res. Commun. *61*: 817–824.

Koch, G., Bilello, P., Fishman, M., Mittelstaedt, R. and Borriss, E. (1976). Immune RNA in Neoplasia, Academic Press (in press).

Koch, F. and Koch, G. (1974). Res. Commun. in Chem. Pathol. and Pharma. *9*: 291–298.

Koch, G., Kubinski, H. and Koch, F. (1974). Hoppe Seyler's Z. für Phys. Chemie. *385*: 1218.

Koch, G. and Oppermann, H. (1975). Virology *63*: 395–403.

Laemmli, U. K. and Favre, M. (1973). J. Mol. Biol. *80*: 575–599.

Laskov, R. and Scharff, M. D. (1970). J. Exp. Med. *131*: 515–541.

Lawrence, C. and Thach, R. E. (1974). J. Virol. *14*: 598–610.

Lodish, H. (1971). J. Biol. Chem. *246*: 7131–7138.

Lodish, H. (1974). Nature *251*: 385–388.

MacDonald, C. and Gibbs, J. (1969). Biopolymers 7: 707–725.

MacDonald, C., Gibbs, J. and Pipkin, A. (1968). Biopolymers 6: 1–25.

Mans, J. R. and Novelli, G. D. (1961). Arch. Biochem. Biophys. 94: 48–54.

Matthews, T. J., Butterworth, B. E., Chaggin, L. and Rueckert, R. R. (1973). Fed. Proc. 32: 461.

McDowell, M. J., Wolfgang, K. J., Villa-Komaroff, L. and Lodish, H. F. (1972). Proc. Nat. Acad. Sci. USA 69: 2649–2653.

Mudd, J. A. and Summers, D. F. (1970). Virology 42: 328–340.

Nuss, D. L. and Koch, G. (1976a). J. Mol. Biol. (in press).

Nuss, D. L. and Koch, G. (1976b). J. Virol. (in press).

Nuss, D. L. and Koch, G. (1976c). J. Virology (submitted).

Nuss, D. L., Oppermann, H. and Koch, G. (1975). Proc. Nat. Acad. Sci. USA 72: 1258–1262.

Oppermann, H. and Koch, G. (1976a). Arch. of Virol. (in press).

Oppermann, H. and Koch, G. (1976b). J. Gen. Virol. (in press).

Oppermann, H., Saborio, J. L., Zarucki, T. and Koch, G. (1973). Fed. Proc. Fed. Amer. Soc. Exp. Biol. 32: 53.

Pong, S.-S., Nuss, D. L. and Koch, G. (1975). J. Biol. Chem. 250: 240–245.

Racevskis, J., Kerwar, S. and Koch, G. (1976). J. Gen. Virol. (in press).

Saborio, J. L. and Koch, G. (1973). J. Biol. Chem. 248: 8343–8347.

Saborio, J. L., Pong, S.-S. and Koch, G. (1975). J. Mol. Biol. 85: 195–211.

Saborio, J. L., Wiegers, K. J. and Koch, G. (1975). Arch. Virol. 49: 81–87.

Sefton, B. M. and Rubin, H. (1970). Nature 227: 843–845.

Srere, P. A. (1974). In, Seventh Annual Miami Winter Symposia on "Biology and Chemistry of Eucaryotic Cell Surfaces", 7: 21–47 (Lee, E. Y. C. and Smith, E. E., eds.).

Wright, P. J. and Cooper, P. D. (1974). Virology 59: 1–20.

List of Participants

Dolf Aarsen

Radiobiological Institute
Institute for Experimental Gerontology
Primate Center
151 Lange Kleiweg
Rijswijk, The Netherlands

Marcel A. Baluda

UCLA Cancer Center
Dept. of Microbiology and Immunology
924 Westwood Boulevard, Suite 940
Los Angeles, California 90024, USA

Hertha Beckmann

Universitäts-Kinderklinik
Martinistrasse 52
D-2000 Hamburg 20, W. Germany

Peter Bentvelzen

Radiobiological Institute
Institute for Experimental Gerontology
Primate Center
151 Lange Kleiweg
Rijswijk, The Netherlands

Marcel C. Bessis

Institut de Pathologie Cellulaire
et de Cancérologie Expérimentale
Hôpital de Bicêtre
Le Kremlin-Bicêtre, France

Ronald Billing

Department of Surgery
School of Medicine
University of California
Los Angeles, California 90024, USA

Jean-Claude Brouet

Hôpital Saint-Louis
2, Place du Docteur-Fournier
F-75475 Paris Cedex 10, France

Arsene Burny

Faculté des Sciences Agronomiques de l'Etat
Chaire de Zootechnie
Gembloux, Belgium

Eugene P. Cronkite   Brookhaven National Laboratory
                        Medical Department
                        Upton, L. I., N. Y. 11973, USA

Karel A. Dicke   Visiting Professor
                        Developmental Therapeutics
                        M. D. Anderson Hospital and Tumor Institute
                        Houston, Texas 77025, USA

Volker Diehl   Hämatologie – Onkologie
                        Medizinische Hochschule
                        Karl-Wiechert-Allee 9
                        D-3000 Hannover, W. Germany

Peter Dörmer   Institut für Hämatologie
                        Gesellschaft für Strahlen- und Umweltforschung mbH.
                        Landwehrstraße 61
                        D-8000 München 15, W. Germany

Peter Duesberg   Virus Laboratory
                        Wendell M. Stanley Hall
                        University of California
                        Berkeley, California 94720, USA

Theodor M. Fliedner   Abteilung für Klinische Physiologie der Universität Ulm
                        Oberer Eselsberg M 24, Niveau 3
                        D-7900 Ulm/Donau, W. Germany

Bernard G. Forget   The Children's Hospital Medical Center
                        Division of Hematology-Oncology
                        300 Longwood Avenue
                        Boston, Massachusetts 02115, USA

Robert C. Gallo   National Cancer Institute
                        Laboratory of Tumor Cell Biology
                        Building 10, Room 6N119
                        Bethesda, Maryland 20014, USA

Thomas Graf   Max-Planck-Institut für Virusforschung
                        Biologisch-Medizinische Abteilung
                        Spemannstrasse 35
                        D-7400 Tübingen, W. Germany

Mel F. Greaves   Department of Zoology
                        University College London
                        Tumour Immunology Unit
                        Gower Street
                        London WC1E 6BT, U. K.

Rudolf Gross   Medizinische Universitätsklinik
D-5000 Köln-Lindenthal, W. Germany

Kurt Hannig   Max-Planck-Institut für Biochemie
D-8033 Martinsried b. München, W. Germany

Boyd A. Hardesty   The University of Texas at Austin
Department of Chemistry
Clayton Foundation Biochemical Institute
Austin, Texas 78712, USA

Erhard Haus   Department of Laboratory Medicine and Pathology
Chronobiological Laboratories
University of Minnesota Medical School
Minneapolis, Minnesota 55455, USA

Harald zur Hausen   Institut für Klinische Virologie der
Universität Erlangen-Nürnberg
Loschgestrasse 7
D-8520 Erlangen, W. Germany

Rüdiger Hehlmann   Medizinische Universitäts-Poliklinik
Pettenkoferstrasse 8a
D-8000 München 2, W. Germany

Klaus-Peter Hellriegel   Medizinische Universitätsklinik
Joseph-Stelzmann-Strasse 9
D-5000 Köln 41, W. Germany

Edward S. Henderson   Medicine A
Roswell Park Memorial Institute
666 Elm Street
Buffalo, N. Y. 14203, USA

Ronald B. Herbermann   National Cancer Institute
Laboratory of Immunodiagnosis
Bethesda, Maryland 20014, USA

Paul Höcker   Ludwig-Boltzmann-Institut für Leukämieforschung und
Hämatologie im
Hanusch-Krankenhaus
Heinrich-Collin-Strasse 30
A-1140 Wien, Austria

Dieter Hoelzer   Abteilung für Klinische Physiologie
der Universität Ulm
Oberer Eselsberg M 24, Niveau 3
D-7900 Ulm/Donau, W. Germany

Peter H. Hofschneider   Max-Planck-Institut für Biochemie
D-8033 Martinsried b. München, W. Germany

Nicole Hulin   Département de Biologie Moleculaire
Laboratoire de Cytologie et Embryologie moléculaire
Rue des Chevaux, 67
F-1640 Rhode-St.-Genèse, France

Tim Hunt   Department of Biochemistry
Level 4, BU4
New Addenbrooke's Hospital
Hills Road
Cambridge, U. K.

Norman N. Iscove   Friedrich Miescher Institut
CH-4402 Basel, Switzerland

Rudolf Jaenisch   The Salk Institute for Biological Studies
P. O. Box 1809
San Diego, California 92112, USA

Marshall Kadin   School of Medicine
Department of Clinical Pathology and
Laboratory Medicine
University of California
San Francisco, California 94143, USA

Françoise Kelly   Institut Pasteur
25, Rue du Docteur Roux
Paris, France

Sven-Aage Killmann   Medicinsk Afedeling A
Rigshospitalet
Blegdamsvej 9
Kopenhagen, Denmark

Gisela Kramer   The University of Texas at Austin
Department of Chemistry
Clayton Foundation Biochemical Institute
Austin, Texas 78712, USA

Bernhard Kubanek   Zentrum für Innere Medizin und Kinderheilkunde
der Universität Ulm
Steinhövelstrasse 9
D-7900 Ulm/Donau, W. Germany

Rainer Laufs   Hygiene-Institut der Universität
                             D-3400 Göttingen, W. Germany

Helmut Löffler   Zentrum für Innere Medizin am Klinikum der JLU
                             Klinikstrasse 36
                             D-6300 Giessen, W. Germany

Klaus Mannweiler   Heinrich-Pette-Institut für Experimentelle Virologie und
                             Immunologie an der Universität Hamburg
                             Martinistrasse 52
                             D-2000 Hamburg 20, W. Germany

Ronald P. McCaffrey   Massachusetts Institute of Technology
                             Center for Cancer Research
                             77 Massachusetts Avenue
                             Cambridge, Massachusetts 02139, USA

Roland Mertelsmann   I. Medizinische Universitätsklinik
                             Martinistrasse 52
                             D-2000 Hamburg 20, W. Germany

Heinz v. Meyersbach   Anatomisches Institut der Medizinischen Hochschule
                             Bischofsholer Damm 15
                             D-3000 Hannover, W. Germany

Nicholas A. Mitchison   Department of Zoology
                             University College London
                             Tumour Immunology Unit
                             Gower Street
                             London WC1E 6BT, U. K.

Karin Moelling   Virologisches Institut der JLU
                             Klinikstrasse 36
                             D-6300 Giessen, W. Germany

William C. Moloney   Harvard Medical School
                             Peter Bent Brigham Hospital
                             Department of Medicine
                             Hematology Division
                             721 Huntington Avenue
                             Boston, Massachusetts 02115, USA

Nicole Müller-Bérat   Statens Seruminstitut
                             Division of Immuno-Hematology
                             Amager Boulevard 80
                             DK-2300 Kopenhagen S, Denmark

Rolf Neth
Universitäts-Kinderklinik
Martinistrasse 52
D-2000 Hamburg 20, W. Germany

Kees Nooter
Radiobiological Institute
Institute for Experimental Gerontology
Primate Center
151 Lange Kleiweg
Rijswijk, The Netherlands

Wolfram Ostertag
Max-Planck-Institut für Experimentelle Medizin
Abteilung Molekulare Biologie
Hermann-Rein-Strasse 3
D-3400 Göttingen, W. Germany

Reza M. Parwaresch
Pathologisches Institut der Universität
Hospitalstrasse 42
Postfach 43 24
D-2300 Kiel, W. Germany

John Paul
Royal Beatson Memorial Hospital
The Beatson Institute for Cancer Research
132 Hill Street
Glasgow G3 6UD, U. K.

Mirca V. Popescu
"S. Nicolau" Institute of Virology
Sos. Mikai Bravu 285
Bukarest, Rumania

Raymond Powles
The Royal Marsden Hospital
Blood Cell Separator and Immunotherapy Unit
Downs Road
Sutton, Surrey, U. K.

Hans Pralle
Zentrum für Innere Medizin am Klinikum der JLU
Klinikstrasse 36
D-6300 Giessen, W. Germany

Martin Raff
Department of Zoology
University College London
Gower Street
London WC1E 6BT, U. K.

Fred Rapp
The Milton S. Hershey Medical Center
College of Medicine
Department of Microbiology
Hershey, Pennsylvania 17033, USA

Félix Reyes

Unité de Recherches sur les Anémies
de l'I.N.S.E.R.M. (U.91)
C.H.U. Henri Mondor
51, Avenue du Maréchal de Lattre de Tassigny
F-94010 Créteil, France

Hansjörg Riehm

Freie Universität Berlin
Kinderklinik und Poliklinik
Kaiserin Auguste Victoria Haus
Heubnerweg 6
D-1000 Berlin 19, W. Germany

Gabriel Rutter

Heinrich-Pette-Institut für Experimentelle Virologie und
Immunologie an der Universität Hamburg
Martinistrasse 52
D-2000 Hamburg 20, W. Germany

Prem Sarin

National Cancer Institute
Laboratory of Tumor Cell Biology
Building 10, Room 6N119
Bethesda, Maryland 20014, USA

Gordon Sato

Department of Biology
University of California
La Jolla, California 92037, USA

Stuart F. Schlossman

Sidney Farber Cancer Center
Harvard Medical School
Department of Medicine
Division of Tumor Immunology
35 Binney Street
Boston, Massachusetts 02115, USA

Johannes Schubert

Zentrum der Inneren Medizin am Klinikum
der JWG Universität
Theodor-Stern-Kai 7
D-6000 Frankfurt/Main 70, W. Germany

Stephen B. Shohet

Department of Clinical Pathology and
Laboratory Medicine
Cancer Research Institute
University of California
San Francisco, California 94143, USA

Joseph V. Simone

St. Jude Children's Research Hospital
Hematology/Oncology
332 North Lauderdale

P. O. Box 318
Memphis, Tennessee 38101, USA

Sol Spiegelman

Institute of Cancer Research
Francis Delafield Hospital
99 Fort Washington Avenue
New York, N. Y. 10032, USA

Peter Starlinger

Institut für Genetik der Universität zu Köln
Weyertal 121
D-5000 Köln 41, W. Germany

Charles D. Stiles

Department of Biology
University of California
La Jolla, California 92037, USA

Armand Tavitian

Institut de Recherches sur les Maladies du Sang
Hôpital Saint-Louis
2, Place du Docteur-Fournier
F-75475 Paris Cedex 10, France

Jim E. Till

The Ontario Cancer Institute
500 Sherbourne Street
Toronto, Ontario M4X 1K9, Canada

George J. Todaro

National Cancer Institute
Bethesda, Maryland 20014, USA

John Tooze

Executive Secretary
EMBO
Postfach 2019
D-6900 Heidelberg, W. Germany

Umberto Torelli

Instituto Di Patologia Speciale Medica
E Metodologia Clinica
Insegnamento Di Ematologia
Via Del Pozzo, 71
I-41100 Modena, Italy

Hermann Träuble

Max-Planck-Institut für Biophysikalische Chemie
Postfach 968
D-3400 Göttingen, W. Germany

Frank Walther

Zentrum der Inneren Medizin am Klinikum
der JWG Universität
Theodor-Stern-Kai 7
D-6000 Frankfurt/Main 70, W. Germany

John F. Watkins

Welsh National School of Medicine
Department of Medical Microbiology
Heath Park
Cardiff CF4 4XN, Wales, U. K.

Ulrich Wiegers

I. Medizinische Universitätsklinik
Martinistrasse 52
D-2000 Hamburg 20, W. Germany

Peter H. Wiernik

National Cancer Institute
Baltimore Cancer Research Center
Section of Medical Oncology
22 S. Greene Street
Baltimore, Maryland 21201, USA

Wolfgang Wilmanns

Zentrum für Innere Medizin
Robert-Bosch-Krankenhaus
Auerbachstrasse 110
D-7000 Stuttgart 50, W. Germany

Kurt Winkler

Universitäts-Kinderklinik
Martinistrasse 52
D-2000 Hamburg 20, W. Germany

Alan M. Wu

Department of Molecular Biology
Litton Bionetic Inc.
7300 Pearl Street
Bethesda, Maryland 20014, USA

Klaus Zeiller

Max-Planck-Institut für Eiweiß- und Lederforschung
Am Klosterspitz
D-8033 Martinsried b. München, W. Germany

Subject Index

virus related marker in human leukemic cells 442
virus related sequences in HL-23 450
Bacteria: chromosome of 481
IS-elements in 481
Basophils: toluidinblue metachromasia in 97
BCG treatment: 275, 297, 301, 307
Blast crisis in CML: 279
B lymphocyte: surface immunoglobulin of 209, 222
see also lymphocytes
Bone marrow: cell differentiation in 10
cells transformed by HEV and AMV 172
culture 5, 21, 45, 79
culture after bone marrow transplantation 88
culture and remission rate 82
culture in leukemia 25, 40, 58, 63, 85
culture in preleukemic disorders 83
growth of electrophoretically separated cells in diffusion chambers 49
growth of virus infected cells 151
Bovine leukemia: 376, 475
DNA polymerase activity 380
hybridization kinetics of virus ³H cDNA 384
virus 375
virus cDNA probe 382
virus genome sequences 384
Burkitt's lymphoma: 202, 457
DNA sequences related to recylcled Hodgkin's ³H DNA 405
simultaneous detection in 405

Calf-thymus terminal nucleotidyl transferase: 491, 503
Carcinoma: fusion experiments with 177
Carcinoembryonic antigen: 112
Cat: leukemia 368
type C virus, endogenous 363
Cell culture: of human lymphocytes 472
see also bone marrow

see also cell line in culture
Cell differentiation: erythroid 108, 125
hemopoietic 33, 51
in leukemia 10, 49
of Friend virus leukemia cells 126 140, 161, 531
of leukemic cells in culture 26, 64
Cell kinetics: 4, 10
in AML 12, 93
in preleukemia 91
Cell lines in culture: 186
Friend virus leukemia 140, 161, 543
human tumor 177
mouse plasmacytoma 546
myelogenous leukemia (HL 23) 442
Raji 202
tumorigenic – in nude mice 186
Cell-mediated immunity: 195
and tumor growth 199
assays of 201
in experimental models 196
in human leukemias 202
to leukemia associated antigens 201
Cell proliferation: 1
in leukemia 16
Cell separation: of colony forming cells by bouyant density distribution 81, 84
see also cell sorter and electrophoretic
Cell sorter: fluorescence activated 138, 247
Cell surface: antigen 196,207, 223, 229, 237, 245, 261
antigen of viral origin 261
cholera toxin binding sites 249
differentiation antigen 245
membrane associated factors 39
of Hodgkin's cells 232
phenotype of human leukaemic cells 257
Cell transformation: by cytomegalovirus 466
by herpes simplex virus 462
Cervical tumor: herpes simplex virus DNA in 461
Chemotherapy in leukemia: 265, 298, 306